Pharmaceutical Statistics

Pharmaceutical Statistics

David S. Jones

BSc, PhD, CEng CChem, FIM, FRSS, MRSC, MPDSNI

Professor of Biomaterials Science
School of Pharmacy
Queen's University of Belfast
Belfast, UK

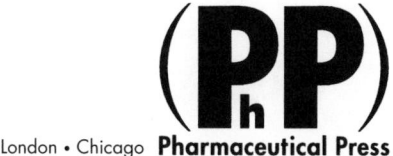

London • Chicago **Pharmaceutical Press**

Published by the Pharmaceutical Press
Publications division of the Royal Pharmaceutical Society of Great Britain

1 Lambeth High Street, London SE1 7JN, UK
100 South Atkinson Road, Suite 206, Grayslake, IL 60030-7820, USA

© Pharmaceutical Press 2002

First published 2002

Text design by Barker/Hilsdon, Lyme Regis, Dorset
Typeset by MCS Ltd, Salisbury, Wiltshire
Printed in Great Britain by TJ International, Padstow, Cornwall

ISBN 0 85369 425 7

A catalogue record for this book is available from the British Library

For Linda, Dary and Holly

Contents

Preface

'The essence of life is statistical improbability on a colossal scale.'
Richard Dawkins

Statistics is a fundamental discipline within the pharmaceutical and related sciences. In spite of this importance, however, it frequently receives limited attention and is often disliked by researchers and students alike. Many scientists view the discipline of statistics with caution and mistrust, and frequently design their investigations around their knowledge of the subject, limited as this may be. Similarly, many undergraduate students of pharmacy view statistics as merely a barrier to the successful completion of a scientific experiment or report. Indeed, the mystique that surrounds statistics may be summarised in the famous quote accredited to Benjamin Disraeli, in which statistics is viewed as a misunderstood discipline.

However, the practical applications of statistics are obvious in everyday life, ranging from working out the odds associated with gambling to assessing performance in a particular sporting event. The advertising industry employs statistics to inform the public of the popularity of a particular product, whereas the government cites its performance in statistical terms, reminding voters of the reductions in unemployment, mortgage rates, and so on. As a scientific discipline, statistics impinges upon the theory and application of all other sciences. Within the pharmaceutical sciences, knowledge of statistics is required to interpret data generated from all types of physical and biological investigations. Examples include comparisons of the pharmacological activities of therapeutic agents, investigation of the agonist/antagonist activities of therapeutic agents, pharmacokinetic calculations and estimations, evaluation of the physicochemical properties of dosage forms, examination of the quality of dosage forms, and validation of analytical methods. These topics are essential components of the undergraduate pharmacy degree and many hours are dedicated to their laboratory examination. However, an essential component of the understanding of any of these experiments is the interpretation of the outcome. After all, this is the 'take home message' for the students.

Although the concept of basic probability is now taught to schoolchildren at primary school level, the teaching of statistics to students of science disciplines is demanding. In particular, the teaching of statistics to undergraduate students of pharmacy is often a challenging task, as, to the vast majority of students, statistics is a mathematical discipline and has little relevance to the pharmacy degree. Many students visualise statistics in a purist sense and fail to realise that, although it is indeed a discipline steeped in mathematical theory, the applications of this theory affect all aspects of scientific judgement. This misapprehension is confounded not only by an aversion to mathematics but also by the style of many currently available statistics textbooks. To obviate these difficulties, the coverage of statistical theory in this textbook has been restricted to providing an understanding of the associated methods, whilst ensuring that all the associated mathematical processes have been explicitly described. Furthermore, the focus of this text involves the application of statistical methods to experimental design and interpretation and, accordingly, although the mathematical foundations and principles are preserved, this text is not a mathematical treatise of statistical theory. Derivations of statistical formulae are not given, but in all cases the reasoning, importance and application of each equation are fully discussed. Therefore, this text will particularly appeal to those who wish to gain a basic comprehension of statistical processes and concepts.

The statistical content of this book has been designed to appeal to both undergraduate students of pharmacy and postgraduate pharmaceutical scientists. No prior knowledge of statistics is required. The text has been structured to enable a gradual understanding of statistical principles before demonstrating the application and execution of specific statistical methods. It may be conveniently divided into two sections. The first section (Chapters 1–4) outlines basic statistical principles, including qualitative measurements, visualisation of data, probability theory and distributions. The second section (Chapters 5–12) details methods by which statistical hypotheses may be mathematically examined and validated. More specifically, Chapter 1 introduces the different types of variable that the pharmaceutical scientist may encounter and also describes different data sampling techniques. In Chapter 2, the commonly used measurements of central tendency and variation of data are illustrated. Here the reader will encounter the mean, median, mode, standard deviation, variance, standard error of the mean, accuracy and precision, amongst other measurements. In Chapter 3, the basis of data presentation is described. Chapter 4 presents an introduction to probability and probability distributions. This is a fundamental chapter that outlines both the basic principles of probability and the properties of commonly employed probability distributions. These probability distributions are employed in the remaining chapters to examine the statistical outcome of experiments. Particular emphasis has been placed on the theory and applications of the normal, t, χ^2 and F distributions. In Chapter 5 the basic principles of statistical hypothesis testing are introduced. This chapter forms the platform for the introduction and understanding of subsequent chapters and details important principles, including the null and alternative hypotheses, one-tailed and two-tailed outcomes, definition of the critical acceptance region for a statistical method, errors in statistical decision-making, and the power of statistical tests. These features are consistently employed in all subsequent chapters and their knowledge is reinforced by use of statistical examples. In this chapter, the concept of parametric and non-parametric statistical tests is introduced and the basis for the use of each of these categories of statistical test is discussed. The theory and application of confidence intervals associated with a variety of statistical parameters (mean, differences between means, standard deviation, proportions, difference between proportions) using both the normal and t distributions are examined in Chapter 6. In Chapters

7–11, the theory and applications of statistical tests to evaluate one, two and multiple hypotheses are discussed in depth.

Uniquely, in this text parametric and non-parametric tests are discussed in parallel (Chapters 7, 8 and 9) or, to avoid excessively long chapters, in adjacent chapters (10 and 11). Another important concept that has been introduced is the rational selection of parametric or non-parametric tests. In many statistical texts, parametric and non-parametric methods are discussed separately: in other words, the choice of whether to apply a parametric or non-parametric statistical test to examine a defined statistical hypothesis has been predetermined. This is not the case here. There are no preconditions in any of the examples, and the reasons for the use of each statistical method are explicitly stated. In particular, straightforward methods have been employed to select whether parametric or non-parametric methods are applicable, in which the normality of the distribution of the population (from which the data was sampled) is initially assessed by numerical comparison of the mean, the median and (where applicable) the mode. I fully appreciate that this estimation is not the definitive measure of normality, but this approach does serve two purposes: it reinforces the principles of the use of parametric and non-parametric tests, and it illustrates how the appropriate type of test may be selected. These points are illustrated in each worked example. More specifically, the theory and applications of one-sample statistical tests (both parametric and non-parametric), namely the one-sample z test, the one-sample t test, the one-sample χ^2 test, the binomial test and the Kolmogorov–Smirnov test, are described in Chapter 7. Chapter 8 presents the theory and applications of statistical tests for two independent samples. Here, parametric tests (two-independent-samples z test, two-independent-samples t test) and non-parametric tests (Mann–Whitney U test, χ^2 analysis and Fisher exact probability tests) are discussed simultaneously, allowing the reader to understand how these two categories of test are selected. In Chapter 9 the theory and application of statistical tests for two related (paired) samples are presented, and this chapter may be considered as the paired equivalent of Chapter 8. Here the theory and mechanics of parametric tests (paired t test) and non-parametric tests (McNemar's test and the Wilcoxon signed-rank test) are discussed concurrently. The calculation of power associated with two independent and two related samples is discussed in Chapters 8 and 9. The theory and applications of analysis of variance (ANOVA) for the evaluation and validation of multiple-sample hypotheses are described in Chapter 10. This chapter comprehensively describes the mechanics of one-way and two-way ANOVA and repeated-measures ANOVA, and illustrates these principles by the use of several examples. Furthermore, this chapter provides a detailed discussion on the theory and application of a-priori and *post-hoc* comparisons associated with ANOVA, and, in addition, calculations of the power, sample size and minimum detectable difference. Chapter 11 presents the mechanics associated with non-parametric multiple-sample statistical tests, namely χ^2 analysis, the Kruskal–Wallis test and Friedman's test, and also describes the theory and applications of some commonly employed non-parametric multiple comparison tests. Finally, Chapter 12 provides a detailed description of linear regression analysis and statistical correlation. Comprehensive descriptions of the theory and applications of these techniques to the pharmaceutical sciences are provided, including both parametric and non-parametric methods for the determination of correlation between two variables.

I sincerely hope that this textbook will inspire pharmaceutical scientists to adopt statistics as an important tool in their academic armoury. Knowledge of statistics will allow a greater understanding of all scientific disciplines. I have attempted to include many examples of the use of statistical methods that are directly relevant to all aspects of the pharmaceutical sciences. Many students have commented to me that this has enhanced their comprehension of statistics and its relevance to the pharmacy degree course.

This textbook is the outcome of 15 years of statistical experience, and I am indebted to many people for assisting and guiding my statistical development throughout this period. From my experiences at the University of Otago I wish to thank Dr George Spears of the Otago Medical School for answering all my statistical questions with enthusiasm and patience, and Professor Ian Tucker (University of Otago) and Professor David Collins (University of Manitoba) for introducing me to the vast array of statistical methods available to the pharmaceutical scientist and filling me with enthusiasm for this subject. I would also like to acknowledge the comments of the numerous students to whom I have had the pleasure of teaching pharmaceutical statistics over several years. These comments have helped to fashion the direction of this book and indeed, informed me of the need for a textbook on this subject. Finally, I am indebted to Dr Colin McCoy for the many hours spent meticulously proofreading this text and providing me with many helpful suggestions about the direction and clarity of the book, and to Ms Cherith Glenn for the time spent typing and compiling statistical tables for the appendix section.

On a personal level I wish to acknowledge the support of Professor Sean Gorman and Professor David Woolfson at the School of Pharmacy, QUB, for their words of encouragement during the preparation of this book, particularly during those periods whenever the end seemed distant.

Finally, this book would not have been completed without the support, patience, love and encouragement of my wife, Linda, and our children, Dary and Holly. This book is dedicated to them.

David Jones
Queen's University, Belfast
November 2001

About the author

David Jones gained a BSc (1st class honours) in Pharmacy in 1985 and a PhD (Pharmaceutics) in 1988. He registered with Pharmaceutical Society of Northern Ireland in 1989 and took up a lectureship in Pharmaceutics and Pharmaceutical Technology in the School of Pharmacy, University of Otago, New Zealand. In 1992, he was appointed as the Head of Formulations at Norbrook Laboratories Ltd. In 1994, he was appointed to a lectureship in Pharmaceutics and was subsequently promoted to a senior lectureship (1997) and to a personal Chair (in Biomaterial Sciences) in 1999. His research concerns the characterisation, formulation and engineering of pharmaceutical systems and biomedical devices. He is the author of approximately 270 research papers and has been awarded the Lilly prize for pharmaceutical research (1997) and the British Pharmaceutical Conference Science Award (1997). Professor Jones is both a Chartered Engineer and a Chartered Chemist and is a Fellow of the Institute of Materials, a Fellow of the Royal Statistical Society and a Member of the Royal Society of Chemistry. He is the co-editor of the *Journal of Pharmacy and Pharmacology* and is also a director and founding member of two campus companies, Xiomateria Ltd. and Carapacics, which are both involved in Medical Device and Pharmaceutical applications of novel polymeric systems.

1

Basic concepts and definitions

The term *statistics* may be conveniently described as the science of collecting, analysing and interpreting data relating to an aggregate of individuals (Kendall and Buckland, 1982). From this definition, it may be appreciated that statistics is an integral part of all scientific and science-related disciplines. Hence, it is important for students who are studying such disciplines to have a basic understanding of the principles and applications of statistics. Interestingly, we have all been exposed to, and indeed have used, statistical inferences as part of normal society. For example, in sport, reference may be made to the relative attributes of one team in comparison to their competitors. In another example, descriptive statistics are frequently used in the language of advertising, in terms such as 'nine out of ten people prefer ...'. Therefore, at a basic level, the use of statistics is not a foreign concept.

Statistics may be conveniently divided into two sub-categories, *descriptive* and *inferential*.

- *Descriptive statistics* provides general information about the fundamental statistical properties of data, e.g. mean, median, standard deviation, coefficient of variation. Traditionally, the use of descriptive statistics has been considered to be relatively limited; however, it is important to realise that proper consideration of data using descriptive measures is an essential factor in the entire process of data analysis.
- *Inferential statistics* is involved in the formulation of conclusions based on information derived from experimental procedures, e.g. the antihypertensive effect of drug A was 'significantly' greater than that of drug B and so on.

Therefore, in scientific studies, statistics may be usefully employed in a number of ways, including:

- collection of data
- numerical description of data
- formulation of a hypothesis concerning the nature of the data
- understanding the relevance of the data by the use of appropriate statistical methods
- the design of experiments to test the hypotheses, or indeed, to further consolidate or reject the hypothesis.

Undergraduate and postgraduate students of pharmacy often ask why they need to study statistics, because highly trained statisticians are already available. A metaphorical reply to this question is that one may be trained to use a computer in order to perform basic functions such as word processing or setting up spreadsheets. However, to perform more complex tasks using computers, one would have to consult a trained computer scientist or systems analyst. Similarly, for statistics, a basic training will allow the student to understand key principles that are relevant to scientific research. Examples include:

- the nature and extent of variation of chemical and biological data
- the relevance and meaning of key statistical terms (e.g. significance, p-values, standard deviation, variables)
- the proper interpretation of data generated during a research study (or data reported in a published manuscript)
- the rational design of scientific studies.

Indeed, a final application of a basic statistical training is the understanding of when, and for what purpose, a trained statistician is required!

1.1 Variation in scientific studies

A *variable* may be described as a property with respect to which individuals in a sample differ in some ascertainable way (Sokal and Rohlf, 1981). Examples of variables include:

- the height of men in a particular region
- the weights of tablets derived from the same batch
- the concentrations of drug in plasma of clinical subjects following administration of a defined dose of drug
- concentrations of cholesterol in the plasma of male subjects.

The information described within such variables may then be manipulated, presented and statistically analysed to provide a complete picture of the properties of that variable.

Inherent to the process of performing biological and chemical measurements is the state of *variability*, i.e. replicate measurements of a particular property will exhibit different numerical outcomes. The presence of such variability is the main reason for the need for inferential statistics. For example, consider two pharmaceutical analysts performing a spectrophotometric assay to determine the concentration of a therapeutic agent in a given solution. The outcomes of the assays will vary for a number of reasons, including:

- the relative analytical skills of the two analysts
- the instrument employed for the analysis

- the quality (and cleanliness) of the cuvettes
- inaccuracy of dilutions of the original solution.

In the absence of variation, it would be straightforward to comment on differences between groups of data because each value would be absolute. However, as such situations do not exist in scientific experiments, statistical methods are required to allow conclusions to be made concerning experimental data.

1.2 Types of variables

Before carrying out any statistical procedure, whether descriptive or inferential, it is important to characterise the nature of the variable in question, as this will have a direct bearing on the choice of the most appropriate statistical technique. Typically, variables may be described as one of the following:

- measurement variables (continuous and discrete)
- ranked variables
- attributes.

1.2.1 Measurement variables

Measurement variables are those that may be described in a numerically ordered fashion. There are two types, *continuous* and *discrete* variables.

1.2.1.1 Continuous variables

Continuous variables can assume an infinite number of numerical values between the lowest and highest points on a scale. An example is the concentration of therapeutic agent in a pharmaceutical product. Typically, a pharmaceutical product is required by the licensing authorities to contain between 90 and 105% of the nominal amount over the period of storage. Thus, in a tablet containing nominally 100 mg of active agent, the specified limits are 90–105 mg. The drug content of tablets from this batch is thus considered as a continuous variable, because the tablets from this batch can assume an infinite number of possible masses within the specified limits. In practice, however, the sensitivity of the chemical assay for the therapeutic agent imposes restrictions on the number of possible observed concentrations. Thus, if the sensitivity of the assay is 1 μg, the number of possible values within the specified concentration range is of the order of 15×10^3.

1.2.1.2 Ranked variables

Ranking scales are also examples of continuous variables because, although they do not represent physical measurements, such scales represent numerically ordered systems. One example of this is illustrated in a paper by Keane *et al.* (1994), in which the amount of inorganic salts (encrustation) deposited on ureteral stents in vivo was examined visually following surgical removal of the stents, and the following ranking applied:

0   no encrustation
1   microscopic deposits on <50% of the stent
2   microscopic deposits on >50% of the stent
3   small macroscopic deposits on <50% of the stent
4   small macroscopic deposits on >50% of the stent
5   heavy macroscopic deposits.

Thus, although the values described do not offer an exact measurement, it may be observed that as the amount of encrustation increases so does its numerical representation.

1.2.1.3 Discrete (discontinuous, meristic) variables

Discrete variables are variables that have a fixed number of values. Examples include:

- the number of asthma attacks recorded in a group of patients
- the number of colonies of microorganisms
- the number of fatalities associated with a particular operation.

Discrete variables always have integer values (whole numbers).

1.2.1.4 Nominal variables (attributes)

Nominal variables cannot be measured, because of their qualitative nature. Examples include gender, age group, religious affiliation, side-effects associated with the use of therapeutic agents, clinical effects of treatment and placebo. Unlike ranked variables, nominal variables are not associated with numerical values. Typically, whenever attributes are combined with frequencies, they are referred to as *enumeration data* (see Table 1.1).

Table 1.1 Incidence of oral candidosis in a regional hospital in a single month

Nominal variable (gender)	Reported incidence
Male	59
Female	82
Total number of cases	141

1.3 **Statistical samples and populations**

Two important terms that the reader should be fully acquainted with are *samples* and *populations*.

- The population may be defined as the entire number of observations that constitute a particular group; any particular property associated with a population is termed a *parameter*.
- Samples are generally a relatively small group of observations that have been taken from a defined population.

Pharmaceutical examples of populations and samples are given in Table 1.2.

As may be imagined, characterising the properties of a particular population requires measuring all the constituents of that population. Thus to fully characterise the weights of tablets in a particular batch, every tablet in that batch should be weighed. For some products, this

Table 1.2 Examples of populations and samples

Example (task)	Population parameter	Sample
Characterisation of the weights of tablets in a particular batch	All tablets that constitute the batch	100 tablets removed for weighing
Measurement of the incidence of heart disease in Scotland in patients over 45 years of age	All inhabitants of Scotland over the age of 45	300 patients attending GP clinics at specified geographical locations throughout Scotland
Evaluation of the IQ of schoolchildren in Northern Ireland in year 7	All schoolchildren in Northern Ireland in year 7	100 children in year 7 attending selected schools in Northern Ireland
Evaluation of the incidence of asthma in a certain chemical company employing 500 workers	All employees of the company	50 named workers at the company
Evaluation of the worldwide incidence of head injury in professional boxers	All professional boxers worldwide	Examination of the medical records of all professional boxers in the UK

could involve the weighing of a million tablets! It is impractical to do this routinely, so small samples are randomly removed from the population and characterised in terms of a particular property. On the basis of information derived from the random sample, assumptions about the nature of the population may be formulated. Thus, to use an example from Table 1.2, by measuring the weights of a sample of tablets removed from a batch, we can make assumptions about the weights of all tablets in the batch.

As described previously, population parameters are fixed values, i.e. non-variable. Thus, the weight or drug content of a batch of tablets is definite because these parameters have been determined by measurement of all members of the batch. Conversely, information concerning a particular parameter that is derived from a sample is referred to a *sample statistic*. It is worth further highlighting that sample statistics are variable. Thus, successive samples from a population will have different numerical values of the parameter in question. These differences may be attributed, at least in part, to differences in the properties of each batch of sample and variability in the analytical procedure employed to quantify the designated property, as described in the introductory section of this chapter.

1.4 Samples and sampling techniques

In the preceding section, the use of sample data to provide information on population parameters was introduced. In the light of this, it is not surprising that one of the most important components of any experiment or procedure is the process of sampling. At first sight, sampling may appear to be rather a straightforward procedure; however, failure to select the most appropriate sampling method may lead to bias and possibly incorrect statistical conclusions. The availability of several different sampling methods illustrates the need for careful selection of the most appropriate method. *Random sampling* and *stratified sampling* are examples of typical sampling methods.

1.4.1 Random sampling

Most readers will have a basic knowledge of random sampling. In this process, specific procedures are followed to ensure that each member of the chosen population has an equal chance of being selected. An everyday example of random sampling is the choice of numbers (as balls) in bingo or lottery events. The procedure ensures that there is no bias and, consequently, estimation of population parameters from the sample statistics will be accurate. It has been proposed (Snedecor and Cochran, 1980) that the efficacy of random sampling procedures is enhanced when the variability of the population is small and homogeneous. The concept of homogeneous variability is considered in later chapters (8–11).

The experimental procedure by which random sampling is performed may be as simple as assigning numbers to each member of a population and then randomly selecting samples from an enclosed container (e.g. box, bag) or a mechanical selector. In the selection of a large number of samples, however, it is more appropriate to employ a random number generator; such programs are readily available for personal computers.

1.4.2 Stratified sampling

Stratified sampling is a more complex procedure in which the population under examination is subdivided into strata (groups), and then samples are randomly removed from each designated stratum. Typically, this type of sampling is performed to reduce sampling error or natural bias. Furthermore, it is accepted that this method is particularly successful whenever the within-observation variability is markedly less than the between-observations variation between strata. Stratified sampling techniques have been successfully used in the pharmaceutical and medical sciences. For example, in the investigation of the effects of salivary substitutes on the lubricity of the oral cavity in patients suffering from xerostomia, it is appropriate to segregate patients into different strata

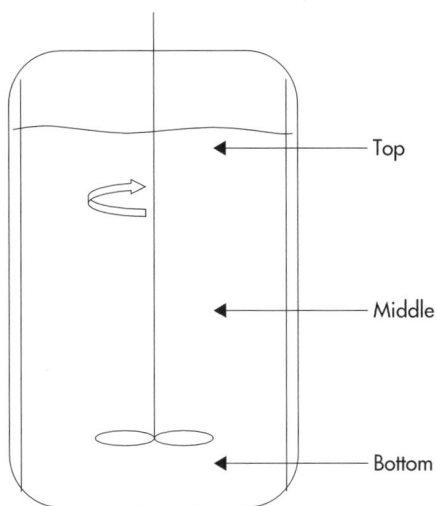

Figure 1.1 Sampling regions in a filling vessel.

according to aetiology, i.e. Sjögren's syndrome, head and neck radio-therapy, patients prescribed tricyclic antidepressants, etc. Patients in these categories will all present with xerostomia, but the aetiologies are different and hence failure to employ stratified sampling will enhance the error associated with the experimental procedure.

In the pharmaceutical industry, stratified sampling is employed at certain points during different steps of the manufacturing process. For example, in the manufacture of a liquid formulation, samples of the product are removed from the top, middle and bottom of the filling vessel before filling, the locations within the vessel becoming the strata (Figure 1.1). Similarly, in the filling process, samples of the finished product are removed at predetermined intervals for routine analysis; in this case the sampling times are the strata.

1.5 Conclusions

In this introductory chapter two main concepts have been described: the nature of statistical data and the methods by which data may be sampled from a population. Both of these concepts are important in the design, execution and statistical analysis of pharmaceutical and related studies. The type of sampling influences the design of an experiment; the nature of the data directly influences both the experimental design and the type of statistical test that may be applied to examine the similarities or differences between populations or samples. In the following chapters the importance of these concepts will be illustrated.

References

Keane P F, Bonner M C, Johnston S R, *et al.* (1994). Characterisation of biofilm and encrustation on stents *in vivo*. *Br J Urol* 73: 687–91.

Kendall M G, Buckland W R (1982). *A Dictionary of Statistical Terms*, 4th edition. London: Longman.

Snedecor G W, Cochran W G (1980). *Statistical Methods*, 7th edition. Ames: Iowa State University Press.

Sokal R R, Rohlf F J (1981). *Biometry*, 2nd edition. New York: W H Freeman.

2

Measurement of central tendency and variation of data

After data have been collected in an experiment or study, the statistical analyst will be asked to summarise the properties of the data set. This will allow the analyst to examine the nature of the data. The two properties that are most frequently employed to describe the properties of a set of data are the *central nature* (tendency) and *variability*. The importance of these parameters, and the methods by which they may be mathematically described, are considered in this chapter.

2.1 Measurement of central tendency

Estimation of the central nature of data is perhaps the most common statistical calculation that most students will perform. Typically, the central nature of data may be conveniently described by a number of methods and terms, including the mean (e.g. arithmetic, weighted), median and mode. These various terms, their calculation and the rationale for their use are described in this section.

2.1.1 Arithmetic mean

Most readers will be familiar with the term 'average', or *mean* as it is known by statisticians. The mean is the most popular method for describing the central nature of data, and refers to the centre of a distribution of data. Indeed, the use of the mean is most appropriate whenever the data is symmetrically distributed around the mean value, i.e. a Gaussian distribution. Mathematically, the arithmetic mean is described as follows:

$$\frac{\sum_{j=1}^{N} X_j}{N}$$

where $\sum$ is the notation for 'the sum of', X_j refers to all data from $j = 1$ to $j = N$ and N is the number of data contributing to the calculation.

To illustrate a calculation of the arithmetic mean, consider the following example.

EXAMPLE 2.1 *The reduction in blood pressure (mmHg) in 6 patients 4 hours after administration of a standard dose of a novel antihypertensive agent is shown in Table 2.1. Calculate the mean reduction in blood pressure reduction in the 6 patients.*

Substituting the figures from Table 2.1 into the equation for the arithmetic, we obtain:

$$\frac{\sum_{j=1}^{N} X_j}{N} = \frac{(20 + 25 + 21 + 34 + 41 + 37)}{6} = \frac{178}{6} = 29.67 \text{ mmHg}$$

Typically, in current usage, the term 'arithmetic mean' is abbreviated to simply the 'mean' and is denoted by the symbols $\bar{X}$ (sample mean) or μ (population mean).

2.1.2 Weighted (arithmetic) mean

The weighted (arithmetic) mean is a special example of the mean in which each datum point in the distribution does not contribute equally to the overall calculation of the mean. In the calculation of the mean describe above, the reduction in blood pressure exhibited by each patient contributed equally to the overall calculation, i.e. each patient contributed equally. Weighted means are therefore commonly employed whenever the data is divided into groups, each of which possesses different weighting (i.e. importance). The use and calculation of weighted means is illustrated in Example 2.2.

EXAMPLE 2.2 *The effect of a defined dose of a commercially available analgesic to suppress pain following a painful stimulus was evaluated in 20 volunteers using a visual analogue scale. The results are*

Table 2.1 Effect of an antihypertensive drug on blood pressure lowering in six patients

Patient number	Reduction in blood pressure (mmHg)
1	20
2	25
3	21
4	34
5	41
6	37

Table 2.2 Recorded assessment of pain by 20 volunteers following administration of a commercially available analgesic and exposure to a painful stimulus

Number of volunteers	Pain assessment by volunteers
2	3 (extreme pain)
12	2 (moderate pain)
6	1 (slight pain)

presented in Table 2.2. Calculate the mean of the pain assessment by the 20 volunteers.

In this clinical example, the three sub-groups describe different clinical effects and are therefore not equal in magnitude (weighting). The calculation of the weighted average employs the following equation:

$$\frac{\sum_{j=1}^{N} w_j X_j}{N}$$

where X_j denotes all data from $j = 1$ to $j = N$, N is the number of data that contribute to the calculation and w_j is the weighting (frequency) of each group or series. Therefore, the (weighted) mean of the above example is calculated as follows:

$$\frac{\sum_{j=1}^{N} w_j X_j}{N} = \frac{(2 \times 3) + (12 \times 2) + (6 \times 1)}{20} = \frac{36}{20} = 1.8$$

It is worthwhile noting that the calculated mean does not have any dimensions, as a direct result of the analogue scale used to assess pain.

A further example of the use of weighted means involves the calculation of final examination marks for undergraduate and postgraduate student courses. Frequently such courses include a contribution from both written examinations and coursework (e.g. assignments, marked tutorials, practicals, etc.), each of these contributing unequally to the final calculation of marks. Consider a scenario in which a student has achieved 75% and 70% in the examination and coursework components, respectively, of a university course, and that these courses contribute unequally to the final mark, e.g. 80% and 20% respectively in this example. The final mark (weighted mean) achieved by the student is calculated as follows:

$$\frac{\sum_{j=1}^{N} w_j X_j}{N} = \frac{(80 \times 75) + (70 \times 20)}{100} = 74\%$$

2.1.3 Median

As described previously, it is particularly appropriate to use the mean for the description of the central nature of a set (distribution) of data when the data are distributed in a Gaussian fashion, i.e. distributed equally on either side of the mean. The median is an alternative method of describing the central nature of data which is relatively unaffected by the nature of the spread of data. In simple terms, the median is the central value, or the mean of the two middle values, of a set of data arranged in order of magnitude. The calculation of the median, and its comparison with the mean of a set of asymmetrical data (data unequally distributed around the mean) is illustrated in Example 2.3.

EXAMPLE 2.3 *The adherence of the opportunistic pathogen* Candida albicans *to 10 buccal epithelial cells (BEC) in vitro was examined and is shown in Table 2.3. Calculate the mean and median values for the adherence profile of this pathogen.*

Step 1 Calculation of the mean

$$\frac{\sum_{j=1}^{N} X_j}{N} = \frac{(2+0+0+6+4+24+9+6+1+0)}{10} = 5.2$$

blastospores of C. *albicans* per buccal epithelial cell.

Step 2 Calculation of the median
First, arrange the data in order of magnitude:

$$0, 0, 0, 1, 2, 4, 6, 6, 9, 24$$

Determine the *central value*, i.e. the mean of values in positions 5 and

Table 2.3 Number of blastospores of *Candida albicans* adherent to a defined number of buccal epithelial cells, as examined using an in-vitro method

Epithelial cell number	Number of adherent C. albicans
1	2
2	0
3	0
4	6
5	4
6	24
7	9
8	6
9	1
10	0

6. Thus, the calculated median is 3 adherent blastospores of C. *albicans* per buccal epithelial cell.

Step 3   Conclusions
The description of the central nature of data using the mean and median can therefore yield different numerical outcomes. This is because extreme values in a particular set of data, e.g. 24 in the above study, have a greater effect on the calculated value of the mean than of the median. Hence the greater suitability of the median in describing the central nature of data containing extreme values.

The calculation of the median containing an odd number of data is performed as follows.

EXAMPLE 2.4   *The weights of 11 tablets, removed from a batch for quality control purposes, are presented in Table 2.4. Calculate the mean and median values of the tablet weights.*

Step 1   Calculation of the mean

$$\frac{\sum_{j=1}^{N} X_j}{N}$$

$$= \frac{(251 + 255 + 250 + 245 + 265 + 260 + 231 + 225 + 250 + 275 + 300)}{11}$$

$$= 255.2 \text{ mg}$$

Step 2   Calculation of the median
First, arrange the data in order of magnitude:

225, 231, 245, 250, 250, 251, 255, 260, 265, 275, 300

Table 2.4   Individual weights of 11 tablets removed from a production batch

Tablet number	Tablet weight (mg)
1	251
2	255
3	250
4	245
5	265
6	260
7	231
8	225
9	250
10	275
11	300

The median is defined as the central value, i.e. the value in position 6. Therefore, the calculated median is 251 mg.

In terms of frequency distributions (Chapter 4), the median represents the 50th percentile (quartile), i.e. the number of observations greater than the median is equal to the number lower than the median. Furthermore, in a symmetrical distribution, the value of the mean is equal to that of the median.

2.1.3.1 *Choice of the mean or median to describe the central tendency*

A discussion of the use of the mean and median for the description of the central nature of data will be helpful to the reader at this point.

For data that is distributed in a normal fashion, the numerical values of the mean and median should be identical and so either term may successfully be used to accurately describe the central point of the distribution. However, the choice of which parameter to use becomes more problematic when the data exhibits non-normality. The common misconception amongst students of statistics is that the mean is exclusively used to describe the central nature of data that are normally distributed, whereas the median is exclusively used to describe the central nature of data that are non-normally distributed. This is not specifically the case and, indeed, both the mean and median may be used to describe the central properties of moderately skewed (i.e. non-normal) distributed data. In these cases, the values of the mean and median will be different and will be more diverse as the skewness of the distribution increases. If the data is positively skewed (i.e. distributed towards the y-axis), the mean will be numerically greater than the median; the converse is true for negatively skewed distributions. The use of the median is preferable to the use of the mean for the description of distributions that are particularly skewed, i.e. those that possess extreme values. In these cases, the value of the mean is unacceptably distorted, whereas the value of the median is relatively unaffected.

2.1.4 Mode

The mode may be described as the most commonly occurring measurement in a set of data. To illustrate the calculation of the mode, consider the set of data given in Table 2.5.

EXAMPLE 2.5 *The concentrations of therapeutic agent (mg/mL) in 10 vials of a commercially available parenteral product have been deter-*

Table 2.5 Concentration of a therapeutic agent in 10 vials of a commercially available product

Vial number	Concentration of therapeutic agent (mg/mL)
1	200
2	205
3	205
4	201
5	199
6	195
7	202
8	205
9	205
10	207

mined using a chromatographic method. Calculate the mode of the observed concentrations.

The most common (popular) value in the above set of data is 205 mg/mL (four occurrences) and consequently, this value is the mode.

Data sets may contain more than one mode. If two modes are present in a data set, the data is said to be *bimodal*. Thus, in the following data set:

20, 22, 23, 25, 25, 25, 25, 28, 29, 29, 30, 31, 31, 31, 31, 31, 33

two modes exist: 31 (termed the *major mode*) and 25 (termed the *minor mode*). A distribution in which each observation occurs with equal frequency is assumed to possess no mode.

With reference to frequency distributions, the mode is numerically equal to the mean and the median in symmetrical distributions. In asymmetrical distributions, an empirical relationship exists between the mean, median and mode:

mean – mode = 3 (mean – median)

The mode is less frequently used than the mean and median for the description of the central nature of data. However, it may be useful to describe the number of modes in a distribution, particularly if more than one exists.

2.2 Measurement of the variation of data

In the previous section, methods were introduced that describe the central nature of data, but these methods provided no information about the variability of the data from which such central measures were obtained. Therefore, in addition to knowledge of the central nature of data, it is desirable to possess a measure of the variability or dispersion of data. Such information provides a measure of the relative proximity of the data set. This concept may be illustrated by a comparison of the two sets of data provided in Table 2.6. Just by looking at the central nature (mean) of each set of data, one might assume that the two sets of data were similar in nature. However, it is clear from Table 2.6 that the data sets are dissimilar. Therefore, it is commonplace in statistics to present the central nature of results in conjunction with a measure of variation of data. The following sections will describe various methods by which the variation of data may be calculated and presented.

2.2.1 Range

The range may be defined as the difference between the largest and smallest values in a set of measurements. The ranges of data sets A and B in Table 2.6 are as follows:

data set A: range = 30 − 10 = 20

data set B: range = 30 − 28 = 2

The use of the range to accurately describe data variation is limited, as its calculation involves only two measurements from the set of data (i.e. the highest and lowest data points). Therefore, the range does not truly describe the variation of the entire data set. Furthermore, in the estimation of the variability of populations from sample data, the range is considered inappropriate, as it is unlikely that a sample will contain both the highest and the lowest values in a population. Therefore, the sample range is considered to be a poor estimation (i.e. an underestimation) of the range associated with a population.

Table 2.6 Individual values associated with two sets of data possessing identical means

Data Set A	Data Set B
10	28
20	29
30	30
20	29
10	28
Mean = 30	Mean = 30

The major use of the range is to define the variability associated with non-normally distributed data.

2.2.2 Mean deviation

The mean deviation, formally termed the first absolute moment, is a measure of data variation that is calculated as the average deviation from the mean. Given the usefulness of the mean as a measure of central tendency, a term that describes the deviation around this central parameter may be of direct statistical relevance.

In mathematical terms, the mean deviation is described as follows:

$$MD = \frac{\Sigma(X_j - \overline{X})}{N}$$

where $(X_j - \overline{X})$ is the absolute value of the deviation (difference) of the values in the data set from the mean of the data set and N is the number of observations in the data set.

The following example illustrates the calculation of the mean deviation.

EXAMPLE 2.6   *A solution of tetracycline hydrochloride has been sent to the quality control laboratory of a pharmaceutical company for analysis. The drug content of aliquots from this solution has been assayed using ultraviolet spectroscopy and the results are tabulated in Table 2.7. Calculate the mean deviation of the drug content of the solution.*

Step 1   Calculate the mean

$$\frac{\sum_{j=1}^{N} X_j}{N} = \frac{(100.6 + 98.3 + 98.9 + 95.1 + 104.5 + 105.5)}{6} = 100.5 \text{ mg/mL}$$

Step 2   Calculate the mean difference

$$MD = \frac{\Sigma(X_j - \overline{X})}{N}$$

$$= \frac{\left[\begin{array}{l} (100.6 - 100.5) + (98.3 - 100.5) + (98.9 - 100.5) \\ + (95.1 - 100.5) + (104.5 - 100.5) + (105.5 - 100.5) \end{array} \right]}{6}$$

$$= \frac{\Sigma[(0.1) + (2.2) + (1.6) + (5.4) + (4.0) + (5.0)]}{6} = 3.1 \text{ mg/mL}$$

The mean deviation is calculated using the absolute values of the

Table 2.7 Content of tetracycline hydrochloride in six aliquots of a solution

Aliquot number	Content of tetracycline hydrochloride (mg/mL)
1	100.6
2	98.3
3	98.9
4	95.1
5	104.5
6	105.5

difference between the measurement and the mean, i.e. no reference is made to the algebraic sign. The use of absolute values for the calculation of mean deviations has led some authors to suggest that the term *mean absolute deviation* is a more appropriate terminology for this statistical parameter. Finally, it is worth commenting that the term *median deviation* is also appropriate and is defined as the sum of the absolute deviations from the median.

2.2.3 Variance

In the calculation of the mean deviation, the algebraic sign was ignored in order to provide a positive numerical outcome. One further method that may be used to avoid the algebraic charge generated from the subtraction of the mean from certain measurements is to square their difference (deviation). The addition of the successive squared differences generates a fundamental statistical term, the *sum of squares*. This term will be further encountered in Chapters 10 and 12. Mathematically, the sum of squares is described as

$$SS = \Sigma(X_j - \bar{X})^2$$

where X_j and $\bar{X}$ have the same definitions as before.

The variance is often referred to as the *mean sum of squares* and can be written as

$$\sigma^2 = \frac{\Sigma(X_j - \mu)^2}{N}$$

where σ^2 is the variance of a population, X_j is the numerical value of each measurement, μ is the population mean value and N is the number of observations.

Furthermore, the variance of a sample (s^2), i.e. the most appropriate estimation of the population variance (σ^2), is described by

$$s^2 = \frac{\Sigma(X_j - \bar{X})^2}{N-1}$$

where $\bar{X}$ is the mean of the sample data and N is the number of observations in the sample.

It is important to consider the implications of the equations that
describe variance.

- First, the notation of variance – σ^2 or s^2 – depends on whether population or
  sample data is under consideration.
- Secondly, the equations that describe the variances of population and sample
  data differ principally in the denominator term, i.e. N for the population variance and $N-1$ for the sample variance.

The primary reason for the differences between the two equations
relates to the relative inaccuracy of the estimation of the population
variance from the sample variance when the latter equation includes
simply N, the number of observations, as the denominator. In this situation, the sample variance is considered to be a biased estimate of the
population variance, and the term $(N-1)$ acts to remove this bias.

At this point it is worthwhile for the reader to consider the relationship between the sample and population variances. Unlike the population variance, the sample variance is a variable measurement.
Therefore, if a random sample is removed from a population, e.g. if 100
tablets are removed from a batch of 1 000 000 tablets (the population)
and their individual weights determined, the variance of the sample (the
group of 100 tablets) will not exactly equal the population variance.
Indeed, if repeated samples are removed from the batch of 1 000 000
tablets and the variances of the weights of each sets of sample measured,
the variances of each of these different samples will be slightly different.
These differences are a direct consequence of the variable nature of the
sample variance, which itself is due to factors described in the first chapter (e.g. differences in weights of each batch, variability due to inaccuracies in the balance, operator inaccuracies, etc.). However, if samples of
size N were repeatedly randomly removed from the population and their
variances determined (using $N-1$ as the denominator), the average of
all the calculated sample variances would equal the population variance.
In this scenario, the modified equation to calculate the sample variance
has provided a good estimate of the population variance. The concept
of the importance of the use of $N-1$ in the denominator for the
calculation of sample variances is described below.

Consider a population to be composed of three data points, 3, 5
and 7. From this information, the population variance may be derived
using the following equation:

$$\sigma^2 = \frac{\Sigma(X_j - \mu)^2}{N}$$

Individual values (X_j)	$X_j - \mu$	$(X_j - \mu)^2$
3	-2	4
5	0	0
7	+2	4

Therefore:

$$\sigma^2 = \frac{\Sigma(X_j - \mu)^2}{N} = \frac{(4 + 0 + 4)}{3} = 2.67$$

From the population above, nine individual samples, each composed of two values, are removed by repeated sampling. On each occasion the samples are replaced prior to resampling, thus ensuring that each individual value has an equal chance of being selected. The outcome of the sampling, i.e. the various pairs of data that may be achieved, is as follows:

Sample	Values	$(X_j - \bar{X})^2$	$\Sigma(X_j - \bar{X})^2/N - 1$	s^2
1	3, 3	$(3 - 3)^2 = 0$ $(3 - 3)^2 = 0$	$(0 + 0)/1$	0
2	5, 5	$(5 - 5)^2 = 0$ $(5 - 5)^2 = 0$	$(0 + 0)/1$	0
3	7, 7	$(7 - 7)^2 = 0$ $(7 - 7)^2 = 0$	$(0 + 0)/1$	0
4	3, 5	$(3 - 4)^2 = 1$ $(5 - 4)^2 = 1$	$(1 + 1)/1$	2
5	5, 7	$(5 - 6)^2 = 1$ $(7 - 6)^2 = 1$	$(1 + 1)/1$	2
6	5, 3	$(5 - 4)^2 = 1$ $(3 - 4)^2 = 1$	$(1 + 1)/1$	2
7	7, 5	$(7 - 6)^2 = 1$ $(5 - 6)^2 = 1$	$(1 + 1)/1$	2
8	3, 7	$(3 - 5)^2 = 4$ $(7 - 5)^2 = 4$	$(4 + 4)/1$	8
9	7, 3	$(7 - 5)^2 = 4$ $(3 - 5)^2 = 4$	$(4 + 4)/1$	8

The average sample variance can then be calculated:

average $s^2 = (0 + 0 + 0 + 2 + 2 + 2 + 2 + 8 + 8)/9 = 2.67$

This numerical exercise has further highlighted the following points:

- The sample variances of groups of random samples removed from a population may not be exactly equal to one another, because of the variable nature of the sample variance.

- The variance of a single random sample of measurements does not provide a good estimation of the variance of the population from which the sample was derived.
- A good estimation of the population variance may be achieved from sample data, provided that the denominator of the equation used to calculate sample variance is modified to $N - 1$, and, additionally, an average of several sample variances is calculated.

Finally, it is interesting to consider the relative merits of the mean deviation and the variance for describing the variability of data. These terms provide similar information about the spread of data around a central point (the mean). However, the variance can be related to probability (and hence, statistical hypothesis testing), and is therefore considered to be a more relevant parameter. This fundamental difference is sufficient to ensure that the variance (and the related parameter, standard deviation) is the parameter of choice for the description of data variability. The relationship of variance to probability and statistical hypothesis testing is described in more detail in later chapters.

2.2.4   Standard deviation

The *standard deviation* is a commonly used measure of the dispersion of data that is defined as the positive square root of the *variance*. The standard deviation may be written mathematically as follows:
Standard deviation of a population

$$\sigma = \sqrt{\frac{\Sigma(X_j - \mu)^2}{N}}$$

Standard deviation of a sample

$$s = \sqrt{\frac{\Sigma(X_j - \bar{X})^2}{N - 1}}$$

Again the denominators employed in the calculations of the standard deviations of the population and sample are N and $(N - 1)$, respectively.

Most calculators and computers can calculate standard deviations rapidly, but it is still a good idea for the reader to know how to calculate this parameter manually because this gives a greater understanding of the basis of this term. To facilitate such manual calculations, shorter methods are available for calculation of the standard deviation (and also the variance). The modified methods for the calculation of the standard deviation are based on the following equations:

$$\Sigma(X - \bar{X})^2 = \Sigma X^2 - \frac{(\Sigma X)^2}{N}$$

This leads to the following expansions for the standard deviation:
Standard deviation of a population

$$\sigma = \sqrt{\frac{\Sigma(X_j - \mu)^2}{N}} = \sqrt{\frac{\Sigma X^2 - ((\Sigma X)^2/N)}{N}}$$

Standard deviation of a sample

$$s = \sqrt{\frac{\Sigma(X_j - \overline{X})^2}{N-1}} = \sqrt{\frac{\Sigma X^2 - ((\Sigma X)^2/N)}{N-1}}$$

An illustration of the use of these equations for the calculation of the standard deviation of a sample is provided in the following example.

EXAMPLE 2.7 *A batch of bolus tablets has been prepared and is awaiting release from the quality control laboratories of a pharmaceutical company. One of the properties of the bolus tablets that must be quantified is the time required for the release of 50% of the original drug loading of the bolus ($t_{50\%}$) using the dissolution test described in the British Pharmacopoeia (1998). Table 2.8 shows the $t_{50\%}$ of 15 boluses randomly sampled from the batch. Calculate the mean and standard deviation of the time required for the release of 50% of the original drug loading of the bolus.*

Table 2.8 Time taken for dissolution of 50% of the original mass of drug from 15 bolus tablets derived from a single batch

Bolus number	$t_{50\%}$ (h)
1	20.2
2	21.6
3	24.5
4	28.6
5	22.6
6	24.0
7	21.9
8	22.0
9	26.1
10	25.3
11	23.4
12	20.1
13	23.5
14	24.0
15	25.9

Step 1 *Calculate the mean*

$$X = \frac{\begin{pmatrix} 20.2 + 21.6 + 24.5 + 28.6 + 22.6 + 24.0 + 21.9 \\ + 22.0 + 26.1 + 25.3 + 23.4 + 20.1 + 23.5 + 24.0 + 25.9 \end{pmatrix}}{15}$$

$$= \frac{353.7}{15} = 23.6 \text{ h}$$

Step 2 *Calculate the sample standard deviation*

$$s = \sqrt{\frac{\sum X^2 - ((\sum X)^2/N)}{N-1}}$$

X	X^2
20.2	408.0
21.6	466.6
24.5	600.3
28.6	818.0
22.6	510.8
24.0	576.0
21.9	479.6
22.0	484.0
26.1	681.2
25.3	640.1
23.4	547.6
20.1	404.0
23.5	552.3
24.0	576.0
25.9	670.8
$\sum X = 353.7$ h	$\sum X^2 = 8415.3$ h^2

Thus:

$$s = \sqrt{\frac{\sum X^2 - ((\sum X)^2/N)}{N-1}} = \sqrt{\frac{8415.3 - ((353.7)^2/15)}{14}} = 2.3 \text{ h}$$

So, the mean and standard deviation of the $t_{50\%}$ of the sample removed from a batch of bolus tablets is 23.6 ± 2.3 h.

One practical point in such calculations is the numerical relationship between the standard deviation and the range. Usually, the standard deviation is approximately a fifth to a sixth of the numerical value of the range. This may be considered as a 'rule of thumb' relationship and should be recalled whenever the reader is checking calculations. If such an approximate relationship is not observed, then it is strongly advised that all the calculations should be re-checked.

2.2.4.1 General comments on the standard deviation

The standard deviation is the most commonly used measure of the dispersion of data, because it may be related to the probability of a measurement occurring within certain regions on the frequency distribution. Thus, in normal (symmetrical), and indeed in moderately skewed (asymmetrical) distributions:

- 68.27% of all values are included within the numerical range described by $\bar{X}$ + s and $\bar{X}$ – s, namely one standard deviation around the mean.
- 95.45% of all values are included within the numerical range described by $\bar{X}$ + $2s$ and $\bar{X}$ – $2s$, namely two standard deviations around the mean.
- 99.73% of all values are included within the numerical range described by $\bar{X}$ + $3s$ and $\bar{X}$ – $3s$, namely three standard deviations around the mean.

In the example described above concerning the time required for the release of 50% of the original loading of therapeutic agents, the mean and standard deviation were calculated to be 23.6 ± 2.3 h. Consequently

- 68.27% of all values are included within the numerical range described by 21.3 h (i.e. 23.6 – 2.3 h) to 25.9 h (i.e. 23.6 + 2.3 h).
  Therefore, in the current example, 10 out of 15 values were distributed within this range.
- 95.45% of all values are included within the numerical range described by 19.0 h (i.e. 23.6 – 4.6 h) to 28.2 h (i.e. 23.6 + 4.6 h).
  Therefore, in the current example, 14 out of 15 values were distributed within this range.
- 99.73% of all values are included within the numerical range described by 16.7 h (i.e. 23.6 – 6.9 h) to 30.5 h (i.e. 23.6 + 6.9 h).
  Therefore, in the current example, all values were distributed within this range.

The standard deviation (and indeed the variance) is dramatically affected by extreme values in a population, a point that should be considered whenever the variation of a set of data is under discussion. The effects of extreme values on the variance is illustrated in the following example.

EXAMPLE 2.9 *The concentrations (mg/5 mL) of a penicillin antibiotic in five separate bottles of a paediatric suspension have been examined using an iodometric technique. Calculate the mean and standard deviation and consider the contribution of each observation to the sample variance.*

Table 2.9 Concentrations of a penicillin antibiotic in each of five bottles of a paediatric suspension

Bottle number	Concentration of penicillin
1	125
2	124
3	121
4	123
5	16

Step 1 Calculate the mean

$$\bar{X} = \frac{(125 + 124 + 121 + 123 + 16)}{5} = 101.8 \text{ mg/5 mL}$$

Step 2 Calculate the variance

$$s^2 = \frac{\Sigma(X_j - \bar{X})^2}{N - 1}$$

$$= \left[\frac{(125.0 - 101.8)^2 + (124.0 - 101.8)^2 + \cdots + (16.0 - 101.8)^2}{4} \right]$$

$$= 2302.7 \text{ (mg/5 mL)}^2$$

Step 3 Calculate the standard deviation
Remembering that the standard deviation is the square root of the variance, the standard deviation may be easily calculated as $\sqrt{2302.7} = 48.0$ mg/5 mL.

Step 4 Consider the contribution of each observation to the sample variance

The contribution of each observation to the overall variance (bottles 1, 2, 3, 4 and 5), and hence standard deviation, may be easily computed using the standard formula:

$$s^2 = \frac{\Sigma(X_j - \bar{X})^2}{N - 1}$$

For example, in bottle 1, the recorded concentration of penicillin was 125 mg/5 mL.

$$s_1^2 = \frac{(125 - 101.8)^2}{4} = 134.56 \text{ (mg/5 mL)}^2$$

Thus, we have the data shown in Table 2.10.

Table 2.10 Concentrations of a penicillin antibiotic in each of five bottles of a paediatric suspension, illustrating the individual contributions of each vial to the total variance

Bottle number	Concentration of penicillin (mg/5 mL)	Contribution to the overall variance
1	125	134.5
2	124	123.2
3	121	92.2
4	123	112.4
5	16	1840.4
		$s^2 = 2302.7$ (mg/5 mL)^2

As individual values deviate further from the sample mean, their effects on the variance are greater than for values in which this deviation is not as marked. Consequently, in some data, large standard deviations may be attributed to one or more extreme (outlier) sample values. In the above example, the concentration of penicillin in bottle 5 represents an outlier, and may indicate a problem with either the manufactured batch or the analytical method.

As previously stated, distributions in which the mean is numerically greater than the median are positively skewed. The data described represents such a distribution (mean = 132.4 mg/5 mL; median 123 mg/5 mL).

2.2.5 Standard deviation (error) of the mean

The standard deviation of the mean, sometimes referred to as the standard error of the mean (SEM), is a term that is commonly used (and unfortunately misused) in statistics. As a result of this use and misuse, students of statistics should be fully acquainted with this term. To gain a proper understanding of the SEM, it is first necessary to compare and contrast the meaning of the standard deviation of the mean and the standard deviation, as described in section 2.2.4. As outlined previously, the standard deviation describes the variability (dispersion) of a set of data around a central value, and an estimate of the variability of the data in a population may be derived from it. The standard deviation of the mean, however, is a measure of the variability of a set of mean values, calculated from individual groups of measurements (samples) that have been derived from a population. The differences between these two terms are illustrated in the following example.

EXAMPLE 2.10 *A batch of amoxicillin trihydrate paediatric suspension has been manufactured. Before filling, the manufacturer wishes to*

ensure that the concentration of the suspended drug is uniform within the batch. To check this, five individual aliquots (100 mL) are removed and the concentration of each aliquot determined five times using a chromatographic method. The results are shown in Table 2.11. Calculate the standard error of the mean of these data sets.

The standard error of the mean is calculated using the individual mean values of each aliquot, as follows:

$$s = \sqrt{\frac{\sum X^2 - ((\sum X)^2/N)}{N-1}} = \sqrt{\frac{2875.59 - ((119.9)^2/5)}{5-1}} = 0.31 \text{ mg/mL}$$

Therefore, as illustrated above, the mean and standard deviation of each aliquot may be easily calculated, providing a measure of variability of each individual aliquot. However, on some occasions, the variation associated with individual mean values is of greater interest than the variability of the individual values that comprise each sample. Therefore, an overall mean and standard deviation of the five aliquots described above may be calculated using the formula for standard deviation. In the above example, the mean and standard deviation may be calculated as 24.0 ± 0.31 mg/mL. The standard deviation so calculated is referred to as the standard deviation of the mean and may be considered as a measure of the precision of the mean.

The observant reader may have noticed that the magnitude of the standard deviation of the mean is lower that that of the individual standard deviations associated with each aliquot. Once more this may be easily explained by consideration of the nature of the observations that are included in the calculation of each of these deviation terms. Remember that the standard deviation is particularly susceptible to

Table 2.11 Concentration of amoxicillin in five aliquots, removed from a batch for the purpose of quality control

Concentration of amoxicillin trihydrate (mg mL^{-1})				
Aliquot 1	Aliquot 2	Aliquot 3	Aliquot 4	Aliquot 5
25.1	27.6	24.3	23.9	25.7
25.4	25.5	26.4	24.9	23.5
21.9	25.6	25.1	26.1	24.2
24.5	25.0	27.1	27.0	25.7
23.1	24.2	25.0	25.2	24.3
$\bar{X} = 24.0$	$\bar{X} = 24.2$	$\bar{X} = 24.3$	$\bar{X} = 23.9$	$\bar{X} = 23.5$
$s = 1.5$	$s = 1.3$	$s = 1.1$	$s = 1.2$	$s = 1.0$

extreme values. Therefore, if such values are present in an individual data set, the standard deviation of that set will increase. Conversely, the magnitude of the mean is relatively unaffected by the inclusion of extreme data. These two effects are exhibited in Table 2.12. We can see that the mean suppresses the effects of extreme values, and consequently, the standard deviation of a series of such means will be lower as a result of this suppressive effect:

$$s = \sqrt{\frac{\sum X^2 - ((\sum X)^2/N)}{N-1}} = \sqrt{\frac{433.44 - ((34.8)^2/3)}{3-1}} = 3.86$$

It is possible to calculate the standard deviation of the mean by repeatedly sampling a population, as outlined in Example 2.10, but in practice this is not required as there is sufficient information available within one set of data (sample) to perform the appropriate calculation. Therefore, although the variation of the population is unknown, the standard deviation of an individual set of data (sample) can be used to estimate this parameter. Statistical theory states that the SEM may be calculated by dividing the standard deviation of a set of data by the square root of the number of observations in the data set (N):

$$SEM = (s/\sqrt{N})$$

This equation allows us to predict the variation of the mean of the population; i.e. if many means were gathered by random sampling of sets of data, their variation would vary to the extent predicted by the above equation. It is worth remembering that the calculated value of the standard deviation of the mean using the standard deviation of a sample from a population will not exactly equal the true standard deviation of the mean. This is because the standard deviation of a sample is a random variable and will differ from sample to sample.

Table 2.12 Hypothetical sets of data, illustrating the effects of extreme values on the standard deviation and mean

Data set A	Data set B	Data set C
5	5	5
7	7	7
8	8	8
9	9	9
15	21	51
$\bar{X} = 8.8$	$\bar{X} = 10.0$	$\bar{X} = 16.0$
$s = 3.8$	$s = 6.32$	$s = 19.6$

2.2.5.1   General comments on the standard deviation and the standard error of the mean

By this point, the reader should have identified the major differences between the standard deviation and the standard deviation (error) of the mean. Despite the fear of repetition, the following section is intended as a summary of the major characteristics of each term.

- The *standard deviation of a sample* derived from a population is employed as an estimate of the variability of the population. As a result, the value of the standard deviation would not be expected to reduce if the number of observations in the sample increases. However, a greater confidence of population variability may be obtained by making a larger numbers of observations of the standard deviation of samples.
- The *standard deviation of the mean* is a measure of the variability (precision) of the estimation of a defined population parameter, i.e. the mean. The numerical value of the standard error of the mean depends on the number of observations included in its calculation. In particular, as the size of the sample increases to increase the precision of measurement, the magnitude of the standard error of the mean decreases. This is reflected by the inclusion of the term $\sqrt{N}$ in the denominator of the equation to calculate this parameter.

In the introductory paragraph of this section, reference was made to the possible misuse of the standard deviation of the mean in reported scientific studies. This occurs when authors have gathered data that vary widely, i.e. the standard deviation is high. Examples of the sources of this variation have been outlined in Chapter 1. Typically, the authors have decided that such a large variation may offer (generally to referees of submitted manuscripts) a reason to question experimental technique, types of methods employed, etc., and consequently, the standard errors of the means have been reported instead. The equation describing the standard error of the mean is lower than the standard deviation by a factor of $\sqrt{N}$, and hence the apparent variability of the data is effectively decreased (i.e. the study appears to be more precise). Reporting of standard deviations is of particular interest if one wishes to describe the nature of data, e.g. the type of distribution or the variability (particularly in the case of biological experiments), or to calculate probabilities. On the other hand, if the author aims to describe the properties of an experimentally derived parameter, e.g. cholesterol blood levels in a group of men aged 45 years, weight of tablets in a batch, viable microbial counts in pharmaceutical products, etc., then the use of the standard error of the mean is preferable.

2.2.6 Coefficient of variation

The coefficient of variation (CV) is a statistical term that expresses the variability of a set of data and is defined as the ratio of the standard deviation (s) to the mean of the data set ($\bar{X}$):

$$CV(\%) = \frac{s}{\bar{X}} \times 100$$

This term allows the variation of data sets of differing magnitude to be directly compared. Thus, if the means ± standard deviations of two data sets are (A) 2500 ± 125 and (B) 50 ± 35, at first glance one may be deceived into believing that the variation of data set B (standard deviation = 35) is less than that of data set A (standard deviation = 125). However, such a comparison is meaningless and deceptive because the magnitudes of the values of the means for the two groups have not been considered. To correctly evaluate the variability of the two data sets, their coefficients of variation should be calculated and compared. The coefficients of variation of the two data sets are:

$$\text{data set A: } CV(\%) = \frac{s}{\bar{X}} \times 100 = \frac{125}{2500} \times 100 = 5\%$$

$$\text{data set B: } CV(\%) = \frac{s}{\bar{X}} \times 100 = \frac{35}{50} \times 100 = 70\%$$

Therefore, the coefficient of variation of data set A is markedly less than that of data set B, illustrating the greater variability associated with the latter.

The magnitude of the coefficient of variation depends on the nature of the data concerned. Typically in pharmaceutical analytical experimentation the coefficient of variation is low (<3%) because the variability associated with such measurement is usually low. Conversely, the coefficient of variation of biological experiments, e.g. measurement of the plasma concentration of a drug in volunteers, may be quite large (up to 100%) because the variability of such measurements is often high.

2.3 Accuracy and precision

The terms *accuracy* and *precision* are frequently used to describe the nature of data and data variability. Given their particular use in certain aspects of the pharmaceutical sciences, e.g. pharmaceutical analysis, it is useful at this stage to compare and contrast these various terms and to describe their most appropriate applications.

2.3.1 Accuracy

Accuracy may be appropriately defined as the closeness of a measured value to the true value, i.e. the value that would be expected in the absence of error. In pharmaceutical analysis, it is commonplace to describe the accuracy of an analytical method as the closeness of the observed (analysed) and expected values. A number of methods may be used to describe the difference between observed and expected values, and some of these are described below.

2.3.1.1 Absolute error

Mathematically, the absolute error is calculated using the formula

$$error_{abs} = O - E$$

where $error_{abs}$ is the the absolute error, O is the observed value, or alternatively, the observed mean of a set of values, and E is the expected (true) value. The use of the absolute error is illustrated in the following example.

EXAMPLE 2.11 *A solution of quinine sulfate has been analysed using three analytical methods, and the results are shown in Table 2.13. Calculate the absolute error associated with these methods.*

The most accurate method may be defined as that which possesses the lowest value of absolute error, namely HPLC with ultraviolet detection (absolute error = +0.01 mg/mL). The least accurate method, ultraviolet spectroscopy, is associated with the largest value of absolute error.

The absolute error is a useful method by which the accuracy of a measurement may be determined, but unfortunately it is affected by the magnitude of the measurement. Thus, in the above example, the fluorescence spectroscopic method may be assumed to be relatively accurate (2.19 compared with 2.50 mg/mL), with an absolute error value of −0.31 mg/mL. However, consider an example in which the concentra-

Table 2.13 Concentration of quinine sulfate in a solution, as determined using three analytical methods

Analytical method	Observed value (mg/mL)	Expected value (mg/mL)	Absolute error (mg/mL)
HPLC with ultraviolet detection	2.51	2.50	+0.01
Ultraviolet spectroscopy	3.53	2.50	+1.03
Fluorescence spectroscopy	2.19	2.50	−0.31

tion of quinine sulfate in a second solution was 0.5 mg/mL and the concentration of the solution as measured by fluorescence spectroscopy was 0.19 mg/mL. In this example, the absolute error is −0.31 mg/mL, identical to the absolute error associated with the use of fluorescence detection for the determination of the concentration of the more concentrated quinine sulfate solution (2.50 mg/mL). However, it is apparent to the reader that, although the calculated absolute errors of these two methods are identical, the measured value (0.19 mg/mL) is not an accurate representation of the true value (0.5 mg/mL). This is the major disadvantage associated with the use of absolute errors.

2.3.1.2 Relative error

This term was developed to overcome the problem described in the preceding paragraph and describes the error as a proportion of the true (expected) value. In the calculation, the sign of the difference (positive or negative) is ignored. Thus,

$$error_{rel} = \frac{error_{abs}}{E} = \frac{O-E}{E}$$

The relative error may also be expressed as a percentage value:

$$\%error_{rel} = \frac{error_{abs} \times 100}{E} = \frac{(O-E) \times 100}{E}$$

As before, greater numerical values of relative error are indicative of decreased accuracy.

The advantage of the use of relative error may be observed by consideration of the previous example. From the last column in Table 2.14 we can see that the accuracy of a measurement may be easily determined by calculation of the relative error. In addition, the relative error may be employed to compare the accuracies of different measurements (values). Thus, the comparative accuracies of the two fluorimetric analyses of two solutions of quinine sulfate, possessing identical absolute errors, may be meaningfully compared (Table 2.14).

2.3.2 Precision

Precision is a statistical term that describes the dispersion (variability) of a set of measurements. However, unlike accuracy, precision provides no indication of the closeness of an observation to particular expected quantity. Typically, high precision is associated with a low dispersion of values around a central value, i.e. low standard deviations. The

Table 2.14 The concentrations of quinine sulphate in solution, as determined using three analytical methods

Analytical method	Observed value (mg/mL)	Expected value (mg/mL)	Absolute error (mg/mL)	Relative error (%)
HPLC with ultraviolet detection	2.51	2.50	+0.01	0.40
Ultraviolet spectroscopy	3.53	2.50	+1.03	41.20
Fluorescence spectroscopy	2.19	2.50	−0.31	12.40
Fluorescence spectroscopy	0.19	0.50	−0.31	62.00

differences between precision and accuracy are further explained in the following example, which describes the final fill volume of an antacid suspension (nominal, i.e. expected, volume 50 mL).

EXAMPLE 2.12 *In a quality control laboratory the fill volumes of three samples of an antacid suspension have been measured and recorded (Table 2.15). Comment on the accuracy and precision of the fill volumes of the three samples.*

The relative errors associated with samples A and B are identical and these samples are therefore considered to be equally accurate measurements of the true (expected) fill volume. Conversely, the accuracy of the mean fill volume of sample C is poor (43.6% relative error) and this is therefore considered to be a poor representation of the true fill volume.

Table 2.15 Fill volumes of selected samples of an antacid formulation

Fill volume of sample A (mL)	Fill volume of sample B (mL)	Fill volume of sample C (mL)
47	29	28
48	39	26
49	49	27
50	59	30
51	69	30
$\bar{X} = 49.0$	$\bar{X} = 49.0$	$\bar{X} = 28.2$
$s = 1.6$	$s = 15.8$	$s = 1.80$
Error$_{rel}$ of mean = 2.0%	Error$_{rel}$ of mean = 2.0%	Error$_{rel}$ of mean = 43.6%

Consideration of the standard deviations associated with the data from which the mean values of each sample are derived may be employed to evaluate the precision of the measurements. The data set associated with sample A has a low standard deviation (and hence a low coefficient of variation, 3.3%), denoting a small extent of dispersion of the data set around the mean. Therefore, this data set is said to be precise. Similarly, the data associated with sample C has low standard deviation (and a low coefficient of variation, 6.4%), and is also considered to be precise. Conversely, the standard deviation of the data included in sample B is high, denoting large variability around the mean (coefficient of variation is 32.2%), and hence this data set is considered to be imprecise, i.e. exhibits low precision. Therefore, to conclude:

- sample A exhibits *high* accuracy and *high* precision
- sample B exhibits *high* accuracy and *low* precision
- sample C exhibits *low* accuracy and *high* precision.

This example illustrates the main differences between accuracy and precision and has also shown that a sample may possess high accuracy and low precision and vice versa. Therefore, these two terms are not necessarily related.

2.4 Conclusions

In this chapter various methods that are employed to illustrate the central tendency and variation of a set of data or a population have been described. These measurements are referred to as descriptive statistics and form an integral part both of the description of data or populations and of the analysis of data using parametric statistical methods. In subsequent chapters the applications of these measurements will be fully illustrated and, as a reflection of their importance, the reader will gain further experience in the calculation of the mean, standard deviation, standard error of the mean and variance.

3

Presentation of data

The previous two chapters have provided an overview of the types of data generated from experimental procedures and various mathematical descriptions of this data, in terms of central tendency and variation. The reader may have observed that the data in Chapter 2 was presented in tabular form. This is one of the most common methods of data presentation, and usually follows collection and refinement of experimental outputs. Another way in which data may be presented is by the use of graphs (plots). Graphical data presentation is a powerful tool, employed by scientists in all disciplines. The use of a graphical format may indicate trends both to the experimenter and to the reader of a scientific report. This chapter is devoted to the important topic of graphical data presentation, the types of graphs that may be employed to present scientific data, and their construction.

3.1 Basic rules for construction of graphs

The construction of graphs is a relatively simple process if some simple rules are remembered.

3.1.1 Title and key

All graphs should be considered as complete units of information. The title should inform the reader of the nature of the data described: it must be concise, informative and relevant to the information contained within the graph. For graphs that contain two or more plots, a key that identifies the symbols of each plot should be provided.

3.1.2 Axes

The axes are important in the construction of graphs, because they define the spatial (pictorial) basis of the presentation of data. Graphs are composed of sets of data that describe the relationship between (usually) a fixed variable and a random variable. To ensure optimum graphical presentation of data, the choice of the range of numerical values of each axis is important. This is demonstrated here in an example from the scientific literature, which graphically presents the effects of biological fluids on the adherence of the urinary pathogen *Staphylococcus epidermidis* to polyurethane and silicone continuous ambulatory dialysis catheters. (For the reader who is not acquainted with this type of research, it is sufficient to understand that as infection related to the use of medical devices such as catheters leads to patient morbidity, and possibly mortality, it is important to identify and understand the microbial adherence process.) Figure 3.1 graphically displays the effect of a biological fluid, artificial spent dialysate, on the adherence of this organism to commercially available continuous ambulatory dialysis catheters. There are two major points that should be recognised from these graphs:

- First, the information provided on the axes is concise and explanatory, and is sufficient for the reader to understand the nature of the experiment.
- Secondly, as one of the purposes of the investigation was to compare the effects of the biological fluid on the adherence of *S. epidermidis* to catheters of different polymeric composition, it was important to select an identical numerical range on the axes of the different graphs. As may be observed from Figure 3.1, important differences are apparent between the resistance of each biomaterial to the adherence of the test microorganism and, additionally, the effect of the biological fluid on the adherence process is visually evident.

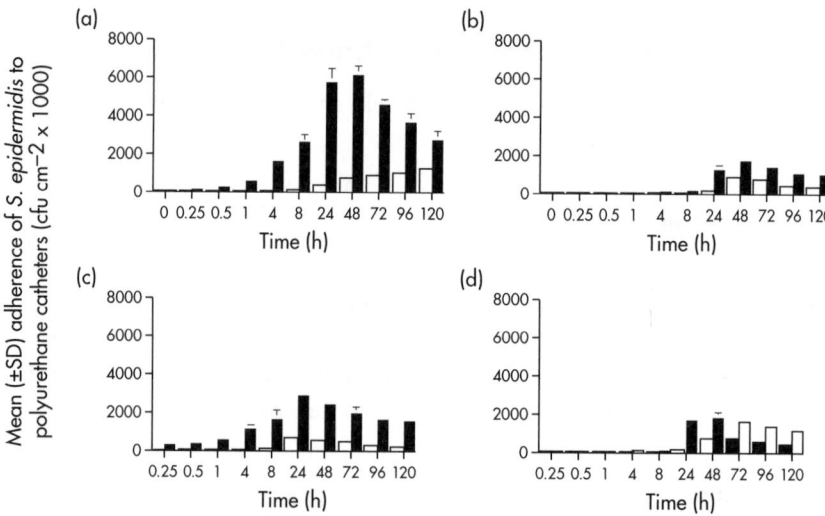

Figure 3.1 Adherence of hydrophobic (black bars) and hydrophilic (white bars) isolates of *Staphylococcus epidermidis* to (a) polyurethane peritoneal catheters pre-treated with phosphate buffered saline, (b) polyurethane peritoneal catheters pre-treated with artificial spent dialysate, (c) silicone peritoneal catheters pre-treated with phosphate buffered saline, (d) silicone peritoneal catheters pre-treated with artificial spent dialysate (from Gorman *et al.*, 1997a, reproduced with kind permission from Kluwer publishers).

It is important to select the numerical range of the axes of graphs and label them carefully to ensure clarity of data presentation.

One point of caution in selecting a numerically restricted *y* axis concerns misinterpretation of data. For example, consider the following comparison of the monthly costs to a general practitioners' practice of three types of dosage form containing a drug designed for the treatment of cardiovascular disease (Table 3.1). As may be observed, the greatest cost was associated with the use of the transdermal patch, followed by the conventional tablet and lastly the sustained release dosage form. The difference between the transdermal patch and the sustained release form is a factor of 2.2. This numerical difference is correctly highlighted in Figure 3.2a in which the height of the bar associated with the transdermal dosage form is visibly twice as great as that of the sustained release dosage form. In Figure 3.2b, the data has been plotted using an abridged *y* axis, i.e. the *y* axis numerically ranges from 2800 to 6800. Visual consideration of the heights of the bars associated with the transdermal patch and sustained release dosage forms reveals that the former now appears to be approximately 10 times greater than the latter. This is, of course, erroneous, but highlights the dangers of inappropriate selection of the numerical values of the *y* axis.

The spacing of the values of each axis must be selected according to their magnitude, to ensure that the resulting plot is proportional.

3.1.3 Estimates of variability

In certain circumstances, e.g. whenever the author wishes to illustrate statistical differences in two sets of data, it is important to include estimates of the variability of data in graphs. In so doing, it is important first to document the mathematical basis of the plotted variability, e.g. standard deviation, standard error, and secondly to ensure that the error bars do not overlap one another as this may confuse the reader.

Table 3.1 Monthly costs to a general practitioners' practice of three types of dosage form containing a drug designed for the treatment of cardiovascular disease

Type of dosage form	Average monthly cost (£)
Sustained release	3000
Transdermal patch	6500
Conventional tablet	3800

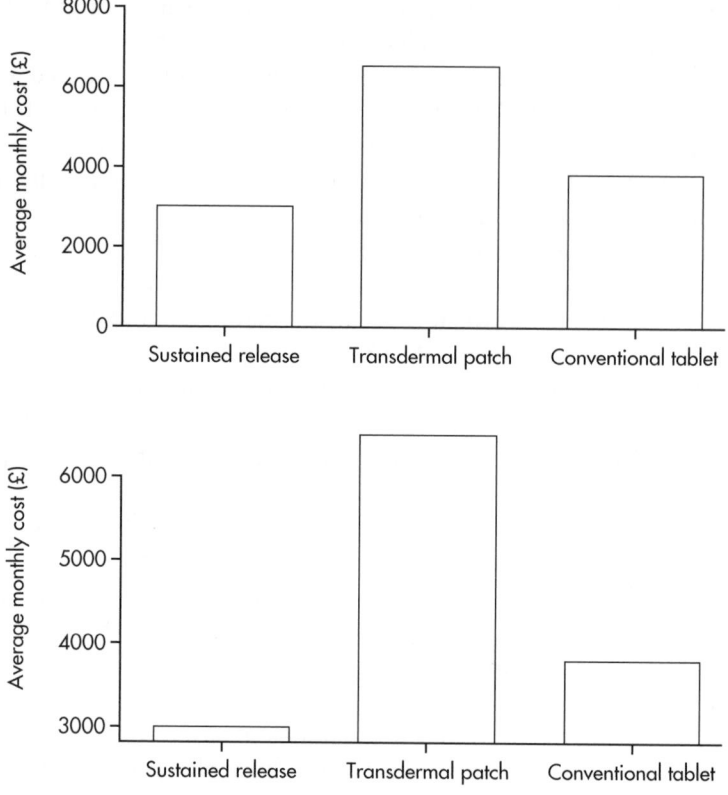

Figure 3.2 Monthly costs to general practitioners' practice of three types of dosage form containing a drug designed for the treatment of cardiovascular disease (data taken from Table 3.1).

3.2 Types of graphs and plots

There are several types of graphs or plots that are commonly employed to display scientific data, and these may be subdivided into major categories, namely:

* graphs or plots that are employed to describe relationships between a fixed (independent) variable and a dependent variable
* graphs that are employed to pictorially describe distributions of data.

3.2.1 Graphs and plots that are employed to describe relationships between a fixed (independent) variable and a dependent variable

This category is commonly used within the pharmaceutical and related sciences: examples are shown in Table 3.2. There are various formats

Table 3.2 Pharmaceutical examples of dependent and independent data sets

Dependent variable (y axis)	Independent variable (x axis)
Analytical response, e.g. fluorescence intensity, ultraviolet radiation absorbance, light scattering	Concentration of an analyte
Concentration of therapeutic agent in a biological fluid following administration of a dosage form	Time
Concentration of a therapeutic agent in a dosage form following storage	Time
Stress required to maintain the rate of shear	Rate of shear of a pharmaceutical sample
Hardness of a tablet	Force of compression during manufacture

may be used to plot such relationships between data, including line graphs, scatter graphs and bar graphs (Figure 3.3). The author has the final choice of graph format, but it is worth remembering that the chosen graph should present the data eloquently and clearly without undue clutter.

Some types of graph are employed specifically for the presentation of certain types of data. For example, scatter plots are commonly employed to display the correlation between data sets. The mathematical and practical bases of correlation will be described in Chapter 12; at this point it is enough to say that scatter plots are employed to show the existence (or not) of a linear relationship. An example is given in Figure 3.4, which shows the (lack of) relationship between the ultimate tensile strength of polyurethane ureteral stents (a measure of their resistance to fracture) and their duration of implantation in vivo in patients. The absence of a significant linear relationship between these two random variables is indicative of their low correlation.

Conversely, pie charts are commonly used to present data in the form of percentages. They are circular in design. The total area of the circle is allowed to represent 100%, i.e. the total frequency, and the chart is divided into sections according to the proportion of the data set. An example of a pie chart, depicting the prescribing costs associated with four antibiotics, is shown in Figure 3.5. Pie charts are employed primarily for the display of qualitative data; however, many authors prefer to use bar charts for this purpose because they are easier to construct and they can display quantitative data (e.g. mean and standard deviation).

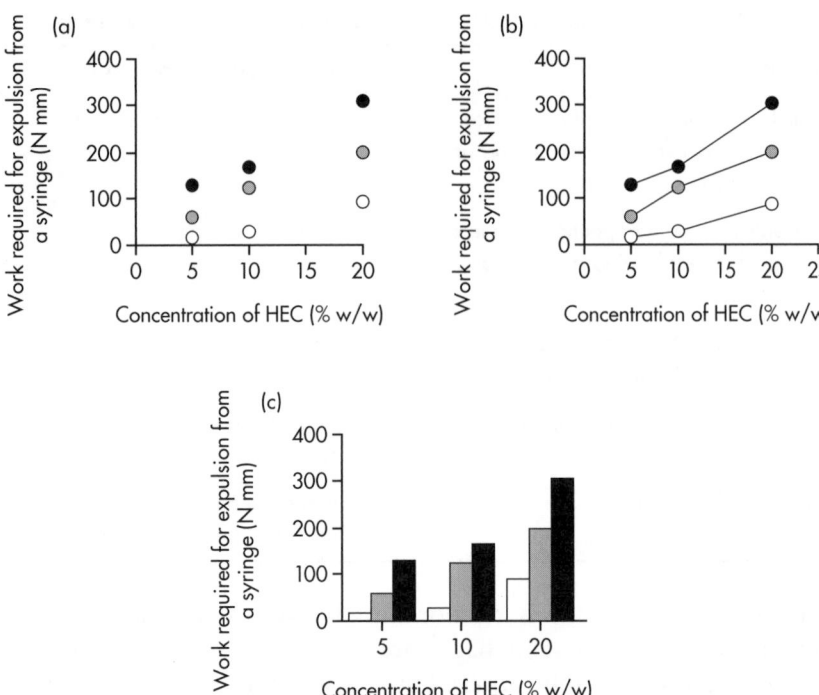

Figure 3.3 Effects of concentration of hydroxyethylcellulose (HEC) on the work required to expel bioadhesive periodontal formulations from a syringe: (a) scatter graph, (b) line graph, (c) bar graph. Open circles/bars, formulations contain 5% w/w polyvinylpyrrolidone (PVP) and 1% w/w polycarbophil (PCP); shaded circles/bars, formulations contain 10% w/w PVP and 1% w/w PCP; black circles/bars, formulations contain 20% w/w PVP and 1% w/w PCP (data taken from Jones *et al.*, 1996).

3.2.2 Graphs that are employed to pictorially describe distributions of data

Frequently, scientific data describes a distribution, e.g. the heights of men in a particular geographical region. Different procedures are adopted for the graphical presentation of this data, the most common of which are frequency and cumulative frequency distributions, histograms and stem and leaf displays. The use of these is described in the following sections.

3.2.2.1 *Frequency distributions*

As outlined, the basis of formation of frequency distributions involves the collection of data (observations), the assignment of the data into either discrete or designated categories and the presentation of this data,

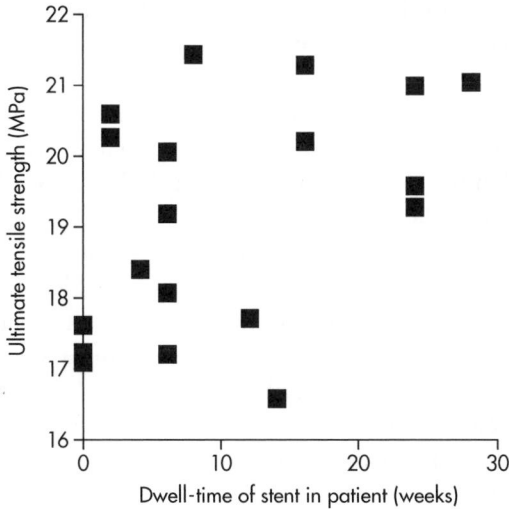

Figure 3.4 Effect of dwell-time in patients on the ultimate tensile strength of polyurethane ureteral stents (data taken from Gorman *et al.*, 1997b).

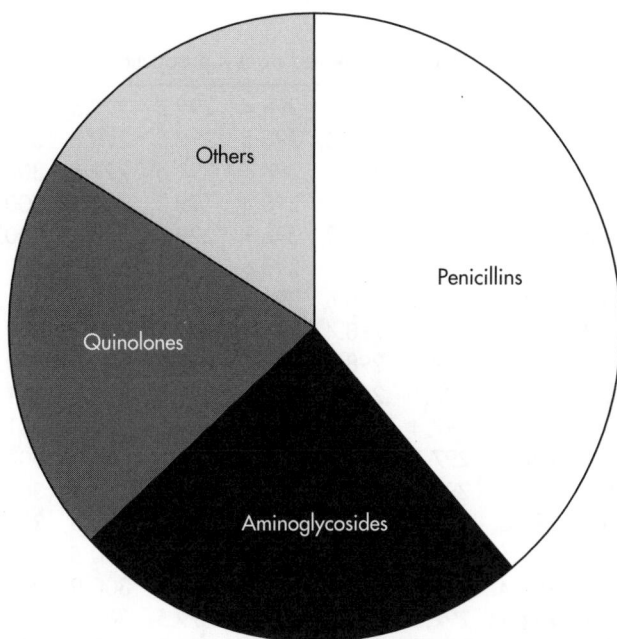

Figure 3.5 Pie chart of the prescription habits associated with four antibiotics in a general hospital: pencillins (white area) 39%; aminoglycosides (black) 24%; quinolones (dark shading) 21%; others (light shading) 16%.

e.g. in the form of a table or a graph. Frequency distributions are commonly employed to find out about the shape of the data distribution.

Suppose 210 tablets have been removed at random from a production batch of tablets and weighed (to one decimal place). The recorded weights are presented in Table 3.3. These weights have then been classified into various intervals (Table 3.4), to allow graphical presentation of this data.

Table 3.4 presents the frequency distributions for a quantitative variable, namely tablet weight. The weights of tablets is a continuous variable and can theoretically assume an infinite number of numerical values between the lowest and highest points on a scale, in this case 290–310 mg. Of course, as described in Chapter 1, the actual number of values that may be included within this category is restricted by the sensitivity of the analytical equipment (a balance, in this case). The choice of groupings shown in Table 3.4 is arbitrary and is selected by the person responsible for the collation of the data. In this case, on the basis of the objectives of the study, the sensitivity of the balances, quality control requirements etc., it has been decided that 20 groupings should be selected to represent 900-μg increments in weight. Two important terms are frequently employed in statistics to describe the

Table 3.3 Weights of 210 tablets removed from a production batch

290.2	294.1	296.4	297.5	298.5	298.4	299.5	299.5	300.2	303.9
290.5	295.4	296.5	297.6	298.6	298.5	299.5	299.8	300.4	303.8
291.5	295.6	296.8	297.4	298.5	298.6	299.6	299.9	300.4	304.1
291.8	295.4	296.5	297.5	298.7	298.4	299.3	300.1	300.5	304.5
292.4	295.8	296.4	297.1	298.3	298.1	299.8	300.1	300.5	304.6
292.8	295.6	296.8	297.4	298.4	298.6	299.4	300.2	300.8	305.1
292.6	295.1	296.1	297.5	298.6	298.3	299.8	300.5	301.2	305.9
292.7	295.3	296.1	297.6	298.4	298.4	299.1	300.4	301.5	305.6
293.4	295.8	296.5	297.1	298.6	298.5	299.2	300.5	301.4	305.4
293.5	295.5	296.4	297.1	298.2	299.1	299.6	300.5	301.5	306.9
293.6	296.5	297.2	297.4	298.2	299.2	299.5	300.9	301.5	306.8
293.8	296.1	297.5	297.7	298.1	299.8	299.6	300.8	301.8	307.1
293.7	296.5	297.7	297.8	298.4	299.5	299.4	300.9	301.6	307.6
293.8	296.4	297.8	297.6	298.2	299.6	299.5	300.8	301.5	308.5
294.1	296.8	297.6	297.4	298.6	299.8	299.4	300.5	301.6	302.1
294.5	296.9	297.4	297.8	298.5	299.4	299.3	300.9	303.1	302.5
294.6	296.9	297.1	297.5	298.5	299.8	299.5	300.9	303.2	302.5
294.8	296.9	297.3	297.5	298.3	299.3	299.8	300.8	303.6	302.7
294.6	296.2	297.6	297.3	298.3	299.3	299.4	300.8	303.5	302.8
294.8	296.5	297.4	298.4	298.3	299.6	299.5	300.4	303.5	302.2
294.3	296.8	297.1	298.3	298.1	299.4	299.1	300.2	303.4	302.7

extreme values of each class interval. The smallest value that may be included within a certain interval is termed the *real lower limit*; the *real upper limit* is the largest value that may be included in a class. Together, these two categories form the *true class limits*. It is interesting to comment on the differences between the true class limits and the values tabulated in Table 3.4. Table 3.4 has recorded defined class limits, e.g. 290, 291, 292 mg, etc., but these values do not consider the accuracy (sensitivity) of measurement of the data. In the table the weights are given to the nearest milligram. However, in the assignment of these categories, decimal values that fall equidistant between the top of one class and the bottom of another must be considered, as these form the true class limits. One of the classes in our current example is 290–291 mg. Tablets weighing 289.5 mg and 291.4 mg would have been recorded as 290 and 291 mg, respectively. Hence, these tablets would have been classified as residing within the class 290–291 mg. The true class limits of a frequency distribution are therefore dependent on the accuracy (sensitivity) of measurement or collection of data.

The data presented in Table 3.4 may be presented as a frequency distribution to visualise the distribution of data (Figure 3.6). The data

Table 3.4 The weights in Table 3.3 classified into intervals

Weight of tablet (mg)	Number (frequency)
290.1–291.0	2
291.1–292.0	2
292.1–293.0	4
293.1–294.0	6
294.1–295.0	8
295.1–296.0	9
296.1–297.0	21
297.1–298.0	30
298.1–299.0	32
299.1–300.0	36
300.1–301.0	24
301.1–302.0	9
302.1–303.0	7
303.1–304.0	8
304.1–305.0	3
305.1–306.0	4
306.1–307.0	2
307.1–308.0	2
308.1–309.0	1
309.1–310.0	0

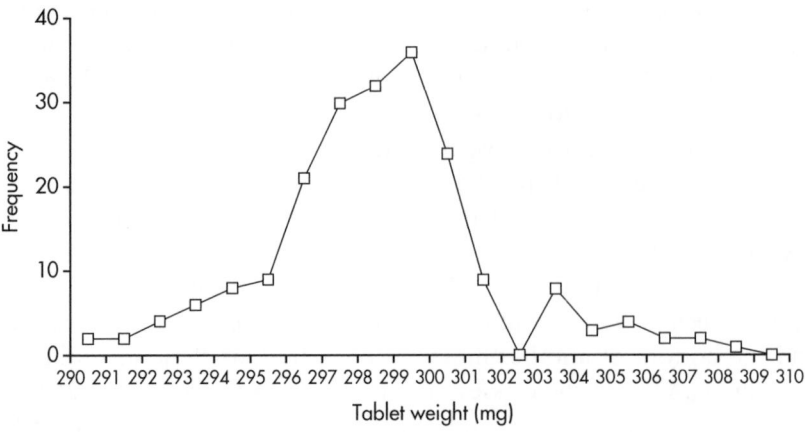

Figure 3.6 Frequency distribution (polygon) of the weights of 210 tablets removed from a production batch (data derived from Table 3.4).

described in Table 3.5 may also be presented as a frequency distribution. In this, the number of side-effects is a defined quantity and is therefore termed a *discrete variable*.

3.2.2.2 Histograms

The frequency distribution of a data set may also be conveniently presented using a *histogram*. Histograms look similar to bar charts: both consist of a set of rectangles, both have their bases on the *x* axis with centres at the class marks and, in both cases, the areas are proportional to class frequency. However, histograms are used primarily to graphically present frequency distributions and, in addition, the individual bars are adjacent (joined) to one another to form a continuous data display. An example of a histogram is shown in Figure 3.7, using the data presented in Table 3.4.

Table 3.5 The incidence of side-effects associated with the clinical use of a new antihypertensive agent in 80 patients: an example of a frequency distribution that employs a discrete variable (number of side-effects)

Side-effects	Number (frequency) of patients
1	12
2	20
3	24
4	12
5	12

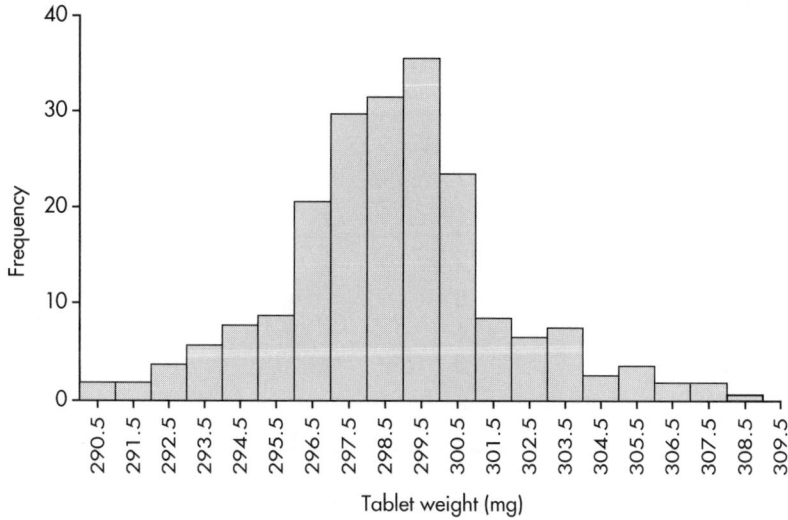

Figure 3.7 Histogram of weights of 210 tablets removed from a production batch (data derived from Table 3.4).

In histograms, class intervals are typically chosen to be of the same size, e.g. in the above figure the class interval is 1 mg. In these circumstances, the heights of the rectangles are therefore directly proportional to the class frequencies and, consequently, height is frequently employed to define the number of observations in a particular class interval. If the class intervals are not all the same size, it is important to adjust the data accordingly, as in the following example.

EXAMPLE 3.1   *As part of the quality control procedures in a pharmaceutical company, the concentration of oxytetracycline in an injection formulation has been analysed in 30 vials. The results are recorded in Table 3.6.*

In the above example, the class intervals are of equal magnitude and therefore the height of the bars in the histogram will be directly proportional to their areas. However, if the data is presented in a different format, e.g. if the class intervals from 101.0–101.9 (six observations) and 102.0–102.9 mg/mL (three observations) were combined, we would have a new class interval, 101.0–102.9 mg/mL, with nine observations. To ensure that the histogram is constructed correctly, the total number of observations in this new class interval should be divided by two, as the new interval is twice the size of the other intervals. When the histogram is plotted, the width of the new class interval will be twice

Table 3.6 Concentration of oxytetracycline in parenteral vials that have been removed from a production batch

Concentration (mg/mL)	Number of vials
95.0–95.9	1
96.0–96.9	1
97.0–97.9	2
98.0–98.9	3
99.0–99.9	4
100.0–100.9	8
101.0–101.9	6
102.0–102.9	3
103.0–103.9	1
104.0–104.9	1

that of the others and the associated frequency (on the y axis) will be 4.5, so the total area of the histogram will remain constant.

3.2.2.3 Construction of frequency distributions and histograms

There are several points that should be remembered concerning the optimal presentation of data as a frequency distribution.

- Initially, the largest and smallest values in the set of collected data, and hence the range of data, should be identified. For example, in Table 3.3 the range is 290.2–308.5 mg.
- The range of data should then be divided into an appropriate number of intervals, called *class intervals*. These intervals should be of the same size, where possible. The size of the class interval is dependent both on the data and on the type of information for presentation, but usually between 5 and 20 class intervals are chosen. In Table 3.4, 20 class intervals were chosen to provide comprehensive information about the weight distribution of tablets in a production batch, an important quality control concern.
- In histograms, it is important that mathematical corrections are carried out to compensate for class intervals of unequal sizes.
- Once the class intervals have been chosen, the number (frequency) of observations falling within each interval is recorded. The product is a frequency distribution.

3.2.2.4 Cumulative frequency distributions

Another method of graphical presentation of data may be as a cumulative frequency distribution. In this, the data are typically presented in terms of the total frequency of all observations that are less than the upper class boundary of a class interval. This is conveniently termed a 'less than' cumulative frequency distribution. Alternatively, the data may be presented in terms of the total frequency of observations that are greater than or equal to the lower class boundary of a particular class interval, i.e. a *'more than'* cumulative frequency distributions. An example of each of these types of cumulative frequency distribution is presented below, using the data described in Table 3.7.

The class intervals used in Table 3.7 commence at one tenth of a unit and go up to the next full unit, e.g. from 290.1 to 291.0. In the generation of cumulative frequency information and plots, it is important to correctly state the cumulative frequency less than each upper class limit, or alternatively, more than the lower class limit for each of the class intervals. This correction has been performed in Table 3.7 by calculating the average, i.e. the true upper or lower class limits, of the upper value of one class interval and the lower value of the next interval. In the example above, the upper class limits have been calculated as 0.05 mg greater than the tabulated limits.

The main use of cumulative frequency plots is in the estimation of the total number of observations occurring either below or above a

Table 3.7 Cumulative frequency distribution data describing the weights of 210 tablets selected from a production batch

Weight of tablet (mg)	Cumulative frequency (less than)	Weight of tablet (mg)	Cumulative frequency (more than)
<290.05	0	>290.05	210
<291.05	2	>291.05	208
<292.05	4	>292.05	206
<293.05	8	>293.05	202
<294.05	14	>294.05	196
<295.05	22	>295.05	188
<296.05	31	>296.05	179
<297.05	52	>297.05	158
<298.05	82	>298.05	128
<299.05	114	>299.05	96
<300.05	150	>300.05	60
<301.05	174	>301.05	36
<302.05	183	>302.05	27
<303.05	190	>303.05	20
<304.05	198	>304.05	12
<305.05	201	>305.05	9
<306.05	205	>306.05	5
<307.05	207	>307.05	3
<308.05	209	>308.05	1
<309.05	210	>309.05	0
<310.05	210	>310.05	0

particular class interval. For example, if you have been asked by the quality control division of your company to estimate the number of tablets that weighed below 300.05 mg, you can easily do so using the graph in Figure 3.8 by drawing a vertical line from the specified value (300.05 mg) until it contacts the 'less than' cumulative frequency plot. At this intersection, a horizontal line is drawn and extended until it intersects the y axis. The numerical value at this intersection reflects the number of tablets that weigh less than the specified value (150). The same approach may be used to calculate of the number of tablets that weighed above a specific value, but of course in this instance; the 'more than' cumulative frequency plot should be used.

Cumulative frequency plots may also be employed to estimate the number of observations occurring within defined class intervals. For example, the quality control manager may request information about the total number of tablets that weighed less than 295.05 mg but more than (or equal to) 292.5 mg. The solution to this problem is similar to the previous example. First, a vertical line is drawn from the defined value on the x axis (295.05) until it intersects with the 'less than' cumulative frequency plot, and then a horizontal line is drawn until it intersects the y axis. The numerical value, an estimate of the number of tablets that weigh less than 295.05 mg, is then recorded. This approach

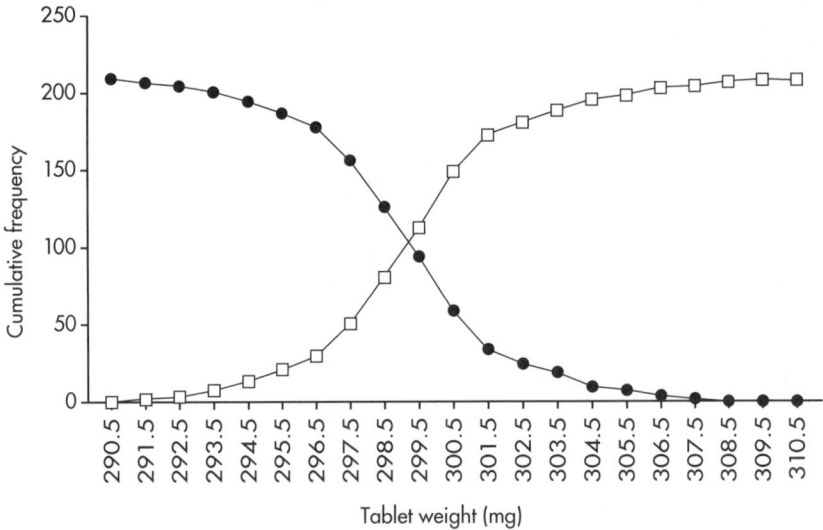

Figure 3.8 Cumulative frequency distributions of weights of 210 tablets removed from a production batch (data derived from Table 3.4). Open squares depict a *less than* cumulative frequency distribution, black circles represent a *more than* cumulative frequency distribution.

is then repeated using 292.5 mg as the starting point on the x axis. The corresponding value on the y axis provides an estimate of the number of tablets that weighed more than 292.5 mg. The latter value (>292.5 mg) is then subtracted from the former value (<295.05 mg) to determine the number of tablets that weighed within the specified limits.

Finally, *percentage cumulative frequency polygons* may also be employed to display data. In these, the conventional y axis (frequency) is transformed to a percentage by dividing by the total frequency. This allow us to calculate the percentage of observations occurring less than (or more than) a defined class interval to be calculated in the fashion described above. The understanding and interpretation of percentage cumulative frequency distributions, e.g. the *cumulative normal distribution*, is an important concept in statistics and we will return to it in subsequent chapters.

3.2.2.5 Stem and leaf plots

Although histograms and frequency distributions are commonly employed for the presentation of data, these methods do have some disadvantages. For example, the quality of the information presented is dependent on the operator's choice of class intervals. Poor choice of such intervals may result in an inadequate summary of data. Furthermore, in histograms where the data is grouped, the individual numerical values of each datum are lost. One method that does not suffer from these disadvantages is the stem and leaf plot. In this approach, each datum is numerically divided into two portions, referred to as the stem and leaf. The *stem* is composed of a vertical arrangement of integers; the *leaves* are formed by adding a unit to the integers. In contrast to the vertical arrangement of the stem, the leaves are arranged horizontally, adjacent to the parent integer. The generation of a stem and leaf plot may be further explained using the data presented in Table 3.8, which describes the systolic blood pressure of a group of 30 men aged between 40 and 50.

The first step in the formation of a stem and leaf plot involves the selection of the stem, i.e. the backbone of the plot. The integers chosen

Table 3.8   The systolic blood pressure (mmHg) of 30 men aged 40–50 years

145	148	133	171	144	158
165	156	138	154	140	146
124	158	150	178	157	138
149	160	142	125	164	175
154	161	168	131	120	162

for the stem usually consist of the first digits of the data. For example, for the first value in Table 3.8 (145 mmHg), a suitable stem is 14 and for the last datum point in the table, i.e. 162 mmHg, the stem would be 16. The stem values are then arranged vertically in ascending order. For the data set described in Table 3.8, the stems are as follows:

| 12 |
| 13 |
| 14 |
| 15 |
| 16 |
| 17 |

To complete the stem and leaf plot, the last digit of each number (the leaf) is placed horizontally adjacent to the corresponding stem grouping. The completed stem plot for the data in Table 3.8 is as shown in Figure 3.9. The stem plot has provided a visual representation of the data set. Indeed, it may be observed that the data is reasonably symmetrical. Estimating the shape (symmetry) of the data set is one of the main uses of the stem and leaf plot.

Before leaving the concept of stem and leaf plots, there are a couple of further points that require clarification:

- The selection of the numerical value of the stem is dependent on the size range of the data pool. For example, the stem associated with the data presented in Table 3.4, whose range is 290.2–308.5 mg, is 290, 291, 292 mg, etc., and the leaves are the decimal place. Thus the stem of the value 290.2 is 290 and the associated leaf is 0.2 mg.
- In the example relating to Table 3.8, the choice of stem has ensured that the class interval is 10 mmHg. Under certain circumstances, it may be appropriate to subdivide the class intervals to gain a greater understanding of the

Stem	Leaf						
12	0	4	5				
13	1	3	8	8			
14	0	2	4	5	6	8	9
15	0	4	4	6	7	8	8
16	0	1	2	4	5	8	
17	1	5	8				

Figure 3.9 Stem and leaf plot for the data described in Table 3.8 concerning the systolic blood pressure of 30 men aged 40–50 years. In this figure a class interval of 10 mmHg has been employed

distribution of data within smaller limits of the data. Once more, using the data presented in Table 3.8, the stem and leaf plot may be redrawn to encompass a smaller class interval, such as 5 mmHg (Figure 3.10).

One interesting application of stem and leaf plots is in the comparison of two distributions, in which either distribution is plotted on either side of the stem. An example of this is shown in Table 3.9, which presents the blood cholesterol levels in 20 male and female patients aged between 50 and 60 years. Assuming a class interval of 10 mg%, the stem and leaf plot for the above data sets would appear as in Figure 3.11.

As may be observed, the stem and leaf plot is particularly useful in describing the distribution in blood cholesterol levels and, additionally, for visual comparison of the cholesterol concentration in the two sets of volunteers.

3.2.3   Common morphologies of frequency curves

One of the main themes of this chapter has been the use of graphical methods for the visual representation of frequency data. In the examples considered so far, the distributions have been similar in shape; however, it is important for the reader to understand that frequency distributions may adopt a number of different morphologies. Indeed, as will be described in subsequent chapters in this book, the shape of the

Stem	Leaf			
12a	0	4		
12b	5			
13a	1	3		
13b	8	8		
14a	0	2	4	
14b	5	6	8	9
15a	0	4	4	
15b	6	7	8	8
16a	0	1	2	4
16b	5	8		
17a	1			
17b	5	8		

Figure 3.10   Stem and leaf plot for the data described in Table 3.8 concerning the systolic blood pressure of 30 men aged 40–50 years. In this figure a class interval of 5 mmHg has been employed.

Table 3.9 Cholesterol blood levels (mg%) in male and female volunteers aged 50–60 years

Males	Females
200	190
210	185
195	174
184	196
220	182
236	200
210	165
235	199
240	210
200	202
199	200
189	190
236	186
240	179
250	190
243	184
230	182
225	201
237	191
215	180

			Leaf (Males)	Stem	Leaf (Females)				
				16	5				
				17	4	9			
			9	4	18	0	2	2	4	5	6
			9	5	19	0	0	0	1	6	9
			0	0	20	0	0	1	2
	5	5	0	0	21	0
				0	22	
7	6	6	5	0	23	
		3	0	0	24	
				0	25	

Figure 3.11 Stem and leaf plot for the data described in Table 3.9 concerning the cholesterol blood levels in male and female volunteers aged 50–60 years. In this figure a class interval of 10 mm% has been employed.

frequency distribution directly affects the choice of statistical method that may be applied to the data.

In this chapter, examples of frequency distributions have been described and illustrated, e.g. Figure 3.6. These graphs are rather jagged in nature, as a direct result of the class intervals used to describe the data and, additionally, the (limited) number of recorded observations. As a result of these limitations, such plots are termed *frequency polygons*. The jagged nature of the frequency polygons may be reduced, i.e. smoothed, by increasing the number of observations and by decreasing the class interval. The weights of 210 tablets were listed in Table 3.3, and their weight distributions were displayed in Figure 3.6. The shape of this plot would have been much smoother if, for instance, 2500 tablets had been weighed and characterised into class intervals of 0.1 mg.

Whenever distributions are derived from a large sample size and plotted using restricted class intervals, a number of different morphologies may result. It is possible to categorise the shapes of the distribution in the following ways:

- They may be *unimodal* (one peak), *bimodal* (two peaks) or *multimodal*.
- For unimodal distributions, is there *symmetry* or *asymmetry* (a *skewed* distribution)? An important example of a symmetrical, unimodal distribution is the *normal distribution*, which is discussed in more detail in subsequent chapters.
- For asymmetrical distributions, is the distribution skewed to the left (*positive*) or to the right (*negative*)?

There are other distributions that do not conform to the above classification, such as the J-shaped and reverse J-shaped distributions, in which there is a maximum at one end of the distribution. An interesting example of (skewed) J-shaped distributions was reported by Gorman *et al.* (1996). In this study the authors examined the effects of a non-antibiotic antimicrobial agent, chlorhexidine gluconate, on the adherence of the opportunistic pathogen *Candida albicans* to buccal epithelial cells, an important virulence attribute. In Figure 3.12 it may be observed that the distribution of adherence of blastospores (control and treated) to buccal epithelial cells follows a reverse J-shaped distribution. One other interesting observation may also be made from these curves. In both cases, the frequency distributions of the treated *C. albicans* blastospores were shifted towards the *y* axis. These shifts were due both to a decrease in the mean number of adherent blastospores per buccal epithelial cell and, importantly, to an increased number of buccal epithelial cells with few or no adherent blastospores of *C. albicans*. These observations provide an insight into the potential usefulness of chlorhexidine gluconate for the prevention of infection.

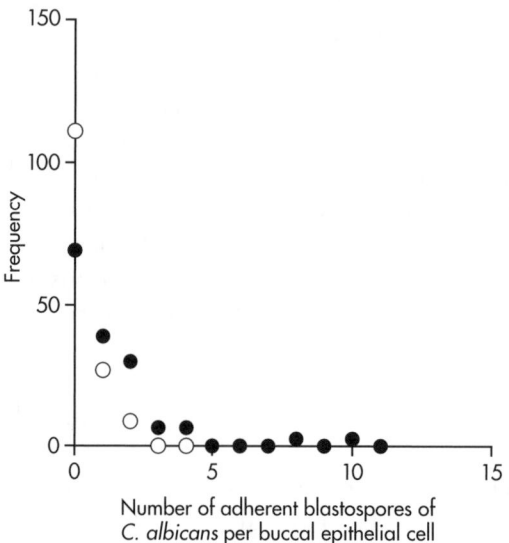

Number of adherent blastospores of
C. *albicans* per buccal epithelial cell

Figure 3.12 Effects of chlorhexidine gluconate (0.005% v/v) treatment of blastospores of *Candida albicans* on their subsequent adherence to buccal epithelial cells in vitro. Open circles represent the adherence of viable blastospores following treatment with chlorhexidine gluconate; black circles represent the adherence of control (deionised-water treated) viable blastospores (data taken from Gorman *et al.*, 1996).

3.2.3.1 Skewness and kurtosis

Two further important terms that are used to describe many frequency distributions are *skewness* and *kurtosis*. Skewness is employed to quantify the degree of asymmetry of a distribution and there are several methods by which it may be calculated. The first method, termed *Pearson's first coefficient of skewness*, is as follows:

˙skewness = (mean − mode)/standard deviation

As the mean and mode are equal in a normal distribution, the skewness coefficient of a normal distribution is equal to zero.

Another method to estimate asymmetry (skewness), which avoids the use of the mode, is termed *Pearson's second coefficient of skewness*, and is defined as follows:

skewness = 3(mean − median)/standard deviation

Other measures of skewness, including the moment coefficient of skewness, are also used in statistics, but these are more complex and are outside the remit of this text.

Kurtosis is a characterisation of the density of observations residing within different regions of a distribution.

- The standardised normal distribution is a defined frequency distribution and is described as *mesokurtic*. The properties of this distribution are described in more detail in the next chapter.
- If the shape of the peak of the normal curve is flattened, i.e. data has been transposed from the centre and tails into the shoulder regions of the curve, the distribution is said to be *platykurtic*.
- A *leptokurtic* curve is one in which the centre region has been elongated and the density of the tails increased.

3.3 Conclusions

In this chapter various methods for the graphical presentation of scientific data have been described. The type of graph selected is primarily the choice of the author of the study; however, regardless of the actual choice made, it is important that the graph accurately presents the data. Sufficient detail should accompany each graph to ensure its interpretation by other scientists.

In addition, this chapter introduced the concept of frequency distributions and related plots and their construction. The use and interpretation of frequency distributions is an integral aspect of statistics and will be continued in subsequent chapters.

References

Gorman S P, Jones D S, Adair C G, *et al.* (1997a). Conditioning fluid influences on the surface properties of silicon and polyurethane peritoneal catheters: implications for infection. *J Mat Sci: Mat Med* 8: 631–5.

Gorman S P, Jones D S, Bonner M C, *et al.* (1997b). Mechanical performance of polyurethane ureteral stents in vitro and ex vivo. *Biomaterials* 18(20): 1379–83.

Gorman S P, Jones D S, McGovern J G, Woolfson A D (1996). Frequency distribution of *Candida albicans* blastospores adhered to mucosal epithelial cells in-vitro. *J Pharm Pharmacol* 48(12): 1315–19.

Jones D S, Woolfson A D, Djokic J, Coulter W A (1996) Development and physical charaterisation of bioadhesive semi-solid, polymeric systems containing tetracycline for the treatment of periodontal diseases. *Pharm Res* 13(11): 17321–6.

4

Probability and probability distributions

Probability may be generically defined as the aspect of mathematics that is concerned with calculating the likelihood of the occurrence of an event. Despite the overtly mathematical nature of probability, the use of the term has become an integral part of modern conversation. Consequently, it is not uncommon to hear or use phrases such as 'I have a 50% chance of passing this exam' or 'There is a 70% chance of rain today', 'The player has a 30% chance of being passed fit for the match', and so on. Because of the widespread use of this most basic aspect of probability theory, most people have some basic understanding of the principles involved. One of the most common applications of probability theory in a 'non-scientific' discipline is in gambling, and indeed, this application was largely responsible for the development of the science of probability.

The importance of probability theory to statistical analysis cannot be overemphasised. In Chapters 1–3, the concepts of variables and the mathematical and graphical descriptions of sets of data have been explained. These chapters have therefore provided an introduction to descriptive statistics. The sub-discipline of statistics known as *inferential statistics* is of great importance, as this provides the various methods by which the comparative analysis of sets of data may be performed. Inferential statistics allows information about a large population to be estimated on the basis of the statistical analysis of a smaller sample from that population. Central to the operation of inferential statistics is a knowledge of probability. It is often said that a thorough knowledge of probability theory is required in order to fully understand statistics. The present author endorses this, but to provide a full coverage of probability theory would not fall within the remit of this textbook, and therefore only a basic introduction to the topic, sufficient for the understanding of the latter chapters of the textbook, is provided.

4.1 Basic probability theory

In the introductory section of this chapter, the general public awareness of probability was highlighted. Most people possess the ability to calculate some basic aspects of probability; for instance, everyone is aware that when a coin is tossed there are only two outcomes, heads or tails. Therefore, the chance of obtaining a head following a single toss of an unbiased (fair) coin is 50%. (Note the use of the term 'unbiased': this enables us to assume that the outcome of the procedure is dominated by the laws of chance and not, for example, by a defect in the manufacture or geometry of the coin that will predispose to a particular experimental outcome.) Other examples that are frequently used to illustrate probability theory include the probability of obtaining a particular number following the rolling of a die, or the chance of picking a particular card from a shuffled pack.

Probability theory is also employed in pharmaceutically relevant situations. For example, the performance of a new injection filling machine may be ascertained by removing 500 vials of filled product from the first production batch of a product and measuring their fill volumes to examine whether or not the final volume is within the specification for the product. If 496 vials, i.e. 0.992 or 99.2%, are found to be within specification, the probability of the fill volume passing the finished product specification is 0.992. This is not an exact value but rather an estimate of the probability of the filling performance of the new machine. To determine an exact value is impractical because it would require analysis of every vial in the batch. Therefore, in this scenario, the probability of an event in a population has been estimated by measuring the probability of the event associated with a sample that has been removed from the population.

4.1.1 Basic rules of probability

Having described some simple examples, we can now state some basic rules that are employed to calculate probability.

4.1.1.1 *Range of values*

The probability of an event occurring must fall between 0 and 1. Therefore, a probability of 1 indicates that an event *will* occur, whereas a probability of 0 indicates that an event *will not* occur.

4.1.1.2 *Calculation of probability*

The probability of an event is calculated by dividing the number of ways or times an event occurs by the way all possible outcomes can occur. Hence the probability of rolling a 2, 3 or 6 in one throw of an unbiased die is 3/6 = 0.5.

4.1.1.3 Mutually exclusive events

The probability of the occurrence of two or more mutually exclusive events may be calculated by the addition of the individual probabilities for each event. Hence, in a situation where there are two events (A and B), the probability (P) of either event occurring may be described by:

$$P(A \text{ or } B) = P(A) + P(B)$$

The term *mutually exclusive* implies that if one event occurs, then the other events do not occur. To illustrate this principle, consider a scenario in which 10 coloured beads – 5 red, 4 green and 1 blue – have been placed into an opaque box. The probability of randomly withdrawing a red or green bead from the box may be calculated by adding together the individual probabilities associated with the withdrawal of either coloured bead. Therefore,

$$P(\text{red or green}) = P(0.5) + P(0.4) = 0.9$$

i.e. there is a 90% chance of withdrawing either a red or a green bead from the box. This is a mutually exclusive situation. If a red bead was selected it cannot be green or blue at the same time. It is essential not to overlook the selection of mutually exclusive events; careful consideration must be given to experimental details. For example, consider the situation in which you have been asked to calculate the probability of selecting a Jack or a spade from a pack of playing cards. These two events are not mutually exclusive, as one can select the Jack of spades card.

4.1.1.4 Independent events

The probability of two independent events both occurring may be mathematically described using the multiplication rule:

$$P(A \text{ and } B) = P(A) \times P(B)$$

The use of this rule may be easily demonstrated by considering the above example of the selection of coloured beads from an opaque box. What is the probability of removing a green and a blue bead from the box? In fact there are two answers to this problem, depending on the experimental method employed. In the first scenario, the first bead may be removed, its colour noted and the bead then replaced into the box. Under these circumstances, the probability is calculated using the equation described above. Hence:

$$P(\text{green and blue}) = P(\text{green}) \times P(\text{blue}) = 0.4 \times 0.1 = 0.04$$

i.e. there is a 4% chance of picking a green bead and a blue bead. This equation is therefore used whenever the occurrence of the first event does not affect the probability of the second or subsequent events.

The observant reader may by now have identified the scenario in which the multiplication rule, in the form shown above, may not be employed for the calculation of the probability of the joint occurrence of two independent events. In the example above, the probability of removing a green bead is 0.4. Suppose that following its removal, the green bead is placed to one side, i.e. it is not replaced in the box. The probability of removing a blue bead is now 1/9 (0.11) and not 0.1. In this situation, the probability of removing a green and blue bead, in that order is calculated using the following equation:

$$P(\text{green and blue}) = P(\text{green}) \times P(\text{blue following green})$$
$$= 0.4 \times 0.11$$
$$= 0.044$$

A further example of this type of problem may be found in the lottery draws that are now commonplace in many countries. Imagine a hypothetical example in which the lottery game is composed of 40 numbers and the draw consists of removing 6 numbers randomly without replacement. You may wish to calculate the probability of drawing 6 numbers in a specific order. The answer is quite sobering and is calculated as in Table 4.1. Fortunately, in the real world lotteries only ask for 6 numbers to be selected and no sequential ordering is required. To calculate the probability of winning the lottery, the probability of the above event is multiplied by the number of different ways in which the 6 numbers may be drawn, i.e. 6! (720). Therefore, the probability of winning the jackpot in a 50-ball lottery is (only!) 2.6×10^{-7} $(3.61 \times 10^{-10} \times 720)$.

Table 4.1 Probability of selection of six numbers in a specific order in a typical lottery draw

Event	Number of possible outcomes	Probability
P(first number)	40	1/40 = 0.0250
P(second number)	39	1/39 = 0.0256
P(third number)	38	1/38 = 0.0263
P(fourth number)	37	1/37 = 0.0270
P(fifth number)	36	1/36 = 0.0278
P(sixth number)	35	1/35 = 0.0286

Total probability = [(0.0250) × (0.0256) × (0.0263) × (0.0270) × (0.0278) × (0.0286)] = 3.61×10^{-10}

4.1.1.5 *Events that are not mutually exclusive*

To calculate the probability of two events that are not mutually exclusive, the addition law of probability described in section 4.1.1.3 may be employed, but this must be applied in corrected form to account for the overlap of the two events. A good example of a scenario in which two events are not mutually exclusive is the calculation of the probability of drawing either a King or a diamond from a pack of cards. Mathematically, an equation may be written for such problems:

$$P(A \text{ and } B) = P(A) + P(B) - P(AB)$$

where A is the probability of drawing a King, i.e. 4/52 (0.077); B is the probability of drawing a diamond, i.e. 13/52 (0.25); and AB is the probability of drawing the King of diamonds, i.e. the non-mutually exclusive event. The probability of this is 1/52 (0.019), so the overall probability may be calculated as:

$$P(A \text{ and } B) = (0.077) + (0.25) - (0.019) = 0.308$$

To further highlight this problem, consider the following typical pharmaceutical example.

EXAMPLE 4.1 *The labelling of pharmaceutical products is an essential component of their finished product specification as the contents of the label provide information concerning the chemical composition of the product, and the use (and safety) and accountability of the product. Imagine that you are in charge of the quality control section of a large pharmaceutical company and you have recently being asked to assess the quality of labels of a new product that has been supplied by an external source. To assess the quality of the new source of labels, 1000 labels have been removed from the quarantine area and their appearance recorded. The findings are displayed in Table 4.2. Calculate the probability of finding a label that is defective either because of illegibility of wording (due to a printing error) or poor adhesion.*

Table 4.2 Quality control assessment of a sample of labels from a batch

Defect (if any)	Number of observation (frequency)
None	905
Illegibility of wording	45
Illegibility of company's logo	25
Poor adhesion	15
Illegibility of wording and poor adhesion	10

This problem may be addressed as follows:

P(illegibility of wording or poor adhesion)

$= P$(illegibility of wording)

$+ P$(poor adhesion) $- P$(illegibility of wording and poor adhesion)

$= (45/1000) + (15/1000) - (10/1000)$

$= 0.05$

i.e. 50 labels were defective in terms of either illegibility of wording or poor adhesion.

4.2 Probability distributions

The reader should now be acquainted with the basic rules concerning the calculation of the probabilities associated with an event. Inferential statistics employs probability theory to make assumptions about the properties of populations on the basis of data recorded from smaller samples taken from a population. An instrumental component of such estimations is the use of probability distributions, i.e. the relationships between particular variables and their probability of occurrence. In examples where the variable is discrete, the relationship between the set of variables and their associated probabilities is referred to as a *discrete probability distribution*; if the variable is continuous in nature, the resultant distribution is termed a *continuous probability distribution*. In many scientific disciplines, e.g. pharmaceutical sciences, physics, chemistry or biology, it is often possible to theoretically predict (calculate) the outcome of experiments on the basis of a knowledge of the scientific principles underlying the experiment. For example, the probability associated with a particular genetic trait may be predicted. In the pharmaceutical sciences or engineering, mathematical modelling techniques may be employed to provide an estimation of the outcome of an experiment. When the outcomes from experiments differ from these expected distributions, a researcher will often conclude that the initial assumptions were, at least in part, incorrect and will therefore require amendment.

4.2.1 Discrete probability distributions

As previously described, discrete probability distributions are those in which the probability of the occurrence of discrete events is calculated and graphically portrayed. To illustrate these, consider firstly the numerical outcome following the rolling of one die and then two dice (Table 4.3).

Table 4.3 Probabilities associated with defined numerical values obtained following the rolling of one or two dice

One die		Two dice	
Variable (numerical outcome)	Probability	Variable (numerical outcome)	Probability
1	0.167	2	0.038
2	0.167	3	0.056
3	0.167	4	0.083
4	0.167	5	0.111
5	0.167	6	0.139
6	0.167	7	0.167
		8	0.139
		9	0.111
		10	0.083
		11	0.056
		12	0.038

The plot of theoretical probabilities against defined variables is referred to as a *probability distribution*. The reader will probably have noticed the similarities between probability distributions and frequency distributions. Typically, probability distributions are generated either following theoretical considerations (as described in Table 4.3) or, alternatively, following the collection of a large number of observations. In general terms, frequency distributions represent the distribution of data derived from the analysis of a sample taken from a population, whereas probability distributions reflect the distribution of a variable in a population. Two further points are worth mentioning here:

- In a probability distribution, the sum of all the individual probabilities is always 1 (i.e. the area under the plotted distribution is 1).
- The distribution shown in Figure 4.1 is a discrete probability distribution because the variable can adopt a countable number of values.

  A second example of a discrete probability distribution is shown in Table 4.4.

4.2.2 Binomial distribution

One of the distributions most commonly employed in the pharmaceutical and life sciences is the binomial distribution. This distribution is used whenever the outcome of an event consists of only two categories. An example of a binomial event has been described previously, namely tossing of a coin. Other examples of binomial data include:

- the outcome of a quality control assessment, which is either a *pass* or a *fail*

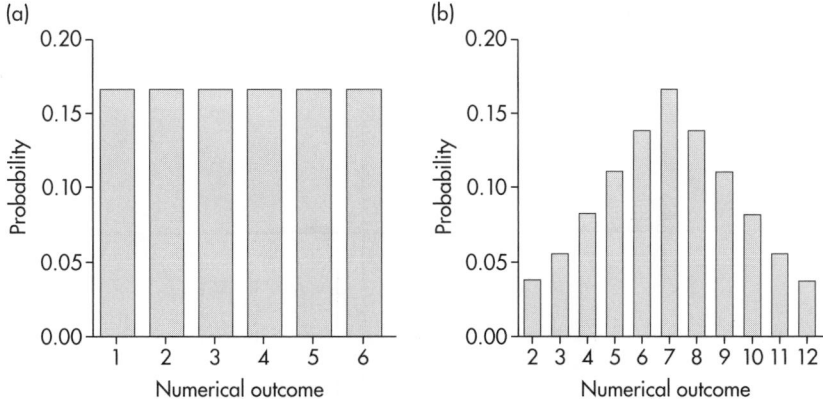

Figure 4.1 Probability distributions for the numerical values shown in Table 4.3 after rolling one die (a) and two dice (b).

Table 4.4 The incidence of side-effects in 8500 patients associated with the clinical use of a new antihypertensive agent

Number of side-effects	Number (frequency) of patients	Probability
1	1200	0.15
2	2000	0.25
3	2400	0.30
4	1700	0.20
5	1200	0.15

- a new formulation may produce side-effects: the outcomes is either *positive* or *negative* (no effects)
- the gender distribution in a population, with only two outcomes – *male* or *female*
- the prevalence of disease in a population: the disease is either *present* or *absent*
- a new pharmaceutical agent is either clinically *efficacious* or *non-efficacious*.

In addition to the requirement for only two possible outcomes, each binomial trial must be independent, i.e. the occurrence of one event must not influence subsequent events. This general concept has been described in section 4.1.1.

In the generation of the binomial distribution, it is assumed that the proportion of observations (or individuals) in one category is p and, consequently, the proportion of observations in the other category is $1 - p$, i.e. q. (Remember that the sum of the probabilities of all events must equal 1.) To illustrate this principle further, consider the following example.

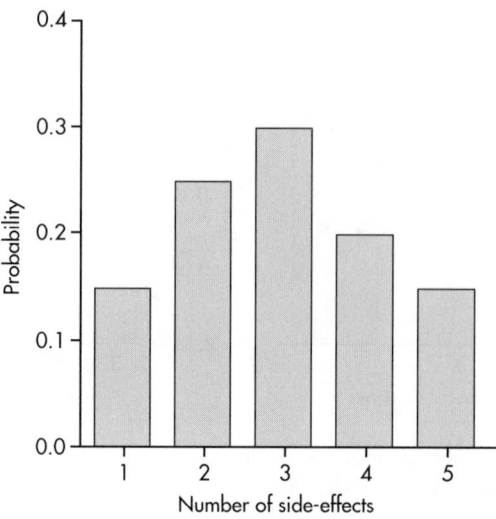

Figure 4.2 Probability histogram showing the number of side-effects associated with the clinical use of a new anti-hypertensive agent.

EXAMPLE 4.2 *In pharmaceutical manufacturing, tablets from a batch may be categorised into those that pass or those that fail quality control. As part of the quality control process for a batch of tablets, the probability associated with the pass category was 0.95 whereas the probability associated with the fail category was 0.05. Calculate the probability of selecting (a) two defective tablets, (b) two non-defective tablets and (c) one defective and one non-defective tablet, each in a sample of two tablets.*

(a) The probability of selecting two defective tablets in a sample of two may be calculated using the multiplication rule (section 4.1.1), i.e. $(0.05) \times (0.05) = 0.0025$.

(b) Similarly, the probability of selecting two tablets that have passed quality control is $(0.95) \times (0.95) = 0.9025$.

(c) The same principles may be employed to calculate the probabilities of selecting two dissimilar events, i.e. the probability of selecting a defective and a non-defective tablet from the above batch. To perform this, the probability of all possible outcomes must first be considered as follows:
   - two defective tablets (p^2)
   - one defective tablet and one 'non-defective' tablet (pq)
   - one non-defective tablet and one defective tablet (qp)
   - two non-defective tablets (q^2)

The overall probability is $p^2 + pq + qp + q^2 = 1$

The probability of selecting one defective and one non-defective tablet in a sample of two is therefore

$$2pq = 2(0.05 \times 0.95) = 0.095$$

This example may be extended to consider the scenario in which three samples are removed from the batch of tablets and the probability of each event is calculated. The outcomes following the removal of three sample tablets are:

- three defective tablets, i.e. $p^3 = (0.05)^3 = 0.000125$
- two defective tablets and one non-defective tablet, i.e. ppq, pqp, $qpp = 3p^2q = 0.007125$
- one defective tablet and two non-defective tablets, i.e. pqq, qpq, $qqp = 3pq^2 = 0.135375$
- three non-defective tablets, i.e. $q^3 = (0.95)^3 = 0.857375$

Once more, $p^3 + 3p^2q + 3pq^2 + q^3 = 1$

As this example has illustrated, the complexity of calculating the probability of events using binomial data increases as the number of samples increases, and the calculation of such events using the above method of calculation becomes difficult. However, the difficulty may be overcome by the expansion of the binomial term, $(p + q)^N$, in which N denotes the sample size, p is the probability of the occurrence of the first event, i.e. the selection of a defective tablet in the example above, and, q is the probability of the occurrence of the second event, i.e. the selection of a non-defective tablet.

Written in full, the probability of X observations (in a particular category) in a sample of size N that has been removed from a binomial distribution may be mathematically described as follows:

$$P(X) = \binom{n}{X} p^X q^{n-X}$$

where p^X denotes the probability of a sample composed of X observations possessing a probability p and q^{n-X} denotes the probability of a sample composed of $N - X$ observations possessing a probability q.

The above equation can be rewritten as

$$\binom{n}{X} = \frac{n!}{X!(n-X)!}$$

$$P(X) = \frac{n!}{X!(n-X)!} p^x q^{n-X}$$

The term $\binom{n}{X} p^x q^{n-X}$ is generally referred to as the Xth term in the expansion of $(p + q)^N$. The use of this equation is illustrated in Example 4.3.

EXAMPLE 4.3 *Using the binomial expansion and referring to Example 4.2, calculate the probability of selecting three defective tablets in a sample of three.*

In Example 4.2, the probabilities were p (defective) = 0.05, q (non-defective) = 0.95. Furthermore, the number of observations (X) is 3 and the sample size (N) is 3. Therefore,

$$P(X) = \frac{3!}{3!(0!)} (0.05)^3(0.95)^0 = 0.000125$$

This is in agreement with the calculation in Example 4.2.

This equation may also be used to calculate the probability of selecting one defective tablet in a sample size of three. Thus,

$$P(X) = \frac{3!}{1!(3-1)!} (0.05)^1(0.95)^2 = 0.135375$$

Once more, this is in agreement with the calculation that was based on basic probability theory.

One simple method for the expansion of the binomial term is by the use of Pascal's triangle (Table 4.5). This provides the coefficients that form an integral component of the binomial expansion.

Table 4.6 describes various expansions of the binomial from $N = 1$ to $N = 8$, based on the coefficients presented in Table 4.5. Using the above expansion, one can calculate, for example, the probability of selecting four non-defective tablets in a sample of four, remembering that the probability associated with sampling a non-defective tablet (q) is 0.95. From Tables 4.5 and 4.6, the appropriate expansion of the binomial expression is

$$p^4 + 4p^3q + 6p^2q^2 + 4pq^3 + q^4 = 1$$

Here q^4 denotes the probability of selecting four non-defective tablets, i.e. $(0.95)^4 = 0.815$.

Table 4.5 An excerpt from Pascal's triangle

n	Pascal's triangle (coefficients for binomial expansions)															
1								1		1						
2							1		2		1					
3						1		3		3		1				
4					1		4		6		4		1			
5				1		5		10		10		5		1		
6			1		6		15		20		15		6		1	
7		1		7		21		35		35		21		7		1
8	1		8		28		56		70		56		28		8		1

Table 4.6 Expansion of the binomial term, $(p + q)^n$, for defined values of the exponent, n

n	Expansion of $(p + q)^n$
1	$p + q$
2	$p^2 + 2pq + q^2$
3	$p^3 + 3p^2q + 3pq^2 + q^3$
4	$p^4 + 4p^3q + 6p^2q^2 + 4pq^3 + q^4$
5	$p^5 + 5p^4q + 10p^3q^2 + 10\,p^2q^3 + 5pq^4 + q^5$
6	$p^6 + 6p^5q + 15p^4q^2 + 20p^3q^3 + 15p^2q^4 + 6pq^5 + q^6$
7	$p^7 + 7p^6q + 21p^5q^2 + 35p^4q^3 + 35p^3q^4 + 21p^2q^5 + 7pq^6 + q^7$
8	$p^8 + 8p^7q + 28p^6q^2 + 56p^5q^3 + 70p^4q^4 + 56p^3q^5 + 28p^2q^6 + 8pq^7 + q^8$

The effects of sample size on the probability of the outcome of a particular event in a binomial event are interesting. For example, assume that the probability of an event (p) is 0.3 (and hence q, the probability of the other outcome, is 0.7). The series of graphs shown in Figure 4.3 illustrate the effects of sample sizes ($N = 1, 2, 3, 4, 5$ and 10) on the resultant binomial distributions.

It is perhaps helpful at this stage to explain the concepts associated with the above calculations to ensure that the reader has fully grasped the concept of the binomial distribution. The situation described in Table 4.7 refers to binomial events, i.e. events in which there are two outcomes. We wish to assess the probability of observing one of the two

Table 4.7 Calculation of the probability of observing or selecting an event in a binomial distribution over a range of sample sizes, assuming that the probability of the event is 0.3

Number of successes	Sample size					
	1	2	3	4	5	10
0	0.7	0.490	0.343	0.240	0.168	2.822×10^{-2}
1	0.3	0.420	0.441	0.411	0.360	0.121
2		0.090	0.189	0.265	0.309	0.233
3			0.027	0.076	0.132	0.267
4				0.008	0.028	0.200
5					0.002	0.103
6						0.0368
7						9.00×10^{-3}
8						1.447×10^{-3}
9						1.378×10^{-4}
10						5.904×10^{-6}

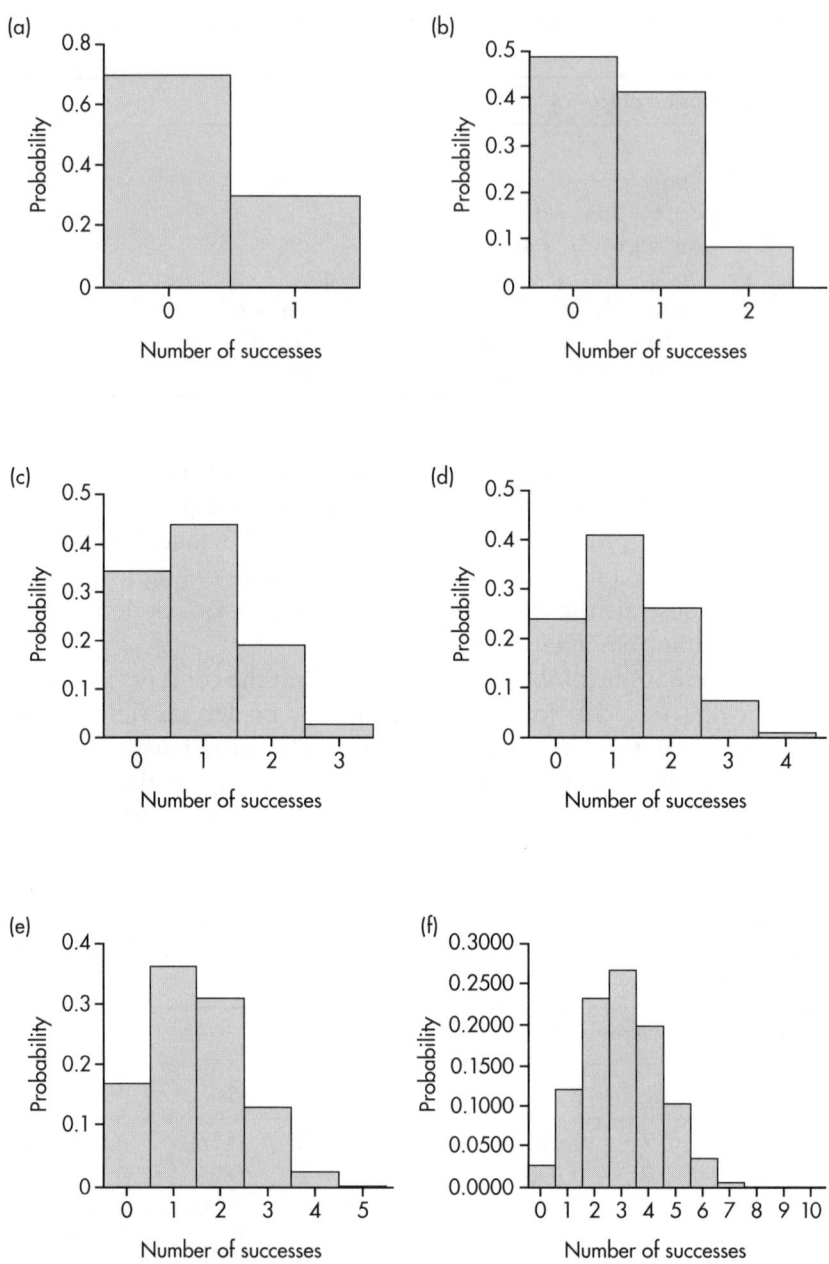

Figure 4.3 Binomial distributions of defined probabilities ($p = 0.3$) and different sample sizes (n) (data derived from Table 4.7): (a) $p = 0.3$, $q = 0.7$, $n = 1$; (b) $p = 0.3$, $q = 0.7$, $n = 2$; (c) $p = 0.3$, $q = 0.7$, $n = 3$; (d) $p = 0.3$, $q = 0.7$, $n = 4$; (e) $p = 0.3$, $q = 0.7$, $n = 5$; (f) $p = 0.3$, $q = 0.7$, $n = 10$.

outcomes whose probability is 0.3. A typical example of this is the probability of observing a man with a particular disease state in a population. If a man is selected at random from the population, the probability that he will exhibit symptoms of the disease state is 0.3, and, conversely, the probability that he will not exhibit symptoms of the disease state is 0.7. Plotting this as a bar chart produces the rather amorphous distribution shown in Figure 4.3 ($N = 1$). If two men are removed from the population, what are the probabilities of both of them exhibiting symptoms of the disease, one of them exhibiting symptoms of the disease, or both being disease free? Once more, this may be calculated using the binomial expansion for $N = 2$ and plotted as shown in Figure 4.3 ($N = 2$). This has been repeated for other examples of N, i.e. other sample sizes, and also plotted in this figure. Note that the shape of the resulting probability distribution depends on the sample size. Furthermore, in the example where the sample size is 10, the shape of the curve is becoming symmetrical, i.e. it is converging to the normal (Gaussian) distribution. As a general rule, the binomial distribution approximates a normal distribution whenever the product of the probability of success of an event and the number of samples is $\geqslant 5$.

In the current example when N is 10 and p is 0.3, their product $np = (10) \times (0.3)$ is equal to 3 and the distribution is not normal. On close inspection of the data, one can see that this is indeed the case, as there is a significant tail associated with larger numbers of successes. In particular, the graph suggests that there is zero probability associated with 8 or more successes, but reference to Table 4.7 shows that this is not really the case.

4.2.2.1 Summary of the characteristics of the binomial distribution

Two possible outcomes
The binomial distribution is a probability distribution that describes the probability of the occurrence of a successful event whenever there are only two possible outcomes.

Effect of sample size
The probability of success is dependent on the probability of the event (p) and the sample size (N). These two parameters define the binomial distribution and, additionally, may be employed to calculate the probability of a specified outcome of a number of binomial trials. Examples of these calculations have been provided in the previous section.

Sum of probabilities
The sum of all probabilities of a binomial experiment is equal to 1, as in all probability calculations.

Theoretical and observed values

The binomial distribution is a theoretically calculated probability distribution. The calculated probability of success of an event is referred to as the *true mean*. The observed values that have been obtained following experimentation are sample proportions (means) and are estimates of the true mean.

Variability and standard deviation

The variability of a random variable in a binomial event may be calculated and is usually expressed as a standard deviation. Consider firstly the calculation of the standard deviation associated with the number of heads observed following two tosses of an unbiased coin. The possible outcomes are as follows:

0 heads: probability 0.25
1 head: probability 0.5
2 heads: probability 0.25

To calculate the *mean*, the number of successes is multiplied by the probability and all components added:

$$(0 \times 0.25) + (1 \times 0.5) + (2 \times 0.25) = 1$$

Therefore, the average number of heads per toss of a coin is 1.

The variance is calculated by multiplying the probability of each event by the squared difference of the event from the mean and then adding all components together. Thus,

$$[\{(0-1)^2 \times 0.25\} + \{(1-1) \times 0.5\} + \{(2-1)^2 \times 0.25\}] = 0.5$$

The *standard deviation* is the square root of the variance, i.e. $\sqrt{0.5} = 0.71$.
Expressed mathematically:

(a)   mean = Np
where N is the sample size and p is the probability of a binomial event. In the coin-tossing example above, $N = 2$ and $p = 0.5$, so

mean = 2×0.5
  = 1

(b)   variance = Npq
where q is the probability of the other binomial event $(1 - p)$. In the above example,

variance = $2 \times 0.5 \times 0.5$
  = 0.5

(c)   standard deviation = $\sqrt{(Npq)}$
In the above example,

standard deviation = $\sqrt{(2 \times 0.5 \times 0.5)} = \sqrt{0.5}$
  = 0.71.

Minimising variance
The variance of a binomial distribution will be minimised whenever the difference between p and q is large, i.e. $\geqslant 0.6$. To demonstrate this, consider a (binomial) experiment in which the probabilities were (a) $p = 0.1$, $q = 0.9$ and (b) $p = 0.5$ and $q = 0.5$, and there were 10 samples in each experiment. The standard deviations for each experiment may be calculated using the above equation:

(a) $\sqrt{(Npq)} = \sqrt{(10 \times 0.1 \times 0.9)} = 0.95$
(b) $\sqrt{(Npq)} = \sqrt{(10 \times 0.5 \times 0.5)} = 1.58.$

Use of proportions
The standard deviation (and variance) may also be calculated using proportions, using the following equation:

$$s = \sqrt{\frac{pq}{n}}$$

where the mathematical terms have the same meaning as before. Using the same examples as before, the standard deviation may be calculated:

(a) $\quad s = \sqrt{\dfrac{pq}{n}} = \sqrt{\dfrac{0.1 \times 0.9}{10}} = 0.095$

(b) $\quad s = \sqrt{\dfrac{pq}{n}} = \sqrt{\dfrac{0.5 \times 0.5}{10}} = 0.158$

It is worthwhile pointing out that the numerical values of the standard deviation calculated using numbers and proportions are not the same. This is to be expected, as the former value refers to absolute values whereas proportions refer to relative values. Furthermore, the numerical value of the standard deviation of proportions is inversely proportional to the number of samples, and hence the variability may be decreased by increasing the sample size. In general, binomial data obtained from large sample sizes provide information that approximates the (true) population data. Hence, to use a pharmaceutical example, the information collected from a representative sample concerning a binomial outcome, e.g. the presence or absence of side-effects, will provide information relevant to the entire population.

Effect of the probability of an event
We have already seen that the sample size directly affects the shape of the binomial distribution, with large sample sizes generating distributions that approximate to the normal distribution. In addition, the

probability of an event also affects the shape of the binomial. Consider the following distributions:

$$p = 0.01, q = 0.99, n = 6$$
$$p = 0.10, q = 0.90, n = 6$$
$$p = 0.30, q = 0.70, n = 6$$
$$p = 0.50, q = 0.50, n = 6$$

Using the appropriate expansion of the binomial term, $(p + q)^6$, the following data may be generated (Table 4.8):

$$p^6 + 6p^5q + 15p^4q^2 + 20p^3q^3 + 15p^2q^4 + 6pq^5 + q^6$$

This data is illustrated in Figure 4.4. The probability distributions become more symmetrical as the difference between the probabilities of the event occurring and not occurring is reduced to zero.

4.2.2.2 Examples of calculations using the binomial distribution

As most of material in this chapter will be new to many readers, some further examples of calculations using a binomial distribution may prove useful. Some of these have been described in the previous section, but it may be useful to recap on some of the principles involved in determining probabilities.

EXAMPLE 4.4 *An injection has been formulated containing sulfamethoxazole and trimethoprim. It is known that the probability of precipitation within the formulation is 1%. Calculate the chance of observing 2, or fewer than 2, vials containing precipitate in a sample of 100 vials.*

First, it is important to note that the question has asked for the chance of observing $\leqslant 2$ vials. Therefore, three separate probabilities must be calculated ($P(0)$, $P(1)$, $P(2)$) and the values combined.

Table 4.8 Binomial distribution of data from outcomes with different probabilities but identical sample sizes

p	q	p^6	$6p^5q$	$15p^4q^2$	$20p^3q^3$	$15p^2q^4$	$6pq^5$	q^6
0.01	0.99	1.0×10^{-12}	5.9×10^{-10}	1.5×10^{-7}	1.9×10^{-5}	0.001	0.057	0.941
0.10	0.90	1.0×10^{-6}	5.4×10^{-5}	1.2×10^{-3}	1.5×10^{-2}	0.098	0.354	0.531
0.30	0.70	7.3×10^{-4}	0.010	0.060	0.185	0.324	0.303	0.118
0.5	0.5	0.016	0.094	0.234	0.313	0.234	0.094	0.016

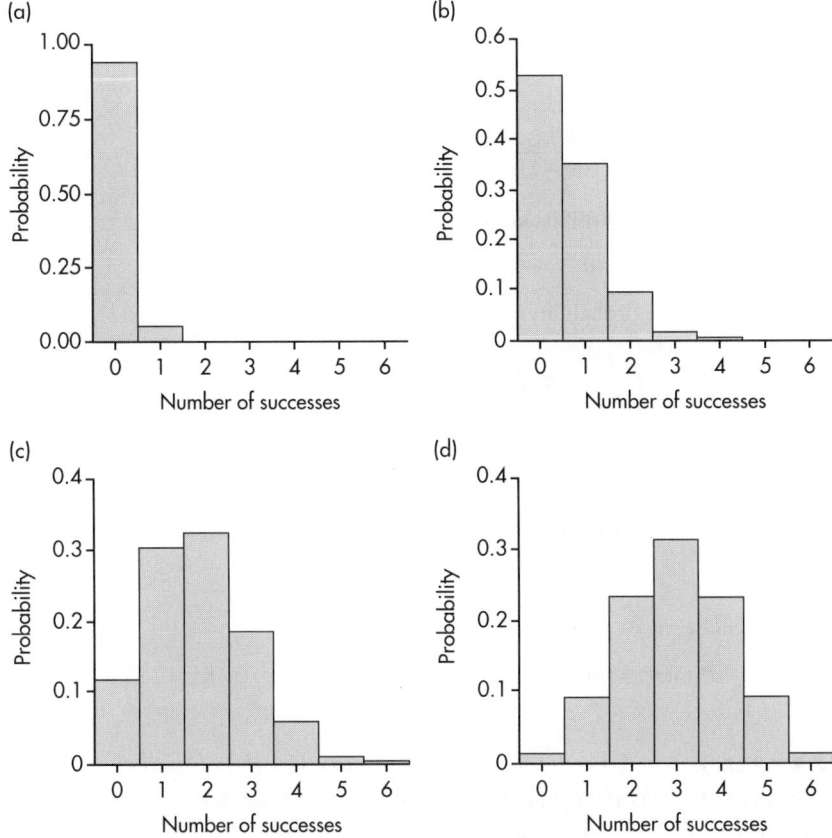

Figure 4.4 Binomial distribution of data from outcomes with different probabilities but similar sample sizes: (a) $p = 0.01$, $q = 0.99$, $n = 6$; (b) $p = 0.1$, $q = 0.9$, $n = 6$; (c) $p = 0.3$, $q = 0.7$, $n = 6$; (d) $p = 0.5$, $q = 0.5$, $n = 6$.

* Calculate the probability of observing precipitate in zero vials, $P(0)$:

$$P(0) = \binom{100}{0} p^0 q^{100-0}$$

$$= \left[\frac{100!}{0!(100-0)!} \right] (0.01)^0 (0.99)^{100}$$

$$= (1)(1)(0.366)$$

$$= 0.366$$

• Calculate the probability of observing precipitate in one vial, $P(1)$

$$P(1) = \binom{100}{1} p^1 q^{100-1}$$

$$= \left[\frac{100!}{1!(100-1)!}\right](0.01)^1(0.99)^{99}$$

$$= (100)(0.01)(0.37)$$

$$= 0.370$$

• Calculate the probability of observing precipitate in two vials, $P(2)$

$$P(2) = \left[\frac{100}{2}\right] p^2 q^{100-2}$$

$$= \left[\frac{100!}{2!(100-2)!}\right](0.01)^2(0.99)^{98}$$

$$= (4950)(0.0001)(0.373)$$

$$= 0.185$$

• Calculate the overall probability:

$$P(\text{total}) = P(0) + P(1) + P(2) = 0.366 + 0.370 + 0.185 = 0.921$$

EXAMPLE 4.5 *A medical device company has developed two proto-type formulations designed to aid the retention of dentures within the oral cavity. One formulation has been designed to provide a greater adhesion, and hence retention, than the other. A panel of volunteers has been recruited to examine and compare the relative adhesive strengths of the two denture formulations. In a typical experiment, each recruit samples batches of each denture adhesive six times and then records the relative adhesive strengths of the formulations. One individual in particular has correctly ranked the adhesive strengths of the denture adhesives in five out of six occasions. Has this individual been trained to evaluate the comparative adhesive strengths of denture adhesives?*

In answering this question, we first assume that the two formulations do not differ in texture, colour or taste. Bearing this in mind, the probability of selecting each formulation is 0.5.

To answer the posed question, the probability of the individual choosing five correct outcomes in six trials must be calculated. As there are only two outcomes to the clinical trial, this is an example of a binomial event:

$$P(5) = \binom{6}{5} p^5 q^{6-5}$$

$$= \left[\frac{6!}{5!(6-5)!} \right] (0.5)^5 (0.5)^1$$

$$= (6)(0.0313)(0.5)$$

$$= 0.009\ 39$$

Therefore, the probability of the individual selecting five successful outcomes out of a possible six experiments by chance alone is 0.009 39. This indicates that the individual has been trained to discern between differences in the adhesive strength of denture formulations.

EXAMPLE 4.6 *Urethral catheters are employed to assist in the drainage of urine from the bladder to the external environment. One of the clinical problems associated with their clinical use is blockage, an event that requires removal of the blocked catheter and insertion of a new one. The probability of blockage occurring in a named clinical practice with conventional urethral catheters is 0.8 following insertion in vivo for a period of 2 months. A new catheter has been developed and evaluated in 10 patients. After 10 months, 7 catheters were observed to be free from blockage. Does this provide evidence of a possible development in catheter design?*

As before, there are two outcomes to this clinical evaluation: the catheters are either blocked or free from blockage after 2 months. Therefore, this represents a binomial event.

To evaluate the possible importance of this clinical investigation, it is first necessary to calculate the probability of observing 7 'clean' catheters in a trial of 10 patients using the binomial distribution. It may be assumed that p (the probability of observing a clean catheter) is 0.2, and therefore q, the probability of observing a blocked catheter, is 0.8:

$$P(7) = \binom{N}{X} p^X q^{N-X}$$

$$= \left[\frac{N!}{X!(N-X)!} \right] p^X q^{N-X}$$

$$= \left[\frac{10!}{7!(10-7)!} \right] (0.2)^7 (0.8)^3$$

$$= (120)(0.000\ 0128)(0.512)$$

$$= 0.000\ 79$$

The probability of observing 7 clean catheters out of a sample size of 10 is extremely low (0.000 79), so this indicates that the new catheter is highly efficacious and that this does represent an advance in catheter design.

4.2.3 Poisson distribution

The Poisson distribution is another discrete data distribution that is commonly employed to describe random occurrences when the probability of observing an event is small. The Poisson distribution approximates to the binomial distribution when the sample size is large and the probability of a specified event is small. Mathematically, the Poisson distribution is described by

$$P(X) = \frac{e^{-\mu}\mu^X}{X!} = \frac{\mu^X}{e^{\mu}X!}$$

where $P(X)$ is the probability of an event occurring in a single observation and μ is the mean number of occurrences (number of observations × probability, Np).

The above equation may be expanded to enable calculation of the probabilities of occurrence of an event or events (Table 4.9).

In biological systems, Poisson distributions are typically employed to describe the occurrence of rare events either in a spatial mode, e.g. the distribution of microorganisms over a defined area or number of epithelial cells, or in a temporal mode, i.e. as a function of time. The variable must exhibit two major characteristics:

- the mean must be small relative to the possible number of events that can occur per sampling unit (space or time), i.e. the event must be rare
- the event must be independent.

To illustrate the use of the Poisson distribution, consider the data shown in Table 4.10 describing the adherence of blastospores of

Table 4.9 Expansion of the equation that defines the Poisson distribution

Number of occurrences	Expansion
0	$P(0) = e^{-\mu}$
1	$P(1) = e^{-\mu}\mu$
2	$P(2) = e^{-\mu}\mu^2/2!$
3	$P(3) = e^{-\mu}\mu^3/3!$
4	$P(4) = e^{-\mu}\mu^4/4!$

Table 4.10 Adherence of blastospores of *Candida albicans* to vaginal epithelial cells, as defined using the Poisson distribution

Number of adherent blastospores per epithelial cell	Recorded frequency	Theoretical probability	Expected frequency (N × P)
0	21	$P(0) = e^{-\mu} = 0.135$	$0.135 \times 172 = 23.22$
1	50	$P(1) = e^{-\mu}\mu = 0.271$	$0.271 \times 172 = 46.61$
2	51	$P(2) = e^{-\mu}\mu^2/2! = 0.271$	$0.271 \times 172 = 46.66$
3	28	$P(3) = e^{-\mu}\mu^3/3! = 0.180$	$0.180 \times 172 = 30.96$
4	14	$P(4) = e^{-\mu}\mu^4/4! = 0.090$	$0.090 \times 172 = 15.40$
5	5	$P(5) = e^{-\mu}\mu^5/5! = 0.036$	$0.036 \times 172 = 6.13$
6	2	$P(6) = e^{-\mu}\mu^6/6! = 0.011$	$0.011 \times 172 = 2.03$
7	1	$P(7) = e^{-\mu}\mu^7/7! = 0.003$	$0.003 \times 172 = 0.58$

Candida albicans to vaginal epithelial cells in vitro. A Poisson distribution would be expected to adequately describe the frequency of microbial adherence to epithelial cells for a number of reasons:

- The mean number of adherent blastospores per epithelial cell is low despite the epithelial cell possessing a markedly greater surface area than the yeast cell. The average diameter of a yeast cell is 4 μm whereas the average diameter of a vaginal epithelial cell is about 70 μm.
- The adherence of blastospores to epithelial cells is an independent event, i.e. it is not reliant on the presence of other blastospores. In addition, the adherence of blastospores to epithelial cells is not prohibited by the presence of previously adherent blastospores.

First, the mean number of blastospores per epithelial cell is calculated:

$$\bar{X} = \frac{344}{172} = 2.0$$

In the Poisson equation the mean value (2.0) is denoted by the term μ and this is employed to calculate the theoretical probability and the expected frequency (Table 4.10). The observed frequencies match the expected frequencies, calculated using the Poisson equation. To be statistically correct, it is necessary to check that the observed frequencies match the expected frequencies using a goodness-of-fit test, which will be described in Chapter 7. Assuming that there is a good match between the observed and expected frequencies, one can conclude that adherence of *C. albicans* to vaginal epithelial cells is an independent event.

The Poisson distribution is therefore usefully employed to calculate the probability of the occurrence of rare events. Many of these occur in a pharmaceutical context, e.g. the selection of a defective item from a production batch of a pharmaceutical product, drug-induced mortalities, or fracture of indwelling medical devices (e.g. ureteral stents). An example of the use of the Poisson equation to calculate the probabilities of such events is given below.

EXAMPLE 4.7   *The propensity of ureteral stents to fracture in vivo is reported as 0.5%. Calculate the probability that one ureteral stent will fracture in vivo in a clinical trial of 500 patients.*

First, the mean value is calculated, i.e.

$$Np = 500 \times 0.005 = 2.5.$$

Using the Poisson distribution, the probability for the occurrence of one event is determined:

$$P(1) = e^{-\mu}\mu = e^{-2.5} \times 2.5 = 0.205$$

Therefore, the probability that one ureteral stent will fracture in a clinical trial of 500 patients is 20.5%.

Interestingly, this calculation may also be performed using the binomial distribution, and, as may be observed, similar results are obtained:

$$P(1) = \left[\frac{N!}{X!(N-X)!}\right]p^X q^{N-X}$$

$$= \left[\frac{500!}{1!(500-1)!}\right](0.005)^1(0.995)^{499}$$

$$= (500)(0.005)(0.082) = 0.205$$

These calculations highlight the close relationship between the binomial and Poisson distributions.

4.2.3.1 Summary of the characteristics of the Poisson distribution

The main characteristics of the Poisson distribution are as follows:

- mean = Np (number of observations × probability)
- variance = Np
- standard deviation = $\sqrt{Np}$

Note that in the Poisson distribution the mean and variance are identical. This is not a mistake, but a true characteristic of this distribution.

4.2.4 Continuous probability distributions

The probability distributions that have been described so far in this chapter are examples of discrete probability distributions because the variable under examination was finite, i.e. was divided into a number of countable intervals. Many distributions cannot be described in this manner because the variable is continuous in nature. In such examples, the variable may adopt an infinite number of outcomes and, as a result, the probability of any single event occurring is zero. (Hint: probability is the ratio of the number of times an event occurs to the total (infinite) number of outcomes.) Furthermore, because of the continuous nature of the distribution, it is impossible to assign a probability to an exact value of the variable. For example, in the continuous distribution described in Table 3.3, it is impossible to calculate the probability that a tablet will weigh 300.9 mg as the value of this probability is infinitely small. However, it is possible to calculate the probability of an event occurring within a range. Thus, in Tables 3.3 and 3.4, it is possible to calculate the probability of finding a tablet within the range 300.1–302.0 mg.

There are many pharmaceutical and biomedical examples of continuous probability distributions. The following example describes the weight loss of 11 700 patients after a 12-month treatment period with a new therapeutic agent (Tables 4.11 and 4.12).

EXAMPLE 4.8 *A new obesity treatment has been developed and has been clinically evaluated in 11 700 patients. The weight loss in each patient after a 12-month treatment period with the novel treatment has been recorded and is tabulated in Table 4.11 and 4.12. Present the data in Tables 4.11 and 4.12 graphically both as frequency distributions and as probability density functions.*

The information described in these two tables has been derived from the same clinical study, but the description of the data differs, i.e. different

Table 4.11 Frequency data distribution of the weight loss in 11 700 subjects 12 months after administration of a new therapeutic agent

Mid-point of range (kg)	Observations	Relative frequency	Relative frequency density
4.5	806	0.0689	0.0115
10.5	6682	0.5711	0.0952
16.5	4143	0.3541	0.0590
22.5	69	0.0059	0.0010

Table 4.12 Frequency data distribution of the weight loss in 11 700 patients 12 months after administration of a new therapeutic agent

Mid-point of range (kg)	Observations	Relative frequency	Relative frequency density
2.5	15	0.0013	0.0006
4.5	101	0.0086	0.0043
6.5	690	0.0600	0.0300
8.5	1621	0.1385	0.0692
10.5	2411	0.2061	0.1030
12.5	2650	0.2265	0.1132
14.5	2129	0.1820	0.0910
16.5	1193	0.1020	0.0510
18.5	821	0.0702	0.0351
20.5	65	0.0056	0.0028
22.5	4	0.0003	0.0002
24.5	0	0	0

class intervals have been selected in the two tables: 6 kg in Table 4.11 and 2 kg in Table 4.12.

The data from these tables is displayed in two forms in Figure 4.5: as a conventional relative frequency distribution (Figures 4.5a and c), and as the relative frequency density (sometimes referred to as the *probability density function*) in Figures 4.5b and d. The relative frequency density may be defined as the relative frequency per unit value of the x ordinate. For example, in Table 4.11, the relative frequency density may be obtained by dividing the relative frequency by 6, hence reflecting the relative frequency per kilogram. Conversely, the relative frequency may be derived from the relative frequency density by multiplying by the class interval.

The data described in Tables 4.11 and 4.12 is derived from the same clinical study, but organised into different class intervals in order to illustrate the effects of class interval, and hence sample size, on the shape of the resultant distribution. As may be observed, the shape of the distribution in Figure 4.5d is smoother than that in Figure 4.5b. Furthermore, if the sample size is increased even further, i.e. the class interval is reduced, a smooth (continuous) curve may be obtained. Eventually, as the sample size approaches the size of the population, the relative frequency density is referred to as the *probability density function*, as this describes the probability distribution of the variable. Interestingly, the relative frequency density (or indeed the probability density function) may be employed to quantify the probability of an event occurring. In this example, calculation of the area under the curve

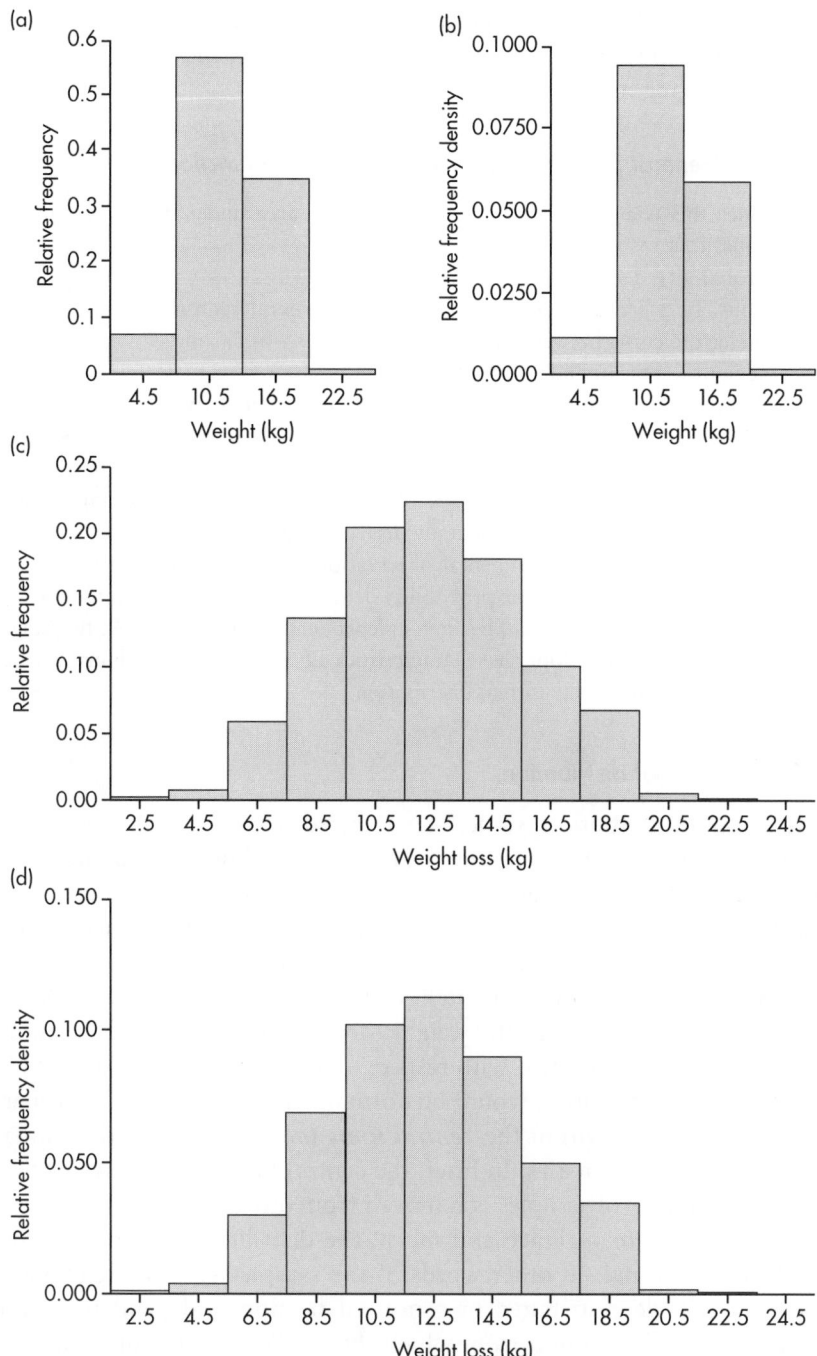

Figure 4.5 Graphical illustrations of the weight loss in 11 700 subjects 12 months after administration of a new anti-obesity treatment.

between two defined limits on the x variable (weight loss) will provide information about the probability of this event, i.e. the probability of a patient showing a particular weight loss.

4.2.4.1 General properties of probability density functions

- Since this is a probability function, the total area under the curve must be equal to 1.
- Probability density functions possess means, variances and standard deviations. In general, the mean lies within the general central region. The area under the curve between two defined limits may be calculated with a knowledge of the mean and standard deviation.
- Although some probability density functions may be derived from theoretical probability calculations, in general the variables that are studied in the pharmaceutical and related sciences are not the result of simple probability situations. Therefore, the exact shape of the probability curve is obtained only after the plotting of experimentally derived data.
- As the number of experimental observations increases (i.e. the sample size increases), the shape of the probability density function and magnitude of key parameters, e.g. the mean, become independent of sample size. At this stage, the observations adopt the characteristics of a defined probability density function, namely the normal distribution.

4.2.4.2 Normal distribution

The normal distribution, sometimes referred to as the *Gaussian distribution*, is arguably the most important theoretical distribution in statistics and, as a result, is employed in many inferential statistical tests. Furthermore, many variables that are encountered in the pharmaceutical and related sciences are assumed to display a normal distribution, e.g. the weight of tablets in a batch, the concentration of active agent in a pharmaceutical product, the weights or heights of people. If the entire population were examined with respect to a certain attribute (variable), the resultant distribution would be normal. Many of the above properties are contained within the *central limit theorem*, one of the fundamental results of statistics. In brief, the central limit theorem states that if a large number of samples is removed from any distribution (i.e. variable) with a finite variance and mean, the distribution of the variable tends to be normal. In other words, if the sample size is large enough, the data will de distributed in a normal fashion, independent of the nature of the distribution from which the samples were removed. Two examples of this have already been shown in this chapter. In the first (Figure 4.1), it was shown that the shape of the probability density plot approached normality as the sample size was increased (the class interval was decreased). In the second example (Figure 4.3), the effects of sample size on the shape of the binomial distribution were illustrated. Once more, as the sample size increased, the shape of the distribution became 'normal' in appearance. An important consideration in the central limit theorem is the concept of sample size. The sample size required to show normality is dependent on the nature of the original distribution. If the original distribution is normal, then the size of sample is relatively unimportant, but if the distribution is particularly skewed, then a large number of samples is required to generate a normal distribution.

Before leaving this discussion of the central limit theorem, it is important to reiterate that the approximation of the binomial distribution (and indeed the Poisson distribution) to the normal distribution is a special example of the central limit theorem. As stated previously, this approximation holds true when the sample size is large and neither p (nor q) is close to zero (i.e. the distribution is not heavily skewed). Mathematical examples of the approximation of the binomial distribution to the normal distribution are given in subsequent sections of this text.

Properties of the normal distribution

The shape of the normal distribution (illustrated in Figure 4.6) is distinctive and has the following properties:

- it is symmetrical
- it is bell-shaped
- it extends from $-\infty$ to ∞
- it contains an infinite number of observations
- the shape is defined by the mean and the standard deviation
- the mean, median and mode are numerically equal (see Chapter 2).

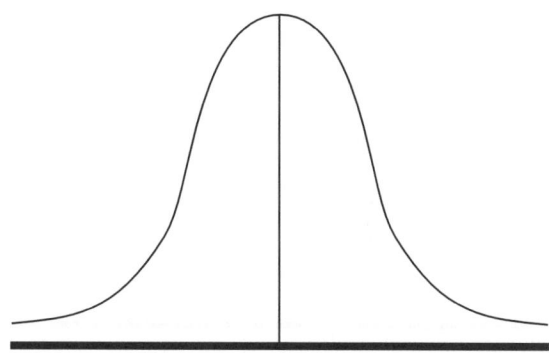

Figure 4.6 Normal distribution.

There are two other important points to note about the normal distribution.

- It is a *theoretical* distribution, i.e. experimental data will not exactly fit all of the above criteria, but they will conform to the description of normality. For example, experimental data is finite, not infinite.
- Every normal distribution is *numerically* unique. Hence, the normal distribution of heights of men in a population will differ from the normal distribution of the weights of tablets in a batch of tablets. However, although the values of the mean and standard deviation will differ from one experiment to another, the curve will retain its shape, i.e. it will be bell-shaped and symmetrical.

These points are highlighted in Figures 4.7 and 4.8.

Figure 4.7 displays three distributions that possess normal characteristics, i.e. they are bell-shaped and symmetrical. The means of all three distributions are identical, as indicated by the vertical line. However, the spreads at each end of the distributions differ, i.e. the standard deviations of each distribution are not equal. The distribution (a) has the greatest standard deviation, and (c) has the lowest.

Conversely, Figure 4.8 displays three normal distributions that possess identical variability (standard deviations) but differ in mean values. The distribution (a) has the lowest value of the mean and (c) the highest.

Mathematically, the normal distribution is described by the following equation:

$$f(X) = \frac{1}{\sigma\sqrt{2\pi}} \, e^{-(X-\mu)^2/2\sigma^2}$$

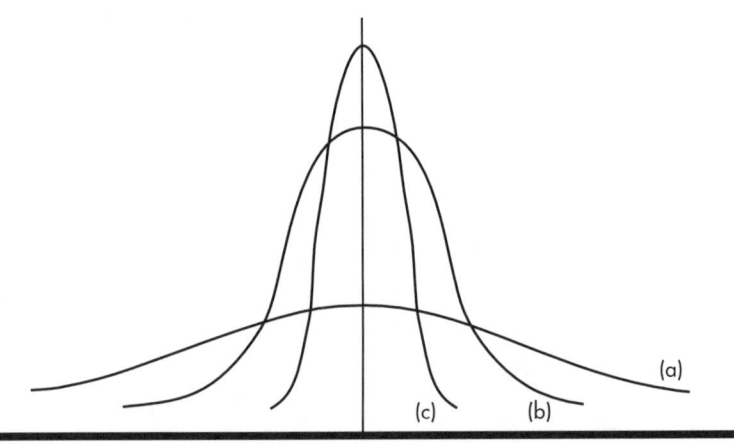

Figure 4.7 Normal distributions with the same mean values but differing in the numerical values of standard deviations.

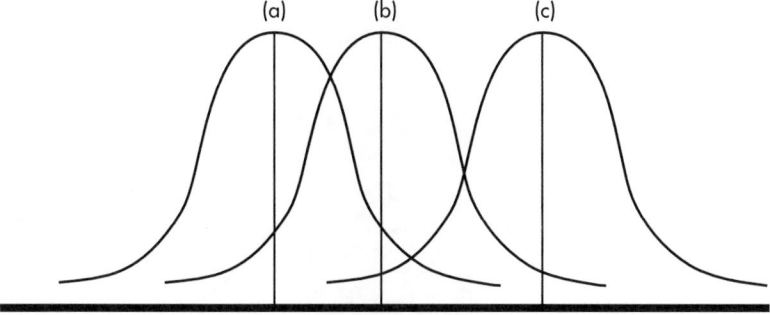

Figure 4.8 Normal distributions with the same standard deviation but different mean values.

where μ is the mean, σ is the standard deviation and e is the base of the Naperian or natural logarithms, i.e. 2.71828. This equation therefore states that the normal distribution may adopt an infinite number of curves, all bell-shaped and symmetrical in nature, because there is an infinite number of mean and standard deviation values that may be adopted. In addition, this equation also confirms that, providing the mean and standard deviation of a distribution are known, the ordinate $(f(X))$ may be calculated for any value of X. In this manner, the normal distribution plot may be generated. In addition, the mathematically astute reader may have realised that to determine the probability of observing (sampling) a value between two values on the x axis (e.g. X_2 and X_1), the area under the curve between these values may be calculated by integration $(\int_{X_1}^{X_2}(X))$. It is extremely useful to remember the following values for the relationships between the standard deviations and the areas under the curve:

- mean ± one standard deviation contains 68.27% of all values
- mean ± two standard deviations contains 95.45% of all values
- mean ± three standard deviations contains 99.73% of all items.

These three statements are illustrated in Figures 4.9a, b and c, respectively.

Conversely, it may be easier to remember the following:

- 50% of all values lie between the mean ± 0.67 standard deviations
- 95% of all values lie between the mean ± 1.96 standard deviations
- 99% of all values lie between the mean ± 2.57 standard deviations.

This information has already been introduced in Chapter 2.

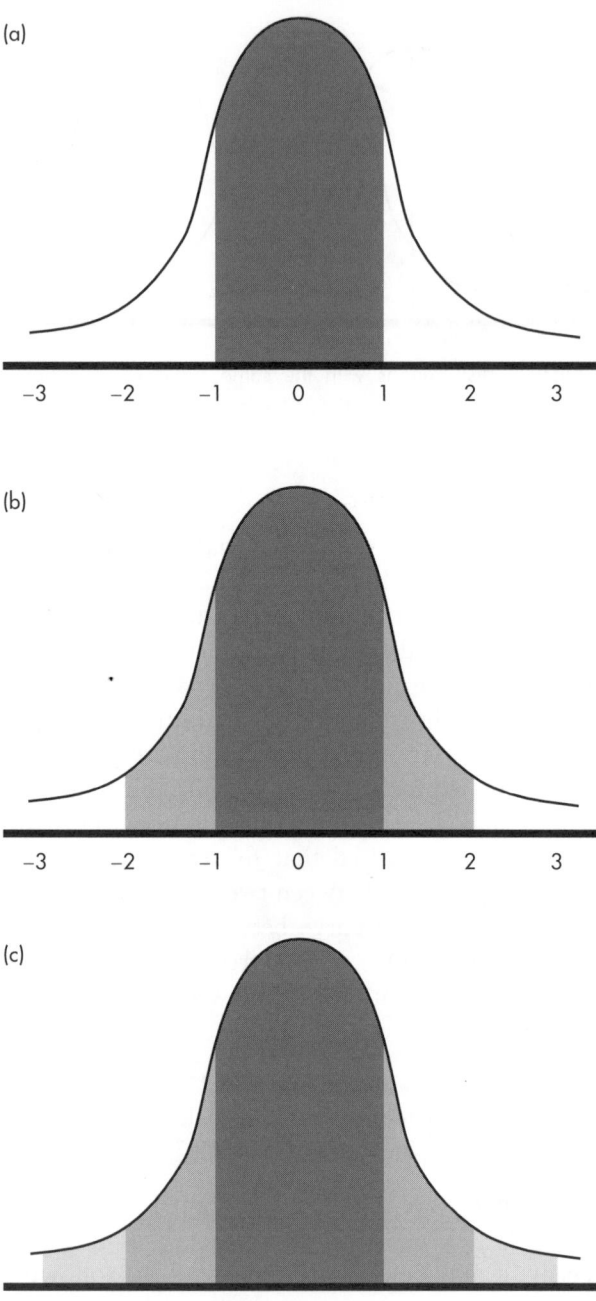

Figure 4.9 Areas enclosed within (a) ±1 standard deviation, i.e. 68.27%; (b) ±2 standard deviations, i.e. 95.45%; and (c) ±3 standard deviations, i.e. 99.73%. In all cases, 0 denotes an arbitrary mean value.

4.2.4.3 Standard normal distribution

One point that was highlighted in the previous section is that each normal distribution is unique, possessing a unique mean and standard deviation. Therefore, to calculate the probability of an event occurring using each unique distribution would require calculation of the probability density function for that variable, an arduous task indeed. To overcome this apparent difficulty the *standard normal distribution*, a generic distribution that possesses a mean value of 0 and a standard deviation of 1, is employed. The areas under the curve associated with this distribution have been calculated and may be used to estimate the probability of occurrence of an event whose full normal distribution has not been calculated. The method by which this is performed is commonly referred to as a *z transformation*. The following examples explain the mechanism by which the *z* transformation may be employed to define the (normal) probability distribution of a variable (*X*).

EXAMPLE 4.9 *A batch of 5000 tablets has been produced and the concentration of active agent assayed in all tablets. The mean (±σ) of the batch is 200 ± 10 mg and the distribution of concentrations of active agent is normally distributed. Calculate the proportion of the batch that contains 180 mg or less of active agent.*

This question may be rephrased as 'What proportion of tablets lie in the region of the normal probability density function that is shaded in Figure 4.10, i.e. that region depicting 180 mg or less?'

The difficulty in answering this question is that we have no prior information concerning the nature of the normal distribution, i.e. the exact probability density function relating to the concentration of active agent in each tablet is unknown. To acquire this knowledge would require inputting hundreds of possible *X* values (drug concentrations) into the equation that describes the normal distribution (see page 84), setting $\mu = 200$ mg and $\sigma = 10$ mg, and calculating the resultant probabilities ($f(X)$) and plotting them against the *X* variable. Clearly this would be extremely time consuming. Therefore, to overcome this problem, the first step in answering this question involves the transformation of the normal distribution of mean (±σ) equal to 200 ± 10 mg to a standard normal distribution possessing a mean (±σ) equal to 0 ± 1. Then, as we have access to a table that describes the cumulative areas under the standard normal distribution (Appendix 1), the probability associated with a defined event may be calculated.

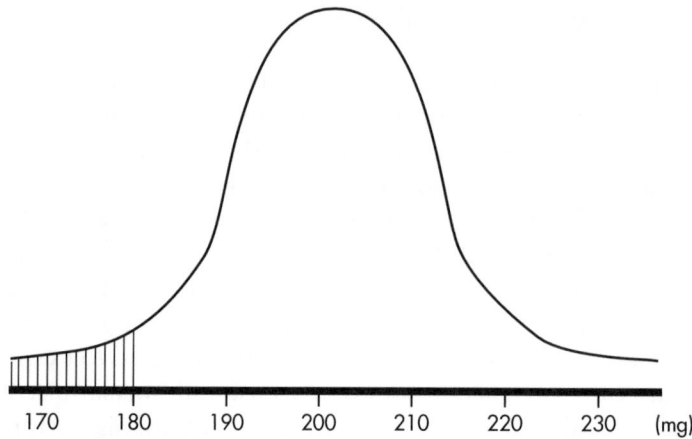

Figure 4.10 Normal distribution of drug concentration (per tablet) within a batch of tablets ($n = 5000$, $\mu = 200$ mg, $\sigma = 10$ mg).

In performing the z transformation, two identifiable mathematical steps must be performed:

- The mean must be transformed from the actual value (200 mg in this example) to 0.
- The standard deviation must be transformed from the actual value (10 mg in this example) to 1.

Full descriptions of the mean and standard deviation were provided in Chapter 2 and it is assumed here that the reader understands the basis of their calculation. One important point to note about the mean that is relevant in the transformation process is that the numerical value of the mean may be reduced by a constant value if the constant is subtracted from each member of the data set. To confirm this, consider the following data set:

12	15	16	14	18	19	17	16	14	14	mean = 15.5

Subtract 6 from each value:

−6	−6	−6	−6	−6	−6	−6	−6	−6	−6	
6	9	10	8	12	13	11	10	8	8	mean = 9.5

Therefore, in a similar fashion, if the mean is subtracted from each data set, i.e. $X - \mu$, the data set is converted to an arbitrary scale with a mean of 0. The transformation of the mean values, $X - \mu$, is shown in Figure 4.11.

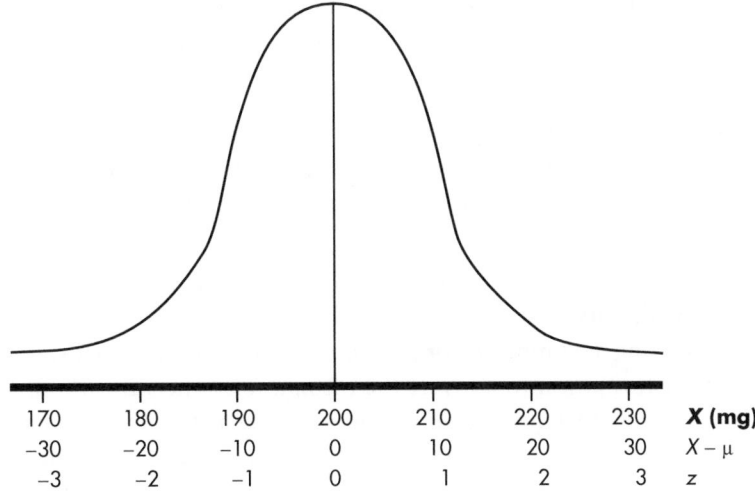

170	180	190	200	210	220	230	**X (mg)**
−30	−20	−10	0	10	20	30	$X - \mu$
−3	−2	−1	0	1	2	3	z

Figure 4.11   z transformation of a normal distribution concerning drug concentration (per tablet) within a batch of tablets ($n = 5000$, $\mu = 200$ mg, $\sigma = 10$ mg) to a standard normal distribution ($\mu = 0$, $\sigma = 1$).

The second part of the calculation involves the transformation of the standard deviation from 10 mg to a value of 1. This is performed by dividing the standard deviation (10 mg) by itself to provide a value of unity.

Therefore, the total z transformation may be described mathematically as:

$$z = \frac{X - \mu}{\sigma}$$

where z is the transformed value of the x axis, X is a defined value from the original data set, μ is the mean of the original data set and σ is the standard deviation of the original data set. The implementation of this equation may be explained by consideration of the original problem, i.e. calculation of the proportion of tablets that contain $\leqslant 180$ mg of active agent.

Employing the equation for z transformation, a z value may be generated:

$$z = \frac{X - \mu}{\sigma} = \frac{180 - 200}{10} = -2.00$$

To interpret this value, one must consult the table describing the areas under the standard normal distribution (Appendix 1) and record the probability that is associated with a z value of –2.00, namely 0.0228. This is the probability that a tablet randomly sampled from the batch will contain 180 mg or less of active agent. By the use of the z transformation, information about the probability density of a unique distribution has been rapidly generated.

EXAMPLE 4.10 *The concentration of an ion in the plasma of humans is 150 ± 7 mmol/L in healthy subjects. Calculate the proportion of the population whose plasma ion concentration is ≥159 mmol/L.*

This question may be rephrased as, 'What proportion of the population have a plasma ion concentration that lies in the region of the normal probability density function that is shaded in Figure 4.12, i.e. that region depicting 159 mmol/L or greater?' Once more, the first step is to use a z transformation to convert the plasma ion concentration normal distribution ($\mu = 150$ mmol/L, $\sigma = 7$ mmol/L) to a standard normal distribution ($\mu = 0$, $\sigma = 1$). This will then allow the shaded area under the curve in Figure 4.12 to be calculated, on the basis of the area under the standard normal distribution.

Using the z transformation,

$$z = \frac{X - \mu}{\sigma} = \frac{159 - 150}{7} = 1.286$$

From Appendix 1, it may be observed that this z value corresponds to an area of 0.0985. Therefore, 9.85% of the population have a plasma ion concentration of 159 mmol/L or greater.

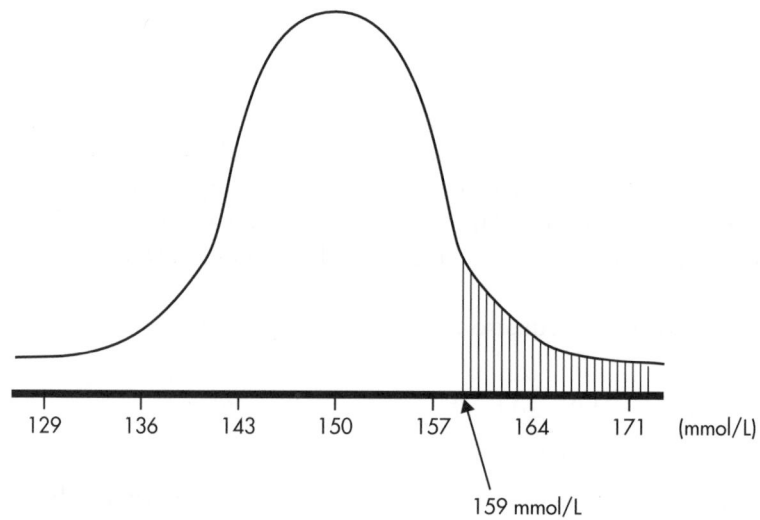

Figure 4.12 Normal distribution of plasma ion concentration within a population ($\mu = 150$ mmol/L, $\sigma = 7$ mmol/L).

EXAMPLE 4.11 *A pharmaceutical company has purchased a new fill-ing machine for sterile parenteral formulations. A batch of a solution has been prepared and filled in 100 mL injection vials. Following analy-sis of the batch (N = 2500), the volume of fluid in each vial was deter-mined and the mean and standard deviation calculated as 100.19 ± 0.61 mL. The quality control department of the company has specified that the volume of fill of the solution should be 100 ± 2 mL in 99.5% of all vials and between 100 ± 2.5 mL in 99.9% of all vials, to comply with the licence specifications of the product. Has the batch fulfilled these specifications?*

This is another example in which a z transformation may be used to address the problem. The example above has posed two questions, which should be addressed independently. In the first, it has been asked whether the fill volume in 99.5% of all vials lies between 98 and 102 mL. As before, we have no information concerning the area under the normal distribution relating to the fill volume of the parenteral product and, although this could be mathematically generated, it is eas-ier to transform the normal distribution into the standard normal dis-tribution, whose area has been fully characterised.

Figure 4.13 illustrates the distribution of fill volumes in the batch of injection vials. The central bar refers to the mean of the distribution (100.19 mL), the x axis depicts the standard deviations around the

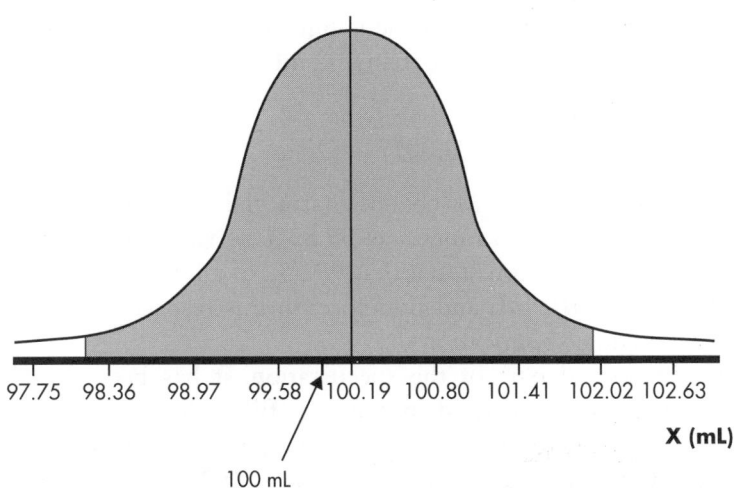

Figure 4.13 Normal distribution of injection fill volume (μ = 100.19, σ = 0.61). The shaded region depicts the probability of selecting a vial with a volume in the range 98–102 mL.

mean (-4σ to $+4\sigma$) and the shaded area refers to the region of interest, i.e. the probability of observing a vial whose fill volume is between 98 and 102 mL.

To calculate the area of the shaded region and also the area of the rejection region, i.e. the areas of either tail of the distribution, a z transformation is performed:

$$z = \frac{X - \mu}{\sigma} = \frac{102.00 - 100.19}{0.61} = 2.97$$

Referring to the table of areas under the standard normal distribution (Appendix 1), it may be observed that a z value of 2.97 corresponds to an area of 0.9985, i.e. the probability (area under the curve) of observing a vial possessing a volume ranging from $-\infty$ to 102.00 mL is 0.9985. Therefore, the area of rejection ($>$102.00 mL) is

$$1 - 0.9985 = 0.0015$$

Similarly, to calculate the second area of rejection, i.e. the probability of observing an injection vial whose volume is less than 98.00 mL, again a z transformation is employed:

$$z = \frac{X - \mu}{\sigma} = \frac{98.00 - 100.19}{0.61} = -3.59$$

A z value of -3.59 corresponds to an area of 0.0002, i.e. the probability of rejection of a vial is 0.0002.

The total probability that the volume of fluid within the vial was either less than 98 mL or more than 102 mL is then obtained by adding the individual probabilities:

$$P = 0.0015 + 0.0002 = 0.0017$$

Therefore, there is a 0.17% chance that a vial will contain a volume that is outside the stated range, i.e. 99.83% of vials are within range. The original specification stated that 99.5% of all vials should contain between 98 and 102 mL and therefore, in this respect, the batch has passed fill volume specifications.

In the second part of the specification, it has been stated that 99.9% of all vials should possess a fill volume in the range 97.5–102.5 mL. Once more, this question may be answered using a z transformation. To calculate the area above 102.5 mL, the following equation is employed:

$$z = \frac{X - \mu}{\sigma} = \frac{102.50 - 100.19}{0.61} = 3.79$$

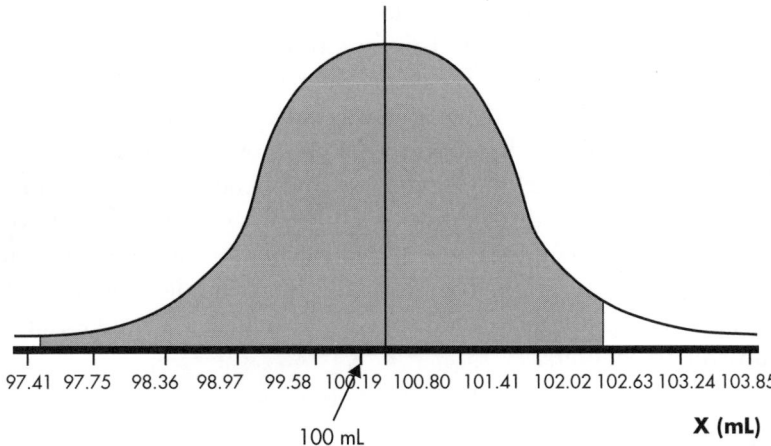

97.41 97.75 98.36 98.97 99.58 100.19 100.80 101.41 102.02 102.63 103.24 103.85

100 mL

X (mL)

Figure 4.14 Normal distribution of injection fill volume ($\mu = 100.19$, $\sigma = 0.61$). The shaded region depicts the probability of selecting a vial with a volume in the range 97.5–102.5 mL.

From Appendix 1, the z value of 3.79 corresponds to an area of 0.999, i.e. the probability of a vial possessing a fill volume of 102.5 mL or less. Therefore, the probability of a vial possessing a fill volume of 102.5 mL or greater is

$$p = 1 - 0.999$$
$$= 0.0001$$

The area below 97.5 mL is calculated in a similar fashion:

$$z = \frac{X - \mu}{\sigma} = \frac{97.50 - 100.19}{0.61} = -4.41$$

The area below 97.5 mL is therefore approximately 0.000 01.

The total probability of a vial possessing a fill volume of either less than 97.5 mL or more than 102.5 mL is once again found by addition of the individual probabilities:

$$P = 0.0001 + 0.000\ 01 = 0.000\ 11$$

Therefore, there is a 0.011% chance that a vial will contain a volume outside the stated volume range, i.e. 99.99% of vials are within range. The original specification stated that 99.9% of all vials should contain between 97.5 and 102.5 mL and therefore, in this respect, the batch has passed fill volume specifications.

The batch therefore has passed quality control specifications, i.e. at least 99.5% of vials contained between 98 and 102 mL and at least 99.9% of vials contained between 97.5 and 102.5 mL.

These examples have been selected to illustrate the main types of problem that may be addressed using z transformations. In Examples 4.9 and 4.10, the probability of an event occurring either below or above a defined value on the x axis was calculated. As in these examples there was only one direction to the question, e.g. below the specified value, this is a one-tailed outcome and hence, calculation of the area of one tail of the distribution is sufficient to answer the question. In Example 4.11, the question required calculation of the areas below and above a defined region. Therefore, this is a two-tailed outcome. The importance of the number of tails in statistical analyses will be clarified in subsequent chapters.

4.2.4.4 Student's t distribution

Student's t distribution, commonly termed the t distribution, was first described by in 1908 William Sealy Gossett (who used the pseudonym of Student) and has since found widespread use in statistical analysis. The t distribution is commonly used in statistical analyses when the sample size is small, as the distributions of means after sampling do not correctly conform to the normal distribution. The t distribution may be calculated by removing samples of defined size (N) and applying the following equation to the data so obtained:

$$t = \frac{\bar{X} - \mu}{s/\sqrt{N}}$$

where $\bar{X}$ is the mean of the sample, μ is the mean of the population, s is the sample standard deviation and N is the number of observations per sample.

In his original work Gossett transcribed the heights of 3000 criminals on to separate pieces of card, and selected 750 samples, each containing 4 cards. The equation above was applied to each sample to provide 750 values of t. The t distribution was then visualised by plotting the relative frequency density against the calculated t statistic.

To fully understand the basis of the t distribution, it is important to consider the derivation of this statistic and its relationship to the normal distribution. As described previously, in the normal distribution the population mean and standard deviation are denoted by μ and σ. If a sample is removed from the normal distribution, one may calculate the mean ($\bar{X}$) and the sample standard deviation (s) and employ these values as good estimates of the corresponding population parameters. Furthermore, if several samples are taken from this normal distribution, then a series of means will be generated whose standard deviation may be calculated. The standard deviation of the mean (standard error) has already been encountered in this text (section 2.2.5) and is calculated using the following equation:

$$\text{SEM} = \frac{s}{\sqrt{N}}$$

where s is the sample standard deviation and N is the number of observations.

When the sample size is large, the following points may be observed:

- The sample mean ($\bar{X}$) is derived from a normal population (as defined in the central limit theorem).
- The standard deviation (error) of the mean (SEM = $s/\sqrt{N}$)) is a reliable estimate of the population standard deviation.
- Application of the equation describing the t statistic would result in a normal distribution with a mean and standard deviation of 0 and 1 respectively, i.e. the standardised normal distribution.

Conversely, for small sample sizes, the mean ($\bar{X}$) is also derived from a normal distribution; however, the sample standard deviation will vary from one sample to another and therefore $s/\sqrt{N}$ is not a good estimate of the standard deviation (error) of the distribution. Thus, whenever the sample standard deviation is large, the t statistic is small and, conversely, whenever the sample standard deviation is small the t statistic is large. The overall effect of these differences is to produce a distribution that is morphologically different from the standardised normal distribution. In particular, the tails of the t distribution may be markedly longer, i.e. occupy a greater area. As a result of the variation from one sample to another, the t distribution is normally employed to calculate confidence intervals and to compare mean values for small samples in preference to the normal distribution.

Main characteristics of the t distribution
- It is symmetrical (like the normal distribution).
- The tails (the area occupied by the extremes of the distribution) are longer than for the standardised normal distribution. For example, when the sample size is 10, the t statistic for 95% probability is 2.26 (Appendix 2), whereas the corresponding z statistic is 1.96.
- The shape of the distribution is dependent on the sample size (see Figure 4.15). Samples of small size may produce a range of sample standard deviations. The variations from sample to sample decreases as the sample size is increased and hence, the extreme values of the t statistic are less probable. This results in a reduction in the areas occupied by the tails of the distribution.

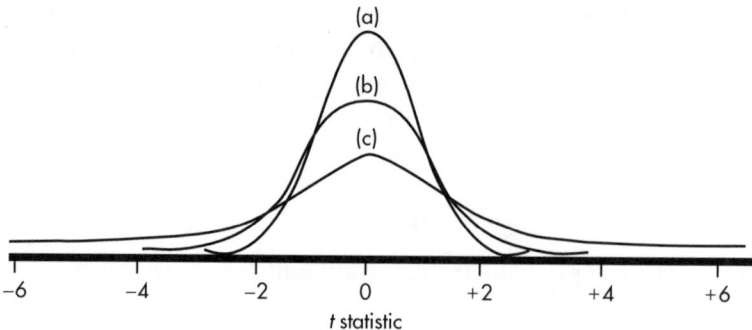

Figure 4.15 Effects of degrees of freedom on the shape of the *t* distribution: (a) 20 *df*, (b) 4 *df*, (c) 1 *df*.

- As the sample size increases, the shape of the *t* distribution becomes more similar to that of the standardised normal distribution. This may be illustrated by comparison of areas under the *t* distribution ($n = 120$) and the *z* statistic corresponding to 95% probability, i.e. 1.98 and 1.96, respectively.
- A parameter related to the sample size which is commonly employed in statistics concerning the *t* distribution is the *degrees of freedom*. In the case of a one-sample test, e.g. the calculation of the *t* statistic after random sampling from a population (as described in this section), the number of degrees of freedom is defined as:

$$df = N - 1$$

where N is the sample size.

- Because of the effects of the sample size on the shape of the *t* distribution, it is time consuming to report the areas under each *t* distribution corresponding to different probabilities for each degree of freedom. Therefore, the *t* distribution is normally reported as the *t* statistic corresponding to defined probabilities and different degrees of freedom (Appendix 2).

The application of the *t* distribution to the examination of similarities (or differences) between treatments is described in Chapters 7 and 8.

4.2.4.5 Chi (χ^2) distribution

The χ^2 (pronounced ky squared) distribution is another important distribution that forms an integral part of several statistics procedures, e.g. the χ^2 test, goodness of fit tests. This distribution may be defined mathematically as

$$Y = Y_0(\chi^2)^{0.5(v-2)}e^{-0.5\chi^2} = Y_0\chi^{v-2}e^{-0.5\chi^2}$$

where v is the number of degrees of freedom $(N - 1)$, Y_0 is a constant that is dependent on v and χ^2 is the chi-squared statistic. As before, the total area under the curve is equal to 1. The equation is mathematically too complex to be explained here. However, one important point to note is that the equation contains one variable parameter (v), the rest being either a constant or the value of χ^2 from which the corresponding ordinate is being calculated. Therefore, the χ^2 distribution is described by this one parameter (degrees of freedom), whereas the normal and t distributions are two-parameter distributions, their shapes being defined by the mean and standard deviation. The number of degrees of freedom directly influences the shape of the χ^2 distribution, as illustrated in Figure 4.16.

It is useful at this stage for the reader to gain experience in the interpretation of the χ^2 distribution, particularly in light of the changing nature of the distribution. The areas under the χ^2 distribution are described in Appendix 3. Consideration of the following example will provide the reader with useful information about the χ^2 distribution.

EXAMPLE 4.12   *From the χ^2 distribution relating to 6 degrees of freedom, provide the following information:*

- *the critical value of χ^2 relating to an area of 0.10 to the right of the distribution*
- *the critical value of χ^2 relating to an area of 0.10 to the left of the distribution*
- *the critical value of χ^2 relating to a total area of 0.10.*

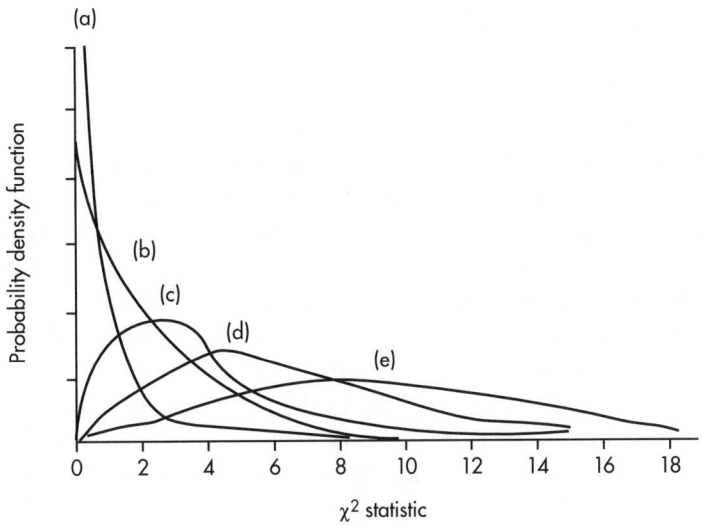

Figure 4.16 χ^2 distribution for different degrees of freedom: (a) 1 *df*, (b) 2 *df*, (c) 4 *df*, (d) 6 *df*, (e) 10 *df*.

In the answers to all the above questions, it is important to refer to the areas under the χ^2 distribution that relate to 6 degrees of freedom.

- *Critical value of χ^2 relating to an area of 0.10 to the right of the distribution.* An area of 0.10 to the right of the distribution implies that the area to the left of the distribution is 0.90. Therefore, the critical value of χ^2 is obtained by obtaining the value that relates to $\chi^2_{0.90}$ and 6 degrees of freedom, i.e. 10.64.
- *Critical value of χ^2 relating to an area of 0.10 to the left of the distribution.* An area of 0.10 refers to $\chi^2_{0.10}$ (and 6 degrees of freedom), i.e. 2.20.
- Critical value of χ^2 relating to a *total area of 0.10*. The corresponding critical value for an area of 0.10 under the distribution may theoretically be achieved in a number of ways, because the distribution is not symmetrical. For example, an area of 0.10 may be satisfied by an area to the right of the distribution of 0.06 and an area to the left of 0.04, or by 0.07 to the right and 0.03 to the left, and so on. However, it is usual to assume that the two areas are equal, i.e. 0.05 under both the left and right tails of the distribution. From this the critical values may be calculated as before. Thus, the critical value relating to an area of 0.05 under the left tail is $\chi^2_{0.05}$ (with 6 degrees of freedom), i.e. 1.64. The critical value relating to an area of 0.05 under the right tail, i.e. the upper 95th percentile, is $\chi^2_{0.95}$ (with 6 degrees of freedom), i.e. 12.59. Therefore, the critical values are 1.64 and 12.59.

z values and the χ^2 distribution

Interestingly, z values, derived from a normal distribution, are related to χ^2 values. If a sample ($N = 1$) is removed from a normal distribution, the z^2 value may be calculated as before:

$$z^2 = \frac{(X - \mu)^2}{\sigma^2}$$

where X is the numerical value of the sample, μ is the mean of the population and σ^2 is the variance of the population. If this process is repeated a large number of times, then a plot of the probability density of z^2 values may be generated, the shape of which is identical to the χ^2 distribution (with 1 degree of freedom). Therefore, in this example $z^2 = \chi^2_1$ (the subscript 1 refers to the number of degrees of freedom).

To expand this example further, assume that the sample size was increased to a defined number of observations (N). If the z^2 value for each observation from the sample is calculated and the values summed (Σz^2) and plotted as a probability density function, the resultant distribution is identical to the χ^2 distribution with N degrees of freedom, i.e.

$$\chi^2_N = \sum \frac{(X - \mu)^2}{\sigma^2}$$

It is worth noting that whenever the number of degrees of freedom is large (>30), then the standard normal distribution and χ^2 distribution are comparable. In this, the z value (from the standard normal distribution) and the χ^2 value are related by the following equation:

$$\sqrt{2\chi_p^2} - \sqrt{2v - 1} = z_p$$

where χ_p^2 is the critical χ^2 value relating to a particular percentile p, and z_p is the z value relating to a particular probability density.

The use of the standard normal distribution to predict critical χ^2 values is illustrated in the next example.

EXAMPLE 4.13 *Calculate the critical values of χ^2 relating to a probability of 0.975, assuming 100 degrees of freedom, using the standard normal distribution and the χ^2 distribution.*

From Appendix 3 (the areas under the χ^2 distribution), it may be observed that the critical value relating to a probability of 97.5% and 100 degrees of freedom is 129.56.

Using a rearrangement of the equation described above, the value of $\chi_{0.975}^2$ may be calculated using the standard normal distribution:

$$\chi_{0.975}^2 = \tfrac{1}{2}(z_{0.975} + \sqrt{2v - 1})^2$$
$$= \tfrac{1}{2}(1.96 + \sqrt{(2 \times 100) - 1})^2 = 129.07$$

The similarities of the two estimates are apparent. The full extent and use of these relationships will be further discussed in conjunction with the χ^2 test.

The application of the χ^2 distribution to the examination of similarities (or differences) between treatments is described in Chapters 7 and 9.

4.2.4.6 F distribution

The F distribution is another important distribution in inferential statistics. It is derived from the sampling distribution of the ratio of two independent estimations of the variance from normal distributions. In particular, consider two samples of known sizes that have been removed from two normal distributions of defined variances; the F statistic may be defined as

$$F = \frac{N_1 s_1^2 / (N_1 - 1)\sigma_1^2}{N_2 s_2^2 / (N_2 - 1)\sigma_2^2}$$

where N_1 and N_2 denote the sample sizes, s_1^2 and s_2^2 denote the variances of the two samples and σ_1^2 and σ_2^2 denote the variances of the normal distributions from which the samples were removed.

The F distribution is therefore acquired in a similar fashion to the t distribution, by a series of repeated samplings and plotting the probability associated with each calculated F statistic.

The shape of the F distribution is dependent on two factors, namely the degrees of freedom that are associated with each sample. These are termed the *numerator* and the *denominator*. The F distribution is employed to test the equality of two variances and, in addition, for multiple hypothesis testing (ANOVA). The use of the F distribution for these purposes is discussed in detail in subsequent chapters.

4.3   Conclusions

This chapter has provided an introduction to probability theory and has also described the properties of some specific probability distributions. The reader should remember that all statistical decision-making is based on probability theory, and anyone who wants to apply statistical methods to experimental situations must have a basic understanding of the principles. The amount of probability theory that has been included in this text is designed to fulfil these needs, but the inquisitive reader may wish to pursue this topic further in more specialised texts (e.g. DeGroot, 1986; Lindgren, 1993; Ross, 1997).

Several probability distributions have been described in this chapter, including the binomial, Poisson, normal, Student's t, χ^2 and F distributions. It is important that the reader should be acquainted with these distributions, because they form an essential component of statistical decision-making and the calculation of the probability of occurrence of an event. The reader needs to understand the information provided in this chapter in order to appreciate the applications of probability distributions which are introduced in subsequent chapters and illustrated by the use of statistical examples.

References

DeGroot M H (1986). *Probability and Statistics*, 2nd edition. London: Addison-Wesley Longman.

Lindgren B W (1993). *Statistical Theory*, 4th edition. London: Chapman & Hall.

Ross S (1997). *A First Course in Probability*, 5th edition. Englewood Cliffs, NJ: Prentice Hall.

5

Statistical hypothesis testing

In the preceding chapters, several examples of methods by which data may be statistically described were explained; these are known as *descriptive statistics*. Typically, descriptive statistics are employed to provide general statistical information concerning the properties of a data set, i.e. a sample or a population. However, descriptive statistics cannot be directly used to answer many of the problems encountered by scientists on a daily basis. For example, in a clinical study, one may wish to compare the bioavailability of a proprietary product and its generic equivalent using the appropriate pharmacokinetic parameters, e.g. area under the curve, C_{max}, t_{max}, etc. In this study, the sponsor is inquiring whether or not there is a difference in the pharmacokinetic properties of the two preparations (other than the difference due to experimental error). The purpose of the study is to examine whether the difference in the means of the various pharmacokinetic properties is substantial enough to represent a valid difference between the clinical effects of the two preparations. The difference in means may be small enough to be a result of natural experimental variation, i.e. the difference has occurred by chance alone. This phrase, 'occurred by chance alone' is one that is frequently used in statistics, so it is necessary to reflect on the relevance of this concept, once more using a pharmaceutical example. Consider a study in which a pilot batch of tablets ($N = 5000$) has been prepared and the weight of each individual tablet examined immediately after compression using an automated balance. Subsequently, the analyst has removed two samples of tablets ($N = 10$) from the pilot batch and has once more weighed each tablet. The descriptive statistics associated with each group are presented in Table 5.1.

The difference in the magnitude of the population statistics and the sample statistics may be attributed to variability. The population statistics are definite (fixed), because they have been determined with reference to each member of the entire population. Conversely, sample statistics are unique to that sample, i.e. the groups of 10 tablets in the above example. The observed discrepancy between the sample statistics and population statistics is a result of variability due to chance and is referred to as the *sampling error*. It is important to highlight that, in this context, error does not infer incorrect sampling technique or poor

Table 5.1 Descriptive statistics for tablet weights within an entire (population) batch of tablets and for two samples derived from the population batch

Group	Mean (mg)	Standard deviation (mg)
Population ($N = 5000$)	250.0	4.5
Sample 1 ($N = 10$)	253.5	4.9
Sample 2 ($N = 10$)	252.6	4.1

experimental technique but often reflects the effect of individual results on the descriptive statistics associated with a sample. Typically, as highlighted above, the focus of many statistical analyses is to elucidate mathematically whether the differences in the statistical properties of two or more samples may either be explained by statistical error, or alternatively, may reflect true inter-group differences. In statistical tests, the demarcation between these two categories is defined by reference to probability distributions, and, for this reason, the fundamental aspects and characteristics of several commonly employed probability distributions have been described in Chapter 4. However, before discussing the range of available statistical tests relevant to the comparison of data derived from pharmaceutical studies, it is important to introduce the basic theory of hypothesis testing.

5.1 Basic theory of statistical hypothesis testing

In statistical hypothesis testing, assumptions are established concerning the likelihood of an event and then, using appropriate methodology, the validity of these assumptions is examined. For example, consider a manufacturing process for a pharmaceutical product that has been in operation for several years and has been validated in conjunction with the US Food and Drug Administration (FDA) guidelines. This is a well-controlled manufacturing process that produces a pharmaceutical dosage form to a required specification. In this scenario, one may *assume* that the batch of product will pass quality control analysis. If, however, a batch does not conform to the finished product specification, then the assumption concerning the quality of the batch was incorrect and hence an alternative proposal was valid. The failure of the batch to meet the finished product specification may be due to a problem with the manufacturing process, e.g. the automated production process may have information technology problems leading to incorrect times of mixing, drying, etc. This example has been cited to illustrate the basis of statistical hypothesis testing. First an assumption is established and then the data are collected from which conclusions concerning the validity of the initial assumption may be formulated.

To illustrate these principles further, we can use the example described in the introduction to this chapter in which the weights of two samples of tablets derived from a batch and, additionally, the weights of all tablets in the batch were determined (Table 5.1). It is clear from the data that the sample means and standard deviations are not identical to the mean and standard deviation associated with the population, i.e. the true population parameters. Consequently, one question that may be raised concerns the validity of the sample data, e.g. are the mean values associated with the samples different to the population mean? Alternatively, one may assume that the sample means are representative of the population mean and therefore the observed differences between the sample means and the population mean may be accredited to error. To confirm (or reject) this assumption, it is necessary to examine the sampling distribution of the mean. The population statistics state that the population mean and standard deviation are 250.0 mg and 4.5 mg, respectively. The sampling distribution of the mean is established by sampling a large number (theoretically an infinite number) of samples from the population, each containing 10 members (tablets). The mean of each sample is calculated and a frequency distribution established by plotting frequency against the continuous variable, in this case sample mean. Typically, the plot shown in Figure 5.1 may be observed.

The above frequency distribution provides information about the probability of sampling a defined mean tablet weight and is consequently employed to determine the probability of removing a sample

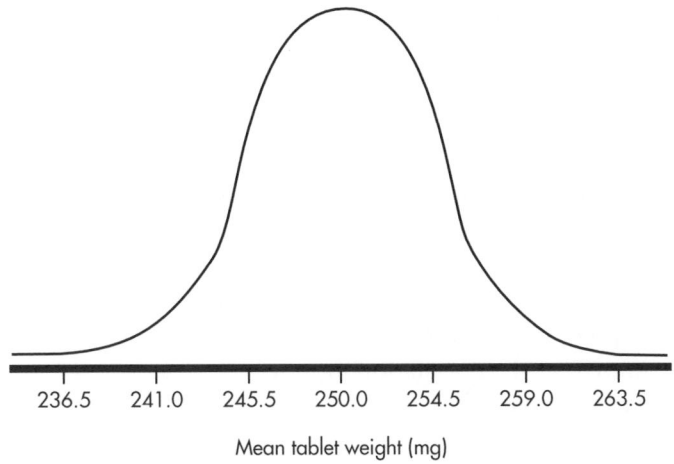

| 236.5 | 241.0 | 245.5 | 250.0 | 254.5 | 259.0 | 263.5 |

Mean tablet weight (mg)

Figure 5.1 Sampling distribution of tablet weights.

from the population with a defined sample mean. In practice, it is impractical to remove an infinite number of samples from a population, sample their mean weights and generate a probability distribution. The z transformation is employed to overcome this problem, as described in Chapter 4. The z value describes to the probability of observing an event based on the standardised normal distribution. This statistic is a measure of sampling error as it calculates the difference between an observed value that has been randomly sampled from a population and the population mean. The equation that is used to calculate the z statistic is

$$z = \frac{X - \mu}{\sigma}$$

where X is the mean of the sample, μ is the mean of the population and σ is the standard deviation of the population. The sampling error in the z transformation $(X - \mu)$ is divided by the standard deviation of the population, as this relates the error to the variability. The reader should remember that the normal distribution is described by two parameters, the mean and the standard deviation. The former provides information concerning the location of the central point of the observation, whereas the latter refers to the variability, i.e. the percentage of observations resident within an area under the probability distribution that is associated with a range of X values.

Returning to our example concerning tablet weights, the questions that were raised regarding the significance of the difference between the population mean and each of the sample means may now be assessed using the z transformation. Thus, the probabilities of observing sample means of 253.5 mg and 252.6 mg are as follows.

For sample 1,

$$z = \frac{253.6 - 250}{4.5} = 0.8$$

From tables of the standardised normal distribution (Appendix 1), it may be observed that a z value of 0.8 has an associated probability of 0.7881. Consequently, as the probability of observing a sample mean of 253.6 mg or less is 78.81%, it may be concluded that this is a likely event or, in other words, it is reasonable to assume that the sample mean is representative of the population mean.

Similarly, for sample 2,

$$z = \frac{252.6 - 250}{4.5} = 0.58$$

From the standardised normal distribution, a z value of 0.58 relates to a probability of 0.72. This denotes the probability of observing a sample mean of 242.5 mg or less. Once more, it is reasonable to assume that the sample mean is a good reflection of the population mean.

Now, consider the scenario in which a third sample of tablets was removed at the finishing stages of the tableting process and the weight of the tablets in the sample determined, as before. In this sample the mean tablet weight was recorded as 235.7 mg. Is this sample mean representative of the population mean? This question may be answered in a similar fashion to the two previous examples by the use of a z transformation:

$$z = \frac{235.7 - 250}{4.5} = -3.18$$

From the standardised normal distribution it may be observed that this calculated z statistic is associated with a probability of approximately 0.0008. This implies that the likelihood that a sample of 10 tablets possessing a mean weight of 235.7 mg being removed from a population of mean 250.0 ± 4.5 mg is 0.08%. In light of the low probability associated with this event, it may be concluded that this sample is not representative of the population mean of the batch of tablets, or alternatively, the sample was effectively derived from another population! This outcome may seem unusual to the reader, as it has been stated in the example that the sample was derived from the same batch of tablets as the previous two samples. The third sample is, however, not representative of the population (i.e. it is not a representative sample) and, in light of what we have been told about the time of sampling, it is perhaps indicative of a particular flaw in the manufacturing process that becomes apparent as the batch nears completion of manufacture.

5.1.1 Assumptions in statistical hypothesis testing

The scenario described above concerning the similarities and differences between sample and population statistics takes us into the mechanics of statistical hypothesis testing. Before collection of the three samples from the batch of tablets, it was assumed that the means of the three samples should be representative of the population mean. This assumption is commonly referred to as the *null hypothesis*, and is the starting position in statistical hypothesis testing. The reasons for this position are twofold:

- First, it is extremely difficult to prove that something is true, but it is easier to prove that something is false. For example, one may assume that, in a sporting event, a particular team will always win, as this team has not been beaten in 5 years. However, it is possible that the team will perform poorly on a particular day and lose, thus invalidating the original assumption.

- The second reason for adopting a null hypothesis is that it is a straightforward starting point for any subsequent analysis and, indeed, is a hypothesis that is established for the sole purpose of being rejected. Consequently, it is easier to assume that the sample means are representative of the population mean, and are therefore statistically similar to the population mean, than to assume that the means are not representative and thus differ from the population mean by a defined amount.

In the first two samples that were removed from the batch of tablets, it was confirmed that their mean values were representative of the population mean and, therefore, the null hypothesis was accepted in both cases. Conversely, it was concluded that the mean of the third sample was unrepresentative of the population mean and, therefore, the null hypothesis was not accepted. This outcome raises another problem. How do you interpret a non-acceptance of the null hypothesis? In statistics this is performed by accepting the *alternative hypothesis*, i.e. the opposite of the null hypothesis. In the current example, the null hypothesis has been rejected and therefore, the alternative hypothesis, i.e. the third sample mean is not representative of the population mean, is accepted. Interestingly, a confusing concept, shared by statisticians and students alike, is the interpretation of an accepted null hypothesis. In essence, this difficulty has been presented in the preceding example. On the basis of the results obtained from either sample 1 or sample 2, it was concluded that the null hypothesis was accepted. However, removal and analysis of the third sample yielded a different outcome, i.e. the null hypothesis was rejected. Hence, samples from the same population may yield different statistical outcomes. For this reason, statisticians frequently argue that one can never directly prove the null hypothesis and therefore, terms such as 'fail to reject the null hypothesis' are commonly used. For the purpose of this book, however, we shall be more decisive in statistical hypothesis testing and consequently, the null hypothesis will be either rejected or accepted!

Statistical hypothesis testing is a measure of whether the null hypothesis is accepted or rejected. If the null hypothesis is rejected, the alternative hypothesis is accepted. The alternative hypothesis is generally the operational basis of the research hypothesis. To return to the example concerning tablet weights, we have been asked to identify whether the sample means are different from the population mean. Therefore, the null hypothesis and alternative hypothesis may be expressed as follows:

- *null hypothesis (H_0):* there is no difference between the sample means and the population mean
- *alternative hypothesis (H_a):* there is a difference between the sample means and the population mean

Once the statistical analysis (appropriate to the experimental design) is complete, the results are therefore stated in terms of the acceptance or rejection of the null hypothesis.

5.1.2 Defining the level of significance and the critical regions of acceptance and rejection of the null hypothesis

In advance of the collection of data, it is necessary to state the level of significance as this defines the terms of acceptance and rejection of the null hypothesis. Conventionally, statisticians use a value of 0.05 to define the probability (or improbability) of an event. Thus, if a probability value of 0.05 or less is associated with an event, there is sufficient evidence to conclude that the null hypothesis is not acceptable and that the alternative hypothesis is therefore valid. In statistical convention, the level of significance is generally written as a proportion and is denoted by the Greek letter alpha (α). The choice of α is completely arbitrary, although 0.05 is frequently used in statistical hypothesis testing. In some cases different α values are employed, but it should be remembered that as the level of significance is increased, e.g. $\alpha = 0.01$, it becomes more difficult to reject the null hypothesis. This is particularly important as scientific experiments are generally designed to reject the null hypothesis.

The perceptive reader may have anticipated the next part of the discussion concerning identification of the regions of acceptance and rejection of the null hypothesis. Having established the level of probability, the regions of acceptance and rejection of the null hypothesis associated with defined probability distributions are employed. In Chapter 4, the properties of several probability distributions, e.g. the Student's t distribution, the (standardised) normal distribution, the χ^2 distribution and the F distribution were identified. These test statistics are associated with specific statistical procedures, the calculation of which will be explained in subsequent chapters. However, the calculation of a test statistic, namely the z statistic, has been demonstrated and it is sufficient to note at this point that the calculation and interpretation of other test statistics is similar in many ways. The reader will recall that the calculated z statistic is associated with a defined probability. If this probability is equal to or less than the chosen level of significance, then the null hypothesis is rejected. Conversely, if the calculated level of significance is greater than the α value, the null hypothesis is accepted. To clarify this procedure, let us return to the example concerning tablet weights. In this example, the null hypothesis stated that 'there is no difference between the sample mean and the population mean', whereas the alternative hypothesis stated that 'there is a difference between the sample mean and the population mean'. In the case of sample 1, the z statistic was calculated as 0.8, reflecting a probability of 0.7881. As this value exceeded 0.05, the null hypothesis was accepted. For sample 3, the z value was calculated as -3.18 and was associated with a probability of 0.0008. As this value was less than 0.05, the null hypothesis was rejected and the alternative hypothesis accepted.

Although the approach described above is perfectly valid, it is usual in statistical hypothesis testing to define the critical regions of acceptance or rejection of the null hypothesis, respectively, before calculating the test statistic. In other words, the values of the test statistic associated with null hypothesis rejection and acceptance are defined. To do this, the possible outcomes of the statistical test must be considered before the collection of data. This is discussed in the next section.

5.1.3   One-tailed and two-tailed tests (outcomes)

In the process of statistical hypothesis testing, it is customary to state the null and alternative hypotheses and the level of significance, and to define whether the experimental design (test) is one- or two-tailed. This concept of one- and two-tailed tests refers to the possible outcomes of the study. If there are two possible statistical outcomes in the study, then a two-tailed test must be used; conversely, if there is only one outcome of interest to the investigator, the test statistic must be interpreted using a one-tailed outcome. The discrete differences between these two types of outcomes are illustrated in the following scenario.

The quality control section of a pharmaceutical company has advised that several batches of the company's antacid preparation have failed the preservative efficacy test, as defined by the British Pharmacopoeia. The formulation section has been advised to reformulate the product such that the new product should contain less than 1×10^2 microorganisms/mL, after storage at $20\,°C$ for 2 weeks. Accordingly, the formulation section has produced a new formulation to be assessed for preservative efficacy assessment. The results, presented as the number of surviving microorganisms in 10 bottles, are shown in Table 5.2.

In this situation, the null hypothesis is established before the collection of data, and may be stated as follows: there is no difference

Table 5.2 Microbial content (number of microorganisms/mL) in each of 10 bottles of an antacid preparation

Bottle number	Number of surviving microorganisms/mL
1	75
2	80
3	101
4	82
5	84
6	98
7	93
8	100
9	78
10	89

between the expected mean (100 microorganisms/mL) and the sample mean, i.e. $H_0 = 100$ microorganisms/mL. Conversely, the alternative hypothesis states that there is a negative difference between the observed sample mean and the expected mean, and the new product passes the British Pharmacopoeia specifications, i.e. $H_a < 100$ microorganisms/mL.

The only interest to the investigator in this analysis is whether the mean microbial content of the new formulation was lower than the defined (expected) mean. As there is only one outcome of interest, this is a *one-tailed test*.

Alternatively, the formulation scientist in the above experiment may want to find out more about the performance of the formulation. In this case, it is important to know if the new formulation passes or fails the Pharmacopoeial recommendation. Obviously, if the microbial content is greater than the standard, the product has failed the approved specifications. This will still provide useful information about the direction of the reformulation programme, potentially identifying ineffective preservatives. The null hypothesis in this situation is identical to the previous example, i.e. there is no difference between the expected mean (100 microorganisms/mL) and the sample mean, i.e. $H_0 = 100$ microorganisms/mL. The alternative hypothesis has changed, however, and is now be defined as: there is a difference between the expected mean (100 microorganisms/mL) and the observed mean, i.e. $H_a \neq 100$ microorganisms/mL. The sources of the difference are twofold, i.e. the difference may be a result of the sample mean being either greater or less than the expected mean. Under these circumstances, the outcome of this analysis is *two-tailed*, because there are two possible outcomes that will result in the rejection of the null hypothesis.

The decision as to whether the calculated test statistic should be evaluated as a one-tailed test or a two-tailed test is crucial. An incorrect choice may result in the incorrect interpretation of the statistical analysis, because a significant difference between treatments may be declared insignificant and vice versa.

5.1.4 Defining the critical region for a statistical method

As previously outlined, when a statistical analysis is performed, the sampling distribution and the conventional probability distributions (Chapter 4) are conveniently divided into two regions which enable the interpretation of the importance of the calculated test statistic to be performed. The values of the test statistic associated with the acceptance of the null hypothesis reside within the first region, the so-called *region of non-significance*. The second region defines the values of the test statistic that are associated with the rejection of the null hypothesis and acceptance of the alternative hypothesis. This is the *region of significance*. For all probability distributions associated with test statistics, the magnitudes (and hence the numerical boundaries) of these regions are dependent on two factors: the level of significance (α) and whether the test is one- or two-tailed. For many distributions, e.g. the F distribution, the t distribution and the χ^2 distribution, the number of degrees of freedom associated with the experimental design also defines the boundaries of the regions of acceptance and rejection. The calculation of the number of degrees of freedom for each statistical test will be described in subsequent chapters, in conjunction with an overall description of the statistical tests that employ these statistics. For the purpose of this section, the discussion concerning identification of the critical regions will concentrate on the normal distribution.

Assuming $\alpha = 0.05$, the critical region of the standardised normal distribution may be defined (visualised) in three ways, as illustrated in Figures 5.2, 5.3 and 5.4. In all three cases, the chosen level of significance is 0.05, as denoted by the shaded region. Calculated values of the z statistic (the test statistic that relates to the standardised normal distribution) that reside within these regions allow the analyst to reject the null hypothesis. The reader will notice that one-tailed and two-tailed tests differ in their distribution of the region of rejection. In a two-tailed test, the rejection region is equally divided into two sections, each relating to a single tail that resides at either extreme of the probability distribution. As $\alpha = 0.05$, each tail occupies 2.5% of the distribution. In the case of the standardised normal distribution, the critical regions are denoted by z values of either $\geq +1.96$ or ≤ -1.96. Conversely, in the one-

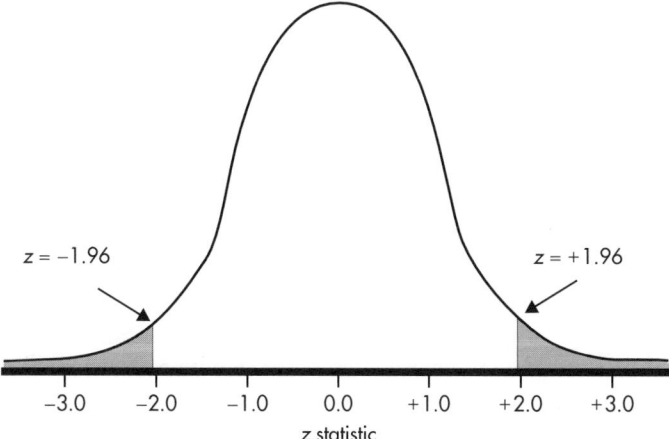

Figure 5.2 Standardised normal distribution showing the critical (shaded) regions of the z statistic for a two-tailed test.

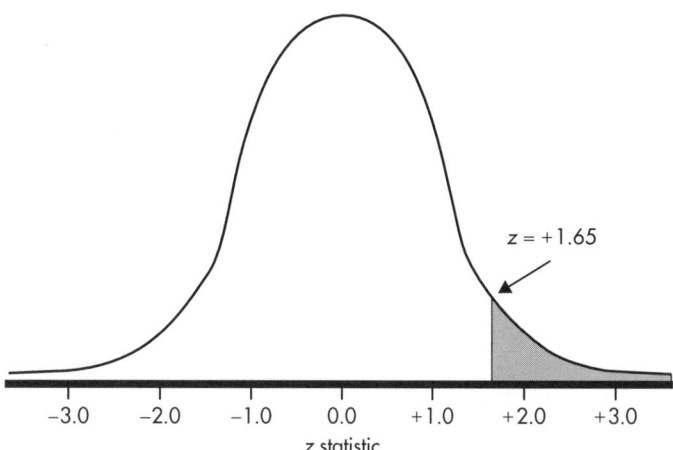

Figure 5.3 Standardised normal distribution showing the critical (shaded) regions of the z statistic for a positive one-tailed test.

tailed test, the rejection region is distributed at either tail of the distribution. If the alternative hypothesis states, for example, that 'the mean of a treatment group is greater than the mean of another group or an expected value', then the critical value of z is $\geqslant 1.65$ and the test is referred to as a *positive one-tailed test*. In the standardised normal distribution, a z value of 1.65 divides the distribution into two regions in which 95% of all observations resides in the region below 1.65 and 5% in the region above 1.65. When the alternative hypothesis declares, for

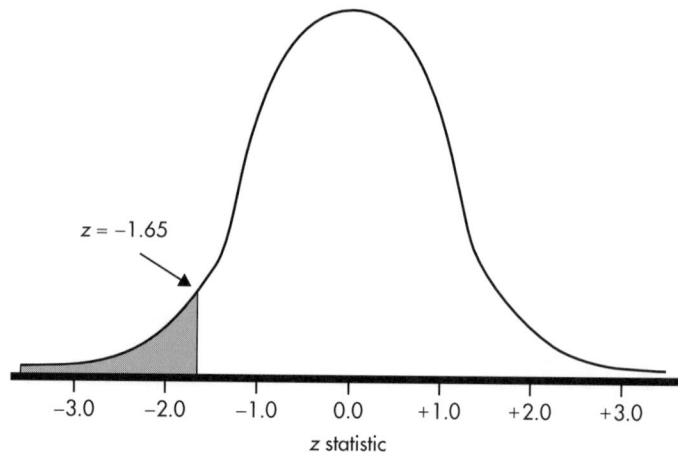

Figure 5.4 Standardised normal distribution showing the critical (shaded) regions of the z statistic for a negative one-tailed test.

example, that the mean of a treatment group is lower than the mean of another group or an expected value, the rejection region resides at the left-hand (negative) side of the standardised normal distribution and is defined by z values that are $\leqslant -1.65$. Analogous to the positive one-tailed distribution, 5% of all observations lie in the critical region $(z \leqslant -1.65)$ and 95% lie in the region > -1.65.

The importance of the selecting the number of tails in a test correctly should now be obvious. Within the region of z values > -1.65 and $< +1.65$ there is no ambiguity, because these values would allow the null hypothesis to be accepted in both one-tailed and two-tailed tests. Similarly, no problems will arise if the z statistic lies within the regions $z \geqslant +1.96$ or $z \leqslant -1.96$, as in both tests these regions are associated with rejection of the null hypothesis and, by inference, acceptance of the alternative hypothesis. The problems arise when the calculated z statistic lies within the regions $+1.65 \leqslant z < 1.96$ and $-1.96 < z \leqslant -1.65$. If the statistical analysis has been incorrectly designed as a one-tailed test and a value of z is returned that resides within these regions, the analyst would therefore have to conclude (incorrectly) that the null hypothesis should be rejected and the alternative hypothesis accepted. Similarly, if analyst had assumed that the test was a two-tailed test, and it was in fact a one-tailed test, then a calculated z value within these regions would result in a false acceptance of the null hypothesis when the true outcome should have been to reject the null hypothesis.

In summary, if the null hypothesis $H_0 = 200$ (a hypothetical value), then the alternative hypotheses are as follows:

- $H_a \neq 200$, for a two-tailed test, in that H_a may be significantly less or significantly greater than 200. The regions of rejection of the null hypothesis are $z \leqslant -1.96$ or $z \geqslant +1.96$ within the standardised normal distribution.
- $H_a < 200$, for a negative one-tailed test. The region of rejection is $z \leqslant -1.65$ within the standardised normal distribution.
- $H_a > 200$, for a positive one-tailed test. The region of rejection is $z \geqslant +1.65$ within the standardised normal distribution.

So far we have used the z statistic to identify the critical regions. In subsequent chapters, identification of the critical regions of other probability distributions will be described in conjunction with the details of how the appropriate test statistics, e.g. χ^2, t, F, are calculated.

5.2 Errors in decision-making (type I and type II errors)

One of the important aspects of statistical decision-making is that the analyst should have confidence in the outcome and interpretation of the statistical analysis. In everyday life we make decisions using an inherent sense to select the correct decision for that particular moment. As we are painfully aware, some of these decisions can go badly wrong. In statistics, decisions are also taken involving the acceptance or rejection of the null hypothesis. However, we do not rely on an 'inherent sense' to define the outcome; instead, the probability of making the wrong decision can be calculated statistically. For example, it is possible to determine the probability of rejecting the null hypothesis when it was in fact true, and conversely, the probability of erroneously accepting the null hypothesis. The methods by which these probabilities are calculated form the basis of this section.

There are two types of error, termed *type I* and *type II*, that may be made in determining the outcome of statistical experiments. The differences between these two categories of error and their importance may be illustrated by reference to the following hypothetical situation. In a clinical study, the effect of a β-blocker on the reduction in diastolic blood pressure reduction of 100 patients was examined. The mean reduction ($\pm$ SD) was 30 ± 3 mmHg, and the sampling distribution of blood pressure reduction is shown in Figure 5.5. In this figure the null hypothesis is defined by the non-shaded region. The shaded region denotes the upper 5% of the distribution. Conventionally, in statistical hypothesis testing, any sample recorded in this region would lead to a rejection of the null hypothesis. However, this is somewhat unusual, as it is known that this is a normal response, i.e. every distribution of a particular variable will have an upper and lower tail. Consequently, if a patient is sampled who presents with a blood pressure reduction of 34.95 mmHg or greater, even though that patient is part of a normal sampling distribution, the statistical analyst would automatically reject the null hypothesis. In so doing, it is therefore assumed that the patient was not derived from the original distribution (mean ± SD, 30 ± 3 mmHg) but from another statistical distribution possessing a different mean value. In effect, a statistical error has been made, in which the null hypothesis has been rejected when it is, in fact, true. This is a *type I error*, the probability of which is the area of the rejection region (0.05 in Figure 5.5). The probability of committing a type I error is denoted by α. Therefore, the probability of committing a type I error is actually the probability of rejecting the null hypothesis.

Conversely, if the null hypothesis is accepted when it is in fact false, a *type II error* has been committed. As a result of this, it is common to calculate the probability of making a type II error whenever the null hypothesis has been accepted. A reciprocal relationship exists between types I and II errors. Thus, if the probability of committing a type I error is reduced (by increasing the α value), the probability of committing a type II error will increase. This relationship is illustrated in Figure 5.6. Figure 5.6a illustrates the sampling distribution of mean blood pressure lowering after administration of a β-blocker. This is a normal distribution, possessing a defined mean and standard deviation (30 ± 3 mmHg). Assuming a significance level of 0.05 (one-tailed), the critical value of the z statistic that defines the rejection of rejection of the

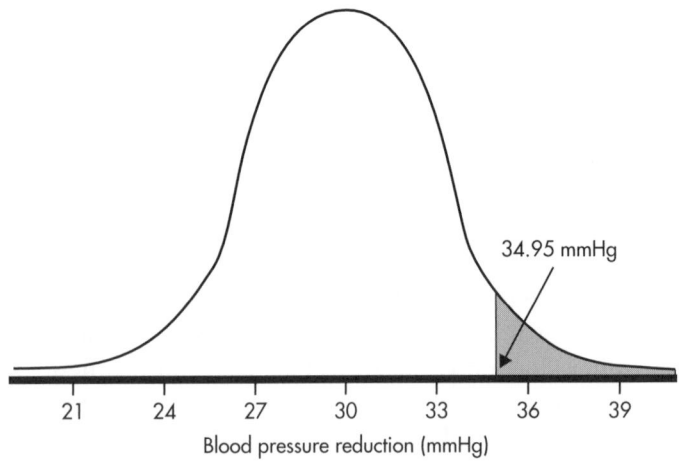

Figure 5.5 Sampling distribution of the reduction in diastolic blood pressure (μ = 30 mmHg, σ = 3 mmHg).

null hypothesis may be calculated as follows:

$$z = \frac{X - \mu}{\sigma} = 1.65 = \frac{X - 30}{3}$$

$$X = (1.65 \times 3) + 30 = 34.95 \text{ mmHg}$$

Therefore, at the defined level of significance, any value observed to be ⩾ 34.95 mmHg will result in a rejection of the null hypothesis.

If it is then assumed that the null hypothesis is false and, accordingly, the alternative hypothesis is accepted, the problems associated with type II errors may be illustrated. In Figure 5.6b we can see a sampling distribution that describes the alternative hypothesis, with a mean and standard deviation of 37 ± 3 mmHg. Remember that in the practical situation we have no knowledge of the sampling distribution of the

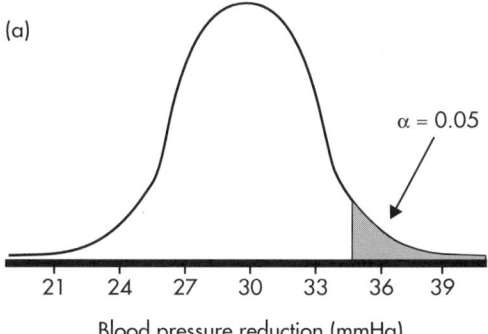

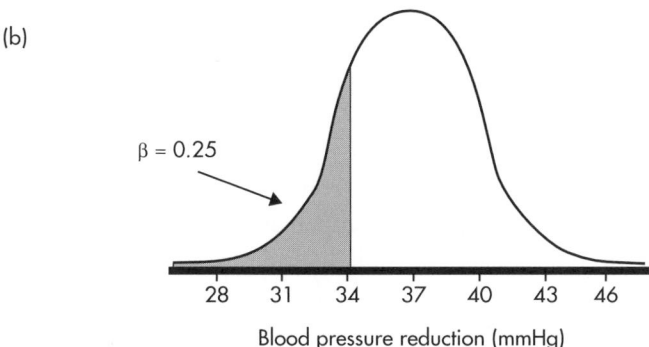

Figure 5.6 Sampling distributions of the mean lowering of blood pressure after administration of a β-blocker: (a) Lowering of blood pressure for the null hypothesis, the shaded area defining the probability associated with a type I error ($\alpha = 0.05$). (b) Lowering of blood pressure for the alternative hypothesis, the shaded area defining the probability of a type II error (β).

second group. In the example provided, the alternative hypothesis will only state that the observed reduction in blood pressure is greater than that defined by the null hypothesis. The sampling distribution of the alternative hypothesis is provided to illustrate the interplay between type I and type II errors, because in the real situation we will not know the mean and standard deviation of the alternative hypothesis. Returning to the example, the alternative hypothesis is normal, possessing tails at each side of the distribution. In Figure 5.6a, the probability of making a type I error, i.e. rejecting the null hypothesis when the null hypothesis is true, is denoted by the shaded region. The shaded region in Figure 5.6b denotes the probability of making a type II error, i.e. accepting the null hypothesis when it should be rejected. Consequently, in the sampling distribution associated with the null hypothesis, the shaded region defines the probability of selecting a mean value of reduction in blood pressure that would fall within the region of non-rejection of the null hypothesis, defined as < 34.95 mmHg. Therefore, the shaded region in Figure 5.6b defines the area of the sampling distribution (relating to the alternative hypothesis) that falls below 34.95 mmHg. The area of this region may be calculated using a z transformation, as follows:

$$z = \frac{\bar{X} - \mu}{\sigma}$$

$$z = \frac{34.95 - 37}{3} = -0.68$$

Referring to the standardised normal distribution, we can see that the area (probability) relating to the calculated z value is 0.25. Therefore, in the above example, $\alpha = 0.05$ and $\beta = 0.25$.

A summary of the interplay between types I and II errors, and of their role in the process of statistical decision-making, is shown in Table 5.3.

There are several different consequences of type I and type II errors, reflecting the different outcomes when the null hypothesis is accepted or rejected. If the null hypothesis is rejected, the research hypothesis is therefore accepted and, accordingly, a proposal has been transposed from speculation to observation. However, if the null hypothesis has been rejected when it is in fact true, a type I error has been committed. In this situation, an incorrect (and potentially dangerous) conclusion has been reached. Conversely, acceptance of the null hypothesis when it is in fact false this will result in the rejection of a perfectly acceptable research hypothesis. The following situation highlights the potential hazards of statistical errors in decision-making.

Table 5.3 Summary of the relationships between statistical outcome and statistical errors

Statistical outcome (decision)	Real result	
	Null hypothesis is true (i.e. H_0: $\mu = 30$ mmHg)	Null hypothesis is false (i.e. H_0: $\mu > 30$ mmHg)
Non-rejection of the null hypothesis	**Correct decision**	Type II (β) error
Rejection of the null hypothesis/acceptance of the alternative hypothesis	Type I (α) error	**Correct decision**

A manufacturer of antibiotics has developed a novel patented β-lactam antibiotic that has been designed for the treatment of pneumonia in patients in hospital intensive care units. A clinical trial has been designed to assess whether the antibiotic is more efficacious than the current antibiotics of choice for the treatment of pneumonia. The null hypothesis of this study is that there is no difference between the clinical efficacies of the antibiotics; the alternative hypothesis states that the new antibiotic exhibits greater efficacy than the current antibiotic. As outlined in Table 5.3, there are two possible true outcomes: the null hypothesis may be either correct or incorrect. *If the null hypothesis is correct*, this implies that there is no difference in the abilities of the two antibiotics to resolve pneumonia. However, following completion of the study and the subsequent statistical analysis, there are two possible statistical decisions.

- First, the analyst may have accepted (not rejected) the null hypothesis and hence, the correct decision will have been recorded.

- Conversely, the analyst may have concluded that the null hypothesis should be rejected and thereby committed a type I (α) error. The consequences of this are quite interesting and clinically relevant! Because the alternative hypothesis has been accepted the company now believes that it has provided respiratory medicine with a new wonder drug and, accordingly, would hope that this drug is prescribed for the treatment of pneumonia, at the expense of the other available treatments. In reality, the drug is no better than other currently available antibiotics and, in the current litigious age, the manufacturers of the competitor antibiotics would probably attempt to correct the type I error within the confines of a law court.

If the alternative hypothesis is correct, a type II error will have been made if the statistical analyst concludes that there was no statistical difference between the efficacies of the antibiotics under investigation when, in fact there is a difference between their comparative abilities to resolve pneumonia. The statistical analyst has accepted the null hypothesis when in fact the alternative hypothesis represented the real (truthful) situation. The potential repercussions of this type II error are not as severe as for the type I counterpart. On the basis of the statistical analyst's findings, the company sponsoring the clinical trial would conclude that this drug offers no advantage and would most likely cease further development. The public would therefore not have the opportunity to benefit from this new antibiotic and the manufacturer would not receive the financial reward that it rightly should. This example has hopefully clarified the importance of statistical errors to the decision-making process.

Errors are involved in all statistical hypothesis testing, and by attempting to reduce one type of error one increases the chances of the other. Accordingly, it is appropriate to offer words of wisdom concerning what levels of each type of error are acceptable in statistical hypothesis testing. Conventionally, the type I (α) error is selected to be 0.05 as this is deemed to be a sufficiently small probability of committing this type of error, while not being too small to erroneously increase the probability of a type II (β) error occurring.

5.3 Power of a statistical test

In statistics, the relationship between statistical decision-making and errors is frequently phrased in terms of the *power* of a study. Typically, the power of a statistical test may be defined as the probability that the null hypothesis is rejected when it is indeed false. In other words, the power is a measure of the ability of the statistical test to validate a research hypothesis when the research hypothesis is in fact true. Remembering that a type II error (β) may be defined as the probability of not rejecting the null hypothesis when it should be rejected, the power is quoted as $1 - \beta$. Accordingly, in the blood pressure reduction example, the power of the statistical test was therefore $1 - 0.25$, or 75%. The power, of the statistical test, i.e. probability of avoiding a type II error, increases as the difference between the null hypothesis and the alternative hypothesis increases.

5.3.1 Experimental design factors affecting the power of statistical tests

The power of a statistical test is an important consideration in any experimental design. Maximising the power of the statistical test results in a greater confidence concerning the fidelity of a statistical outcome. The magnitude of the power of a study is influenced by several factors:

- the chosen probability relating to a type I error (i.e. α)
- the magnitude of the difference between the true mean (alternative hypothesis) and the mean associated with the null hypothesis

- the sample size
- the nature of the statistical test.

An understanding of the nature of the effects of the above variables on the power of a statistical test is essential to ensure that the design of experiments is adequately performed. The nature of these effects is now described.

5.3.1.1 Choice of the level of probability of a type I error

As stated previously, there is a reciprocal relationship between the probability of committing a type I error and the probability of committing a type II error. Consequently, if the probability of performing an α error is strategically reduced, for example to ensure a greater control of the critical value relating to rejection of the null hypothesis, then the probability of committing a type II error is increased. The effects of the magnitude of α on the resultant probability of making a type II error may be illustrated with reference to Figure 5.6. As may be recalled, in this example the sampling distribution associated with blood pressure reduction following administration of a β-blocker was normal, possessing a defined mean and standard deviation (30 ± 3 mmHg). In this figure, a type I error was chosen as 0.05 (one tailed), and the critical value of the z statistic that defines the rejection of the null hypothesis was calculated as 34.95 mmHg. Consequently, sampled values equal to or greater than this critical value are assumed to have been derived from a different normal distribution to that described by the null hypothesis.

Selecting α values of 0.10 and 0.01, the critical values of blood pressure reduction that define the rejection of the respective null hypotheses are calculated as follows:

Type I error (α) = 0.10
First, the z statistic associated with the chosen level of significance ($\alpha = 0.10$) is derived from the table of the standardised normal distribution (Appendix 1). The critical value of blood pressure reduction is then calculated using this z statistic:

$$z = 1.282$$
$$= \frac{\overline{X} - \mu}{\sigma}$$
$$1.282 = \frac{\overline{X} - 30}{3}$$
$$\overline{X} = 33.85 \text{ mmHg}$$

Type I error $(\alpha) = 0.01$

Once more, the z statistic associated with the chosen level of significance ($\alpha = 0.01$) is derived from the table of the standardised normal distribution (Appendix 1). The critical value of blood pressure reduction is then calculated:

$$z = 2.326$$

$$= \frac{\bar{X} - \mu}{\sigma}$$

$$2.326 = \frac{\bar{X} - 30}{3}$$

$$\bar{X} = 36.98 \text{ mmHg}$$

As before, assuming that the null hypothesis is rejected and that the mean and standard deviation of the sampling distribution relating to the alternative hypothesis are 37 ± 3 mmHg, respectively, the probability of observing a type II error may be calculated (Figures 5.7. and 5.8). As may be observed, decreasing the magnitude of α, although decreasing the probability of recording a type I error, increases the probability of a type II error. The value of β may be calculated using a z transformation, as previously described.

Calculation of β when $\alpha = 0.10$

$$z = \frac{\bar{X} - \mu}{\sigma}$$

$$= \frac{33.85 - 37.00}{3} = -1.05$$

This z value refers to the probability of observing a mean blood pressure reduction that is less than or equal to 33.85 mmHg, i.e. 0.14. This is the probability of committing a type II error. The power of this study is thus $1 - 0.14 = 0.86$.

Calculation of β when $\alpha = 0.01$

$$z = \frac{\bar{X} - \mu}{\sigma}$$

$$= \frac{36.98 - 37.00}{3} = -0.0007$$

This z value refers to the probability of observing a mean blood pressure reduction that is $\leqslant 36.98$ mmHg, i.e. 0.50. This is the

(a)

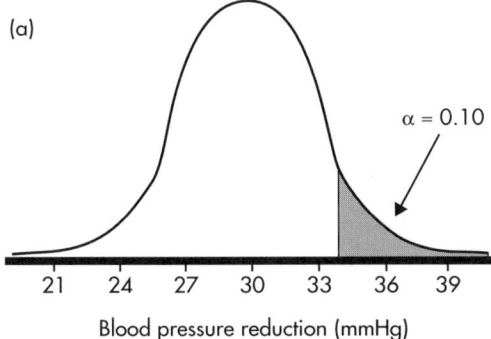

α = 0.10

Blood pressure reduction (mmHg)

(b)

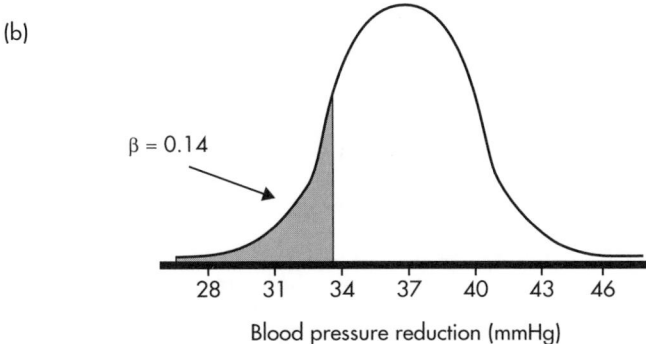

β = 0.14

Blood pressure reduction (mmHg)

Figure 5.7 Sampling distributions of the mean lowering of blood pressure after administration of a β-blocker: (a) Lowering of blood pressure for the null hypothesis, the shaded area defining the probability associated with a type I error ($\alpha = 0.10$). (b) Lowering of blood pressure for the alternative hypothesis 37 ± 3 mmHg (mean ± standard deviation), the shaded area defines the probability of a type II error (β).

probability of committing a type II error. The power of this study is thus $1 - 0.50 = 0.50$.

The effects of choosing a value on the probability of committing a type II error and on power of the study are summarised in Table 5.4.

5.3.1.2 The magnitude of the difference between the true mean (alternative hypothesis) and the mean associated with the null hypothesis

In the previous section power was defined as the probability that the null hypothesis is rejected when it is in fact false. Therefore, the power of a study is directly proportional to the difference between the means of the alternative hypothesis and the null hypothesis. Increasing the differ-

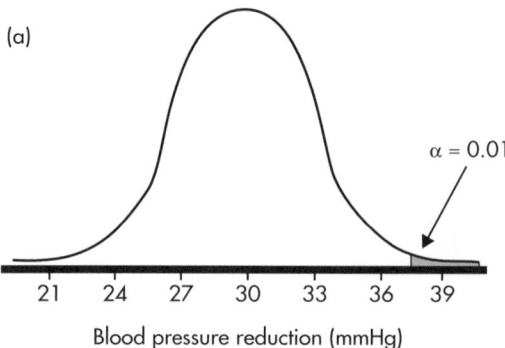

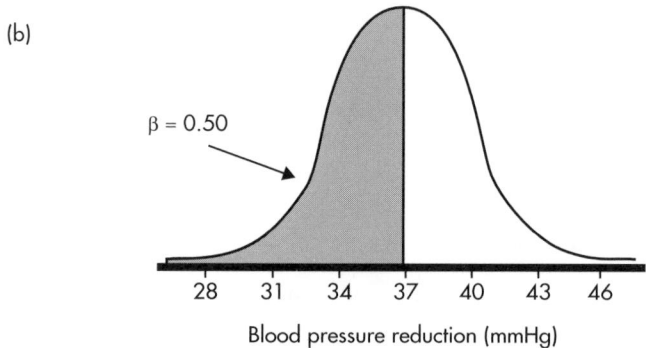

Figure 5.8 Sampling distributions of mean lowering of blood pressure after administration of a β-blocker: (a) Lowering of blood pressure for the null hypothesis, the shaded area defining the probability associated with a type I error ($\alpha = 0.01$). (b) Lowering of blood pressure for the alternative hypothesis (37 ± 3 mmHg mean $\pm$ standard deviation), the shaded area defining the probability of a type II error (β).

ence between these two parameters increases the power of a study. The effects of increasing the difference between the mean values associated with the alternative and null hypotheses on the subsequent power are illustrated in Figures 5.9–5.11. In these figures, the chosen level of significance, i.e. the probability of committing a type I error, has been maintained at 0.05. On the basis of the selected α value, the null hypothesis may be rejected if the observed value is equal to or greater than the critical value of blood pressure reduction, i.e. 34.95 mmHg. In Figures 5.9a, 5.10a and 5.11a, this region is shaded. Furthermore, the probability of committing a type II error may be calculated using a z transformation, as previously outlined.

Table 5.4 Summary of the effects of chosen α level on the probability of committing a type II error and the subsequent power of the study for the example illustrated in Figures 5.6–5.8

Type I (α) error	Type II (β) error	Power
0.01	0.50	0.50
0.05	0.25	0.75
0.10	0.14	0.86

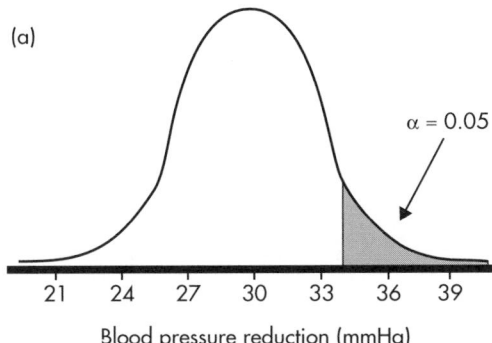

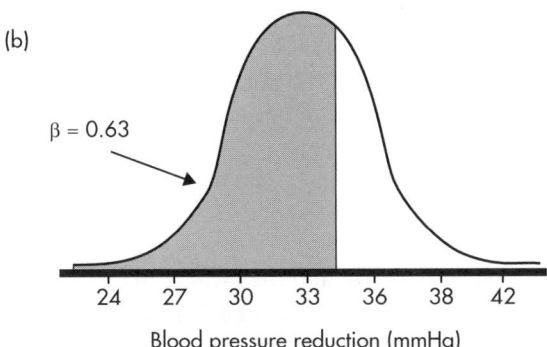

Figure 5.9 Sampling distributions of mean lowering of blood pressure after administration of a β-blocker: (a) Lowering of blood pressure for the null hypothesis, the shaded area defining the probability associated with a type I error ($\alpha = 0.05$). (b) Lowering of the blood pressure for the alternative hypothesis, the shaded area defining the probability of a type II error (β). The mean ±SD values are 30 ± 3 and 34 ± 3 mmHg, respectively.

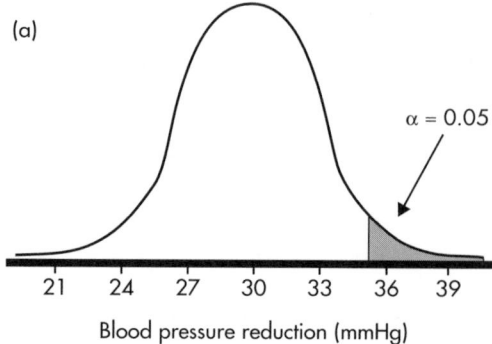

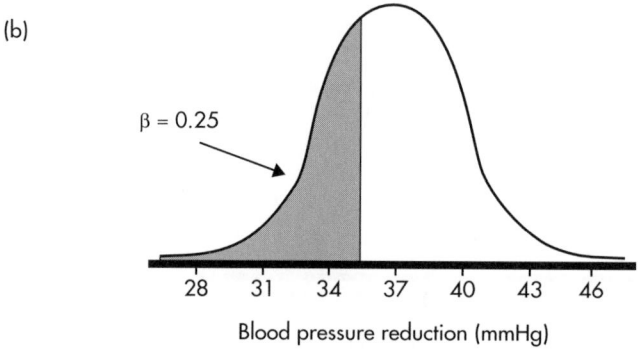

Figure 5.10   Sampling distributions of mean lowering of blood pressure after administration of a β-blocker: (a) Lowering of blood pressure for the null hypothesis, the shaded area defining the probability associated with a type I error ($\alpha = 0.05$). (b) Lowering of the blood pressure, as defined by the alternative hypothesis, the shaded area defining the probability of a type II error (β). The mean ±SD values are 30 ± 3 and 37 ± 3 mmHg, respectively.

Calculation of β when $\alpha = 0.05$ and the mean ± SD values of the null and alternative hypotheses are 30 ± 3 and 34 ± 3, respectively

$$z_\beta = \frac{X - \mu}{\sigma}$$

$$= \frac{34.95 - 34.00}{3} = 0.32$$

The probability of committing a type II error is therefore 0.63 (Figure 5.9). The power of the study is $1 - \beta = 1 - 0.63 = 0.37$.

Calculation of β when $\alpha = 0.05$ and the mean $\pm$ SD values of the null and alternative hypotheses are 30 ± 3 and 37 ± 3, respectively

$$z_\beta = \frac{X - \mu}{\sigma}$$

$$= \frac{34.95 - 37.00}{3} = -0.68$$

The probability of committing a type II error is therefore 0.25 (Figure 5.10), and the power of the study is therefore 0.75, i.e. $1 - \beta = 1 - 0.25$.

Calculation of β when α is 0.05 and the mean $\pm$ SD values of the null and alternative hypotheses are 30 ± 3 and 40 ± 3, respectively

$$z_\beta = \frac{X - \mu}{\sigma}$$

$$= \frac{34.95 - 40.00}{3} = -1.68$$

The probability of committing a type II error is therefore 0.05 and, consequently, the power of the study is $1 - \beta = 1 - 0.05 = 0.95$.

Therefore, it may be concluded that when there is a large difference between the null hypothesis and the alternative hypothesis, the power of a statistical study will be large. This should not be unexpected, as this statement outlines a fundamental statistical concept, i.e. the probability that a difference will be observed is dependent on the magnitude of the difference.

5.3.1.3 Sample size

Although it is understood that both the choice of α and, additionally, the difference between the means of the null and alternative hypotheses are direct determinants of the power of a statistical study, these factors may not be conveniently manipulated to optimise statistical power. For example, although an increase in the value of α may increase power, it also increases the probability of committing a type I error. Furthermore, the differences that exist between the means associated with the null and alternative hypotheses are a function both of the natures of the samples employed in the study and also of the original research hypothesis. They are therefore not amenable to manipulation. However, one easy way of enhancing the power of a statistical design is to increase the number of observations (the sample size). In the scenario concerning blood

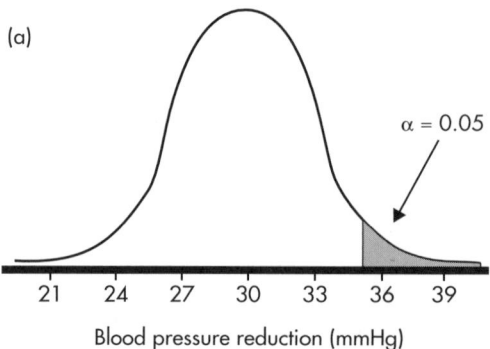

(a)

α = 0.05

21   24   27   30   33   36   39

Blood pressure reduction (mmHg)

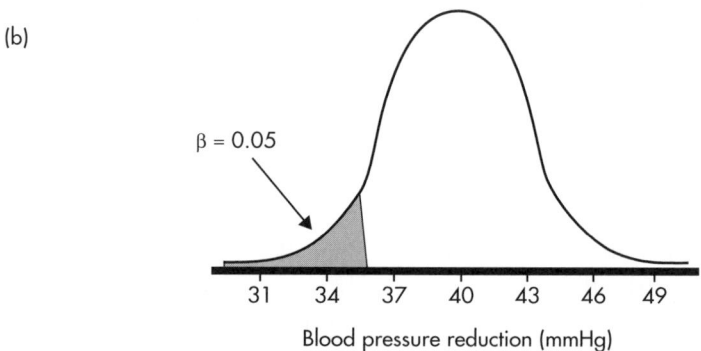

(b)

β = 0.05

31   34   37   40   43   46   49

Blood pressure reduction (mmHg)

Figure 5.11   Sampling distributions of the mean lowering of blood pressure following administration of a β-blocker: (a) Lowering of blood pressure for the null hypothesis, the shaded area defining the probability associated with a type I error ($\alpha = 0.05$). (b) Lowering of the blood pressure for the alternative hypothesis, the shaded area defining the probability of a type II error (β). The mean ±SD values are 30 ± 3 and 40 ± 3 mmHg, respectively.

pressure reductions (and indeed any other variable), the null hypothesis and alternative hypothesis referred to either the similarity or the disparity of mean values. Therefore, the distributions relating to these hypotheses were sampling distributions of mean values. The standard deviation of the sampling distribution of the mean is termed the standard error and has been defined previously (Chapter 2) as

$$\sigma_{\bar{X}} = \frac{\sigma}{\sqrt{N}}$$

Therefore, the standard deviation of the sampling distribution of the mean is decreased as the number of observations is increased. This affects the shape of the resultant sampling distribution by reducing the area of the tails. With reference to the power of a statistical design, the reduced area in the tails decreases the degree (area) of overlap between the sampling distributions associated with the null and alternative hypotheses. It therefore follows that the power of the study, and hence the validity of the outcome of the statistical analysis, is increased.

Statisticians concerned with the design of experiments, particularly clinical trials, are often asked to estimate the number of subjects (samples) that is required to ensure adequate statistical power and therefore confirm that that the conclusions from the study are valid. To perform this estimation, the following information is required:

- Specification of the probability of committing a type I error (α).
- Specification of committing a type II error (β).
- Standard deviation of the method or experiment.
- The difference between the means of the null and alternative hypotheses that is considered to be practically relevant. This is not a randomly chosen value but is carefully selected following consideration of the research hypothesis of the experiment. This value often reflects the minimum value that will ensure clinical efficacy or, alternatively, it may be the minimum difference in the performance of two products that is accepted by a regulatory authority to constitute a real improvement.

The use of the above variables to calculate the number of samples that should be included in a statistical design is relatively straightforward. However, as this depends on the nature of the experimental design, examples of the calculation are reserved for discussion in later chapters, where the mechanics of the various statistical methods that are commonly employed within the pharmaceutical and related sciences are comprehensively described.

5.4 Choice of statistical test

In the process of statistical hypothesis testing, several key stages have been identified:

- statement of the null and alternative hypotheses
- selection of the level of significance (α) and consideration of the probability of committing a type II error
- identification of the nature of the experimental outcome, i.e. whether the result is one-tailed or two-tailed
- identification of the critical statistic that determines the area of rejection of the null hypothesis.

One of the major steps in the process of statistical hypothesis testing involves the choice of statistical test. This is a crucial stage, as the outcome of the analysis will determine the fate of a research hypothesis and, consequently, it is important that the statistical test is selected according to the features of the experimental design. The most appropriate statistical test is chosen according to the desired power of the study, the nature of the population from which the observations were taken and the nature of measurement of the variable. These combined factors are commonly referred to as the *statistical model*. When all these factors have been considered, the correct choice of statistical test may be made and the choice is assumed to be appropriate for the statistical model. In other words, the assumptions of the statistical test are satisfied by the conditions of the experimental design.

5.4.1 Parametric and non-parametric analyses

Typically, statistical tests may be differentiated into two categories, known as *parametric* and *non-parametric analyses*, the choice of which is made according to the statistical model. In many cases, assumptions concerning the statistical model are made, as this information is not readily available to the statistician. Consequently, whenever a particular statistical method is recommended to compare two sets of data, the ability of the test to reject the null hypothesis when it is in fact false is a function of the nature of the assumptions of the statistical model. If there are few assumptions, i.e. the features of the experimental design are fully known, then the conclusions generated by the statistical test are valid and the output of the analysis is conclusive. Conversely, if several assumptions have been made concerning the nature of the statistical model, then it is likely that the output of the statistical analysis will be more general in nature. It is important to ensure that the conditions of the experiment (the statistical model) and the subsequent statistical test are matched, as this will enhance the performance of the analysis.

It should be clear to the reader that whenever there is a substantial amount of information available concerning the statistical model, one can be specific about the choice of statistical test and confident of the reliability of the analysis. Parametric and non-parametric statistical analyses differ primarily in the nature of the assumptions associated with their use. Parametric tests (e.g. t test, F test, z test) may only be used whenever a number of assumptions have been confirmed. If these assumptions are valid, the use of parametric tests is demanded, as this will ensure that the quality of the output from the statistical analysis is optimised. Under these circumstances, the power of the analysis is enhanced because of the high probability of rejecting the null hypothesis whenever it is indeed false. The following experimental conditions (assumptions) should hold before a parametric statistical method is selected and used:

- The samples should be removed from a normally distributed population.
- The samples should be independent, i.e. the process of sampling should not influence the sampling process. This is an assumption for all statistical tests.
- The variances of the populations under examination should be similar. This is termed *homoscedasticity*.
- The variable under examination must be measured on an interval or ratio scale in which the values obtained may be conveniently manipulated using conventional arithmetic. This is an extremely important point that is directly related to the nature of the variable under investigation.

In the normal course of data collection, it is usual for students to collect a small number of replicate samples of a variable for analysis, or alternatively, in clinical studies (e.g. bioequivalence studies), the number of subjects in each group is limited to about 12. In these situations, it is difficult to examine whether the observations (data) were derived from a normal distribution. Consequently, in parametric analyses involving small sample sizes, an assumption is made concerning the nature of the population from which the each data set has been derived. Furthermore, in many cases, the variances of the test populations will not be similar. However, this may not directly prohibit the use of parametric methods as it is generally accepted that these tests are tolerant of minor departures from the above assumptions without invalidating the outcome of the statistical analysis. As the departures from the assumptions become more marked, the results obtained from the analysis will become less powerful and hence incorrect conclusions may follow.

One assumption associated with parametric tests that is well defined is the nature of the data. In parametric analyses, the data (variable) is continuous in nature and may be mathematically manipulated to generate descriptive statistics (mean, variance standard deviation). However, as outlined in Chapter 1, data may fall into other categories, most notably nominal and ordinal scales. Such data may not be statistically analysed using parametric tests and non-parametric analyses must be employed. At this point, it is appropriate to summarise the nature of nominal, ordinal and interval or ratio data.

5.4.1.1 Nominal data

Nominal data is classified into groups that are assigned a name or title. Examples include:

- grouping of patients entered into a clinical study on the basis of age
- grouping of patients in a clinical study on the basis of gender

- categorisation of tablet defects, e.g. capping, chipped, pitting
- categorisation of illness, e.g. bowel cancer, ulcerative colitis, Crohn's disease, diverticulitis
- side-effects associated with a medication, e.g. nausea, vomiting, diarrhoea, headache.

Nominal data is usually expressed in terms of frequencies of observations associated with each category. The statistical analysis of such data may be performed using a χ^2 analysis or a binomial-based test. The mechanics and use of these tests are explained in subsequent chapters in this textbook. Characterisation of the association within nominal data is performed using the contingency coefficient (Chapter 12). The description of nominal data may be successfully performed using frequency, relative frequency or percentages, whereas the mode and range are employed to depict the central tendency and variability respectively.

5.4.1.2 Ordinal data

Ordinal data is considered to represent a higher level of organisation than nominal data. There is a marked similarity between the two types of data in that each are composed of categories; however, the categories in ordinal data are not independent but differ from one another in terms of magnitude. Once more, the nature of ordinal data may be explained by consideration of the following examples:

- categorisation of pain using a visual analogue scale (0 = no pain, 10 = excruciating pain)
- categorisation of inflammation (e.g. gingival inflammation, rheumatoid arthritis, osteoarthritis) using indices
- categorisation of taste (not bitter, moderately bitter, extremely bitter).

In these examples, the data are once more organised into named categories, but there is a relationship between the individual categories that is not present in nominal scales. Hence, categorisation of pain or any of the other examples is a ranking process in which an indication of the relative importance of each category is assumed. Many non-parametric tests are referred to as *ranking tests* and may be employed for the analysis of ordinal data. A prerequisite for the analysis of ordinal data using non-parametric tests is that the data should possess an underlying continuum, i.e. there must be a spread to the typical responses within any category. Hence, if a product is assigned as moderately bitter in the assessment of bitterness of a pharmaceutical preparation, there is the possibility that this category is composed of a series of strata that encompass the term *moderately bitter*. This is the underlying continuum that validates the use of non-parametric methods for the analysis of ordinal data. Parametric statistical tests, whose mechanics involves arithmetic manipulation of data, should not be used to evaluate ordinal data, because successive intervals are unequal and consequently the contributions (weightings) of the different categories are dissimilar.

Characterisation of the association within ordinal data is commonly performed using the *Spearman correlation coefficient* (r_s) (Chapter 12). Ordinal data may be successfully described using frequency, relative frequency or percentages, whereas the median and range are employed to depict the central tendency and variability respectively.

5.4.1.3 Interval and ratio data

Interval and ratio data represent a higher level of organisation than nominal or ordinal data. They may be characterised by knowledge of the distances between two values on any particular scale, i.e. the numerical distance between two values has been defined in terms of a unit of measurement. In an interval scale there is no true zero, but ratio data do possess a defined zero point. A classical example of an interval scale is the measurement of temperature (in either Celsius or Fahrenheit). In each of these scales a zero value does exist, but this is an arbitrary value and does not represent an absence of temperature. As a result of the lack of a true zero value one cannot directly compare two or more values within the temperature scale. Therefore, although it is logical to conclude that the melting point of a prodrug form of ibuprofen (152 °C) is greater than that for ibuprofen itself (76 °C), because of the arbitrary nature of zero on the centigrade scale it is incorrect to state that the melting point of the prodrug is twice that of the parent drug.

The interval scale is referred to as a *quantitative scale* and the information held within this scale may be meaningfully manipulated using arithmetic procedures. As a result of this, interval data may be analysed using parametric statistical tests. Indeed, if all the assumptions of parametric statistics (the statistical model) are valid, statistical comparisons of groups of interval data should be performed using parametric tests, e.g. *t* test, analysis of variance, etc. If, however, there are doubts about fulfilling the assumptions of parametric tests, it is correct to apply non-parametric methods to the analysis of interval data.

The ratio scale is also a quantitative scale, but it differs from the interval scale in one essential property: it possesses a true zero point. Most experiments in the pharmaceutical sciences generate data that is ratio in nature. Examples include mass, height, concentration, blood pressure, glomerular filtration rate, area under the curve, etc. In these examples zero refers to an absence of a measurable value. Similarly, the data derived from ratio scales may be manipulated using conventional arithmetic and may therefore be conveniently analysed using either parametric or non-parametric methods. The final choice of statistical method will once more depend on the relevance of the assumptions in the statistical model.

Interval or ratio data whose distribution is skewed (non-normal) may be successfully described using frequency, relative frequency or percentages, whereas the median and range are employed to depict the central tendency and variability respectively. Interval or ratio data that is normally distributed is described using frequency, relative frequency, percentages or the z score, whereas the mean and standard deviation (or variance) are employed to depict the central tendency and variability respectively. Characterisation of the association within normally distributed interval or ratio data is commonly performed using the correlation coefficient (r) (Chapter 12).

Therefore, it is clear that the choice of either a parametric or non-parametric test for the statistical analysis depends on two major factors: the type of data and the validity of the assumptions of parametric analyses concerning the nature of the population from which the data are derived. More specifically, non-parametric methods are exclusively employed to analyse *nominal* and *ordinal* data, whereas parametric and non-parametric methods may be used to examine *interval* and *ratio* data.

5.4.1.4 Comparisons of the properties and assumptions of parametric and non-parametric statistical tests

In section 5.4.1, consideration has been given to the choice of either parametric or non-parametric statistical tests for the analysis of data. This is an extremely important topic, which has relevance to the outcome (decision-making process) of any defined study. In light of this, it is important to summarise the relative merits, and indeed shortcomings, of these two categories of statistical methods.

- Parametric tests operate within a statistical model in which certain assumptions concerning the nature of the population from which the data have been derived have been made. In particular, parametric tests assume that the data have been removed from a normal (symmetrical) population, that the data are independent and that the variance of the populations under investigation should be similar. In the vast majority of cases of data derived from pharmaceutical studies it is impossible to validate the above conditions and therefore, concomitant with the use of parametric tests is the assumption that the defined conditions are, in fact, operative.
- Fewer assumptions are associated with the use of non-parametric statistics. This is why non-parametric tests have become an important statistical tool.

Non-parametric methods should be employed whenever there is doubt concerning the validity of parametric tests for the analysis of data. As the reader will observe in subsequent chapters, there are non-parametric equivalents for most parametric tests. However, although non-parametric tests are flexible and there are fewer restrictions on their use than for their parametric counterparts, it is incorrect to believe that there are no assumptions associated with the use of non-parametric tests. Non-parametric tests do not assume prior knowledge of the population distribution from which data have been collected, but they do assume that each datum is collected independently and that the measured variable possesses an underlying continuity.

- Greater analytical flexibility is associated with non-parametric tests in terms of the range of types of data that may be analysed using these techniques. Non-parametric tests may be employed to statistically analyse nominal, ordinal, interval and ratio data. Parametric tests may only be used for the analysis of interval or ratio data.

- Non-parametric tests should always be employed to analyse data in which the sample size is small ($N < 6$) unless prior knowledge of the population from which the data are derived is fully understood. The use of parametric statistical methods for the analysis of small sample size data may lead to erroneous conclusions concerning acceptance or rejection of the null hypothesis.

- At this point the reader may be considering the use of non-parametric statistical methods for the analysis of all data. However, to do so without consideration of the nature of the data is incorrect and may lead to the acceptance of the null hypothesis when the null hypothesis is indeed incorrect (increased likelihood of a type II error). It is generally accepted that if a non-parametric test is used when the conditions of the experiment warrant the use of a parametric test, the efficiency of the non-parametric test is approximately 90% that of the parametric test. In other words, to obtain a similar statistical output the size of the sample (e.g. patients recruited into a clinical study) would have to be increased by 10% when the data are analysed using non-parametric methods. Therefore, in addition to increasing the likelihood of failing to reject the null hypothesis, the indiscriminate use of non-parametric methods will have cost implications, i.e. the costs of performing adequate experiments or clinical studies will be increased.

- Experiments based on intricate experimental designs may not be easily statistically evaluated using non-parametric techniques. In particular, the analysis of multifactorial studies in which statistical interactions play an important role is more appropriately performed using (parametric) analysis of variance, or related, methods.

5.5 Conclusions

This chapter has described the considerations that accompany the processes of statistical hypothesis testing and, ultimately, statistical decision-making. All the topics described in this chapter should be considered before beginning an experiment, and the importance of these processes to the successful resolution of the statistical analysis should not be overlooked.

In the following chapters in this book, the use of parametric and non-parametric methods for the analysis of one-sample, two-sample and multisample hypotheses will be described. Parametric and non-parametric methods will be described either within the same chapter or in successive chapters, allowing the relative merits of each method to be highlighted. Finally, the strategies employed in this chapter concerning the mechanics of statistical hypothesis testing will be adhered to, thus emphasising and consolidating the importance of this chapter in the successful completion of the statistical analysis.

6

Statistical estimation using confidence intervals

In Chapter 2, the concept of the central nature and variability of data and the methods by which these two phenomena may be mathematically determined were described. As previously explained, one of the main purposes for calculating the central nature (e.g. the mean) and the variability (e.g. the standard deviation) of a set of sample data is to gain an understanding of the corresponding population statistics. In other words, the mean ($\bar{X}$) and standard deviation (s) of sample data are employed to estimate the true (population) mean and true (population) standard deviation. However, it is reasonable to ask, how reliable are the sample data at representing the population data? Is the sample data a good estimation of the population data?

6.1 The concept of confidence intervals

After calculating the mean and standard deviation of a sample, as is the normal approach in the pharmaceutical and related sciences, we need to provide an indication of the reliability of the data. For example, in a clinical trial ($N = 20$ patients) the volume of urine produced after the administration of a new diuretic drug has been calculated as 5.2 ± 1.9 L. In light of the small sample size, it is unreasonable to predict that the population mean and standard deviation will be identical to these observed sample values, as each sample will produce different mean and standard deviation values. Therefore, when reporting the mean of sample data it is good practice to present some indication of the reliability of the data, i.e. the quality of the estimation of the true mean from the sample mean. This is performed using *confidence intervals*. The confidence intervals are quoted as a mean and range (interval), the latter representing the probability of observing the true mean. The imposed probability is chosen by the person responsible for the statistical manipulation of data; however, the most frequently employed confidence intervals are 90%, 95% and 99%.

Confidence intervals are demonstrated graphically in Figures 6.1 and 6.2. In these, 10 samples, each containing 10 observations, were selected from a normal distribution, whose mean was known to be 50. For each of the 10 samples, the mean and 90% confidence intervals were calculated. (The method for doing this is shown in the following section and does not need to be explained at this stage.) An example of the outcome for each sample is shown in Figure 6.1. The central portion of the bar denotes the mean that has been calculated using the sample data. The regions that extend equally beyond the mean in either direction are the calculated 90% confidence intervals. As for any range, there are upper and lower limits. The calculated mean and (90%) confidence intervals for each sample may be plotted on the one graph, as shown in Figure 6.2. The mean of the population has been included in this graph as a dashed line.

Some features of Figure 6.2 require clarification to enable the reader to fully understand the basis of confidence intervals.

- First, it may be observed that, as expected, the means of all the different samples, although numerically close, are not equal to the population mean. Furthermore, the means of the individual samples are not numerically equal, once more reflecting sample variability.
- Secondly, the confidence intervals of the individual groups also differ in magnitude. These differences may also be logically explained. Confidence intervals are calculated using the standard deviation of the sample and therefore, if the variability of a sample is large, then the size of the confidence interval (i.e. the range) will be larger. Consequently, differences in the sizes of the confidence intervals reflect differences in the standard deviations of the individual samples.
- Finally, it may be observed from Figure 6.2 that, although the individual sample means do not exactly equal the population mean, the 90% confidence intervals in all but one case (denoted by an asterisk) do encompass the population mean. Therefore, the calculated 90% confidence intervals have included the population mean in 9 out of 10 observations, i.e. 90% of observations. If

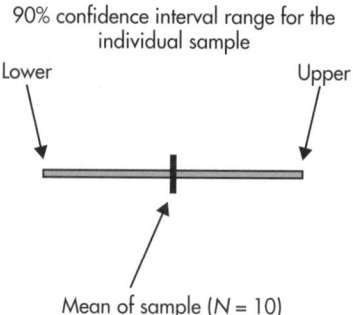

Figure 6.1 Mean and confidence intervals.

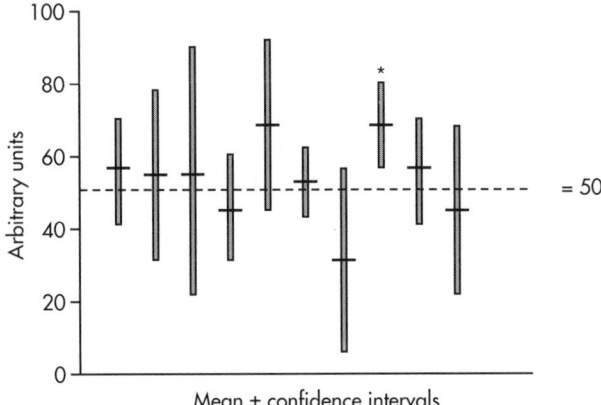

Figure 6.2 Mean and 90% confidence intervals derived from 10 samples (10 observations per sample group).

the 95% confidence intervals had been calculated for each sample and plotted as described in Figure 6.2, the confidence intervals would have encompassed the true mean in 19 out of 20 samples (95%), and so on.

Confidence intervals are therefore calculated to provide the user with the probability that a single sample will contain the true mean (or indeed true standard deviation, etc). It is still possible that if a sample is removed and the mean ± 95% confidence intervals calculated, the true mean will not fall within the range calculated. However, it is also true that if another 19 samples were removed and the mean ± 95% confidence intervals calculated, the true mean would fall within the confidence intervals described by these 19 samples.

The calculation of confidence intervals is performed with reference to a probability distribution, e.g. the normal distribution, t distribution or χ^2 distribution. The mechanism for performing such calculations forms the basis of the remainder of this chapter.

6.2 Confidence intervals for the population mean and the normal distribution

One of the most frequently used methods for calculating confidence intervals involves the use of the normal distribution. If the data conforms to the normal distribution, the two-tailed confidence interval may be calculated using the following equation:

$$P\% = \bar{X} \pm \frac{z_{P\%}\,\sigma}{\sqrt{N}}$$

where P% is the selected confidence interval, i.e. usually 90%, 95% or 99%, $\bar{X}$ is the observed mean, σ is the population standard deviation and $z_{P\%}$ is the z value corresponding to the percentage confidence interval. Remember that the term $\sigma/\sqrt{N}$ refers to the standard error of the mean, previously introduced in Chapter 2.

The z value is therefore an important parameter in the calculation of confidence intervals. Confidence limits are two-tailed events as there are two possible outcomes, i.e. one interval below and one interval above the mean. The z value chosen for inclusion in the equation or calculation of confidence is dependent on the selected value of the probability, as shown in Figure 6.3. Therefore, if we want to calculate the 95% confidence interval, we choose a z value of 1.96 as this value corresponds to the area under the standard normal distribution that encompasses 95% of all values. Similarly, 2.58 and 1.65 are chosen when 99% and 90% confidence intervals are to be calculated. The calculation of confidence intervals based on the standardised normal distribution is shown in the following example.

EXAMPLE 6.1   *A clinical trial (N = 30 patients) has been performed in which the volume of distribution of a new anti-diabetes drug has been calculated as 10.2 ± 1.9 L. Calculate the 95% and 99% confidence limits of the mean value (assuming that the data originated from a normal distribution).*

- 95% *confidence interval*. From the standardised normal distribution, the z statistic associated with 95% probability (two-tailed) is 1.96. Therefore the 95% confidence interval is calculated as follows:

$$P_{95\%} = \bar{X} \pm \frac{z_{95\%}\sigma}{\sqrt{N}} = 10.2 \pm \frac{1.96 \times 1.9}{\sqrt{30}} = 10.2 \pm 0.68 \text{ L}$$

$$= 9.52\text{--}10.88 \text{ L}$$

- 99% *confidence interval*. Similarly, the 99% confidence interval is calculated using a z value of 2.58 (corresponding to 99% probability in a two-tailed outcome):

$$P_{99\%} = \bar{X} \pm \frac{z_{99\%}\sigma}{\sqrt{N}} = 10.2 \pm \frac{2.58 \times 1.9}{\sqrt{30}} = 10.2 \pm 0.89 \text{ L}$$

$$= 9.31\text{--}11.09 \text{ L}$$

Having calculated these values, it is important at this point for the reader to fully comprehend the meaning of confidence intervals. In the clinical example described, the 95% confidence interval was 10.2 ± 0.68 L, i.e. 9.52–10.88 L. The observed mean value (10.2 L) is unlikely to be identical to the population mean value. However, the

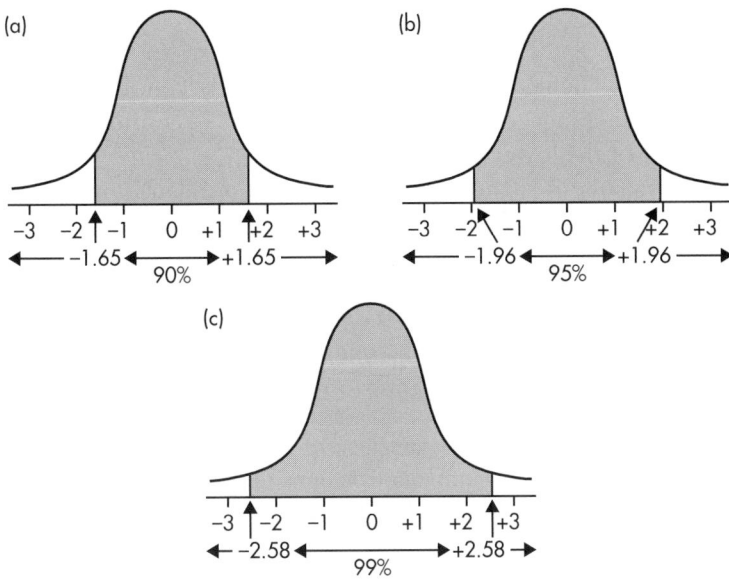

Figure 6.3 Probability functions within the standardised normal distribution.

calculated confidence interval provides an estimation of the reliability of the measured mean. Therefore, we are 95% certain that the true mean will lie within the range defined by the confidence intervals, i.e. 9.52–10.88 L. In other words, if 100 samples were selected and their means and confidence intervals calculated, it is likely that 95 such confidence intervals would contain the true mean. Similarly, in a 99% confidence interval, there is a 99% chance that the true mean will lie within the defined (calculated) range. In general laboratory practice, the mean and confidence intervals of one set of data (sample) are normally calculated, the use of confidence intervals providing sufficient information about the reliability of the mean.

Students often ask why the 99% confidence interval encompasses a greater range of values than the corresponding 95% interval. The answer is quite straightforward and concerns an appreciation of the role of probability in the calculation of confidence intervals. In the calculation of confidence intervals, reference is made to the appropriate probability distribution, the normal distribution in our case. As described previously, the total area under the normal distribution curve is 1 (equal to 100% probability). The area under the curve (and the z value) increases proportionally as the probability of an event increases. Hence the z value associated with 99% probability, i.e. 2.58, is greater than that for the 95% probability (1.96) and accordingly, to ensure 99%

probability of an event, a greater spread of z values is required. Thus in the calculation of 99% confidence intervals a greater area under the normal curve is being considered than with 95% confidence intervals and hence the range of values within the 99% confidence interval exceeds that of the lower interval.

The calculation and applications of confidence intervals are further explored in the following examples.

EXAMPLE 6.2 *The aluminium content of 1000 1-L samples of intravenous fluids was analysed and the mean and standard deviation calculated as 50 ± 3 ppm. Calculate the 95% and 99% confidence limits for estimating the true mean aluminium concentration.*

- 95% *confidence interval.* The sample size is large (1000), so it may be assumed that the aluminium concentration conforms to normality and therefore, the following equation may be employed to calculate confidence intervals:

$$P_{95\%} = \overline{X} \pm \frac{z_{95\%}\, \sigma}{\sqrt{N}}$$

where $z_{95\%}$ denotes the z value corresponding to a probability of 95% (two-tailed), i.e. 1.96, $\sigma = 3$ ppm and $N = 1000$. Thus:

$$P_{95\%} = 50 \pm \frac{1.96 \times 3}{\sqrt{1000}} = 50 \pm 0.19 \text{ ppm}$$

The 95% confidence limits are 49.81–50.19 ppm, i.e. there is a 95% chance that the true population mean will be encompassed within this range.

- 99% *confidence interval.* Once more, the following equation may be used:

$$P_{99\%} = \overline{X} \pm \frac{z_{99\%}\, \sigma}{\sqrt{N}}$$

where $z_{99\%}$ denotes the z value corresponding to a probability of 99% (two-tailed), i.e. 2.58, $\sigma = 3$ ppm and $N = 1000$. Thus:

$$P_{99\%} = 50 \pm \frac{2.58 \times 3}{\sqrt{1000}} = 50 \pm 0.24$$

The 99% confidence limits are 49.76–50.24 ppm, i.e. there is a 99% chance that the true population mean lies within this region.

EXAMPLE 6.3 *100 transdermal patches have been removed from a batch and the stability of the active agent determined at 25 °C. The observed mean (and standard deviation) degradation rate constant for the therapeutic agent was 0.09 ± 0.01 day^{-1}. Calculate the 80% and 95% confidence intervals of the estimates of the mean, and the confidence that the mean degradation rate of the population is 0.09 ± 0.0015 h^{-1}.*

- *80% confidence interval*

$$P_{80\%} = \bar{X} \pm \frac{z_{80\%}\sigma}{\sqrt{N}}$$

From the standardised normal distribution, the z value associated with 80% probability is 1.28 (Appendix 1). Therefore

$$P_{80\%} = \bar{X} \pm \frac{z_{80\%}\sigma}{\sqrt{N}} = 0.09 \pm \frac{1.28 \times 0.01}{\sqrt{100}} = 0.09 \pm 0.001 \text{ h}^{-1}$$

The 80% confidence interval for the estimation of the population mean is $0.089{-}0.091 \text{ h}^{-1}$.

- *95% confidence interval*

$$P_{95\%} = \bar{X} \pm \frac{z_{95\%}\sigma}{\sqrt{N}} = 0.09 \pm \frac{1.96 \times 0.01}{\sqrt{100}} = 0.09 \pm 0.002 \text{ h}^{-1}$$

The 95% confidence interval for the estimation of the population mean is $0.088{-}0.092 \text{ h}^{-1}$.

- *Confidence that the mean degradation rate of the population is $0.09 \pm 0.0015 \text{ h}^{-1}$.* This question offers a different perspective on the use of confidence intervals. In the previous examples we have defined the probability of the confidence interval and then calculated the interval from this. In this example, the interval has been defined and the confidence of that interval is unknown and requires calculation. Once more the generic equation is employed:

$$P\% = \bar{X} \pm \frac{z_{P\%}\sigma}{\sqrt{N}}$$

The known parameters are inserted into this equation:

$$P\% = 0.09 \pm \frac{z_{P\%} \times 0.01}{\sqrt{100}} = 0.09 \pm (z_{P\%} \times 0.001)$$

$$0.09 \pm 0.0015 = 0.09 \pm 0.001 z_{P\%}$$

Therefore:

$$0.0015 = 0.001Z$$
$$1.5 = z_{P\%}$$

The area under the standardised normal curve from $z = 0$ to $z = 1.5$ is 0.4332. Similarly the area under the standardised normal distribution from $z = 0$ to $z = -1.5$ is 0.4332. Therefore, the degree of confidence is 0.8664, i.e. 86.64%.

6.3 Confidence intervals for differences between means

Most frequently, confidence intervals are calculated to provide an estimation of the mean of a population, as described in section 6.2. However, in many cases, it is useful to describe the confidence intervals on the differences between means. Once more, the normal distribution may be employed for this purpose, i.e. it is assumed that the means are derived from a normal distribution. The equation used here is based on the one employed for the calculation of the confidence intervals of a single mean, with two exceptions:

- the difference between the means replaces the mean value
- the standard error of differences between means is used in place of the standard error of the mean (i.e. the square root of the sum of the squares of their standard errors)

The modified equation is:

$$P\% = (\bar{X}_1 - \bar{X}_2) \pm z_{P\%} \sqrt{\frac{s_1^2}{N_1} + \frac{s_2^2}{N_2}}$$

where $\bar{X}_1$ and $\bar{X}_2$ are the means of samples 1 and 2, respectively; s_1^2 and s_2^2 are the variances of samples 1 and 2, respectively; $z_{P\%}$ is the z value relating to the chosen level of probability (e.g. 90%, 95%, 99%), N_1 and N_2 are the sample sizes in samples 1 and 2, respectively and

$$\sqrt{\frac{s_1^2}{N_1} + \frac{s_2^2}{N_2}}$$

is the standard error of the difference between two independent means. The use of this equation is illustrated in the following examples.

EXAMPLE 6.4   *A quality control laboratory wishes to examine and compare the mechanical properties of two wound dressings using tensile analysis. Accordingly, the mean (± standard deviation) tensile strength of a proprietary wound dressing was examined (N = 250) and recorded as 10.35 ± 0.57 MPa. The mean (± standard deviation) of a generic wound dressing was 8.99 ± 0.73 MPa (N = 150). Calculate the 90% and 95% confidence intervals of the difference between the tensile strengths of the two wound dressings.*

- *90% confidence interval.* From the information given, we know that $\bar{X}_1$ and $\bar{X}_2$ are 10.35 and 8.99 MPa, respectively; s_1 and s_2 are 0.57 and 0.73 MPa, respectively; $z_{P\%}$ is the z value relating to the chosen level of probability, i.e. 1.65 for a 90% confidence interval; and N_1 and N_2 are 250 and 150, respectively. Inserting this information into the relevant equation enables us to calculate the 90% confidence interval:

$$P_{90\%} = (\bar{X}_1 - \bar{X}_2) \pm z_{90\%} \sqrt{\frac{s_1^2}{N_1} + \frac{s_2^2}{N_2}}$$

$$= (10.35 - 8.99) \pm 1.65 \sqrt{\frac{(0.57)^2}{250} + \frac{(0.73)^2}{150}}$$

$$= 1.36 \pm 0.12 \text{ MPa}$$

Therefore, the 90% confidence interval for the difference between the mean tensile strength of the two wound dressings is 1.24–1.48 MPa. Therefore, there is a 90% probability that the true mean difference in tensile strengths between the two dressings may be found in the range 1.24–1.48 MPa.

- 95% *confidence interval*. The various parameters in the equation below are identical to those described above with the exception of the z value, which now reflects 95% probability, i.e. 1.96:

$$P_{95\%} = (\bar{X}_1 - \bar{X}_2) \pm z_{95\%} \sqrt{\frac{s_1^2}{N_1} + \frac{s_2^2}{N_2}}$$

$$= (10.35 - 8.99) \pm 1.96 \sqrt{\frac{(0.57)^2}{250} + \frac{(0.73)^2}{150}}$$

$$= 1.36 \pm 0.14 \text{ MPa}$$

Therefore, the 95% confidence interval for the difference between the mean tensile strength of the two wound dressings is 1.22–1.50 MPa and there is a 95% probability that the true mean difference in tensile strengths between the two dressings may be found in this range.

EXAMPLE 6.5 *A new therapeutic agent has been developed to promote diuresis. In a clinical trial, the diuretic effects of this new agent and a commercial agent were assessed. In this the urine was collected over a 12-h period after administration of a single tablet. The mean (± standard deviation) volume of urine collected in the group of patients (N = 65) who received the new therapeutic agent was 48.8 ± 9.1 L, whereas in the control group (who received the commercially available preparation) the volume was 37.9 ± 4.6 L (N = 95). Calculate the 95% and 99% confidence intervals for the difference in urine volume induced by the two therapeutic agents.*

- 95% *confidence interval*. Once more, the equation described at the start of section 6.3 is employed to calculate the required confidence interval, using $z_{95\%} = 1.96$:

$$P_{95\%} = (\bar{X}_1 - \bar{X}_2) \pm z_{95\%} \sqrt{\frac{s_1^2}{N_1} + \frac{s_2^2}{N_2}}$$

$$= (48.8 - 37.9) \pm 1.96 \sqrt{\frac{(9.1)^2}{65} + \frac{(4.6)^2}{95}}$$

$$= 10.9 \pm 2.40 \text{ L}$$

Therefore, the 95% confidence interval for the difference in mean urine volume is 8.50–13.3 L.

- 99% *confidence interval*. Employing $z_{99\%} = 2.58$, the above equation may be written as:

$$P_{99\%} = (\bar{X}_1 - \bar{X}_2) \pm z_{99\%} \sqrt{\frac{s_1^2}{N_1} + \frac{s_2^2}{N_2}}$$

$$= (48.8 - 37.9) \pm 2.58 \sqrt{\frac{(9.1)^2}{65} + \frac{(4.6)^2}{95}}$$

$$= 10.9 \pm 3.16 \text{ L}$$

The confidence intervals for the differences between means is interpreted in the same way as other confidence intervals. Therefore, in this example, there is a 99% probability that the true difference between the two diuretics will fall within the range 7.74–14.06 L.

6.4 Confidence intervals for standard deviations

Determination of the confidence intervals for the standard deviation is most frequently employed to examine the variability of data, e.g. whenever there is unexpectedly high variation in a sample. For this purpose, the χ^2 distribution is used to calculate confidence intervals for the population standard deviation. From Appendix 3, χ^2 values may be obtained that provide information concerning the areas under the probability curve. Hence, to calculate the 95% confidence interval of the population standard deviation, the region under the χ^2 distribution that equates to 95% is found between $\chi^2_{0.025}$ and $\chi^2_{0.975}$. Therefore, 2.5% of observations lie both below $\chi^2_{0.025}$ and above $\chi^2_{0.975}$. With this in mind, the 95% confidence interval is calculated using the following equation:

$$\chi^2_{0.025} < \frac{(N-1)s^2}{\sigma^2} < \chi^2_{0.975}$$

where $N - 1$ is the number of degrees of freedom, i.e. the sample size minus 1, s is the sample standard deviation, σ is the population standard deviation, and $\chi^2_{0.025}$ and $\chi^2_{0.975}$ are the χ^2 statistics relating to probabilities of 2.5% and 97.5%, respectively, for $n - 1$ degrees of freedom.

This equation may be more conveniently rearranged to give

$$\frac{s\sqrt{(N-1)}}{\chi_{0.975}} < \sigma < \frac{s\sqrt{(N-1)}}{\chi_{0.025}}$$

An example of the use of the χ^2 distribution to calculate the confidence intervals associated with the population standard deviation is provided next.

EXAMPLE 6.6 *Before the start of a clinical trial, the weights of 20 healthy male volunteers (aged 21–30 years) were measured and the mean and standard deviation recorded as 76.1 ± 9.4 kg. Calculate the 90%, 95% and 99% confidence intervals of the population standard deviation.*

- *90% confidence intervals*. Using the equation described above,

$$\frac{s\sqrt{(N-1)}}{\chi_{0.95}} < \sigma < \frac{s\sqrt{(N-1)}}{\chi_{0.05}}$$

where N is the number of volunteers (20); s is the sample standard deviation, i.e. 9.4 kg; $\chi_{0.95}$ for 19 degrees of freedom (i.e. 20 volunteers − 1) is $\sqrt{\chi^2_{0.95}}$, i.e. $\sqrt{30.1} = 5.49$; $\chi_{0.05}$ for 19 degrees of freedom is $\sqrt{\chi^2_{0.05}}$, i.e. $\sqrt{10.1} = 3.18$. Therefore:

$$\frac{s\sqrt{(N-1)}}{\chi_{0.95}} < \sigma < \frac{s\sqrt{(N-1)}}{\chi_{0.05}} = \frac{9.4\sqrt{19}}{5.49} < \sigma < \frac{9.4\sqrt{19}}{3.18}$$

$$7.46 < \sigma < 12.88 \text{ kg}$$

Therefore, there is a 90% chance that the true population standard deviation (weights of healthy men aged 21–30 years) will reside within the above limits.

- *95% confidence intervals*. Using the appropriate equation:

$$\frac{s\sqrt{(N-1)}}{\chi_{0.975}} < \sigma < \frac{s\sqrt{(N-1)}}{\chi_{0.025}}$$

where N and s are as before; $\chi_{0.975}$ for 19 degrees of freedom is $\sqrt{\chi^2_{0.975}}$, i.e. $\sqrt{32.9} = 5.74$; and $\chi_{0.025}$ for 19 degrees of freedom is $\sqrt{\chi^2_{0.025}}$, i.e. $\sqrt{8.91} = 2.98$. Therefore:

$$\frac{s\sqrt{(N-1)}}{\chi_{0.975}} < \sigma < \frac{s\sqrt{(N-1)}}{\chi_{0.025}} = \frac{9.4\sqrt{19}}{5.74} < \sigma < \frac{9.4\sqrt{19}}{2.98}$$

$$7.14 < \sigma < 13.75 \text{ kg}$$

and there is a 95% chance that the true population standard deviation falls within the above limits.

- *99% confidence intervals*. As before:

$$\frac{s\sqrt{(N-1)}}{\chi_{0.995}} < \sigma < \frac{s\sqrt{(N-1)}}{\chi_{0.005}}$$

where N and s is the sample standard deviation; $\chi_{0.995}$ for 19 degrees of freedom is $\sqrt{\chi^2_{0.995}}$, i.e. $\sqrt{38.6} = 6.21$; and $\chi_{0.005}$ for 19 degrees of freedom is $\sqrt{\chi^2_{0.005}}$, i.e.

$\sqrt{6.84} = 2.62$. Therefore:

$$\frac{s\sqrt{(N-1)}}{\chi_{0.995}} < \sigma < \frac{s\sqrt{(N-1)}}{\chi_{0.005}} = \frac{9.4\sqrt{19}}{6.21} < \sigma < \frac{9.4\sqrt{19}}{2.62}$$

$$6.60 < \sigma < 15.64 \text{ Kg}$$

and there is a 99% chance that the true population standard deviation (weights of healthy men aged 21–30 years) will lie between 6.60 and 15.64 kg.

It is worth pointing out that the confidence limits of the true (population) standard deviation from the sample standard deviation may be estimated using the normal distribution. In this it is assumed that the population from which the sample data has been derived is normally distributed. When the sample size is large, i.e. greater than 30, the mathematical function $\sqrt{2\chi^2} - \sqrt{2(N-1)} - 1 = z_p$ is appropriate and approximates to a normal distribution. Therefore, by rearrangement of the equation to produce $\chi^2 = \frac{1}{2}(z_p + \sqrt{2(N-1)} - 1)^2$, the χ^2 statistic may be calculated using the normal distribution. From this, the confidence intervals of the true standard deviation may be calculated from the sample standard deviation using the χ^2 statistic, as described previously.

Alternatively, the standard deviation may be directly calculated from the normal distribution using the following equation:

$$P\% = s \pm z_p \frac{s}{\sqrt{2N}}$$

where s is the sample standard deviation, N is the number of samples and z_p is the z value corresponding to the desired level of probability.

The uses of the different methods for calculating the confidence intervals of the standard deviation are described in the next example.

EXAMPLE 6.7 *A solid dosage form containing 100 mg of a thera-peutic agent has been manufactured and stored for 1 year at 37 °C and 75% relative humidity. Analysis of the concentration of therapeutic agent in 101 tablets following this period of storage revealed that the mean (± standard deviation) drug content was 94.13 ± 4.56 mg. Calculate the 95% confidence interval of the population standard deviation of the concentration of therapeutic agent within the tablets.*

- *Use of the χ^2 distribution*

$$\frac{s\sqrt{(N)}}{\chi_{0.975}} < \sigma < \frac{s\sqrt{(N)}}{\chi_{0.025}} = \frac{4.56\sqrt{101}}{\sqrt{129.6}} < \sigma < \frac{4.56\sqrt{101}}{\sqrt{74.2}}$$

$$4.03 < \sigma < 5.32 \text{ mg}$$

Therefore, the 95% confidence interval of the population standard deviation of drug content in solid dosage forms is 4.03–5.32 mg (Note: N is used in place of $N - 1$ as the sample size is large).

- *Use of the normal distribution.* As described above,

$$\chi^2 = \frac{1}{2}(z_p + \sqrt{2(N-1)-1})^2$$

Therefore:

$$\chi^2_{0.975} = \frac{1}{2}(z_p + \sqrt{2(N-1)-1})^2 = \frac{1}{2}(1.96 + \sqrt{2(101)-1})^2$$

$$= 130.21$$

$$\chi^2_{0.025} = \frac{1}{2}(z_p + \sqrt{2(N-1)-1})^2 = \frac{1}{2}(-1.96 + \sqrt{2(101)-1})^2$$

$$= 74.63$$

Note that the values of χ^2 calculated using the normal distribution are numerically similar to the values derived from the χ^2 distribution (Appendix 3).

To calculate the confidence intervals as requested, these χ^2 values are used, as described previously:

$$\frac{s\sqrt{(N)}}{\chi_{0.975}} < \sigma < \frac{s\sqrt{(N)}}{\chi_{0.025}} = \frac{4.56\sqrt{101}}{\sqrt{130.21}} < \sigma < \frac{4.56\sqrt{101}}{\sqrt{74.63}}$$

$$4.02 < \sigma < 5.30 \text{ mg}$$

Results calculated using either method are similar.

6.5 Confidence intervals for proportions

Confidence intervals of proportions may also be calculated using the approximation to the normal distribution and the sample standard deviation. The confidence interval for the population proportion may be calculated using the following equation:

$$P\% = p \pm z \sqrt{\frac{pq}{N}}$$

where p is the proportion of successes, q is the proportion of failures $(1 - p)$, N is the sample size and z denotes the z value relating to a defined probability level.

The use of this equation is described in the following example.

EXAMPLE 6.8 *A healthcare company that specialises in the sterile packaging of disposable gloves has decided to perform a quality audit of the resistance of a batch of packaged disposable gloves to the ingress of unsterile air. Out of a batch of 2500 packages, 200 were removed and* *their sterility examined using the British Pharmacopoeia sterility tests. The results showed that 35 packages failed the sterility tests. On the basis of these observations, calculate the 95% confidence limits for the proportion of defective gloves in the batch (population).*

This problem may be solved using the equation described at the beginning of this section:

$$P_{95\%} = p \pm z_{95\%} \sqrt{\frac{pq}{N}}$$

where $p = 35/200 = 0.175$, $q = 1 - 0.175 = 0.825$, $N = 200$ and $z = 1.96$ (for a 95% probability, two-tailed). Thus:

$$P_{95\%} = 0.175 \pm 1.96 \sqrt{\frac{(0.175) \times (0.825)}{200}}$$

$$= 0.175 \pm 0.053$$

Therefore, the 95% confidence interval for the population proportion is 0.122–0.228, i.e. there is a 95% chance that the true proportion of defective gloves will fall within this range.

Remember that the standard error of the proportion, $\sqrt{(pq/N)}$, may only be used in the calculation of the confidence intervals of a proportion if the sample size is sufficiently large for the normal approximation to be valid. As outlined in Chapter 4, the validity of this assumption may be rapidly estimated by calculating the product of the probability of the event and the sample size. Normality is commonly observed whenever this product exceeds 6.

6.6 Confidence intervals for differences between proportions

The confidence intervals for differences in proportions may be estimated using a similar approach to that described in section 6.3, assuming that the proportions are obtained from a normal distribution. The main difference between the approach outlined in section 6.3 (for the calculation of confidence intervals for the difference between two means) and that required for the calculation of the confidence intervals for the differences in proportions is the mathematical definition of the standard error of the difference between means and proportions. Referring to section 6.3, it may be recalled that the standard error of the differences between two independent means is calculated using the following formula:

$$SE_{(\bar{X}_1 - \bar{X}_2)} = \sqrt{\frac{s_1^2}{N_1} + \frac{s_2^2}{N_2}}$$

Conversely, the standard error of the difference between proportions is mathematically defined as:

$$SE_{(p_1-p_2)} = \sqrt{\frac{p_1(1-p_1)}{n_1} + \frac{p_2(1-p_2)}{n_2}} = \sqrt{\left(\frac{p_1 q_1}{n_1}\right) + \left(\frac{p_2 q_2}{n_2}\right)}$$

Applying the same mathematical approach as that described in section 6.3, the confidence intervals for the difference between two proportions may be defined as:

$$P\% = (p_1 - p_2) \pm (z_\% \times SE_{diff})$$

$$= (p_1 - p_2) \pm \left(z_\% \times \sqrt{\frac{p_1(1-p_1)}{n_1} + \frac{p_2(1-p_2)}{n_2}}\right)$$

where p_1 and p_2 are the two proportions under examination, $z_\%$ is the z value corresponding to the accepted level of probability and SE_{diff} is the standard error of the difference between proportions.

The use (and calculation) of the confidence intervals relating to the difference between two proportions is explained in the following example.

EXAMPLE 6.9   *The relative efficacies of two oral antibiotics for the treatment of bronchial pneumonia have been assessed in a clinical trial. Subjects presenting with bronchial pneumonia at a hospital were divided into two groups, each of which received one or other of the antibiotics. The results from the clinical trial are shown in Table 6.1. Calculate the 95% confidence interval for the difference between the proportions of cured patients in the two groups.*

The equation used to calculate the 95% confidence interval for the difference between the two proportions is

$$P_{95\%} = (p_1 - p_2) \pm \left(z_{95\%} \times \sqrt{\frac{p_1(1-p_1)}{n_1} + \frac{p_2(1-p_2)}{n_2}}\right)$$

where

$$p_1 = \frac{575}{(575+45)} = 0.927$$

Table 6.1   Efficacy of two antibiotics for the treatment of bronchial pneumonia

Cure	Number of patients	
	Antibiotic 1	Antibiotic 2
Yes	575	425
No	45	200

i.e. the proportion of cures associated with antibiotic 1;

$$p_2 = \frac{425}{(425 + 200)} = 0.680$$

i.e. the proportion of cures associated with antibiotic 2; $z_{95\%}$ is 1.96 (95% probability, two-tailed outcome – see Appendix 1); $n_1 = (575 + 45) = 620$; and $n_2 = (424 + 200) = 625$. When these values are substituted into the above equation, the confidence interval for the differences between the proportions of cures resulting from treatment with the two antibiotics may be calculated:

$$P_{95\%} = (0.927 - 0.680)$$

$$\pm \left(1.96 \times \sqrt{\frac{0.927(1 - 0.927)}{620} + \frac{0.680(1 - 0.680)}{625}} \right)$$

$$P_{95\%} = 0.247 \pm 0.042$$

Two further points should be mentioned at this stage.

• No units are associated with the calculated confidence interval of a difference in proportions, because proportions are, by definition, ratios. This is also true of the confidence intervals of a proportion.

• In this example, it has been assumed that the sample size is sufficiently large for the approximation to the normal distribution to apply. This may be easily confirmed by multiplying the number of observations in a particular group (e.g. n_1) by the probability (p_1). Values in excess of 6 confirm the validity of this assumption.

The next example also describes the calculation of the confidence intervals associated with the difference between proportions.

EXAMPLE 6.10 *The effects of treatment of blastospores of* Candida albicans *(stationary phase) with either polyhexamethylenebiguanide (PHMB, 0.1% v/v) or sterile water for 30 min on the number of blastospores adherent to buccal epithelial cells in vitro were examined. The results, expressed as the number of buccal epithelial cells with and without adherent blastospores, are presented in Table 6.2. Calculate the 95% confidence interval for the difference between the proportion of epithelial cells without adherent blastospores following treatment with either PHMB or sterile water.*

The relevant equation to calculate the 95% confidence intervals for the difference between the two proportions is as before:

$$P_{95\%} = (p_1 - p_2) \pm \left(z_{95\%} \times \sqrt{\frac{p_1(1 - p_1)}{n_1} + \frac{p_2(1 - p_2)}{n_2}} \right)$$

Table 6.2 Effects of treatment of blastospores of *Candida albicans* with either PHMB (0.1% v/v) or sterile water on the subsequent adherence to buccal epithelial cells *in vitro*

Outcome	Treatment	
	PHMB	Water
Cells without adherent blastospores	103	54
Cells with adherent blastospores	48	91

where $p_1 = 103/(103 + 48) = 0.682$, i.e. the proportion of epithelial cells devoid of adherent blastospores following treatment with PHMB; $p_2 = 54/(54 + 91) = 0.372$, i.e. the proportion of epithelial cells devoid of adherent blastospores following treatment with sterile water; $z_{95\%}$ is 1.96 (95% probability, two-tailed outcome, Appendix 1); $n_1 = (103 + 48) = 151$; and $n_2 = (54 + 91) = 145$. Substitution of these values into the above equation and computation yields the 95% confidence interval, i.e. $0.31 \pm 0.11 = 0.20$–0.42.

It may sometimes be difficult to fully appreciate the meaning of the calculated confidence interval for the difference between two proportions. Therefore, in medical research, it is commonplace to express the difference between proportions as ratios. In Example 6.10 it may be observed that treatment of blastospores with PHMB is more likely to inhibit adherence to buccal epithelial cells by a factor of 0.682/0.372 = 1.83.

An alternative expression that is commonly employed to relate two ratios is the *odds ratio*. The odds of an event may be defined as the ratio of the probability of the occurrence of an event to that of the non-occurrence of the event. Reverting to Example 6.10, the odds of observing buccal epithelial cells devoid of adherent blastospores following treatment with PHMB is $(0.682/(1 - 0.682) = 2.13$. Similarly, the odds of observing a buccal epithelial cell devoid of adherent blastospores following treatment with sterile water are $(0.373/(1 - 0.372)$. The ratio of these two odds is termed the *odds ratio* or *relative risk*, which for the example described, is 2.13/0.59 = 3.61.

6.7 Confidence intervals and the *t* distribution

As highlighted in the introduction to this chapter, the z statistic is employed to calculate confidence intervals whenever the assumptions of the normal distribution are valid. One requirement is a large sample size. However, the inquisitive reader may ask, how are confidence intervals calculated for sample data? Under these circumstances, the t distribution is employed to calculate confidence intervals, using a similar strategy to that used to calculate the confidence intervals of the true mean for large samples. Thus:

$$P\% = \bar{X} \pm \frac{tS}{\sqrt{N}}$$

where $P\%$ is the chosen probability (usually 90%, 95% or 99%). $\bar{X}$ is the sample mean, t is the t statistic corresponding to the appropriate probability level and degree of freedom and S is the sample standard deviation

The major difference between the above equation and the equation for the calculation of the confidence interval using the normal distribution is the nature of the test statistic. In the normal distribution the value of the z statistic depends only on the chosen probability level and is independent of sample size (the use of the normal distribution implies that the sample size is large). The t statistic, however, is dependent on two parameters: the chosen probability and, additionally, the number of degrees of freedom, which is itself dependent on the size of the sample ($df = N - 1$). It is important that the reader fully understands the nature of the differences between these two methods of calculating the confidence intervals of the population mean.

The use of the t distribution to calculate confidence intervals of the population mean is illustrated in the following examples.

EXAMPLE 6.11   *Table 6.3 shows the concentration of chlorhexidine (mg) in 15 1-mL samples that have been removed from a stock solution (5 L) and assayed by ultraviolet spectroscopy. Calculate the 95% confidence interval of the population mean.*

First, calculate the mean and standard deviation, i.e. 0.207 ± 0.01 mg/mL. As the sample size is small ($N = 15$), the confidence intervals must be calculated using the t distribution, i.e.

$$P_{95\%} = \bar{X} \pm \frac{tS}{\sqrt{N}}$$

The mean and standard deviation have been calculated using the sample data. The final unknown in the equation is therefore the t statistic. Two

Table 6.3 Concentration of chlorhexidine (mg/mL) in 15 samples removed from a stock solution

0.201	0.205	0.203	0.205	0.200
0.212	0.210	0.211	0.209	0.199
0.209	0.211	0.215	0.216	0.205

points should be considered before selecting this value from Appendix 2: the probability level (95%, two-tailed) and the number of degrees of freedom. The latter is calculated by subtracting 1 from the sample size, i.e. $15 - 1 = 14$ *df*. The *t* statistic corresponding to 14 *df* and 95% probability is 2.14 (Appendix 2).

The confidence intervals may then be calculated:

$$P_{95\%} = \overline{X} \pm \frac{tS}{\sqrt{N}} = 0.207 \pm \frac{2.14 \times 0.01}{\sqrt{15}} = 0.207 \pm 0.006 \text{ mg/mL}$$

The confidence interval is therefore 0.201–0.213 mg/mL.

A second example of this calculation is provided below.

EXAMPLE 6.12 *A chemist has developed a synthetic route for the preparation of a compound with antihistamine properties. A 10-kg batch has been prepared, from which 10 100-mg samples have been removed and their purity determined using an analytical method. The results are shown in Table 6.4. Calculate the 95% and 99% confidence intervals of the true purity of the compound.*

The first stage of the calculation involves the calculation of the mean and standard deviation of the data described in Table 6.4, i.e. $96.37 \pm 2.56\%$.

- *95% confidence interval*

$$P_{95\%} = \overline{X} \pm \frac{tS}{\sqrt{N}}$$

    where the mean and standard deviation have been determined as 96.37 and 2.56% and N, the sample size, is 10. The relevant value of the *t* statistic is derived from the table of the critical values of the *t* distribution (Appendix 2) with knowledge of the number of degrees of freedom $(10 - 1 = 9)$ and the chosen level of probability (95%, two-tailed outcome). The *t* statistic is therefore 2.26.

    Consequently, the 95% confidence interval is

$$P_{95\%} = \overline{X} \pm \frac{tS}{\sqrt{N}} = 96.37 \pm \frac{(2.26 \times 2.56)}{\sqrt{10}} = 96.37 \pm 1.83\%$$

- *99% confidence interval.* As the probability associated with the confidence interval has changed, the *t* statistic must be modified. From Appendix 2, the *t*

Table 6.4 Purities (%) of 10 aliquots of an antihistamine removed from a single batch of product

91.2	94.5	97.5	95.6	98.1
96.5	99.8	98.9	97.4	94.2

statistic associated with 9 *df*, two-tailed outcome and 99% probability is 3.25. This knowledge allows calculation of the 99% confidence interval:

$$P_{95\%} = \overline{X} \pm \frac{tS}{\sqrt{N}} = 96.37 \pm \frac{(3.25 \times 2.56)}{\sqrt{10}} = 96.37 \pm 2.63\%$$

6.8 Conclusions

In this chapter the theory and applications of confidence intervals have been outlined. It is important to understand the concept of confidence intervals, because they are frequently employed to provide information about the magnitude of the true statistic from sample data. In particular, the confidence intervals associated with several descriptive statistics have been described, namely the mean, standard deviation, proportions and differences between these parameters. Furthermore, the uses of both the *z* and *t* statistics in the calculation of confidence intervals have been illustrated, and indeed this is the first example of the use of the *t* distribution for the statistical characterisation of small samples. Further examples of this application will be described in subsequent chapters.

7

One-sample statistical hypothesis testing

One-sample hypothesis testing is one of the most straightforward types of statistical analysis. Nevertheless, many of the principles associated with one-sample hypothesis testing, e.g. definition of the null and alternative hypotheses and the associated region of rejection, and interpretation of the outcome of the analytical procedure, are identical to those for two- (and greater) sample hypothesis tests. One-sample hypothesis testing therefore acts as a gentle introduction into the basis of experimental design, the use of statistical tests within a defined experimental design and statistical decision-making.

One-sample testing involves the estimation of whether sample data, generated from an experimental procedure, are (or are not) derived from a defined population. More specifically, many one-sample tests evaluate whether the mean of the sample and the mean of the population are different, or alternatively whether there is a difference between the observed values that constitute the sample and the values that would be expected if the sample was actually derived from the population in question. Before a one-sample test can be carried out, several questions must be answered:

- What is the null hypothesis?
- What is the alternative hypothesis?
- What is the region of rejection of the null hypothesis?
- Is the experimental design one-tailed or two-tailed?
- What is the appropriate (parametric or non-parametric) statistical method?

Throughout the course of this and subsequent chapters, the above questions will be asked before a statistical test is carried out. It is hoped that this structured approach will become second nature to the reader and will enhance the appreciation of statistial hypothesis testing.

As the reader will appreciate, either parametric or non-parametric one-sample tests may be employed for the analysis of experimental data. Two parametric one-sample tests are described in this chapter, the *one-sample z test* and the *one-sample t test*. In addition, this chapter will also describe the use of the non-parametric tests, the χ^2 *one-sample test* and the *Kolmogorov–Smirnov one-sample test* for the analysis of one-sample nominal and ordinal data, respectively. The use of all these analytical techniques will be illustrated using pharmaceutical examples.

7.1 Parametric one-sample statistical tests

As described in Chapter 5, the use of parametric methods for the analysis of experimental data requires careful consideration of the experimental design and, in particular, whether the conditions of the experimental design conform to the statistical model that is necessary for the successful execution of parametric analyses. Assuming that the conditions of the experiment conform to the statistical model, there are two main parametric tests that may be employed to statistically evaluate one-sample tests, the z test and the t test. The use of these tests is considered individually in the next section.

7.1.1 One-sample z test

One-sample z tests are employed for the analysis of one-sample hypotheses when the sample size is large and, in addition, there is sufficient knowledge about the properties of the population with which the experimentally derived sample is being compared. Typically, z tests (and indeed t tests) compare whether the mean of the sample differs from that of a defined population. Furthermore, the z test may also be employed to compare a single (sample) proportion to a hypothesised value. The use of the z test for the above applications is illustrated in the following examples. The reader should pay careful attention to the stepwise nature of the calculations in the following examples, as this strategy will be employed for the remaining examples in this text.

EXAMPLE 7.1 *A pharmaceutical company has purchased a new liquid filling machine for use in its parenteral manufacturing division. The fill properties of the existing filling machine linked to the current manufacturing process are 5.01 ± 0.21 mL per injection vial. A pilot study has been engaged to evaluate whether (or not) the filling performance of the new machine is similar to that of the previous machine using identical process conditions. Therefore, 100 vials of the product were removed from a pilot batch and the mean fill volume was determined gravimetrically to be 5.12 mL. Is there a difference between the performance of the new and existing filling machines?*

Before starting the sampling process, i.e. at the initiation of the study, the following questions will have been raised and the answers documented.

(i) State the null hypothesis

The null hypothesis (H_0) states that there is no difference between the sample mean and the population mean. Therefore, the null hypothesis for the current example states that there will be no difference between the performance of the new filling machine and that of the existing filling machine in terms of fill volume:

$$H_0: \mu = 5.01 \text{ mL}$$

(ii) State the alternative hypothesis

The alternative hypothesis states that there is a difference between the sample mean and the population mean. Therefore, the alternative hypothesis for the current example states that there will be a difference in the performance of the new filling machine and the existing filling machine in terms of fill volume:

$$H_a: \mu \neq 5.01 \text{ mL}$$

(iii) State the level of significance (the rejection region)

The choice of the level of significance (a) is an extremely important consideration in the establishment of the experimental design. Traditionally, a, the probability of rejecting the null hypothesis when it is in fact true, is chosen to be 0.05. However, there may be reasons for not selecting this level, e.g. an experimenter may require a greater confidence associated with a particular observation and, accordingly, select a smaller value of a. However, for the vast majority of examples that will be described in this book, it is assumed that a is 0.05.

(iv) State the number of tails associated with the experimental design

As described in Chapter 5, the number of tails associated with an experimental design is an important determinant of the outcome of the statistical analysis. The number of tails associated with the alternative hypothesis is determined before data collection. In Example 7.1, the null hypothesis may be rejected because the fill volume associated with the new machine may be either higher or lower than that of the existing machine. There are therefore two possible reasons for rejection of the null hypothesis and consequently this example is *two-tailed*. Unfortunately, many students fail to recognise that the number of tails associated with a particular hypothesis must be considered before sampling. If this is carried out after the collection of data, it may be concluded that because the sample mean (5.12 mL) is larger than the mean of the population under comparison (5.01 mL) there is only one possible outcome, i.e. the experiment is one-tailed. I cannot over-emphasise the inaccuracy of this approach.

(v) Select the most appropriate statistical test

The most appropriate statistical test for any experimental design is unique to that design. In the above example there are several attributes that direct the statistical analyst to the most appropriate experimental method, namely:

- It is a one-sample test, as the likelihood of sample data being derived from a defined (historical) population is under examination.
- The sample size is large ($N = 100$) and therefore the distribution of this data is likely to be normal. Generally sample sizes that are greater than 30 conform to the central limit theorem and hence their distributions may be assumed to be normal.

Therefore, a two-tailed parametric, one-sample test may be applied to the statistical question raised in Example 7.1. There are two possibilities that may be selected to resolve this problem: the one-sample z test and one-sample t test. The choice of these is dependent on sample size. As the sample size is large, the z test is the most suitable statistical method to examine the validity of the null hypothesis.

(vi) Perform the statistical analysis

The statistical analysis may be performed in a stepwise fashion.

Step 1   Calculate the test statistic
The z statistic is calculated using the following formula:

$$z = \frac{\bar{X} - \mu_0}{\sigma/\sqrt{N}}$$

where $\bar{X}$ is the observed sample mean, μ_0 is the hypothesised (historical process) mean, σ is the standard deviation of the population (the historical standard deviation of the process) and N is the sample size. Inserting the relevant data into this equation enables the z statistic to be calculated:

$$z = \frac{\bar{X} - \mu_0}{\sigma/\sqrt{N}} = \frac{5.12 - 5.01}{0.21/\sqrt{100}} = \frac{0.11}{0.021} = 5.24$$

Step 2   Define the critical z statistic
The relevance of the calculated z statistic, i.e. whether the null hypothesis is accepted or rejected, is interpreted by defining the critical z sta-

tistic. This value describes the regions of acceptance and rejection of the null hypothesis on the standardised normal distribution. Identification of this critical statistic requires knowledge of the chosen level of significance (α) and the number of tails associated with the experimental design. Therefore, the critical z statistic associated with the specified level of significance (0.05) and a two-tailed design may be derived from the standardised normal distribution as 1.96. The regions of the z distribution associated with the null and alternative hypotheses may now be defined in terms of the z statistic as:

H_0: $-1.96 < z < +1.96$

H_a: $z \geqslant +1.96$ or $z \leqslant -1.96$

(vii) Conclusion

The z statistic associated with Example 7.1 was calculated to be 5.24. As the calculated z value (+5.24) is greater than + 1.96, the null hypothesis is rejected and the alternative hypothesis is accepted. It is therefore concluded that there is a significant difference between the performance of the new and existing filling machines, in terms of fill volumes.

It should be remembered in this example that the variability of the sample measurement is not important in itself. The standard deviation of the process is known and is used in this test. Whenever the population standard deviation is known, as shown in the above example, the z test should be employed.

EXAMPLE 7.2 *A medical device company specialises in the manufacture of silicone urinary catheters by injection moulding. The Young's modulus (elasticity) of the catheters is an important determinant of catheter performance, as it may be related to the ease of catheter insertion into the urethra. Traditionally, the mean and standard deviation of the Young's modulus of silicone catheters when manufactured using the conventional process is 51.6 ± 4.1 MPa. Historically, the medical device manufacturer has purchased the cross-linker for the silicone curing reaction from one supplier; however, this supplier has now announced that it will no longer be involved in the synthesis of this material. The medical device manufacturer has sourced another supplier of the cross-linker and has acquired a sample of this material for the manufacture of a pilot batch of catheters and subsequent assessment of their mechanical properties. To investigate the applicability of the new supplier, 50 catheters have been manufactured using this new source of cross-linker using identical injection moulding parameters to those employed in*

*previous batches. The mean Young's modulus of the 50 catheters was
then determined using tensile analysis and observed to be 49.7 MPa. Is
there a difference between the mechanical properties of silicone
catheters manufactured using the old and new supplies of cross-linker?*

Before sampling begins, the conditions associated with the experimental
design should be established.

(i)   State the null hypothesis

The null hypothesis states that there is no difference between the sample
mean and the population mean. Therefore, the null hypothesis for the
current example states that there will be no difference in the Young's
modulus of silicone catheters prepared using the new and old types of
cross-linker:

$$H_0: \mu = 51.6 \text{ MPa}$$

(ii)   State the alternative hypothesis

The alternative hypothesis states that there is a difference between the
sample mean and the population mean. Therefore, the alternative
hypothesis for the current example states that there will be a difference
in the Young's modulus of silicone catheters prepared using the new and
old suppliers of cross-linker.

$$H_a: \mu \neq 51.6 \text{ MPa}$$

(iii)   State the level of significance (the rejection region)

In this example, it is assumed that the level of significance (α) is 0.05.

(iv)   State the number of tails associated with the experimental design

In Example 7.2, the null hypothesis may be rejected if the Young's
modulus of the pilot batch is greater, or alternatively less, than that of
the Young's modulus of catheters prepared using the traditional supply
of the cross-linker. Therefore, as there are two potential outcomes, this
is a two-tailed study.

(v)   Select the most appropriate statistical test

The most appropriate statistical test to resolve the problem raised in
Example 7.2 is selected after consideration of the features of the statistical model. First, this is a one-sample hypothesis in which the mechanical properties of sample data and historical data are under comparison.

Furthermore, the sample size is large ($N = 50$) and therefore the distribution of this data is likely to be normal (as defined by the central limit theorem). On the basis of this information, a two-tailed parametric, one-sample z test is the most appropriate statistical test to be applied to this problem.

(vi) Perform the statistical analysis

Step 1 Calculate the test statistic
The z statistic is calculated using the appropriate formula:

$$z = \frac{\overline{X} - \mu_0}{\sigma/\sqrt{N}}$$

where $\overline{X}$ is the observed sample mean, i.e. the mean associated with the material produced using the new supplier of cross-linker (49.7 MPa), μ_0 is the hypothesised mean (mean of the historical process, i.e. 51.6 MPa), σ is the standard deviation of the population (the historical standard deviation of the process), i.e. 4.1 MPa, and N is the sample size (50). The test (z) statistic is calculated by inserting this information into the relevant equation:

$$z = \frac{\overline{X} - \mu_0}{\sigma/\sqrt{N}} = \frac{49.7 - 51.6}{4.1/\sqrt{50}} = \frac{-1.9}{0.58} = -3.28$$

Step 2 Define the critical z statistic
Identification of the critical z statistic from the table of the standardised normal distribution (Appendix 1) enables the regions of acceptance and rejection of the null hypothesis to be identified. According to the conditions of the experimental design ($\alpha = 0.05$, two-tailed) the critical z statistic is ± 1.96. The regions associated with the acceptance and rejection of the null hypothesis are therefore:

H_0: $-1.96 < z < +1.96$

H_a: $z \geqslant +1.96$ or $z \leqslant -1.96$

(vii) Conclusion

The z statistic was calculated as -3.28. This is less than -1.96, so the null hypothesis is rejected. Therefore, there is a significant difference between the mechanical performances of silicone catheters prepared using the new supply of cross-linker and those of catheters prepared using the established cross-linker.

This study has specifically identified the inapplicability of the new type of cross-linker for the manufacture of silicone catheters, because the mechanical properties of catherters prepared using it do not meet the mechanical specification.

The following example illustrates the use of the z test to statistically compare a sampled proportion with a hypothesised value.

EXAMPLE 7.3   *In a population the incidence of patients who are hospitalised as a result of asthma attacks and who routinely use a particular β_2 agonist is 25%. A company has introduced a new β_2 agonist that is claimed to reduce the incidence of hospitalisation resulting from asthma attacks. In a clinical trial involving 400 patients the incidence of patients who were hospitalised as a result of asthma attacks and who had been prescribed the new therapy was 21%. Is the claim made by the manufacturer concerning the efficacy of the new β_2 agonist statistically valid?*

At first glance the reader will observe that the data is presented in terms of proportions and therefore the equation that was employed to calculate the z statistic in the previous examples is invalid. However, as in the previous examples, it is important first of all to consider the details of the study design.

(i)   State the null hypothesis

The null hypothesis states that there is no difference between the sampled proportion and the hypothesised proportion. Therefore, the null hypothesis for the current example states that there will be no difference in clinical efficacies (i.e. observed proportions) between the new drug and currently prescribed β_2 agonist therapies.

(ii)   State the alternative hypothesis

The alternative hypothesis states that there is a difference between the sampled proportion and the hypothesised proportion. In particular, the alternative hypothesis (claimed by the manufacturer) states that the clinical efficacy associated with use of the new drug will be greater than that of currently prescribed β_2 agonist therapies. Therefore, the incidence of hospitalisation for patients who were administered the new drug will be less that the incidence associated with the use of the current β_2 agonist.

(iii)   State the level of significance (the rejection region)

In this example, it is assumed that the level of significance (α) is 0.05.

(iv)   State the number of tails associated with the experimental design

The manufacturer has claimed that the efficacy of the new drug is greater than that of other currently available medications. This claim is valid

only if the proportion of hospitalisations is reduced following administration of the new drug. As there is only one outcome of interest to the
drug manufacturer, this is an example of a negative, one-tailed study.

(v) Select the most appropriate statistical test

There are two key points concerning the choice of statistical method:

- The study is an example of a one-sample test in which the proportions of hospitalised subjects following treatment with a new drug and a hypothesised
  value are under comparison.
- The sample size is large ($N = 400$) and therefore the distribution of this data is
  likely to be normal.

Therefore, a one-tailed parametric, one-sample z test for proportions is
the most appropriate statistical test to be applied here.

(vi) Perform the statistical analysis

In this example two discrete categories exist and therefore the data are
binomially distributed. However, the use of the z statistic to interpret such
(discrete) data involves an approximation of the normal distribution.

The z statistic is calculated using the following mathematical
formula:

$$z = \frac{p - \pi_0}{SE(p)} = \frac{p - \pi_0}{\sqrt{\pi_0(1 - \pi_0)/N}}$$

where p is the observed sample proportion, π_0 is the hypothesised proportion that is defined in the null hypothesis, $SE(p)$ is the standard error
of the sample proportion and N is the sample size.

To improve the approximation of binomial data to the normal distribution, a correction factor is commonly employed, termed the *Yates
continuity correction factor*. The use of this correction factor ensures that
the probabilities calculated are similar to those that would have been
obtained if binomial theory had been applied to the problem. This gives us

$$z = \frac{(p - \pi_0) - (1/2N)}{\sqrt{\pi_0(1 - \pi_0)/N}}$$

where $1/2N$ is the Yates continuity correction factor.

The z statistic is calculated by substitution of the appropriate
values into the above equation:

$$z = \frac{(p - \pi_0) - (1/2N)}{\sqrt{\pi_0(1 - \pi_0)/N}} = \frac{(0.21 - 0.25) - (1/2 \times 400)}{\sqrt{0.25(1 - 0.25)/400}}$$

$$= \frac{-0.041\,25}{0.0217} = -1.91$$

One point worth noting concerns the restrictions in the use of the z test for the analysis of proportions. It is accepted that both $N\pi_0$ and $\pi(1 - \pi_0)$ should be greater than 5. In the above example these terms were calculated as 100 and 300 respectively, and thus this assumption is valid.

(vii) Conclusion

The z statistic was calculated as -1.91. From the standard normal distribution it may be observed that for the conditions of this study (one-tailed test, $\alpha = 0.05$), a value of $z \leqslant -1.65$ will result in the rejection of the null hypothesis. As the calculated z value (-1.91) lies within this region, the null hypothesis is rejected. Therefore, the clinical efficacy of the new β_2 agonist is superior to that of currently available β_2 agonists, in terms of prevention of hospitalisation due to asthma attacks.

This example has raised an important issue concerning statistical hypothesis testing. As may be observed, the calculated z statistic was -1.91 and, on the basis of the rejection criteria stipulated at the start of the study, the null hypothesis was rejected. However, if the alternative hypothesis had stated that the clinical efficacy of the new β_2 agonist is dissimilar to the efficacies of currently available β_2 agonists, then the null hypothesis may be rejected if the clinical efficacy of the new drug is either superior or inferior to currently available therapeutic agents. Accordingly, the experimental design would have been a two-tailed test. The region of acceptance of the null hypothesis in this scenario is $-1.96 < z < +1.96$ and, hence, the calculated z value would have led to the acceptance of the null hypothesis. This is a type II error. Although experimentation in the pharmaceutical and clinical sciences usually involves the use of two-tailed statistical tests, there are many cases in which the use of one-tailed statistical designs is valid and these will be illustrated in subsequent chapters.

EXAMPLE 7.4 *In a consumer panel 100 volunteers were asked to comment on the visual acceptability of two tablet formulations, one oval and the other hexagonal. Before introducing the new tablet shape (oval), the manufacturers wish to ascertain whether there is a preference for it. After data collection, it was observed that 78% of panel members questioned preferred the oval tablet. Is there a statistically valid preference for the oval shape?*

This example is similar in design to Example 7.3 and involves the analysis of proportional data as a one-sample experimental design. As before, the following questions should be answered before collecting data.

(i) State the null hypothesis

The null hypothesis states that there is no difference between the sampled proportion and the hypothesised proportion. Therefore, the null hypothesis for the current example states that there will be no preference for either tablet shape, i.e. the probability of preferring either tablet will be 0.5 (50%).

(ii) State the alternative hypothesis

The alternative hypothesis states that there is a difference between the sampled proportion and the hypothesised proportion and, in particular, there will be a defined preference for the oval tablet shape.

(iii) State the level of significance (the rejection region)

In this example, it is assumed that the level of significance (α) is 0.05.

(iv) State the number of tails associated with the experimental design

In this example the company is not interested in investigating whether the preferences for the two tablet shapes are similar or, indeed whether volunteers preferred the hexagonal tablet. The company wishes to ascertain only whether the oval tablet is preferred to the existing (hexagonal) shape and, accordingly, there is only one relevant outcome to the study. As a result, this is an example of a positive, one-tailed study.

(v) Select the most appropriate statistical test

The key points concerning the choice of statistical method are:

- The study is an example of a one-sample test in which the proportions of subjects who preferred the oval tablet are compared to a hypothesised value (proportion).
- The sample size is large ($N = 100$) and therefore the distribution of this data is likely to be normal.

Therefore, a one-tailed parametric, one-sample z test for proportions is the most appropriate statistical test to be applied to above example.

(vi) Perform the statistical analysis

In this example there are two discrete categories and therefore the data are binomially distributed. However, the use of the z statistic to interpret such (discrete) data involves an approximation of the normal distribution. The z statistic is therefore calculated using the following formula:

$$z = \frac{(p - \pi_0) - (1/2N)}{\sqrt{\pi_0(1 - \pi_0)/N}}$$

where p is the observed sample proportion (0.78), π_0 is the hypothesised proportion that is defined in the null hypothesis (0.50), N is the sample size (100) and $1/2N$ is the Yates continuity correction factor.

The z statistic is calculated by substituting the appropriate values into the above equation:

$$\begin{aligned} z &= \frac{(p - \pi_0) - (1/2N)}{\sqrt{\pi_0(1 - \pi_0)/N}} \\ &= \frac{(0.78 - 0.50) - (1/2 \times 100)}{\sqrt{0.50(1 - 0.50)/100}} = \frac{0.275}{0.05} = 5.50 \end{aligned}$$

(vii) Conclusion

The test (z) statistic was calculated as 5.50. From the standard normal distribution it may be observed that for the conditions of this study (one-tailed test, $\alpha = 0.05$), a value of $z \geqslant + 1.65$ will result in the rejection of the null hypothesis. As the calculated z value (+5.50) is greater than +1.65, the null hypothesis is rejected. Therefore, the subjects who participated in the study preferred the oval tablet.

7.1.2 One-sample *t* test

In the use of the z statistic for the interpretation of one-sample statistical hypothesis testing, it has been assumed that the variance of the population is known. In Examples 7.1 and 7.2, the mean and standard deviation of the process, information that has been accumulated from numerous manufactured batches of product, has been employed to provide a reliable estimate of the central tendency and variability of the process. Subsequently, in these examples, the null hypothesis has examined the probability that data derived from a sample could have originated from the population described by the process parameters. However, in many experiments relevant to the pharmaceutical sciences, it is impossible to obtain knowledge of the relevant population statistics and, accordingly, the only available estimates of the central tendency and variability of the population are the mean and variance that are associated with the sample data. Under these circumstances a one-sample *t* test is employed to calculate the *t* statistic and the relevance of this statistic is interpreted using the *t* distribution (with the appropriate numbers of degrees of freedom). Once more, it is worthwhile reiterating the assumptions of the one-sample *t* test, which is, in fact, another parametric statistical test. These are:

- The sample data is randomly selected.
- The sample data is either in an interval or ratio format (measured in discernible units).
- The population from which the sample data is derived is normally distributed.
- The mean and standard deviation of the sample data are reliable estimates of the central tendency and variability of the population from which the data was derived.

The process for calculation of the one-sample *t* test is analogous to that for the one-sample *z* test and, once more, will be illustrated by the use of examples.

EXAMPLE 7.5   *A pharmaceutical company has developed a new benzodiazepine for the treatment of sleep disorders and wishes to evaluate whether (or not) the number of hours of unbroken sleep experienced by patients who are treated with this drug differs from the national average of 7.3 h. In a subsequent clinical study the effect of this new benzodiazepine on the numbers of hours of unbroken sleep experienced by 20 patients was monitored. The results are shown in Table 7.1. Using an appropriate statistical method, examine whether the new benzodiazepine increased the number of hours of unbroken sleep when compared to the national average.*

Before the start of sampling, i.e. the initiation of the study, the following details should be documented.

(i) State the null hypothesis

The null hypothesis states that there is no difference between the sample mean and the hypothetical mean. Therefore, the null hypothesis for the current example states that there is no difference between the number of hours of unbroken sleep experienced by patients who received a single dose of the new benzodiazepine and the national average of hours of

Table 7.1 Numbers of hours of unbroken sleep experienced by patients who received a single dose of a new benzodiazepine

6.6	6.8	6.6	7.1	7.4
6.7	6.9	7.6	7.0	6.4
6.9	6.9	7.3	6.7	6.9
6.2	7.2	6.7	7.1	6.8

unbroken sleep experienced by the population:

$$H_0: \mu = 7.3 \text{ h}$$

(ii) State the alternative hypothesis

The alternative hypothesis states that the number of hours of unbroken sleep experienced by patients who received a single dose of a new benzodiazepine is greater than the national average of hours of unbroken sleep experienced by the population:

$$H_a: \mu > 7.3 \text{ h}$$

(iii) State the level of significance (the rejection region)

In this example, it is assumed that the level of significance (α) is 0.05.

(iv) State the number of tails associated with the experimental design

There is one potential reason for which the null hypothesis may be rejected, namely, the number of hours of unbroken sleep that was experienced by patients who had received the therapeutic agent may exceed that of the national average. Accordingly, the study is one-tailed.

(v) Select the most appropriate statistical test

The primary underlying assumption for the use of the t test for the analysis of one-sample (and two-sample) data is that the sample data is normally or pseudo-normally distributed. This is also an assumption for the z test; however, in this scenario normality is frequently assured because of the large sample size (central limit theorem). In Example 7.5, the variance of the population is unknown but it may be estimated using the variance calculated from the sample data. Whenever the population variance is unknown, the one-sample t test (and not the one-sample z test) must be used. Before the t test is carried out, it must be proved that the data, representing the population from which it was obtained, is in fact normally distributed. This is a contentious topic within statistics and indeed, several different approaches have been suggested, each with varying degrees of reported success and acceptability. Examples of these include the use of Kolmogorov–Smironov or χ^2 goodness-of-fit procedures and graphical methods. In the latter, the cumulative frequency distribution of a normal distribution will adopt a sigmoid curve. Alternatively, the cumulative frequency distribution may be plotted on a normal probability scale using commercially available probability graph paper. If the data is normally distributed, the plot will be linear with a positive slope. Leptokurtic and platykurtic distributions will present as sigmoid and reverse sigmoid curves, respectively. The shapes of negatively and positively shaped distributions resemble the lower and upper portions of a sigmoid curve, respectively.

Another simple (and useful) measure is to consider the descriptive statistical properties of the data, particularly the relative magnitudes of the mean, median and mode. The descriptive statistics for the data presented in Table 7.1 are as follows:

- mean 6.89 h
- median 6.90 h
- mode 6.90 h

As described in Chapter 2, if these three parameters are similar in magnitude, it is likely that the data are normally distributed. It must be emphasised at this point that the comparison of the mean, median and mode is a simple method that may be used to examine the normality of a set of data, but it is not definitive as other factors must be considered, including measures of skewness and kurtosis. However, because of the simplicity of the method, this text will employ comparisons of the mean, median and mode as a measure of the normality of a distribution. The reader should remember that this text has been designed to explain the mechanics and applications of various statistical methods. To illustrate these methods, normality must be assumed and therefore the comparison of the mean, median and mode offers a degree of comfort in the acceptance of this assumption.

Returning to Example 7.5, it will be assumed that the population from which the data have been removed is normally distributed and furthermore, the data has been measured on a ratio scale. As the sample mean and variance are the only estimates of the associated population parameters, it may be concluded that a one-tailed parametric, one-sample t test is the most appropriate statistical test to assess the validity of the null hypothesis.

(vi) Perform the statistical analysis

The t statistic is calculated using the following mathematical formula:

$$t_{(N-1)df} = \frac{\bar{X} - \mu_0}{S/\sqrt{N}}$$

where $\bar{X}$ is the observed sample mean (6.89 h), μ_0 is the hypothesised population mean (7.3 h), S is the sample standard deviation (0.34 h), N is the sample size (20) and $t_{(N-1)df}$ is the t value associated with $N - 1$

degrees of freedom. These data are then inserted into the equation:

$$t_{(N-1)df} = \frac{\bar{X} - \mu_0}{S/\sqrt{N}}$$

$$t_{19} = \frac{6.89 - 7.3}{0.34/\sqrt{20}} = \frac{-0.41}{0.08} = -5.13$$

(vii) Conclusion

The t statistic was calculated as -5.13. To interpret the relevance of this value the critical value of the t statistic that relates to the conditions of this study must be identified (Appendix 2). This is done after consideration of the design of the experiment and, accordingly, for the current study, the following design parameters determine the magnitude of the critical value of the t statistic:

- $\alpha = 0.05$.
- It is a one-tailed experimental design.
- There are 19 (i.e. $N - 1$) degrees of freedom.

From this it may be observed that, for the conditions of this study, a value of $t \geqslant + 1.73$ would result in the rejection of the null hypothesis. As the calculated t value (-5.13) is less than 1.73, the null hypothesis is accepted. Therefore, it may be concluded that, on the basis of the clinical study, the number of hours of unbroken sleep experienced by patients who received a single dose of a new benzodiazepine did not differ from the national average.

A further example of the use of a t test for one-sample hypothesis testing is given in Example 7.6.

EXAMPLE 7.6 *The first batch (40 L) of a new parenteral suspension formulation containing triamcinolone acetonide (40 mg/mL) has been manufactured for the purpose of registration with the FDA. After filling, 25 vials of product have been removed for analysis of their drug content. The results of the analysis are shown in Table 7.2. Does the mean concentration of drug in the batch conform to the nominal concentration (40 mg/mL)?*

(i) State the null hypothesis

The null hypothesis states that there is no difference between the sample mean and the hypothetical mean. i.e. that the concentration of drug in the pilot batch is statistically similar to the hypothetical (nominal)

Table 7.2 Concentration of triamcinolone acetonide (mg/mL) in 25 vials of product

41.5	40.5	40.5	39.8	40.1
40.2	40.2	40.6	39.8	41.1
40.1	40.1	40.1	40.2	39.7
38.9	40.0	40.4	40.3	39.9
42.1	40.1	38.9	40.8	39.5

concentration of the batch:

$$H_0: \mu = 40 \text{ mg/mL}$$

(ii) State the alternative hypothesis

The alternative hypothesis states that there is a difference between the sample mean and the population mean, i.e. that the concentration of drug in the pilot batch is different and does not conform to the hypothetical (nominal) concentration of the batch:

$$H_a: \mu \neq 40 \text{ mg/mL}$$

(iii) State the level of significance (the rejection region)

In this example, it is assumed that the level of significance (α) is 0.05.

(iv) State the number of tails associated with the experimental design

In Example 7.6, there are two potential reasons for which the null hypothesis may be rejected, i.e. the concentration of drug in the pilot batch may be either lower or higher than the nominal concentration. Accordingly, the test is two-tailed.

(v) Select the most appropriate statistical test

The reader will observe that no knowledge of the population variance has been provided in this example. Therefore, the mean and variance of the population (batch) is estimated using the mean and variance of the sample data. The test is a one-sample test because the hypothesis under evaluation is that the sample data could have belonged to the hypothetical population (defined by the null hypothesis). Initially it is important to examine whether the sample data is normal in nature and, for this purpose, it is useful to compare the mean, median and mode of the data set. The descriptive statistics for the data presented in Table 7.2 are as follows:

- mean   40.22 mg/mL
- median   40.10 mg/mL

- mode   40.10 mg/mL
- standard deviation   0.72 mg/mL

The similarity of the mean, median and mode allow us to assume that a normal distribution does exist and therefore a two-tailed parametric, one-sample t test is the most appropriate statistical test. Remember, the small sample size and lack of available information concerning the mean and variance of the population from which sampling was performed invalidate the use of the z test to examine the validity of the null hypothesis.

(vi) Perform the statistical analysis

The t statistic is calculated as before:

$$t_{(N-1)df} = \frac{\bar{X} - \mu_0}{S/\sqrt{N}}$$

Inserting the relevant data enables calculation of the t statistic:

$$t_{24} = \frac{40.22 - 40.00}{0.72/\sqrt{25}} = \frac{0.22}{0.14} = +1.57$$

(vii) Conclusion

The t statistic was calculated as +1.57. Under the experimental conditions ($a = 0.05$, two-tailed test, 24 degrees of freedom), a value either of $t \leqslant -2.06$ or $t \geqslant +2.06$ would result in the rejection of the null hypothesis. As the calculated t value lies within the region $-2.06 < t < +2.06$, the null hypothesis is accepted. Therefore, the concentration of therapeutic agent in the pilot batch conforms to the specified nominal value and, as a result, it can be confirmed that the product has been successfully manufactured in accordance with the specifications of the product licence.

7.1.3 Sample size and power in one-sample parametric statistical tests

Sample size is an important consideration in the design of statistical experiments. Incorrect selection of sample size may have a number of repercussions, including an invalid outcome of a statistical study and inordinate expense. The latter problem has pushed the issue of sample size to the forefront of any experimental design, as the cost of clinical studies is continually escalating. Although many readers will not be directly involved in such studies, this section will be also of use to those considering the number of replicates to analyse during the course of their undergraduate or postgraduate research programmes.

To successfully calculate the required sample size for an experiment, four parameters must be known (or estimated).

- The level of significance (a). This is the probability of rejecting the null hypothesis when the null hypothesis is indeed true. A value of 0.05 is generally selected.
- *The variability of the experiment.* When dealing with population statistics, the population (historical) standard deviation is employed. However, in experiments where the population variability is estimated using sample data, the sample standard deviation is used.
- *The probability of making a type II error.* The reader may recall that the power of the study is defined as the probability that the statistical method will reject the null hypothesis when it is indeed false, i.e. it is the probability of selecting the true outcome. Conversely a type II error (designated β) is the probability that the null hypothesis is accepted when it is false. In the determination of sample size, β is estimated.
- *The difference between the data set and a hypothesised value (or between two data sets) that is accepted to be experimentally valid.* The chosen value is important and must reflect the difference that is practically valid.

Calculation of both the power and the statistically valid sample size of a study is illustrated in the following examples.

EXAMPLE *7.7* *The nominal fill volume of an antacid suspension is 50 mL. Ten bottles were removed from a filled batch and the fill volume measured gravimetrically as 48.8 ± 2.1 mL (mean and standard deviation). Using appropriate statistical methods, calculate whether the measured fill volume differs from the nominal fill volume and the probability of detecting a true difference of 2.5 mL between the sample mean and nominal mean.*

Does the measured fill volume differ from the nominal fill volume?
We apply the previously defined criteria.

(i) State the null hypothesis

The null hypothesis states that there is no difference between the sample mean and the hypothetical mean. Therefore, the null hypothesis for the current example states that the mean fill volume of product in the batch (48.8 mL) is statistically similar to the hypothetical (nominal) fill volume of the batch (50.0 mL):

$$H_0: \mu = 50 \text{ mL}$$

(ii) State the alternative hypothesis

The alternative hypothesis states that there is a difference between the sample mean and the population mean. Therefore, the alternative hypothesis states that the mean fill volume of product in the batch is statistically dissimilar to the hypothetical (nominal) fill volume of the batch:

$$H_a: \mu \neq 50 \text{ mL}$$

(iii) State the level of significance (the rejection region)

In this example, it is assumed that the level of significance (α) is 0.05.

(iv) State the number of tails associated with the experimental design

The experimental design illustrated in Example 7.7 is two-tailed. Once more, there are two potential reasons for rejecting the null hypothesis, i.e. the product fill volume of the pilot batch may be either lower or higher than the nominal fill volume.

(v) Select the most appropriate statistical test

In this example, no individual datum values have been provided and therefore it is not possible to comment on the type of distribution exhibited by the population from which the individual samples were removed. Therefore, for the purpose of this example, we will assume that the distribution is normal and consequently, an appropriate statistical test for Example 7.7 is a one-sample t test.

(vi) Perform the statistical analysis

The t statistic is calculated, as before, using the following mathematical formula:

$$t_{(N-1)df} = \frac{\bar{X} - \mu_0}{S/\sqrt{N}}$$

where $\bar{X}$ is the observed sample mean (48.8 mL), μ_0 is the hypothesised population mean (50.0 mL), S is the sample standard deviation (2.10 mL), N is the sample size (10) and $t_{(N-1)df}$ is the t value associated with $N-1$ degrees of freedom. Insertion of this information into the equation enables the critical t statistic to be calculated:

$$t_9 = \frac{48.80 - 50.00}{2.10/\sqrt{10}} = \frac{-1.20}{0.66} = -1.81$$

(vii) Conclusion

The calculated t statistic was -1.81. Under the experimental conditions ($\alpha = 0.05$, two-tailed test, 9 df), a calculated value of t which is less than or equal to -2.26, or greater than or equal to $+2.26$, would result in the rejection of the null hypothesis. As the calculated t value lies within the region $-2.26 < t < +2.26$, the null hypothesis is accepted. The mean fill volume of the pilot batch is statistically similar to the nominal fill volume.

What is the probability of detecting a true difference of 2.5 mL between the sample mean and nominal mean?
Answering this question requires calculation of the probability of rejecting the null hypothesis when it is indeed false: in other words, calculation of the *power* of the study. The mathematical equation that may be employed for this purpose is:

$$t_{\beta(df)} = \frac{\delta}{\sqrt{s^2/N}} - t_{\alpha(df)}$$

where s is the sample standard deviation, N is the sample size, δ is the estimated difference between the sample mean and hypothetical value that is accepted to represent a practical difference, $t_{\beta(df)}$ is the t value associated with the type II error at a defined number of degrees of freedom and $t_{\alpha(df)}$ is the t value associated with the desired level of significance at a defined number of degrees of freedom. From the parameters described in Example 7.7, $\delta = 2.5$ mL, $N = 10$, $S = 2.1$ mL, $t_{\alpha(df)} = 2.26$ ($\alpha = 0.05$, two-tailed, 9 df). When these values are substituted into the above equation, the t statistic associated with performing a type II error may be calculated:

$$t_{\beta(df)} = \frac{2.50}{\sqrt{(2.1)^2/10}} - 2.26 = \frac{2.50}{0.66} - 2.26 = 1.53$$

The approximate probability associated with a t value of $+1.53$ may be calculated using the t distribution. The calculated t value associated with a β error is one-tailed in nature as it represents the overlap of the sample distribution with the hypothesised distribution in which the null hypothesis is not rejected (when in fact it should be). For this reason, there can only be one relevant outcome, hence the one-tailed outcome. As the reader will appreciate, the exact probability may not determined from the t distribution, e.g. in the above example, a t value of 5.55 (9 df, one-tailed outcome) corresponds to a probability that lies within the range 0.05–0.10. It should be remembered that to calculate the exact probability a full knowledge of the t distribution with 9 df is required. This is not generally available and will have to be calculated by the analyst. To overcome this problem, it is common to use the standardised normal distribution for the interpretation of the probability associated with the β error. Therefore, assuming that 1.53 corresponds to a z value, the probability of making a β error is 0.07 (one-tailed response, $\alpha = 0.05$). We can therefore conclude that the power of the test $(1 - \beta)$ is 0.93. In other words, there is a 93% chance that a difference of at least 2.5 mL, the defined critical difference, will be observed between the sample mean and the nominal mean.

One further consideration in experimental design is the use of an appropriate sample size, i.e. one that will allow the rejection of a particular null hypothesis. The sample size required to fit the above criterion is calculated using the following equation:

$$ N = \left(\frac{s}{\delta}\right)^2 (t_{\alpha(df)} + t_{\beta(df)})^2 $$

where N is the required sample size, s is the sample standard deviation, δ is the detectable difference between the sample mean and hypothesised value, $t_{\alpha(df)}$ is the t statistic associated with making a type I error (α is usually 0.05, either one- or two-tailed) at a defined number of degrees of freedom and $t_{\beta(df)}$ is the t statistic associated with making a type II error (one-tailed) at a defined number of degrees of freedom.

The reader will appreciate that the number of degrees of freedom for the study depends on the number of samples, which is the unknown factor. In light of this, the sample size is calculated using an iterative method. The most appropriate sample size is selected when the calculated value of N is similar to the estimated value of N. This process may be illustrated using the data presented in Example 7.7.

EXAMPLE 7.8 *The nominal fill volume of an antacid suspension is 50 mL. Calculate the number of bottles that should be assayed to reject the null hypothesis that the true fill volume of the pilot batch equals the nominal fill volume.*

To answer this question, it is important to define the parameters associated with the statistical process:

- $\alpha = 0.05$.
- The standard deviation of the sample as an estimate of the population variability. The standard deviation is not provided in the information above and therefore, before the sample size can be calculated, the standard deviation of a defined number of bottles must be determined. For the purpose of this example, we will assume that 10 bottles are collected and their standard deviation calculated as 2.1 mL
- The probability of making a type II (β) error must be estimated. Generally, it is the power of the study that is estimated and the β error is calculated from this. In this example, we assume a power of 90%, i.e. there is a 90% chance

of detecting a defined numerical difference between the sample mean and a nominal value. Therefore, the β error is 0.1.

- The difference (δ) between the data set and a hypothesised value (or between two data sets) that is accepted to be experimentally valid. For the purpose of this calculation (and to conform with the previous calculations), δ is set at 2.5 mL.

Initially we will assume that the required sample size is 20. Therefore, $N = 20$, $s = 2.1$ mL, $\delta = 2.5$ mL, $\alpha = 0.05$ and, accordingly, $t_{\alpha(df)}$ is 2.09 (19 df, two-tailed test because the difference between the mean values of the sample population and the hypothetical mean may be equal to either $+2.5$ mL or -2.5 mL). $\beta = 0.10$ and, accordingly $t_{\beta(df)}$ is 1.33 (19 df, one-tailed outcome).

Applying the appropriate equation:

$$N = \left(\frac{s}{\delta}\right)^2 (t_{\alpha(df)} + t_{\beta(df)})^2$$

$$= \left(\frac{2.1}{2.5}\right)^2 (2.09 + 1.33)^2 = 8.25$$

The estimated value of N (20) is not similar to the calculated value of N (8) and therefore this is an inaccurate estimate. The sample size is therefore re-estimated ($N = 15$) and the calculation is performed once more using this re-estimated value: $N = 15$, $s = 2.1$ mL, $\delta = 2.5$ mL, $\alpha = 0.05$ and, accordingly, $t_{\alpha(df)}$ is 2.14 (14 df, two-tailed test). $\beta = 0.10$ and, accordingly $t_{\beta(df)}$ is 1.35 (14 df, one-tailed test). Applying the appropriate equation,

$$N = \left(\frac{s}{\delta}\right)^2 (t_{\alpha(df)} + t_{\beta(df)})^2$$

$$= \left(\frac{2.1}{2.5}\right)^2 (2.14 + 1.35)^2 = 8.59$$

The difference in magnitude between the estimated and calculated sample sizes is becoming smaller. This difference may be reduced by employing a further estimation of the sample size ($N = 10$): $N = 10$, $s = 2.1$ mL, $\delta = 2.5$ mL, $\alpha = 0.05$ and, accordingly, $t_{\alpha(df)}$ is 2.26 (9 df, two-tailed test), $\beta = 0.10$ and, accordingly $t_{\beta(df)}$ is 1.38 (9 df, one-tailed test).

Hence:

$$N = \left(\frac{s}{\delta}\right)^2 (t_{\alpha(df)} + t_{\beta(df)})^2$$

$$= \left(\frac{2.1}{2.5}\right)^2 (2.26 + 1.38)^2 = 9.35$$

The calculated and estimated values of sample size are now similar, so we know that a sample size of at least 10 is required to fulfil the specified demands of the test.

The iteration process is time consuming when the t statistic is used to calculate sample size. These problems do not arise when the use of the z statistic is valid, e.g. if the population variability is known or, alternatively, when the power of the study is to be calculated, if the sample size is large (> 30). Under these conditions the terms $t_{\alpha(df)}$ and $t_{\beta(df)}$ are replaced by z_α and z_β and no consideration of the sample size is required. Interestingly, the z statistic may be used to estimate the sample size of experiments that would normally employ the t statistic, but in this scenario a correction factor must be included, as follows:

$$N = \left(\frac{s}{\delta}\right)^2 (z_\alpha + z_\beta)^2 + 0.5(z_\alpha)^2$$

Returning to Example 7.8, we shall once again calculate the number of bottles that should be assayed to reject the null hypothesis that the true fill volume of the pilot batch equals the nominal fill volume. In this case $s = 2.1$ mL; $\delta = 2.5$ mL; $\alpha = 0.05$ and therefore, $z_\alpha = 1.96$ (two-tailed test); and $\beta = 0.10$ and therefore $z_\beta = 1.28$ (one-tailed test). Therefore

$$N = \left(\frac{2.1}{2.5}\right)^2 (1.96 + 1.28)^2 + 0.5(1.96)^2$$

$$= 9.4$$

This value of N, calculated using the z statistic, is in good agreement with the value determined using the iterative process in association with the t distribution.

One final calculation that is often employed in the process of experimental design is the estimation of the smallest difference between the sample mean and the hypothetical value that may be detected using statistical methods. This calculation is based on the previous equations, but now the *minimum difference* (δ) is the subject of the equation and the sample size and power are specified. To illustrate the use of this equation, the following design parameters will be specified (as defined in Examples 7.7 and 7.8): $N = 10$, $s = 2.1$ mL, $\alpha = 0.05$ and, accordingly, $t_{\alpha(df)}$ is 2.26 (9 df, two-tailed test); $\beta = 0.10$ and, accordingly $t_{\beta(df)}$ is 1.38 (9 df, one-tailed test). The minimum detectable difference is calculated as follows:

$$\delta = \left(\sqrt{\frac{s^2}{N}}\right)(t_{\alpha(df)} + t_{\beta(df)})$$

$$= \left(\sqrt{\frac{2.1^2}{10}}\right)(2.26 + 1.38) = 2.42 \text{ mL}$$

Therefore, employing a power of 0.90, the minimum difference is 2.42 mL. Consequently, the minimum difference that will be discriminated in 90% of all cases is 2.42 mL.

7.2 Non-parametric one-sample statistical tests

The choice of a parametric method for the analysis of one-sample data requires that there is prior knowledge of the nature of the data under examination. In particular, the use of parametric methods is restricted to those cases in which the population from which the sample data has been derived is normally distributed and, moreover, the data must be measured on either an interval or a ratio scale. In many cases it is not possible to make these assumptions and accordingly the statistical characterisation of one-sample data should be carried out using non-parametric methods. At this stage, it is important to remind the reader that although non-parametric techniques are less complicated and less restrictive in nature, there are assumptions associated with their use. These have been highlighted in Chapter 5.

Non-parametric one-sample tests are commonly employed for the analysis of data that are measured on either a nominal or an ordinal scale. In this chapter, the mechanics and applications of the one-sample χ^2 test and the binomial test for the analysis of nominal data and the one-sample Kolmogorov–Smirnov test for the analysis of ordinal data will be described.

7.2.1 One-sample χ^2 test

In the one-sample χ^2 test, (nominal) data is collected within two or more different categories of a *single* variable and the relationship between the frequencies within the different categories statistically examined. This is a goodness-of-fit test in which the differences between the observed frequency and expected frequency in each category are examined. The type of data that may be analysed and the mechanics of performing the χ^2 test are explained in the following examples.

EXAMPLE 7.9 *A pharmaceutical company has developed a mouthwash formulation for the treatment and prevention of infection within the oral cavity. The marketing section of the company believes that the colour of the solution is an important consideration in the patient acceptability of the product. To evaluate this principle, four formulations have been prepared that differ only in the identity of the added colouring agent. Two hundred volunteers were asked to select their preferred colour, and the results are shown in Table 7.3. Using an*

Table 7.3 Number of volunteers who preferred various colours of mouthwash

Red	55
Green	73
Blue	36
Yellow	36

appropriate statistical method, comment on whether or not there is a preference amongst the various colours of mouthwash.

The following steps will act as a useful guide for the successful execution of the one-sample χ^2 test.

(i) State the null hypothesis

As before, the null hypothesis states that volunteers demonstrate no preference for colour in the mouthwash formulations. Accordingly, the number of volunteers who prefer each colour will be equal. This is termed the *expected frequency* and this value is calculated and employed in the χ^2 analysis.

(ii) State the alternative hypothesis

The alternative hypothesis is the opposite to the null hypothesis and therefore states that there is a preference for a particular colour or colours. Accordingly, the frequencies of response in each category will not be equal or, alternatively, the observed frequencies will not correspond to the frequencies predicted by the null hypothesis.

(iii) State the level of significance

In this example, it is assumed that the level of significance (α) is 0.05.

(iv) Select the statistical test

In this example, a set of sample data (relating to preference for particular colours) will be compared to a hypothetical population (defined by the calculated expected frequencies). The data are nominal in nature and therefore the most relevant statistical test is a one-sample χ^2 test. Remember, parametric tests may not be used to analyse data that is nominal or ordinal in nature.

(v) Calculate the χ^2 statistic

The χ^2 statistic is calculated using the following formula:

$$\chi^2 = \sum \frac{(O_f - E_f)^2}{E_f}$$

where O_f is the observed frequency for a particular cell within the category and E_f is the expected frequency for a particular cell within the category, as defined by the null hypothesis.

The mechanics of the χ^2 test are relatively straightforward (as indeed are many non-parametric tests). As the deviation of the observed frequencies from the expected frequencies increases, the χ^2 statistic will similarly increase in magnitude. The χ^2 distribution, explained in Chapter 4, is not similar in structure to parametric distributions, e.g. the standardised normal or t distributions. When the observed values equal the expected values, the χ^2 statistic is equal to zero and the null hypothesis is accepted. As for the standardised normal and other parametric distributions, a critical value of χ^2 exists which, when equalled or exceeded allows the analyst to conclude that the null hypothesis cannot be accepted. At this stage, one can no longer conclude that the sample data conforms to the description of frequencies in the population that is described in the null hypothesis. It is apparent from this that the selection of the critical χ^2 value is an important stage in the process of statistical hypothesis testing using the χ^2 test. As in the t and F distributions, the shape of the χ^2 distribution is dependent on the number of degrees of freedom, as described in Chapter 4. In a one-sample χ^2 test, the number of degrees of freedom is calculated by subtracting 1 from the total number of categories described by the variable.

In Example 7.9, a one-sample χ^2 test may be employed to evaluate the effects of colour on the acceptability of a mouthwash formulation. The first step in the calculation process involves the definition of the expected frequency in each category. This value is determined by the null hypothesis, which, in this example, states that there should be no colour preference amongst volunteers. Therefore, according to this hypothesis the number of responses in each category should be equal. In light of this, Table 7.3 may be rewritten to include a row that describes expected frequencies (Table 7.4).

Table 7.4 Observed number of volunteers who preferred various colours of mouthwash and the number of volunteers who would be expected to prefer each colour (according to the null hypothesis)

	Red	Green	Blue	Yellow
Observed frequency	55	73	36	36
Expected frequency	50	50	50	50

The χ^2 statistic is computed as follows:

$$\chi^2 = \sum \frac{(O_f - E_f)^2}{E_f}$$

$$= \frac{(55 - 50)^2}{50} + \frac{(73 - 50)^2}{50} + \frac{(36 - 50)^2}{50} + \frac{(36 - 50)^2}{50} = 18.9$$

(vi) Interpret the outcome of the statistical analysis

The critical value of the χ^2 statistic associated with a significance level of 0.05 and 3 df is 7.81 (Appendix 3). As the calculated value of the χ^2 statistic is 18.9, we may therefore conclude that it is improbable that the observed frequencies could be derived from the population described by the null hypothesis, i.e. the null hypothesis is not accepted. Consequently, there is a preference for colour in the mouthwash formulations among the volunteers who participated in the product acceptability study.

It is important to highlight that, in a one-sample χ^2 test, the expected frequencies of each category do not have to be equal. The calculation of the χ^2 statistic in this scenario simply involves the use of individual expected frequency values. The use of the one-sample χ^2 test under these conditions is described in Example 7.10.

EXAMPLE 7.10 *In a survey commissioned by a local health authority it was reported that the usage of prescribed items for the treatment of gastric disorders was as shown in Table 7.5. As part of an auditing process, general practitioners within an urban practice have instructed the practice manager to perform a similar survey of their prescribing habits for the treatment of gastric disorders. For 200 patients who were prescribed medicines for the treatment of gastric disorders, the data shown in Table 7.6 were recorded. Is there a difference in the pre-scribing habits of the general practitioners in the urban practice and those described in the survey commissioned by the health authority?*

This question may be answered in the following fashion.

Table 7.5 Results from a local survey concerning the prescribing of medicines for the treatment of gastric disorders by general practitioners

Category of medicine	Percentage of prescription items
Antacids	15
H_2 receptor antagonists	30
Antibiotics	18
Proton pump inhibitors	37

Table 7.6 Results from a survey concerning the prescribing of medicines for the treatment of gastric disorders by general practitioners operating within an urban practice

Category of medicine	Percentage of prescription items
Antacids	18
H_2 receptor antagonists	40
Antibiotics	2
Proton pump inhibitors	40

(i) State the null hypothesis

As before, the null hypothesis states that there is no difference in the prescribing habits of the urban practice and those recorded by the health authority. Therefore, the null hypothesis may be expressed in the following way:

H_0:   antacids 15%, H_2 receptor antagonists 30%,
antibiotics 18%, proton pump inhibitors 37%

(ii) State the alternative hypothesis

The alternative hypothesis states that there is a difference in the prescribing habits of the urban practice and those recorded by the health authority. Therefore, the frequencies of response in each category will be statistically dissimilar to those described in the null hypothesis (i.e. the expected values).

(iii) State the level of significance

In this example, it is assumed that the level of significance (α) is 0.05.

(iv) Select the statistical test

In this example, a set of sample data (relating to the prescribing habits of general practitioners in a large urban practice) is being compared to a hypothetical population (the prescribing habits of general practitioners recorded by the health authority). The data are nominal in nature and therefore the most relevant statistical test is a one-sample χ^2 test.

(v) Calculate the χ^2 statistic

The data are first collated into tabular form in terms of the observed and expected frequencies (Table 7.7). Then the χ^2 statistic is computed

Table 7.7 Summary of the observed and expected frequencies described in Example 7.10

Frequency	Antacids	H_2 receptor antagonists	Antibiotics	Proton pump inhibitors
Observed (urban practice)	15	30	18	37
Expected (national survey)	18	40	2	40

as follows:

$$\chi^2 = \sum \frac{(O_f - E_f)^2}{E_f}$$

$$= \frac{(18-15)^2}{15} + \frac{(40-30)^2}{30} + \frac{(2-18)^2}{18} + \frac{(40-37)^2}{37} = 18.39$$

(vi) Interpret the outcome of the statistical analysis

The critical value of the χ^2 statistic associated with a significance level of 0.05 and 3 df is 7.81 (Appendix 3). The calculated value of the χ^2 statistic is 18.39. Therefore, as the calculated χ^2 statistic is greater than the critical χ^2 statistic, it is improbable that the observed frequencies could be derived from the population described by the null hypothesis, i.e. the null hypothesis is not accepted. Accordingly, the prescribing habits of general practitioners in an urban practice differ from the national prescribing habits.

7.2.2 Binomial test

The use of the binomial distribution to calculate the probability of an event has been discussed in Chapter 4 and therefore in this chapter we consider only the use of the binomial test for one-sample statistical hypothesis testing. Typically the binomial test is employed for the analysis of data that has been recorded in two categories, whereas the χ^2 test is used when there are three or more categories. Furthermore, the usefulness of the χ^2 test is limited whenever the expected frequency of one of the categories is ≤5. In these circumstances, the binomial test offers a statistically valid option.

In a binomial analysis there are only two categories and, consequently, whenever the probability of one category is known, the probability of the other category may be easily determined. The use of the binomial test to resolve a one-sample test is illustrated in Example 7.11.

EXAMPLE 7.11 *Masking the taste of solutions of penicillins for oral administration is a problem for the pharmaceutical formulator. A pharmaceutical company has developed a penicillin solution (125 mg per 5 mL) for oral administration and has incorporated sorbitol in the formulation to reduce the bitter taste of the medication. However, following consultation with a manufacturer of food-grade flavours, the pharmaceutical company has been advised to incorporate a flavour in the formulation to enhance the taste-masking properties of sorbitol. Therefore, a second formulation was developed containing an orange flavour. A panel of 12 volunteers was asked to denote their preference for either the formulation containing the orange flavour or the formulation without this flavour. The outcome of the study is shown in Table 7.8. Using an appropriate statistical method determine whether there is a preference for either formulation.*

The above problem may be readily resolved in stepwise fashion.

(i) State the null hypothesis

The null hypothesis states that there is no preference for either formulation. Consequently, the probability of selecting either formulation is the same, i.e.

H_0: $p = 0.5$ (and accordingly, $q = 0.5$).

(ii) State the alternative hypothesis

The alternative hypothesis states that there is a preference for one of the formulations among the volunteers engaged in the study. Therefore, the recorded frequencies in each category will be different:

H_a: $p \neq 0.5$ (and accordingly, $q \neq 0.5$).

(iii) State the level of significance

In this example, it is assumed that the level of significance (α) is 0.05.

(iv) Select the statistical test

In this study the data are organised into two categories and are nominal in nature. Analysis of categorical, nominal data may be performed

Table 7.8 Number of recorded preferences for two penicillin formulations in a taste acceptability study involving 12 volunteers

Orange-flavoured formulation	10
Formulation without orange flavour	2

using, among others, the one-sample χ^2 test and the binomial test. However, the binomial test is preferred for the above example because it involves two discrete categories within a single variable.

(v) Designate the number of tails

The interpretation of the binomial test requires knowledge of the number of tails associated with the experimental design. As in previous examples, a one-tailed test is utilised if there is a predisposition to one outcome of the study, whereas a two-tailed test is used if there are two possible outcomes. In Example 7.11 no preference for a particular outcome has been stated before the collection of data. There are therefore two possible outcomes as the frequency associated with the orange-flavoured formulation may be greater or less than the frequency associated with the unflavoured formulation.

(vi) Conduct and interpret the binomial test

In this example, no calculations are required to determine whether the null hypothesis is accepted or rejected. Only knowledge of the total number of observations (N), the expected probability, p (as defined by the null hypothesis) and the smaller (observed) frequency (x) is required. In this example, $N = 10$, $p = 0.05$ and $X = 2$. The probability of recording 2 observations in one category out of a total of 12 observations is determined from the table that portrays the probability associated with observing defined X values within the binomial test (Appendix 4). One point of caution in the interpretation of probabilities from his table is that the table refers to the probabilities associated with a one-tailed event. To derive the probabilities associated with defined values of x within a two-tailed design, the probabilities in the binomial table are simply multiplied by 2.

In this current example, when $N = 12$ and $X = 2$, the associated probability (derived from the binomial table for $p = 0.5$) is 0.019. As this is a two-tailed test, this value is doubled and consequently, the probability is 0.038. As this is less than the pre-selected level of significance (0.05), the null hypothesis is not accepted and, accordingly, there is a preference for the formulation containing the orange flavour.

The use of the binomial table is an abridged method by which the above data may be statistically analysed in rapid fashion. It may be useful to the reader to explain how the above problem may be answered using the binomial calculation. This method has been described in Chapter 4 and the explanation will therefore serve as useful revision.

The probability of a defined number of observations in one category following sampling from a binomial distribution may be calculated using the following equation:

$$P(X) = \binom{N}{X} p^X q^{N-X} = \left(\frac{N!}{X!(N-X)!}\right) p^X q^{N-X}$$

where $P(X)$ is the probability of recording X observations in one category of the binomial distribution, N is the size of the sample, P^X is the probability of recording X items in a sample and q^{N-X} is the probability of recording a sample with $N-X$ observations.

This is a two-tailed study and therefore we wish to calculate the probability of the data diverging from the expected value in either direction. In this example, this translates to the probability of recording 10, 11 or 12 and additionally, 0, 1, and 2 observations in one category, i.e.

$$P(X \geqslant 10, X \leqslant 2)$$
$$= P(X = 10) + P(X = 11) + P(X = 12)$$
$$+ P(X = 0) + P(X = 1) + P(X = 2)$$

The probability of each of the above events is calculated individually using the binomial equation and these probabilities are then added together to return the overall probability:

- $P(X = 12)$

$$P(12) = \left(\frac{12!}{12!(12-12)!}\right) 0.5^{12} 0.5^{12-12} = 0.000\,24$$

- $P(X = 11)$

$$P(11) = \left(\frac{12!}{11!(12-11)!}\right) 0.5^{11} 0.5^{12-11} = 0.002\,93$$

- $P(X = 10)$

$$P(10) = \left(\frac{12!}{10!(12-10)!}\right) 0.5^{10} 0.5^{12-10} = 0.016\,11$$

- $P(X = 0)$

$$P(0) = \left(\frac{12!}{0!(12-0)!}\right) 0.5^{0} 0.5^{12} = 0.000\,24$$

- $P(X = 1)$

$$P(1) = \left(\frac{12!}{1!(12-1)!}\right) 0.5^{1} 0.5^{12-1} = 0.002\,93$$

- $P(X = 2)$

$$P(2) = \left(\frac{12!}{2!(12-2)!}\right) 0.5^{2} 0.5^{12-2} = 0.016\,11$$

The overall probability of recording both 10 or more observations and 2 or fewer observations with a category of a binomial population is:

$$P(X \geqslant 10, X \leqslant 2)$$
$$= P(0.01611) + P(0.00293) + P(0.00024) + P(0.00024)$$
$$+ P(0.00293) + P(0.01611)$$
$$P(X \geqslant 10, X \leqslant 2) = 0.03856$$

Importantly, when $p = 0.5$ (and hence $q = 0.5$), there is a shortcut formula for the calculation of the above problem, as follows:

$$P(X) = \left(\frac{N!}{X!(N-X)!} \right) p^N$$

The probabilities of observing the individual events may be calculated using this equation and summed, as before.

One further issue that requires clarification is the difference between the hypotheses associated with one- and two-tailed binomial tests. As previously mentioned, the two-tailed test is employed whenever there is no prior knowledge of the preferred outcome of the experiment. Therefore, the study has two possible outcomes. Conversely, in a one-tailed study, there is speculation about the directed outcome of the study, i.e. one particular outcome is under statistical analysis. Example 7.11 could have been designed as a one-tailed study, in which the point under statistical debate was simply whether the inclusion of the orange flavour increased patient acceptability. Indeed, in this example, this would be a more sensible statistical strategy to evaluate. In a one-tailed binomial test, the null and alternative hypotheses are as follows:

$$H_0: \ p \leqslant 0.5$$
$$H_a: \ p > 0.5$$

Under these conditions, it may be observed that the inclusion of an orange flavour increased the acceptability of the solution.

7.2.2.1 Use of the binomial test for large sample sizes

Earlier in this section it was stated that one of the advantages of the binomial test for the analysis of nominal discrete dichotomous data was its usefulness for the analysis of studies involving small sample sizes. It is important to remember that the binomial test may also be applied when the sample numbers are large. To employ the binomial equation under these conditions is extremely tortuous and time consuming and, consequently, a normal approximation to the binomial test is employed. This point has already been discussed in Chapter 4, but here the use of the normal approximation to the binomial test will be illustrated using a pharmaceutically relevant example. In this approach, from knowledge of the number of samples, the expected probability and the number of recorded observations, a z statistic may be calculated and the probability associated with the number of recorded observations interpreted using the standardised normal distribution. To illustrate this approach, the scenario described in Example 7.11 will be employed, but now the output has been modified to include a larger number of volunteers.

EXAMPLE 7.12 *Masking the taste of solutions of penicillins for oral administration is a problem for the pharmaceutical formulator. A pharmaceutical company has developed a penicillin solution (125 mg per 5 mL) for oral administration and has incorporated sorbitol within the formulation to reduce the bitter taste of the medication. However, following consultation with a manufacturer of food-grade flavours, the pharmaceutical company has been advised to incorporate a flavour in the formulation to enhance the taste-masking properties of sorbitol. Therefore, a second formulation was developed containing an orange flavour. A panel of 50 volunteers was asked to denote their preference for either the formulation containing the orange flavour or the formulation without this flavour. The outcome of the study is shown in Table 7.9. Using an appropriate statistical method, determine whether the acceptability of the penicillin solution has been improved by inclusion of the orange flavour.*

The solution to this problem will again be addressed in a stepwise fashion.

(i) State the null hypothesis

The null hypothesis states that there is no preference for either formulation. Consequently, the probability of selecting either formulation is equal, i.e.

$$H_0: \ p \leqslant 0.5$$

(ii) State the alternative hypothesis

The alternative hypothesis states that the volunteers demonstrate a preference for the orange-flavoured formulation. Therefore, the recorded

Table 7.9 Number of recorded preferences for two penicillin formulations in a taste acceptability study involving 50 volunteers

Orange-flavoured formulation	35
Formulation without orange flavour	15

frequencies in the category associated with the orange-flavoured formulation will be greater than for the unflavoured formulation:

$$H_a{:}p > 0.5$$

(iii) State the level of significance

In this example, it is assumed that the level of significance (α) is 0.05.

(iv) Select the statistical test

In this study the normal approximation to the binomial test is employed because the data are nominal, discrete and dichotomous. As a result of the large sample size, the probability is more easily calculated by the use of the normal approximation to the binomial test; however, if sufficient computational facilities are available, the binomial equation may be used to answer this statistical problem.

(v) Designate the number of tails

The alternative hypothesis of this study has been predicated on there being only one outcome of interest to the company that is sponsoring the clinical study, i.e. does the inclusion of an orange flavour increase the preference of volunteers for the formulation. Therefore, this is an example of a one-tailed test.

(vi) Conduct and interpret the binomial test

Mathematically, the normal approximation to the binomial test is described as follows:

$$z = \frac{(X - Np_0)}{\sqrt{(Np_0 q_0)}}$$

where X is the number of recorded observations in a defined category, N is the sample size, and p_0 and q_0 are the probabilities associated with recording observations in each category as defined by the null hypothesis. In the current example, $X = 35$, $N = 50$, $p_0 = 0.5$ and $q_0 = 0.5$. Therefore

$$z = \frac{(X - Np_0)}{\sqrt{(Np_0 q_0)}} = \frac{35 - (50 \times 0.5)}{\sqrt{(50 \times 0.5 \times 0.5)}} = 2.83$$

The critical value of z for a one-tailed test is $+ 1.65$. Therefore, as the calculated z statistic exceeds this critical value, we can conclude that the null hypothesis is invalid. A z value of $+ 2.83$ is equivalent to a probability of 0.0023. Consequently, there is a preference for the formulation containing the orange flavour.

Of course in the above example, in which the size of the recorded

Table 7.10 The number of observed and expected preferences for two penicillin formulations in a taste acceptability study involving 50 volunteers

	Observed	Expected
Orange-flavoured formulation	35	50
Formulation without orange flavour	15	50

sample is large, the one-sample χ^2 test could have been used to resolve the statistical problem. The observed and expected frequencies for this example are shown in Table 7.10. Accordingly (assuming the same null and alternative hypotheses, level of significance, etc.), the χ^2 statistic may be calculated:

$$\chi^2 = \sum \frac{(O_f - E_f)^2}{E_f} = \frac{(35 - 25)^2}{25} + \frac{(15 - 25)^2}{25} = 8.00$$

In this example, the critical value of χ^2 (relating to 1 df, $\alpha = 0.05$) is 3.84. The probability associated with a χ^2 value of 8.00 is between 0.01 and 0.001 and, accordingly the null hypothesis is rejected. Therefore, in both respects, namely the decision to reject the null hypothesis and the calculated probability of recording 35 observations in one category (out of a sample of 50 volunteers), the one-sample χ^2 test is in close agreement with the normal approximation to the binomial test. Of course the χ^2 statistic is a squared term. Consequently, the square root of the calculated χ^2 statistic and the calculated z statistic are identical ($\sqrt{8.00} = 2.83$).

7.2.2.2 Power of the binomial test

The power of the binomial test may be readily calculated if the following information is known: the level of significance, the sample size and whether the experimental design is one- or two-tailed. The calculations of the power for one- and two-tailed situations are different and so they will be described separately, using Example 7.11, in which 12 volunteers were employed in the study, as an appropriate example.

In the one-tailed scenario, the null and alternative hypotheses are as follows:

H_0: $p \leqslant 0.5$

H_a: $p > 0.5$

To calculate the power of the study, the critical value, i.e. the smallest value of the number of recorded observations in one category (X) that is associated with a probability value that is either equal to or less than the specified level of significance (0.05), must be determined. To perform this, it is useful to calculate the probability of recording each value of

X in the study (Table 7.11), using the binomial equation:

$$P(X) = \left(\frac{N!}{X!(N-X)!}\right) p^X q^{N-X}$$

As may be observed in Table 7.11, the smallest value of X that is associated with a probability of 0.05 or less (the defined α value of the experiment) is 10. At this point a question that many students commonly ask is 'Why is 2 not the smallest value of X that has an associated probability of 0.05 or less?'. This is a common misconception and one that is raised without undue attention to the null and alternative hypotheses that are associated with a one-tailed study. It should be remembered that the null and alternative hypotheses stated that $p \leqslant 0.5$ and $p > 0.5$ and therefore, in this study we are concerned with values of X that are greater than half the sample size, i.e. 7–12.

From the above table, the critical value of X is 10. The next step involves the calculation of the probability associated with this X value:

$$p = \frac{X}{N} = \frac{10}{12} = 0.83$$

Using this p value within the binomial equation, the probabilities of recording the critical value and values greater than the critical value are calculated and summed to determine the power of the study.

- $X = 10$

$$P(X) = \left(\frac{N!}{X!(N-X)!}\right) p^X q^{N-X} = \left(\frac{12!}{10!(12-10)!}\right) 0.83^{10} 0.17^2 = 0.296$$

Table 7.11 Probabilities of recording a defined number of observations (X) within a defined category in a binomial test (sample size $N = 12$, $p = 0.05$)

Observed value (X)	Probability of recording the observed value, $P(X)$
0	0.0002
1	0.0029
2	0.0161
3	0.0537
4	0.1209
5	0.1934
6	0.2256
7	0.1934
8	0.1209
9	0.0537
10	0.0161
11	0.0029
12	0.0002

- $X = 11$

$$P(X) = \left(\frac{N!}{X!(N-X)!}\right) p^X q^{N-X} = \left(\frac{12!}{11!(12-11)!}\right) 0.83^{11} 0.17^1 = 0.263$$

- $X = 12$

$$P(X) = \left(\frac{N!}{X!(N-X)!}\right) p^X q^{N-X} = \left(\frac{12!}{12!(12-12)!}\right) 0.83^{12} 0.17^0 = 0.107$$

The overall power of the study is obtained by adding together the individual values, as calculated above. The power of the study is therefore $\geqslant 0.107 + 0.263 + 0.296 = 0.67$.

The power of a two-tailed binomial test may be calculated in a similar way. In this case, there are two critical values at either end of the distribution. Using the calculated probability (e.g. $p = 0.83$), the probabilities of observing X values of 0, 1, 2, 10, 11 and 12 may be calculated and summed to provide an overall power of the test.

The power of a binomial test may also be calculated using the normal approximation whenever the sample size is large and, additionally, whenever p is not close to 0 or 1. Under these circumstances, the power (P) of a one-tailed binomial test is calculated using the following equations:

- when H_0: $p \leqslant p_0$ and H_a: $p > p_0$

$$P = \left[z > \left(\frac{p_0 - p}{\sqrt{pq/N}}\right) + z_\alpha \sqrt{\frac{p_0 q_0}{pq}} \right]$$

- when H_0: $p \geqslant p_0$ and H_a: $p < p_0$

$$P = \left[z < \left(\frac{p_0 - p}{\sqrt{pq/N}}\right) - z_\alpha \sqrt{\frac{p_0 q_0}{pq}} \right]$$

where p_0 and q_0 are the hypothesised probabilities, as defined by the null hypothesis; p and q are the actual probabilities; and z_α is the z statistic at a defined level of probability (α) associated with a one-tailed outcome.

The power (P) of a two-tailed binomial test may be calculated using a combination of the above formulations:

$$P = \left[z < \left(\frac{p_0 - p}{\sqrt{pq/N}}\right) - z_\alpha \sqrt{\frac{p_0 q_0}{pq}} \right] + \left[z > \left(\frac{p_0 - p}{\sqrt{pq/N}}\right) + z_\alpha \sqrt{\frac{p_0 q_0}{pq}} \right]$$

In the above equation, all symbols have been defined previously, but z_α denotes the z statistic at a defined level of probability (α) associated with a two-tailed outcome.

The calculation of the power of the study described in Example 7.12 is described below. In this, the null and alternative hypotheses are

$p \leqslant p_0$ and $p > p_0$, the study is one-tailed and the chosen level of significance is 0.05. Furthermore, the probability associated with the flavoured formulation is 0.7 (35/50) and the probability associated with the unflavoured formulation is 0.3 (15/50). Therefore:

$$P = \left[z > \left(\frac{p_0 - p}{\sqrt{pq/N}}\right) + z_\alpha \sqrt{\frac{p_0 q_0}{pq}}\right]$$

$$= \left[z > \left(\frac{0.5 - 0.7}{\sqrt{(0.7 \times 0.3)/50}}\right) + 1.65 \sqrt{\frac{0.5 \times 0.5}{0.7 \times 0.3}}\right]$$

$$= z > -1.28$$

$$= z < +1.28$$

so the power $\cong 0.90$.

If the study had been two-tailed, the power could have been calculated in a similar fashion, but in this case $z_\alpha = 1.96$ (the value associated with 0.05 in a two-tailed study).

$$P = \left[z < \left(\frac{0.5 - 0.7}{\sqrt{(0.7 \times 0.3)50}}\right) - 1.96 \sqrt{\frac{0.5 \times 0.5}{0.7 \times 0.3}}\right]$$

$$+ \left[z > \left(\frac{0.5 - 0.7}{\sqrt{(0.7 \times 0.3)/50}}\right) + 1.96 \sqrt{\frac{0.5 \times 0.5}{0.7 \times 0.3}}\right]$$

$$= (z < -5.23) + (z > -0.95)$$

This may also be expressed as: $P = (z > 5.23) + (z < 0.95)$, which, by consultation with the standardised normal distribution, may be trans­lated into probability values. Thus, $z > 5.23$ is equivalent to a probability of 0.0000, whereas $z < 0.95$ translates to a probability of approximately 0.83. The overall power of the study is 0.83.

These equations may be employed in a related fashion to calculate the required sample size of a study or, alternatively, the minimum detectable difference that the statistical method may resolve. In the former scenario, the power and α are defined and a knowledge of p and q is derived from a preliminary experiment and consequently, N is determined. Similarly, knowledge of the power, N and α will allow estimation of the minimum detectable difference.

7.2.3 Kolmogorov–Smirnov test

As previously explained, the binomial and one-sample χ^2 tests are used for the analysis of primarily nominal data. The Kolmogorov–Smirnov test is another one-sample test that examines the 'goodness of fit' between sample values and a theoretical distribution, i.e. the test examines whether or not the sample data could have been derived from a theoretical cumulative distribution. Typically, the data that is examined using the Kolmogorov–Smirnov test is ordinal in nature, i.e. there is a hierarchical distribution. In a similar fashion to the previous non-parametric one-sample tests, the null hypothesis defines the nature of the hypothetical population and the test statistically compares the sample data to the theoretical data. Because of the ordered, hierarchical nature of the data, the null hypothesis defines the expected cumulative frequency distribution and, consequently, the observed and expected cumulative frequency distributions are statistically compared using this test. The nature and mechanics of the Kolmogorov–Smirnov one-sample test are illustrated in Example 7.13.

EXAMPLE 7.13 *Pharmaceutically acceptable dyes are frequently included in veterinary aerosol formulations both to visualise the location of the dose on the animal after spraying and, additionally, to enhance the visual acceptability of the preparation to the farmer or veterinary surgeon. An antibiotic-containing aerosol has been formulated for veterinary applications and the company is unsure about the shade of red that would be most acceptable to the end users. Therefore, the aerosol preparation has been formulated to contain different shades of red by the incorporation of a range of concentrations of the dye, Sudan red. Thirty farmers were asked to spray each formulation on to the backs of their pigs and to record their visually preferred formulation. The results of this consumer study are shown in Table 7.12. Using an appropriate statistical method, determine whether the farmers demonstrate a colour preference for different shades of red.*

The above problem may be readily resolved in stepwise fashion.

Table 7.12 Number of recorded preferences for five antibiotic aerosol formulations containing different concentrations of Sudan red

Concentration of Sudan red (μg/mL)	Number of preferences
0.01	6
0.05	14
0.1	4
0.5	5
1.0	1

(i) State the null hypothesis

The null hypothesis states that there is no preference for a particular shade of red. Consequently, the probability of selecting any one formulation is the same, i.e.

H_0: $p = 0.2$

(ii) State the alternative hypothesis

The alternative hypothesis states that there is a preference for defined shades of red in the formulations. Therefore, the recorded frequencies in each category will be different to the hypothesised value.

H_a: $p \neq 0.2$

(iii) State the level of significance

In this example, it is assumed that the level of significance (α) is 0.05.

(iv) Select the statistical test

In this study the data are subdivided into five categories and therefore a non-parametric method is required. Furthermore, the statistical analysis will require a one-sample test as the differences between sample data and a theoretical population are under examination. Importantly, although the data are divided into discrete categories, there is a hierarchical relationship between the categories (increasing dye concentration and increasing the intensity of red colour), indicative of ordinal data. In light of these details, the most appropriate test to evaluate the null hypothesis is the Kolmogorov–Smirnov goodness-of-fit test.

(v) Designate the number of tails

The alternative hypothesis has stated that the probability associated with each of the categories is not equal to 0.2, the hypothetical frequency of each category as specified by the null hypothesis. As before, there are two outcomes by which the null hypothesis may be rejected, i.e. $p > 0.2$ or $p < 0.2$ and, accordingly, this study is two-tailed.

(vi) Perform the Kolmogorov–Smirnov test

The mechanics of the Kolmogorov–Smirnov test are very straightforward. The key steps in the execution of this test are:

- *Calculate the expected frequencies (as defined in the null hypothesis). In this example, the null hypothesis has stated that the likelihood (and hence* probability) of selecting any of the categories is the same ($p = 0.2$). To define the expected frequency of each category, the total number of participants in the study (30) is multiplied by this probability. As in the χ^2 test, the expected number of observations should be tabulated. Furthermore, as the Kolmogorov–Smirnov test involves analysis of the cumulative frequency distribution, the cumulative data should be tabulated.

- *Determine the Kolmogorov–Smirnov test statistic.* If the null hypothesis is valid, the differences between the observed and expected frequencies will be small. The next step in the execution of the test involves subtraction of the expected number of observations from the number of observed values. The largest difference is referred to as the *Kolmogorov–Smirnov test statistic* and is used to evaluate the validity of the null hypothesis. The relevant calculations for Example 7.13 are shown in Table 7.13.

Alternatively, the differences between the observed and expected frequencies may be expressed as a decimal fraction, as illustrated in Table 7.14, in which both the observed and expected frequencies are divided by N, the sample size.

The test statistic is the maximum calculated difference between either the observed and expected cumulative frequencies or, alternatively, between the fractional observed and expected frequencies. From Tables 7.13 and 7.14, the test statistics are 8 and 0.27.

The reader may wonder why two test statistics have been calculated for the one study. The reason is that the table concerning the critical values for the Kolmogorov–Smirnov test for discrete data may be expressed in two ways, and the interpretation of both types of presentation will be discussed.

Table 7.13 Recorded and expected preferences for five antibiotic aerosol formulations containing a range of concentrations of Sudan red

Concentration of Sudan red ($\mu g/mL$)	Frequency				
	Observed (sample)	Expected ($p = 0.2$)	Observed (cumulative)	Expected (cumulative)	Difference[a]
0.01	6	6	6	6	0
0.05	14	6	20	12	8
0.1	4	6	24	18	6
0.5	5	6	29	24	5
1.0	1	6	30	30	0

[a] Difference between the recorded number of observations (sample data) and expected number of observations (defined by the null hypothesis)

Table 7.14 Recorded and expected fractional preferences for five antibiotic aerosol formulations containing a range of concentrations of Sudan red

Concentration of Sudan red ($\mu g/mL$)	Frequency				
	Observed (sample)	Expected ($p = 0.2$)	Observed fraction (cumulative)	Expected fraction (cumulative)	Difference[a]
0.01	6	6	0.20	0.20	0.00
0.05	14	6	0.67	0.40	0.27
0.1	4	6	0.80	0.60	0.20
0.5	5	6	0.97	0.80	0.17
1.0	1	6	1.00	1.00	0.00

[a] Difference between the recorded fraction of observations (sample data) and expected fraction of observations (defined by the null hypothesis)

(vii) Interpret the calculated critical value for the Kolmogorov–Smirnov test

As described above, two critical values for the Kolmogorov–Smirnov test may be calculated. In the first, the 'raw' maximum difference between the observed and expected cumulative was calculated (8). To interpret this value the number of data (sample size), the chosen level of significance and the number of categories (k) are required. With knowledge of these, a critical value may be defined. As before, if the calculated statistic (maximum difference) is equal to or greater than the critical statistic the null hypothesis is rejected in favour of the alternative hypothesis. From Appendix 5 it may be observed that when $k = 5$ and the number of samples is 30 the critical value (when $\alpha = 0.05$) is 7. As the test statistic exceeds this critical value, it may be concluded that the null hypothesis cannot be accepted. Therefore, the participants of the study demonstrate a preference for the intensity of red colour of this pharmaceutical aerosol. Interestingly, it may be observed that in this format the Kolmogorov–Smirnov table provides critical values for data sets in which the number of samples is a multiple of the number of classes. In this current example N is a multiple of k and hence identification of the critical value is relatively straightforward. When N is not a multiple of k, the critical values are obtained for N values that are greater and less than the number of samples employed in the study, and the larger critical value derived from the table is used for the purpose of the analysis. To overcome this inconvenience, the critical values of the Kolmogorov–Smirnov statistic are expressed as the difference in the fractional observed and fractional expected frequencies (Appendix 6). Referring to this table it may be observed that, for a sample size of 30, a fractional difference of 0.24 or greater results in the rejection of the null hypothesis. Therefore, as the calculated fractional difference was 0.27, the null hypothesis presented in Example 7.13 is rejected and the alternative hypothesis accepted.

Theoretically, the data in Example 7.13 could have been statistically analysed using a one-sample χ^2 test. The critical χ^2 statistic calculated is this way is 15.7. The critical χ^2 statistic (4 df) is 9.49 and consequently the null hypothesis is rejected. In certain situations, there may be disagreement between the conclusions derived from the Kolmogorov–Smirnov and χ^2 tests for the analysis of ordinal one-sample data. Typically, the χ^2 test is not as sensitive as the Kolmogorov–Smirnov test and, as a result, the chances of making a type II (β) error, i.e. failing to reject the null hypothesis when it is indeed false, are increased. Consequently, it is important to select the Kolmogorov–Smirnov test for the analysis of ordinal (hierarchical) data.

Another important application of the Kolmogorov–Smirnov test is in the analysis of small samples. As the reader is aware, the use of the χ^2 test is limited by the size of the expected frequencies within each category. It has been stated that when the number of degrees of freedom of a study is 1 the expected frequency in each category should be at least 5, whereas if the number of degrees of freedom is two or greater, the expected frequency should be equal to or greater than 5 in at least 20% of all categories and all expected frequencies should be greater than 1. Under these circumstances, the χ^2 test may only be used if categories are combined to increase the expected frequency; however, in so doing, the nature of the analysis is often altered. The use of the Kolmogorov–Smirnov test is not limited in this fashion, which highlights the fact that it has greater power than the χ^2 test.

One final point of interest concerning the Kolmogorov–Smirnov test is the effect of the order of data on the outcome of the statistical analysis. Consider the case in which the responses from the farmers were different and hence, were organised into a different order (Table 7.15).

The largest calculated difference between the observed and expected fractional frequencies in this case is 0.20. The critical value of the Kolmogorov–Smirnov test statistic for a sample size of 30 and a 0.05 level of significance is 0.24 (Appendix 6). As the calculated value is lower than the critical value it may be concluded that the null hypothesis is accepted. There is no preference for colour of aerosol spray amongst the participants of the study. This highlights the dependence of the Kolmogorov–Smirnov test on the order of the data within each category.

Table 7.15 Recorded and expected fractional preferences for five antibiotic aerosol formulations containing a range of concentrations of Sudan red

Concentration of Sudan red (μg/mL)	Frequency				
	Observed (sample)	Expected ($p = 0.2$)	Observed fraction (cumulative)	Expected fraction (cumulative)	Difference[a]
0.01	6	6	0.20	0.20	0.00
0.05	4	6	0.33	0.40	0.07
0.1	14	6	0.80	0.60	0.20
0.5	5	6	0.97	0.80	0.17
1.0	1	6	1.00	1.00	0.00

[a] Difference between the recorded fraction of observations (sample data) and expected fraction of observations (defined by the null hypothesis)

7.3 Conclusions

In this chapter, the design and mechanics of one-sample statistical hypothesis testing have been described. The main points highlighted in this chapter were as follows:

- One-sample tests are employed to discern whether or not data have been sampled from a hypothetical distribution. In many cases, this theoretical distribution is described using a single parameter, e.g. the mean, however, in other cases, e.g. the Kolmogorov–Smirnov test, the theoretical cumulative frequency distribution forms the basis of the one-sample test. One-sample tests are often referred to as 'goodness-of-fit' tests.
- When the statistical analyst is presented with data from a one-sample experimental design, the most important decision that must be made is the choice of the most appropriate statistical method. One-sample statistical tests may be subdivided into either parametric or non-parametric tests. Where appropriate, the use of parametric tests is preferred over their non-parametric equivalents, as the chances of a type II error will be reduced. However, before selecting a parametric test, the statistical analyst must be assured of the relevance of the data collected during the study to the statistical model associated with parametric tests. In particular, parametric tests require that the data have been independently sampled from a normally distributed population and that the data are measured in an interval or ratio scale. If these assumptions are invalid, non-parametric one-sample statistical tests should be employed.
- There are two parametric one-sample statistical tests, the z test and t test. The z test is used when the variance of the population is known, whereas the t test is employed when the variance of the population is estimated from the sample data. When the sample size is large, the analysis of data using the t test and the z test will produce equivalent results.

- Three non-parametric one-sample tests were described in this chapter: the binomial test, the χ^2 test and the Kolmogorov–Smirnov test. The former two tests are primarily (but not exclusively) employed for the analysis of nominal data whereas the latter test is used for the analysis of ordinal data. The binomial test is preferred whenever there are only two categories and, importantly, may be engaged whenever the sample size is too small for the application of the χ^2 test. The χ^2 test may be used if the data has been collected in discrete categories (two or more), but there are limitations as to the use of this test whenever the expected frequencies in the categories are small. The Kolmogorov–Smirnov test is employed to estimate whether the cumulative frequency of sample data differs from the cumulative frequency distribution estimated from the null hypothesis. Importantly, this test may be used whenever the sample size is small or when the expected frequencies in any category are small enough to prohibit the use of the χ^2 test. The Kolmogorov–Smirnov test is often considered to be the most powerful goodness-of-fit test for the analysis of ordinal (hierarchical) type data.

8

Statistical hypothesis testing for two independent samples

One of the most common statistical procedures employed in the pharmaceutical and related sciences is the examination of differences between two sets of sample data, i.e. whether or not the two populations whose properties are estimated by the sample statistics differ from one another. There are two types of two-sample experimental designs, *independent* and *paired*. Statistical hypothesis testing for two independent samples forms the focus of this chapter; methods using two paired samples are considered in Chapter 9. At this stage it is important to both define and explain the significance of the term *independent*. Independent samples may be defined as sets of data that have no relationship with each other; the converse is true for *paired* samples. As may be expected, statistical hypothesis testing for two independent samples may be performed using either parametric or non-parametric methods. In this chapter, the design and mechanics of two parametric methods – the z test and the t test (frequently referred to as Student's t test) – and three non-parametric methods – the Fisher exact probability test, the χ^2 test and the Mann–Whitney U test – will be explained, again with the aid of pharmaceutical examples.

8.1 Parametric statistical tests for two independent samples

8.1.1 Background

The uses of the z and t tests for two independent samples are in many ways similar in operation and assumptions to their one-sample counterparts. In the one-sample scenario, the sample mean is compared to a hypothetical mean value, whereas in the two-sample tests the magnitude of the difference between two mean values, derived from the sample data, is under investigation. As the size of the difference between the two mean values increases, so does the likelihood that the two sets of data were not derived from a single population. In order to understand the operation of the z and t tests for two independent samples, it is important to be fully aware of the theory and mechanics of the tests and furthermore, the similarities and differences between the one- and two-sample tests should be highlighted.

In the two-sample test, the null hypothesis specifically states that there is no difference between the mean values of each set of data and, accordingly, there is no difference between the mean values of the populations from which the data have been sampled. Unlike the equivalent one-sample tests, the two-sample z and t tests examine differences between sampled means and, as a result, the mathematical manipulations employed in the two-sample tests require knowledge of the sampling distribution of differences between means and not the mean values themselves. This concept is generally quite confusing to undergraduate pharmacy students and requires clarification to ensure an understanding of the operation of the z and t tests. If we consider two populations (termed A and B) whose means are μ_A and μ_B and variances σ_A and σ_B, it is possible to simultaneously remove samples of defined size (N) from each population and calculate the mean of each sample and, additionally, to record the difference between the means of the first and second populations. Typically, if the sample size is sufficiently large, the distribution of means for each population will be normal and, importantly, the distribution of the calculated differences between the means of the pairs of samples will be approximately normal. A graphical representation of the sampling distribution of differences between the means of two populations is shown in Figure 8.1. As this is a normal distribution, the two key parameters that influence the resultant shape are the mean and the variance. The mean of the distribution of differences between the means of two populations can be shown to be equal to the difference between the means of the two individual populations, denoted by $\mu_A - \mu_B$. This may be assumed because in most cases each sample mean will equal the population mean and therefore the difference between the means will be zero. On the other hand, the variance of the difference between two independent variables may be shown to be equal to the sum of the variances of the individual populations. From the central limit theorem, the variance of each population may be mathematically defined as σ^2/N and therefore the variance of the difference between the mean values of the two populations is equal to

$$\sigma_{\text{diff}}^2 = \frac{\sigma_A^2}{N_A} + \frac{\sigma_B^2}{N_B}$$

The square root of the above equation generates the standard error of the differences between means, a parameter that is employed in the calculation of both the z and t statistics.

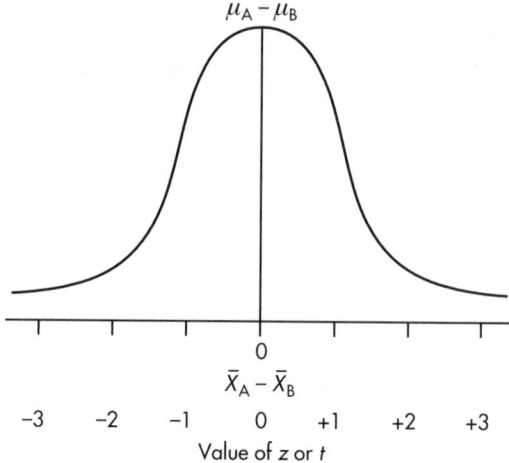

$$\mu_A - \mu_B$$

$$\bar{X}_A - \bar{X}_B$$

Value of z or t

Figure 8.1 Sampling distribution of the differences between means $(\bar{X}_A - \bar{X}_B)$ of two sets of sample data and the relationship with the z or t statistic.

Hopefully it is now clear to the reader that the major difference between one-sample and two-sample parametric tests lies in the nature of the distributions involved in the analysis. However, as may be expected in both types of design, either a z or a t statistic is calculated and, depending on the magnitude of this value, the null hypothesis is either accepted or rejected. In the two-sample tests, the distribution that is examined during the course of the analysis is the sampling difference between the mean values of each population. As this difference increases there is a greater likelihood that the null hypothesis will be rejected. The general equations for the calculation of the z and t statistics are as follows:

- z statistic

$$z = \frac{(\bar{X}_A - \bar{X}_B) - (\mu_A - \mu_B)}{\sigma_{\bar{X}_A - \bar{X}_B}}$$

- t statistic

$$t = \frac{(\bar{X}_A - \bar{X}_B) - (\mu_A - \mu_B)}{s_{\bar{X}_A - \bar{X}_B}}$$

where $\bar{X}_A$ and $\bar{X}_B$ are the two sample means; $\sigma_{\bar{X}_A - \bar{X}_B}$ and $s_{\bar{X}_A - \bar{X}_B}$ are the population and estimated (sample) standard errors of the difference between the sample means, respectively; and $(\mu_A - \mu_B)$ is the mean of the sampling distribution for the differences between the two means.

An understanding of the above description will enable the reader to successfully execute two-sample parametric tests. However, to supplement the above information, individual examples of the uses of the z and t tests will be provided in the following sections.

8.1.2 The z test for two independent samples

The rationale for the use of the two-sample z test is similar to that of the one-sample z test, so the successful application of this test requires knowledge of the variances of the populations under examination. In the vast majority of experiments in the pharmaceutical sciences this information is not readily available. However, two-sample z tests do have applications within the pharmaceutical industry, particularly in the manufacturing sectors. Their use is demonstrated in Example 8.1.

EXAMPLE 8.1 *A pharmaceutical company manufactures an anti-inflammatory solid dosage form using conventional rotary tablet presses at sites in both North America and Great Britain. It has been decided to investigate the productivity of the process at each manufacturing site by comparing the mean number of tablets produced per minute. On the basis of production records covering the last 200 batches manufactured at each site, the process details shown in Table 8.1 were recorded. Is there a difference in the productivity of the two production facilities?*

The following steps should be followed to ensure a methodical resolution of the question.

(i) State the null hypothesis

The null hypothesis states that there is no difference between the mean numbers of tablets produced per minute at each production facility:

$$H_0: \mu_{\text{(Great Britain)}} = \mu_{\text{(North America)}}$$

or alternatively,

$$H_0: \mu_{\text{(Great Britain)}} - \mu_{\text{(North America)}} = 0$$

(ii) State the alternative hypothesis

The alternative hypothesis states that there is a difference between the two mean values. Therefore, the alternative hypothesis for the current example

Table 8.1 Number of tablets of an anti-inflammatory product produced per minute by two manufacturing sites

Manufacturing site	Mean ($\pm$SD) number of tablets produced per minute
North America (NA)	5896.1 ± 108.0
Great Britain (GB)	5921.8 ± 111.8

states that there is a difference in the productivity of the two manufacturing sites, in terms of the number of tablets produced per minute:

$$H_a: \quad \mu_{\text{(Great Britain)}} \neq \mu_{\text{(North America)}}$$

or

$$H_a: \quad \mu_{\text{(Great Britain)}} - \mu_{\text{(North America)}} \neq 0$$

(iii) State the level of significance (the rejection region)

In this example, it is assumed that the level of significance (α) is 0.05.

(iv) State the number of tails associated with the experimental design

In this example, the null hypothesis may be rejected because the productivity of the manufacturing process in the British factory may be either higher or lower than the productivity of the manufacturing process in the American factory. As there are two possible reasons for rejection of the null hypothesis, Example 8.1 is a two-tailed experimental design.

(v) Select the most appropriate statistical test

In this example there are several attributes that direct the statistical analyst to the most appropriate experimental method:

- It is a two-sample test as the similarities or differences between two mean values from two different populations are under investigation.
- The observations are independent.
- Because the sample size is large $(N = 200)$ it may be assumed that the distribution of this data is normal (central limit theorem)
- The variances of the two samples are similar $(\sigma^2_{\text{(North America)}} = 11\,664.0$, $\sigma^2_{\text{(Great Britain)}} = 12\,499.2)$. In this chapter, a method known as the F_{max} test will be described to statistically assess the homogeneity (similarity) of two variances.
- The data have been measured on a ratio scale. The use of parametric two-sample tests requires that the data must be measured on an interval or a ratio scale.
- The data presented in Table 8.1 reflects the historical mean and standard deviation of the processes employed at each manufacturing site. In light of this, this data may be considered to be constant and therefore the variances represent the true (population) variances of the processes.

Therefore, on the basis of the above information, the most relevant statistical method to assess the validity of the null hypothesis, is a two-tailed z test for two independent-samples.

(vi) Perform the statistical analysis

The z statistic is calculated using the following mathematical formula:

$$z = \frac{(\bar{X}_{GB} - \bar{X}_{NA}) - (\mu_{GB} - \mu_{NA})}{\sigma_{\bar{X}_{GB} - \bar{X}_{NA}}}$$

$$= \frac{(\bar{X}_{GB} - \bar{X}_{NA}) - (\mu_{GB} - \mu_{NA})}{\sqrt{(\sigma_{GB}^2/N_{GB}) + (\sigma_{NA}^2/N_{NA})}}$$

where $\bar{X}_{GB}$ and $\bar{X}_{NA}$ are the sampled means of the numbers of tablets produced per minute in the manufacturing sites in Great Britain and North America, respectively; μ_{GB} and μ_{NA} are the true means of the numbers of tablets produced per minute in the manufacturing sites in Great Britain and North America, respectively; σ_{GB}^2 and σ_{NA}^2 are the variances of the numbers of tablets produced per minute in the manufacturing sites in Great Britain and North America, respectively; and N_{GB} and N_{NA} are the numbers of data (batches) sampled for each manufacturing site.

In Example 8.1 the null hypothesis states that there is no difference between the means of the numbers of tablets produced per minute in the manufacturing sites in Great Britain and North America and accordingly, the term $(\mu_{GB} - \mu_{NA})$ is equal to zero. Substituting the appropriate values into the above equation allows the calculation of the z statistic to be carried out:

$$z = \frac{(\bar{X}_{GB} - \bar{X}_{NA})}{\sqrt{(\sigma_{GB}^2/N_{GB}) + (\sigma_{NA}^2/N_{NA})}}$$

$$= \frac{(5921.8 - 5896.1)}{\sqrt{(11\,664.0/200) + (12\,499.2/200)}} = \frac{25.7}{11.0} = 2.34$$

(vii) Conclusion

The z statistic associated with Example 8.1 is 2.34. Under the conditions of the statistical test ($\alpha = 0.05$, two-tailed study), it may be observed that the critical region is $z \geqslant +1.96$ or, alternatively, $z \leqslant -1.96$. As the calculated z value (+2.34) is greater than + 1.96, the null hypothesis is rejected. It is therefore concluded that there is a significant difference in the productivity of the manufacturing sites in Great Britain and North America. More specifically, the productivity of the British facility is significantly greater than that of the North American facility.

In the above example, the sizes of the two samples were identical, but it is worth noting that the sample sizes may be disparate. The sample sizes are entered into the equation above and the z statistic calculated in the normal fashion.

Provided the sample size is large, the z test may be employed to compare proportional values of two-samples. In this scenario, the mechanics of the test are similar to that for the comparison of two mean values. More specifically, the equation that is employed for the calculation of the z statistic relevant to the difference between two proportions is

$$z = \frac{p_A - p_B}{\sqrt{p_0 q_0((1/N_A) + (1/N_B))}}$$

where p_A and p_B are the proportions of sample A and sample B, N_A and N_B are the sizes of sample A and sample B, p_0 is the pooled proportion and $q_0 = 1 - p_0$

The pooled proportion is calculated using the following equation:

$$p_0 = \frac{(N_A \times p_A) + (N_B \times p_B)}{N_A + N_B}$$

The pooled proportion is the most appropriate estimation of the mutual value of the probability, as defined by the null hypothesis. It should be remembered that if the null hypothesis is true, the observed probability is the same for each group. It is more accurate to estimate the proportion, as defined by the null hypothesis, using both sets of data rather than one, and consequently a weighted average of proportions is employed for this purpose.

Example 8.2 illustrates the use of these equations for the comparison of two proportions in a typical pharmaceutical scenario.

EXAMPLE 8.2 *One the acknowledged side-effects associated with chronic use of non-steroidal anti-inflammatory drugs is gastric ulceration. An academic unit is interested in the comparative incidences of gastric ulceration following chronic administration of two non-steroidal anti-inflammatory agents. The incidences of gastric ulceration associated with the uses of drug A and drug B were determined from patient records and were as shown in Table 8.2. Is there a significant difference in the reported incidences of side-effects associated with the use of the two anti-inflammatory drugs?*

Table 8.2 Incidences of gastric ulceration associated with the chronic administration of two non-steroidal anti-inflammatory agents, drug A and drug B

Recorded frequency	Drug A	Drug B
Ulceration	27	44
No ulceration	201	363

(i) State the null hypothesis

The null hypothesis states that there is no difference in the reported incidences of side-effects associated with the use of the two anti-inflammatory drugs:

H_0: incidence of side-effects$_{(drug A)}$ = incidence of side-effects$_{(drug B)}$

or alternatively,

H_0: incidence of side-effects$_{(drug A)}$ − incidence of side-effects$_{(drug B)}$ = 0

(ii) State the alternative hypothesis

The alternative hypothesis states that there is a difference in the reported incidences of side-effects associated with the use of the two anti-inflammatory drugs:

H_a: incidence of side-effects$_{(drug A)}$ ≠ incidence of side-effects$_{(drug B)}$

or

H_a: incidence of side-effects$_{(drug A)}$ − incidence of side-effects$_{(drug B)}$ ≠ 0

(iii) State the level of significance (the rejection region)

In this example, it is assumed that the level of significance (α) is 0.05.

(iv) State the number of tails associated with the experimental design

In this example, there are two possible reasons for rejection of the null hypothesis: the incidence of side-effects associated with the use of drug A may be either greater or less than that associated with drug B, so this is an example of a two-tailed test.

(v) Select the most appropriate statistical test

The key aspects of the experimental design are:

- It is a two-independent-samples test as the similarities or differences between two proportions, representative of two different populations, are under investigation.
- The observations are independent.
- The size of each sample is large and as a result, the normal approximation to the binomial distribution may be used.

Therefore, on the basis of the above information, the most relevant statistical method to compare the proportions from the two independent groups is a z test for proportions with two independent samples.

(vi) Perform the statistical analysis

The z statistic is calculated as described previously:

$$z = \frac{p_{Drug\ A} - p_{Drug\ B}}{\sqrt{p_0 q_0((1/N_{Drug\ A}) + (1/N_{Drug\ B}))}}$$

where p_A and p_B are incidences of side-effects (expressed as proportions) associated with the use of the two anti-inflammatory drugs; N_A and N_B are the sample sizes for each group of patients (228 and 407, respectively); and p_0 is the pooled proportion.

The first step involves the calculation of the proportion of side-effects associated with each drug:

$$p_A = \frac{27}{228} = 0.118$$

$$p_B = \frac{44}{407} = 0.109$$

Calculate the pooled proportion:

$$p_0 = \frac{(N_A \times p_A) + (N_B \times p_B)}{N_A + N_B}$$

$$= \frac{(228 \times 0.118) + (407 \times 0.109)}{(228 + 407)} = 0.112$$

Calculate the z statistic:

$$z = \frac{p_A - p_B}{\sqrt{p_0 q_0((1/N_A) + (1/N_B))}}$$

$$= \frac{0.118 - 0.109}{\sqrt{0.112 \times 0.888((1/228) + (1/407))}} = 0.345$$

(vii) Conclusion

From the conditions of the statistical test ($\alpha = 0.05$, two-tailed study), it may be observed that the critical (rejection) region is $z \geqslant +1.96$ or, alternatively, $z \leqslant -1.96$. The calculated z value is 0.345, and accordingly the null hypothesis is accepted. Therefore, it is concluded that there is no difference in the incidences of side-effects associated with the use of the two non-steroidal anti-inflammatory drugs.

8.1.3 The *t* test for two independent samples

The equation used for calculating the z statistic is similar to that used for the t statistic. The fundamental difference between the two equations lies in the nature of the variance term. In the equation for the calculation of the z statistic the population variance is used, indicating that there is prior knowledge of this parameter. Conversely, in the calculation of the t statistic the variances of the populations from which the samples were drawn are estimated from the variances of the sample data. As highlighted in Chapter 7, the underlying assumptions of the z and t tests are similar and accordingly, the use of the two-sample t test is valid when the following conditions hold:

- The two sets of data are measured on either an interval or a ratio scale.
- The populations from which the two sets of data have been collected are normally distributed. The two-samples t test is employed for the comparison of means of two sets of data that have been determined using small sample sizes. Therefore, the normality of the two populations is assumed, but is not always validated or implied by the central limit theorem. The two-sample t test theoretically requires that the two populations from which the data have been derived are normally distributed, but the test can tolerate small deviations from normality without leading to erroneous statistical conclusions. Under these circumstances, the mean is a logical measure of the central nature of the populations.
- The variances of the populations under examination are unknown. However, the variances of the sample data are assumed to be a valid estimate of the population parameters and are accordingly employed in the calculation of the t statistic.
- The variances of the populations that have been estimated using the appropriate sample data are assumed to be similar.

The following equation for the calculation of the t statistic is valid whenever the size of the samples in each group is equal:

$$t = \frac{(\overline{X}_1 - \overline{X}_2) - (\mu_1 - \mu_2)}{s_{(\overline{X}_1 - \overline{X}_2)}} = \frac{(\overline{X}_1 - \overline{X}_2)}{\sqrt{s_1^2/N_1 + s_2^2/N_2}}$$

However, whenever the sizes of the two sets of data are unequal, this equation must be altered to ensure reliability of the estimation of the population variance. As stated above, one of the assumptions of the t test is homogeneity of variance, which is regardless of the validity of the null hypothesis and independent of equality of sample size. It may be useful for the reader to remember that if the means of the two populations under examination differ, this does not necessarily imply that the variances will change, rather that the central tendency of one population has been shifted away from the other. In light of the assumed equality of sample variances, each individual sample variance may be considered to provide an estimation of the population variance (σ^2). Of course, each sample variance is in fact an estimate of the population variance.

However, if there are two independent estimations of the population variance, an improved estimation of the population variance may be achieved from an average of the two sample variances. Calculation of the average variance is performed using a weighted average in which the sample variances are affected by the associated number of degrees of freedom (and hence sample size). The average variance of the two samples is referred to as the *pooled variance* (s_p^2) and is calculated using the following formula:

$$s_p^2 = \frac{(N_1 - 1)s_1^2 + (N_2 - 1)s_2^2}{N_1 + N_2 - 2}$$

The equation for the calculation of the *t* statistic is subsequently modified to include the pooled variance term:

$$t = \frac{(\bar{X}_1 - \bar{X}_2) - (\mu_1 - \mu_2)}{s_{(\bar{X}_1 - \bar{X}_2)}}$$

$$= \frac{(\bar{X}_1 - \bar{X}_2)}{\sqrt{s_p^2/N_1 + s_p^2/N_2}} = \frac{(\bar{X}_1 - \bar{X}_2)}{s_p\sqrt{1/N_1 + 1/N_2}}$$

where $\bar{X}_1$ and $\bar{X}_2$ are the mean values of the two sets of sample data (termed 1 and 2); N_1 and N_2 are the numbers of observations in the two data sets (termed 1 and 2); s_p^2 is the pooled variance; $(N_1 - 1)$ and $(N_2 - 1)$ are the numbers of degrees of freedom associated with sample 1 and sample 2, respectively; and $(N_1 + N_1 - 2)$ is the total number of degrees of freedom for a two-independent-samples *t* test.

Therefore, in the calculation of the *t* statistic for the two-sample statistical test, the following steps are required.

- First, the mean and variance of each sample are calculated.
- From a knowledge of the sample size (and hence numbers of degrees of freedom) and the sample variances, the pooled variance is calculated.
- The pooled variance is then employed in the determination of the standard error of the differences between means, i.e. the denominator term in the above equation.
- Following determination of the difference between the two mean values, the *t* statistic is calculated by dividing this difference by the standard error.

The use of the *t* test for the statistical assessment of the significance of the difference between sample means is illustrated in Examples 8.3 and 8.4.

EXAMPLE 8.3 *For registration purposes two formulations of a new semi-solid product containing an anti-viral agent have been manufactured and placed on stability testing under controlled storage conditions*

(37 °C). After 3 months, 10 2-g samples of each formulation were removed and the concentration of drug in each sample determined using a validated high performance liquid chromatography (HPLC) method. The analytical results are shown in Table 8.3. Using an appropriate statistical method, determine whether there is a difference in the mean concentration of drug in each formulation following the period of storage.

This is a typical situation that is encountered by both formulation scientists and chemical analysts. In the development of ethical products the stability profile of the formulations must be characterised and presented to the regulatory authorities as part of the registration package of the product. Therefore, this problem is essentially asking whether or not there is a difference in the stability of the drug in the two different formulations. Statistically, this question may be addressed in a stepwise fashion.

The following points are addressed before the collection of data.

(i) State the null hypothesis

The null hypothesis states that there is no difference between the two sample means. Therefore, the null hypothesis for the current example states that there is no difference in the mean concentrations of drug in each formulation:

$$H_0: \quad \mu_{\text{formulation 1}} = \mu_{\text{formulation 2}}$$

Table 8.3 Total concentration of an anti-viral drug in 10 units taken from each of two formulations after storage at 37 °C for 3 months

Total concentration of drug (mg) in each unit	
Formulation 1	Formulation 2
104.1	102.9
108.2	99.6
108.6	98.1
100.8	104.2
106.5	90.2
101.0	101.0
102.6	99.9
99.2	89.5
95.2	95.5
100.8	98.6

(ii) State the alternative hypothesis

The alternative hypothesis states that there is a difference between the two sample means. Consequently, the alternative hypothesis states that there is a difference between the mean concentrations of drug in each formulation:

$$H_a: \mu_{\text{formulation 1}} \neq \mu_{\text{formulation 2}}$$

(iii) State the level of significance (the rejection region)

In this example, it is assumed that the level of significance (α) is 0.05.

(iv) State the number of tails associated with the experimental design

In Example 8.3 the null hypothesis may be rejected for two reasons: the concentration of drug per unit in the first formulation may be either significantly greater or significantly less than that of the second formulation. As there are two possible outcomes to the study, this is a two-tailed experimental design.

(v) Select the most appropriate statistical test

At this stage the analyst must decide whether a two-sample parametric or non-parametric method should be applied to resolve the statistical problem. As previously described the successful use of a parametric method requires that certain criteria should be valid: in particular, the variances of the two groups should be similar and, furthermore, the populations from which the sample data were derived should be normally distributed, or close to it. Therefore, the first step in the choice of statistical method involves an examination of the descriptive statistical properties of each set of data. These are summarised in Table 8.4.

In Chapter 5 the concept of the comparison of the similarity of the mean, median and (where applicable) the mode for the assessment of the normality of a distribution was introduced. This comparison is one

Table 8.4 Descriptive statistics (mean, median, mode, variance and standard deviation) for the concentration of anti-viral agent in two different formulations

Descriptive parameters	Formulation 1	Formulation 2
Mean (mg)	101.70	99.75
Median (mg)	101.30	99.55
Mode (mg)	100.80	Not applicable
Variance (mg^2)	3.01	6.41
Standard deviation (mg)	1.73	2.53

measurement of normality, but not a definitive assessment of this property. However, because of its simplicity, this measurement will be used throughout the book to examine the normality of a distribution, without further comment.

As may be observed from Table 8.4, the mean and median of each formulation are of a similar magnitude and therefore, for the purpose of this analysis, it may be assumed that the populations from which the sample data have been derived are normally distributed. The sample size of each group is small, thus invalidating the use of the z test. Furthermore, the variances of the two batches appear to be similar in magnitude. However, as this is a statistics text, the reader may not be surprised to read that a statistical test is available that allows comparison of variances to be performed. This is referred to as the *homogeneity of variances* (F) test, as the test employs the F distribution for the interpretation of the outcome of the analysis. The mechanics and interpretation of the test will be explained using the data depicted in Table 8.4.

The F test calculates the ratio of two variances as an F statistic. The probability of observing this F statistic is then ascertained using the F distribution. Mathematically, the ratio is defined as:

$$F = \frac{s_1^2}{s_2^2}$$

where s_1^2 and s_2^2 denote the variances of the two sample groups.

In Example 8.3, the two sample variances have been calculated and therefore the F ratio may be easily computed. However, before embarking on this, it is good statistical practice to define the parameters associated with the F test. Accordingly, the *null hypothesis* states that there is no difference between the variances of the two groups, whereas the *alternative hypothesis* claims that the variances of the two groups are different. The *level of significance* (α) is assumed to be 0.05 and the test is *two-tailed* because the null hypothesis may be rejected for two reasons: namely, the variance of the first group may be greater than that of the second, or vice versa. With this information in mind, the F ratio is then computed with the larger of the two variances defined as the numerator:

$$F = \frac{s_1^2}{s_2^2} = \frac{6.41}{3.01} = 2.13$$

To statistically interpret this F statistic, the following information is required:

- The level of significance, $\alpha = 0.05$.
- The number of tails in the experiment: this is a two-tailed experiment.

- The number of degrees of freedom associated with the numerator, calculated by subtracting 1 from the number of observations in this set of data: $(10 - 1) = 9$.
- The number of degrees of freedom associated with the denominator, calculated by subtracting 1 from the number of observations in this set of data: $(10 - 1) = 9$.

By referring to the tables of the F distribution (Appendix 7), it may be observed that the critical value of the F statistic is 4.03 $(F_{\alpha = 0.05, \text{ two-tailed, num } df = 9, \text{ denom } df = 9})$. From Appendix 7, it may be observed that the critical value of the F statistic is 4.03. If the calculated F value is less than 4.03 the null hypothesis is accepted, whereas if the calculated F value is equal to this value, or exceeds it, the null hypothesis is rejected. Accordingly, as the calculated F statistic is 2.13, the null hypothesis is accepted, i.e. the variances of the two groups are statistically similar in magnitude (homogeneous).

Therefore, on the basis of the above information, a two-tailed parametric, two-independent-samples t test is the most appropriate statistical test to resolve the statistical problem described in Example 8.3.

(vi) Perform the statistical analysis

The t statistic that describes the difference between the mean values of each batch is calculated as follows:

$$t = \frac{(\overline{X}_1 - \overline{X}_2) - (\mu_1 - \mu_2)}{s_{(\overline{X}_1 - \overline{X}_2)}} = \frac{(\overline{X}_1 - \overline{X}_2)}{\sqrt{s_p^2/N_1 + s_p^2/N_2}} = \frac{(\overline{X}_1 - \overline{X}_2)}{s_p \sqrt{1/N_1 + 1/N_2}}$$

Firstly, the pooled variance must be calculated. A simplified form of the equation described below may also be used because the sample sizes of the two groups are identical, but at this stage it is good practice for the reader to gain experience in the use of the weighted average to calculate the pooled variance:

$$s_p^2 = \frac{(N_1 - 1)s_1^2 + (N_2 - 1)s_2^2}{N_1 + N_2 - 2} = \frac{(9 \times 3.01) + (9 \times 6.41)}{(10 + 10 - 2)} = 4.71$$

With knowledge of the pooled variance, the number of observations in each group and the mean values of each group, the t statistic may be determined:

$$t = \frac{(\overline{X}_1 - \overline{X}_2)}{\sqrt{s_p^2/N_1 + s_p^2/N_2}} = \frac{(101.70 - 99.75)}{\sqrt{4.71/10 + 4.71/10}} = \frac{1.95}{0.97} = 2.01$$

(vii) Conclusion

To interpret the relevance of this t value (+2.01), the critical t value under the conditions of the experimental design must be identified. The important parameters that define this value are:

- $\alpha = 0.05$
- two-tailed experimental design
- 18 df associated with the study, i.e. $(N_1 + N_2 - 2)$.

On the basis of this information, calculated t values that are either less than or equal to -2.09, or greater than or equal to $+2.09$, will result in the rejection of the null hypothesis. Alternatively, if the calculated t value lies within the region of the t distribution defined as $-2.09 < t < +2.09$, the null hypothesis will be accepted. The calculated t value is located within the region of acceptance of the null hypothesis and therefore it may be concluded that there was no difference in the concentration of antiviral drug in the two formulations after storage for 3 months at 37 °C.

Interestingly, the calculated t statistic was similar in magnitude to the critical value. Therefore, although this study has confirmed that there were no differences in the concentrations of drug in each formulation, it is possible that the magnitude of difference in concentrations of the two formulations may be greater after longer periods of storage. This will subsequently increase the calculated t statistic and may drive this value into the region of rejection of the null hypothesis. In other words, after longer periods of storage, the two formulations may differ in their stability profiles.

The formulation scientist may want to know the magnitude of the difference between the mean concentrations of the two formulations that will result in a rejection of the null hypothesis. In other words, this question may be rephrased as, 'What difference between the mean concentrations will result in a statistically discernible difference in the stability profiles of the two formulations?'. This may be answered by using the critical t statistic, which defines the point of acceptance or rejection of the null hypothesis, and substituting this value into the equation for the two-samples t test. In this application the unknown parameter in the equation is the difference between the two mean values of the sample data sets $(\bar{X}_1 - \bar{X}_2)$.

Employing the same experimental parameters and the critical t statistic ($t = 2.09$ for a two-tailed test with 18 df),

$$t = \frac{(\bar{X}_1 - \bar{X}_2)}{\sqrt{s_p^2/N_1 + s_p^2/N_2}}$$

therefore

$$(\bar{X}_1 - \bar{X}_2) = t_{(19df,\,\text{two-tailed})} \sqrt{\frac{s_p^2}{N_1} + \frac{s_p^2}{N_2}}$$

$$= 2.09 \times \sqrt{\frac{4.71}{10} + \frac{4.71}{10}} = 2.03 \text{ mg}$$

The critical difference in mean concentrations of the two formulations that will result in the rejection of the null hypothesis is thus 2.03 mg. After storage at 37 °C for 3 months the experimentally determined difference between the mean concentrations of the two formulations was 1.95 mg. If the sets of data are representative samples and accordingly estimate the mean concentrations in each formulation, it is highly probable that the differences between the mean concentrations will increase with time of storage. This indicates that there may be a stability problem in one formulation.

In the previous example (8.3), the two-samples t test was applied to data in which the sample size of each data set was equal. The following example describes the use of the two-sample t test for the statistical comparison of two data sets that have dissimilar numbers of observations. There are two reasons for providing this example:

- The two-sample t test is one of the most common statistical tests that is used by pharmaceutical and related scientists and therefore further experience in its use will be helpful to the reader.
- This example provides further experience in the calculation of the pooled variance, often a point of confusion amongst undergraduate students of pharmacy and related disciplines.

EXAMPLE 8.4 *A pharmaceutical company that specialises in the formulation of generic products has developed a solid dosage formulation of an H_2 receptor antagonist for the treatment of gastric and duodenal ulceration. As part of the registration process, a clinical trial has been performed in which the pharmacokinetic profiles of the generic formulation and the proprietary product have been compared in 25 volunteers following administration of a single dose (tablet). The maximum concentrations of drug in the plasma (C_{max}) of the two formulations are shown in Table 8.5. Is there a difference in the generic and proprietary formulations with respect to their C_{max}?*

Adopting a similar strategy to that outlined in the previous example, the following points should be addressed.

Table 8.5 Maximum concentration of an H_2 receptor antagonist in the plasma of patients who received a single dose of either a generic or a proprietary formulation during the course of a bioavailability study

Generic formulation (C_{max}, $\mu g/mL$)	Proprietary formulation (C_{max}, $\mu g/mL$)
5.6	3.9
6.8	3.5
4.9	3.6
5.2	4.2
5.8	4.9
6.4	2.9
6.9	3.4
6.0	3.8
5.8	2.4
5.1	3.8
4.9	4.8
6.8	4.1
7.0	

(i) State the null hypothesis

The null hypothesis states that there is no difference between the two sample means. Therefore, the null hypothesis states that there is no difference in the mean C_{max} values between the generic and proprietary formulations:

$$H_0: \mu_{C_{max} \text{ generic formulation}} = \mu_{C_{max} \text{ proprietary formulation}}$$

or alternatively

$$H_0: \mu_{C_{max} \text{ generic formulation}} - \mu_{C_{max} \text{ proprietary formulation}} = 0$$

(ii) State the alternative hypothesis

The alternative hypothesis states that there is a difference between the two sample means. Consequently, the alternative hypothesis states that there is a difference in the mean C_{max} values for the generic and proprietary formulations:

$$H_a: \mu_{C_{max} \text{ generic formulation}} \neq \mu_{C_{max} \text{ proprietary formulation}}$$

or alternatively

$$H_a: \mu_{C_{max} \text{ generic formulation}} - \mu_{C_{max} \text{ proprietary formulation}} \neq 0$$

(iii) State the level of significance (the rejection region)

In this example, it is assumed that the level of significance (α) is 0.05.

(iv) State the number of tails associated with the experimental design

Once more this is an example of a two-tailed test because the null hypothesis may be rejected for two reasons: the mean C_{max} of the generic formulation may be greater or less than the mean C_{max} of the proprietary formulation.

(v) Select the most appropriate statistical test

In this example there are two groups of data, the means of which will be statistically compared. There is no direct relationship between the data and, accordingly, the two sets of data are independent. The next stage in the selection process involves whether a parametric or non-parametric two-samples statistical method should be employed. Remember that a parametric test should be used whenever the conditions of the experimental design make it possible to do so. To ascertain whether a parametric test may be employed, the following points should be clarified:

- Are the variances of the two groups similar?
- Are the populations from which the sample data were derived normally or pseudo-normally distributed?

These questions may be clarified by inspection of the descriptive statistics of each data set (Table 8.6). Here the mean, median and mode (where applicable) of each sample are similar in magnitude and therefore, we will assume that the populations from which the sample data have been derived are normally distributed.

The variances of the two sets of sample data appear to be similar in magnitude; this similarity may be statistically confirmed by calculating the F ratio. In this, the *null hypothesis* states that there is no difference between the variances of the two groups, whereas the *alternative hypothesis* claims that there is a difference in the variances of the two groups. The *level of significance* (α) is assumed to be 0.05 and the test is two-tailed because the null hypothesis may be rejected because either

Table 8.6 Descriptive statistics (mean, median, mode, variance and standard deviation) for the maximum concentrations of drug in the plasma (C_{max}) of a generic formulation and a proprietary formulation

Descriptive parameters	Generic formulation C_{max}	Proprietary formulation C_{max}
Mean (μg/mL)	5.94	3.78
Median (μg/mL)	5.80	3.80
Mode (μg/mL)	Not applicable	3.80
Variance (μg/mL)^2	0.61	0.50
Standard deviation (μg/mL)	0.78	0.71

$s_1^2 > s_2^2$ or $s_1^2 < s_2^2$. The F ratio is then calculated with the larger of the two variances defined as the numerator:

$$F = \frac{s_1^2}{s_2^2} = \frac{0.61}{0.50} = 1.22$$

The critical value of the F statistic is identified from the table that describes the critical values of the F distribution (Appendix 7) when $\alpha = 0.05$ for a two-tailed design and the numbers of degrees of freedom associated with the numerator and denominator are 12 (=13 – 1) and 11 (= 12 – 1), respectively. Accordingly, the critical value of the F statistic is 3.43 ($F_{\alpha = 0.05,\ \text{two-tailed, num } df = 12,\ \text{denom } df = 11}$). As the calculated F statistic was 1.22, the null hypothesis is accepted, i.e. the variances of the two groups are statistically similar in magnitude. Therefore, on the basis of the above information, a two-tailed parametric, two-sample t test is the most appropriate statistical test. The z test should not be used in this case, because of the small sample size of each group.

(vi) Perform the statistical analysis

The first step in the determination of the t statistic involves the calculation of the pooled variance:

$$s_p^2 = \frac{(N_1 - 1)s_1^2 + (N_2 - 1)s_2^2}{N_1 + N_2 - 2} = \frac{(13 - 1)0.61 + (12 - 1)0.50}{(13 + 12 - 2)} = 0.56$$

With knowledge of the pooled variance, the number of observations in each group and the mean values of each group, the t statistic may be determined:

$$t = \frac{(\bar{X}_1 - \bar{X}_2)}{\sqrt{s_p^2/N_1 + s_p^2/N_2}} = \frac{(5.94 - 3.78)}{\sqrt{0.56/13 + 0.56/12}} = \frac{2.16}{0.30} = 7.20$$

(vii) Conclusion

To interpret the relevance of this t value, the critical t value under the conditions of the experimental design must be identified. The important parameters that define this value are

- $\alpha = 0.05$
- two-tailed experimental design
- 23 df associated with the study, i.e. ($N_1 + N_2 - 2$).

On the basis of this information, the region of rejection of the null hypothesis is either $t \leqslant -2.07$ or $t \geqslant +2.07$. As the calculated t value is +7.20 (and hence $\geqslant +2.07$), the null hypothesis is rejected. Therefore, there is a difference in the clinical performance of the generic and proprietary formulations in terms of the maximum concentration in the plasma following administration of a single tablet. In regulatory terms, the generic formulation does not behave in a similar fashion to the proprietary formulations and cannot be considered to be bioequivalent to the proprietary formulation.

8.1.4 Design criteria in parametric statistical tests for two independent samples

The need and rationale for the calculation of sample size and power have been described previously (section 7.1.3). However, it is worthwhile recalling that the major factors inherent in the experimental design that affect the required sample size are as follows:

- *The level of significance*: if the chosen level of significance (α) is low, the *t* value associated with this value will be large and, accordingly, large sample sizes will be required to detect a significant difference between the means of the two samples. Therefore, whenever a low α value is selected (i.e. to minimise the probability of a type I error), a large sample size should be employed.
- *The power of the test*: this refers to the probability that the null hypothesis will be rejected when it is indeed false. The power of the test is commonly referred to as $1 - \beta$, in which β is the probability of committing a type II error, i.e. accepting the null hypothesis when the null hypothesis is false. If the required power of the test is high, the value of β must therefore be small. As a result, the *t* statistic associated with the β value will be high and the required sample size will be large.
- *The population variance*: this is estimated as a pooled variance using the weighted average of the variances of the two sets of data. If the variances of the two samples are large, a larger sample size is required to discern differences between the mean values of two samples.
- *The minimum detectable difference between the means of the two populations*: A large sample size is required when a small minimum detectable difference between the means of two samples is specified. The situation is reversed when larger minimum detectable differences are specified.

The required sample size for a particular study may be calculated using the following formula:

$$N \geqslant \left(\frac{2s_p}{\delta}\right)^2 (t_{\alpha(df)} + t_{\beta(df)})^2$$

where N is the estimated sample size, $t_{\alpha(df)}$ is the *t* statistic associated with the chosen level of significance (α) and the degrees of freedom of the study, $t_{\beta(df)}$ is the *t* statistic associated with the probability of a type II error (β) and the degrees of freedom of the study, s_p^2 is the (pooled) sample variance (an estimation of the population variance) and δ is the minimum difference between the mean values of the two samples that is considered to be experimentally or clinically relevant.

The form of this equation is similar to that described in section 7.1.3 for the calculation of the sample size of one-sample parametric statistical tests. The use of this equation for the calculation of the required sample size for two-sample *t* tests is demonstrated in Example 8.5.

EXAMPLE 8.5 *The acid stability of two tablet formulations containing identical concentrations of active agent was evaluated under conditions that did not comply with Good Manufacturing Practice (GMP). From this pilot study, the rates of degradation of the active agent in an acidic buffer were calculated and an estimation of the population variance was performed and recorded as 50.61 min^{-2}. As a result of this it has been decided that a full stability study on these two formulations should be performed under the appropriate regulatory conditions. However, the company is unclear as to the number of samples from each batch that should be employed for the purpose of this study to enable a significance difference between the two batches to be observed, if indeed a difference does exist. Using an appropriate statistical method, estimate the sample size of each formulation that should be included in the stability study. The company has declared that it would wish to know if the degradation rates of the two formulations differed by more than 5 min^{-1}.*

This example is analogous to Example 7.8 and therefore a similar (iterative) approach can be employed to estimate the sample size. As before, the parameters of the statistical process must be defined. Thus:

- The chosen level of significance (α) is 0.05.
- The within-sample variability (variance), estimated from a previous pilot study, is 50.61 min^{-2}. This has been calculated as the pooled variance of the two sets of data (formulations).
- The probability of committing a type II (β) error, i.e. accepting the null hypothesis when the null hypothesis is false, is chosen as 10%. Therefore, the power of the study ($1 - \beta$) is 90%, i.e. there is a 90% chance of observing a true difference between the two populations.
- The minimum detectable difference between the two sample means that is under investigation (5 min^{-1}).

Once more, a simple method by which the optimum sample size may be estimated is the iterative approach. This is performed as follows.

Step 1
Assume that sample sizes of 50 are required. Therefore, the sample size may be calculated using the following equation:

$$N \geqslant 2\left(\frac{s_p}{\delta}\right)^2 (t_{\alpha(df)} + t_{\beta(df)})^2$$

or

$$N \geqslant \frac{2s_p^2}{\delta^2}(t_{\alpha(df)} + t_{\beta(df)})^2$$

where N is the estimated sample size, s_p is the pooled standard deviation, δ is the minimum detectable difference (5 min^{-1}). $t_{\alpha(df)}$ is the t statistic associated with the chosen level of significance (0.05), a two-tailed outcome and the number of degrees of freedom associated with the estimated sample size. If there are 50 samples in each group the number of degrees of freedom will be 98. Therefore, from Appendix 2, $t_{\alpha(98df, \text{two-tailed})}$ is 1.984. $t_{\beta(df)}$ is the t statistic associated with the probability of committing a type II error (β), a one-tailed outcome and the number of degrees of freedom of the study. This equates to a β value of 0.1 (1.00 − 0.90). Therefore, $t_{\beta(98df)}$ is 1.290. Inserting these values into the above equation allows the calculation of the estimated sample size:

$$N \geqslant \frac{(2 \times 50.61)}{5^2}(1.984 + 1.290)^2 = 43.40$$

Step 2
With the above knowledge, use 44 as the estimated sample size. The statistics associated with $N = 44$ are

$$t_{\alpha(df)} = t_{(0.05)\,(86df),\,\text{two-tailed}} = 1.988$$

$$t_{\beta(df)} = t_{(0.10)\,(86df),\,\text{one-tailed}} = 1.291$$

$$N \geqslant \frac{(2 \times 50.61)}{5^2}(1.988 + 1.291)^2 = 43.53$$

Therefore, because the two iterations agree, it is concluded that the number of samples in each group should be at least 44.

In some cases, the two sample sizes will not be equal, perhaps as a result of the availability of samples in a particular group. In the scenario in which number of sample sizes in one treatment group is defined, the size of the second treatment group may be calculated using the following equation:

$$N_2 = \frac{n \times N_1}{2N_1 - n}$$

where N_2 is the calculated size of sample for the second treatment group, N_1 is the sample size of the first treatment group and is defined by the conditions of the experiment and N is the estimated sample size of the experiment that has been calculated using the iterative technique.

In Example 8.5, let us assume that the sample size of one treatment group has been limited to 25. To calculate the sample size of the second treatment group the above equation is employed, following calculation of the estimated sample size (determined using an iterative technique, assuming that the two groups were of identical size). Therefore, N_1 is 25 and N (derived from the iteration) is 44. The required size of the second treatment group is

$$N_2 = \frac{n \times N_1}{2N_1 - n} = \frac{44 \times 25}{(2 \times 25) - 44} = 183.3$$

The size of the second treatment group should therefore be at least 184.

One other scenario that is statistically relevant in the experimental design concerns the calculation of the minimum detectable difference between the means of two groups, i.e. the minimum difference that is significant within the conditions of the experiment. The method by which this is performed is related to that described above for the estimation of the sample size. Indeed, the equation used to determine the minimum detectable difference (δ) is a rearranged version of the equation for estimation of sample size, with δ now the subject of the equation:

$$\delta = \sqrt{\frac{2s_p^2}{N}} (t_{\alpha(df)} + t_{\beta(df)})$$

The notation used in this equation has been described above.

The use of this equation for the estimation of the power of the study and the minimum detectable difference between two treatment means is demonstrated in Example 8.6.

EXAMPLE 8.6 *A company has developed a new isotonic drink, which it claims increases endurance in athletes, measured as the time that athletes can continue running, and wishes to examine this hypothesis in a clinical trial. However, before commissioning this trial, the company has asked that the following experimental parameters should be calculated: the minimum detectable difference, the required sample size for the purposes of recruitment of subjects and the power of the study. In a previous pilot study involving a limited number of patients the pooled variance of the two treatment groups was estimated as 5.25 min².*

Calculate the minimum detectable difference between the two treatment groups

To calculate the minimum detectable difference between the two treatment groups the following parameters are required:

- *The chosen level of significance.* We will assume that α is 0.05, i.e. the test for minimum detectable difference is being conducted at the 95% level.
- *The within-sample variability (variance).* This has been estimated as 5.25 min² from the pooled variance using data generated from a previous pilot study.

- *The probability of committing a type II (β) error.* This is the probability of accepting the null hypothesis when the null hypothesis is false, and, for the purpose of this example, this value will be selected as 10%. Therefore, the power of the study (1 − β) is 90%, i.e. there is a 90% chance of observing the true calculated minimum detectable difference.
- *Sample size.* We will assume that the sample size in each group is 10.

Armed with this information, the minimum detectable difference is calculated as follows:

$$\delta = \sqrt{\frac{2s_p^2}{N}}(t_{\alpha(df)} + t_{\beta(df)}) = \sqrt{\frac{(2 \times 5.25)}{10}}(2.10 + 1.33) = 3.51 \text{ min}$$

To ensure a complete understanding of the above calculation it is worthwhile to define the criteria associated with the two t statistics (t_α and t_β). t_α denotes the chosen level of significance under the conditions of the experiment (two-tailed experimental design). In the above example, a probability value of 0.05 has been chosen and associated with this are $(N_1 + N_2 - 2) = 18$ df. The probability of committing a type II error has been set at 0.10 and accordingly the parameters associated with the t statistic are 18 df and a one-tailed outcome. $t_{\beta(0.1, 18)}$ is therefore 1.33, so there is a 90% chance of observing a mean difference of 3.51 min between the two treatments.

Calculate the power of the study

The generic equation (stated above) that describes the relationship between the minimum detectable difference, the standard deviation (or variance) and the sample size may be further rearranged to enable the calculation of the power of the study to be performed. In Example 8.6, the sponsor has requested that power of the experimental design to be calculated. This calculation requires prior knowledge of the minimum detectable difference, the standard deviation and the appropriate t statistics (α and β).

In example 8.6 we will therefore assume the following:

- The level of significance (α) is 0.05.
- The minimum detectable difference is arbitrarily selected as 4 min.
- The estimated pooled variance is 5.25 min².

Rearranging the previous equation in terms of t_β produces the following:

$$t_{\beta(df)} \leqslant \frac{\delta}{\sqrt{(2 \times s_p^2)/N}} - t_{\alpha(df)}$$

Returning to Example 8.6, the numerical value of $t_{\beta(df)}$ may now be calculated:

$$t_{\beta(df)} \leqslant \frac{4.00}{\sqrt{(2 \times 5.25)/10}} - 2.10_{(18df,\,\text{two-tailed},\,\alpha=0.05)} = 1.80$$

To interpret this t statistic in terms of power, two further steps must be performed:

- First, the probability of the t statistic must be interpreted under the conditions of the experiment, i.e. 18 df, one-tailed probability. Accordingly, the probability associated with a t statistic of 1.80 is greater than 0.025 but less than 0.05.
- Secondly, the power is calculated by subtracting these probabilities from 1 (remembering that power is equal to $1 - \beta$). Therefore, the power of the study ranged from 0.95 ($= 1 - 0.05$) to 0.975 ($= 1 - 0.025$). In the above example, the probability of observing a true difference of 4.00 min in running times between the two groups of athletes lies between 95% and 97.5%.

The calculations above assumed that the sample sizes of the two treatment groups were identical (10). In the equation to estimate minimum detectable difference and power a single value of N is employed (which is identical for each treatment group). However, as outlined previously, there may be experimental restrictions on the design of an experiment in which the sizes of samples in the two treatment groups are not identical. Therefore, to determine the minimum detectable difference and the power of a study, a single mean value of the two sample sizes must be employed. This is calculated as the harmonic mean and not the arithmetic mean, using the following equation:

$$N = \frac{2N_1 N_2}{N_1 + N_2}$$

where N_1 and N_2 denote the sample sizes of treatment groups 1 and 2, respectively, and N denotes the calculated mean sample size that is employed in further calculations.

In general, the power of a two-sample t test is increased if the sample sizes of the two treatment groups are identical.

8.2 Non-parametric statistical tests for two independent samples

8.2.1 Background

The use of non-parametric methods for the analysis of experimental data was introduced in Chapters 5 and 7 and therefore only a brief introduction concerning their use for the two-independent-samples data analysis will be provided at this point.

In all statistical analyses, one of the most significant decisions that must be performed is whether to use a parametric or non-parametric method. The most commonly employed parametric method in the pharmaceutical sciences is the two-sample t test, as described in the previous section. However, there are several restrictions on the use of this test. For example, parametric methods are most frequently employed when:

- the data have been measured on an interval or ratio scale
- the sample size is moderately large
- the variances in the treatment groups are equal
- the data have been sampled from populations that are normally distributed.

If these assumptions are valid, then a parametric test should be employed. Non-parametric methods may also be applied in these circumstances, but in so doing the analyst will increase the risk of committing a type II error (failure to reject the null hypothesis when it is actually false) and hence reduce the power of the study. Increasing the sample size may compensate for the reduction in power of the study, but this will have cost implications for the sponsors of the experiment.

In this section four non-parametric methods that may be employed for the comparison of two-sample data are described. As in Chapter 7, the advantages and disadvantages of each of these methods are described, including illustrations of experimental scenarios that warrant their use.

8.2.2 The Mann–Whitney U test

The Mann–Whitney U test is a test that may be employed to statistically compare two sets of independent data that have been measured on an ordinal, interval or ratio scale. Although the mechanics of the test are different, the Mann–Whitney U test is the non-parametric counterpart of the two-independent-samples t test for parametric data. The basic assumption of the Mann–Whitney U test is that the populations from which the two sets of sample data have been derived are similar, i.e. have similar distributions. This is the statement of the null hypothesis. The alternative hypothesis is that the distributions are different, and accordingly the values in one group are larger than those in the other group. Another statement of the null hypothesis is that the magnitudes of the values in the two treatment groups are similar.

8.2.2.1 Mechanics of the Mann–Whitney U test

The Mann–Whitney U test is commonly known as a *ranking* test. Indeed, one of the alternative names for this test is the *Wilcoxon rank sum test*. It is therefore not unexpected that one of the mathematical manipulations in performing this test involves a numerical ranking of the data. In this ranking process, the magnitudes of the values are taken into consideration, and accordingly larger values are allocated greater ranks than smaller values. The same is true whenever the data involves both positive and negative numbers, e.g. −5 is allocated a smaller rank than +5. After the data in the two treatment groups have been ranked, the sum of the ranks in each treatment group is calculated. The Mann–Whitney U statistic may be then be computed and interpreted in terms of the acceptance or rejection of the null hypothesis.

The Mann–Whitney U statistic is conveniently calculated using the following equation:

$$U = (N_1 N_2) + \frac{N_1(N_1 + 1)}{2} - R_1$$

where N_1 is the number of values in treatment group 1, N_2 is the number of values in treatment group 2 and R_1 is the sum of the ranks corresponding to treatment group 1.

Alternatively, the notation in the equation may be altered and the Mann–Whitney U statistic may be calculated using the data associated with treatment group 2:

$$U = (N_1 N_2) + \frac{N_2(N_2 + 1))}{2} - R_2$$

where N_1 is the number of values in treatment group 1, N_2 is the number of values in treatment group 2 and R_2 is the sum of the ranks corresponding to treatment group 2.

It may be apparent to the reader that the two equations will generate two numerically different U statistics. Obviously the interpretation of the calculated statistic will be different according to the choice of equation. The lower value of U is used to determine the outcome of the statistical analysis.

The use of the Mann–Whitney U test and the calculation and interpretation of the Mann–Whitney U statistic are shown in the following examples.

EXAMPLE 8.7   *As a clinical trials manager, you have been asked to design an experiment to evaluate the pharmacokinetic properties of two tablet formulations. For this purpose, a parallel experimental design was selected and 2 groups of 12 patients recruited into the clinical trial. One group received a new formulation in which the therapeutic agent had been micronised (99% of all particles <5 μm) whereas the second* *group received the established formulation (99% of all particles <50 μm). Each patient received one dose of one formulation. The results, expressed as the maximum concentration of drug in the blood (C_{max}), were as shown in Table 8.7. Using an appropriate statistical method, determine whether or not there is a significant difference between the clinical performances of the two formulations.*

Before the clinical trial begins, the following points should have been addressed.

(i) State the null hypothesis

The null hypothesis states that there is no difference between the C_{max} of the two formulations:

> H_0: the new and established formulations have similar pharmacokinetic properties (C_{max})

(ii) State the alternative hypothesis

The alternative hypothesis states that there is a difference between the C_{max} of the two formulations:

> H_a: the new and established formulations have different pharmacokinetic properties (C_{max})

Table 8.7 Pharmacokinetic study of the maximum concentration of a therapeutic agent in plasma (C_{max}) of human volunteers after administration of a single tablet of either a new formulation or an established formulation

Established formulation (C_{max}, μg/mL)	New formulation (C_{max}, μg/mL)
5.6	9.6
6.9	5.7
5.8	7.8
5.8	8.5
6.0	9.4
5.6	7.9
7.1	8.4
5.8	13.7
5.1	26.9
5.7	21.0
5.9	17.5
4.8	19.6

(iii) State the level of significance (the rejection region)

In this example, it is assumed that the level of significance (α) is 0.05.

(iv) State the number of tails associated with the experimental design

This is an example of a two-tailed test because the null hypothesis may be rejected for two reasons: the C_{max} values associated with the new formulation may be either greater or less than the corresponding values of the established formulation.

(v) Select the statistical analytical method

After the data has been collected, a key decision must be made about the most appropriate statistical method for data analysis. In this experimental design the comparative pharmacokinetic performances of two formulations are under examination. There is no direct relationship between the data and, accordingly, the two sets of data are independent. Therefore, the statistical analysis requires a two-independent-samples test.

The next choice for the statistical analyst is whether a parametric or non-parametric statistical method should be employed. If the experimental conditions are suitable for the use of a parametric method, then the two-sample t test should be employed. In particular, the populations from which the data have been derived should be normally distributed, the sample size should be sufficiently large, the variances of the two groups should be similar and the data should preferably be measured on an interval or ratio scale. To clarify the nature of the distributions and secondly the similarity or dissimilarity of variances, further mathematical manipulations of the data are required (Table 8.8).

Table 8.8 Descriptive statistics (mean, median, mode, variance and standard deviation) for the maximum concentrations of drug in the plasma (C_{max}) of a new formulation and an established formulation

Descriptive parameters	Established formulation C_{max}	New formulation C_{max}
Mean (μg/mL)	5.8	13.0
Median (μg/mL)	5.8	9.5
Mode (μg/mL)	5.8	Not applicable
Variance (μg/mL)^2	0.4	44.9
Standard deviation (μg/mL)	0.6	6.7

The mean, median and mode of the data associated with the established formulation are of similar magnitude, and therefore it can be assumed that the population from which this sample data have been derived is normally distributed. Conversely, the mean and median of the data associated with the new (micronised) formulation are dissimilar, raising doubts about the normality of the parent population.

The homogeneity (or heterogeneity) of variances is assessed using the F test. The null hypothesis for this test states that there is no difference between the variances of the two groups; the alternative hypothesis states that there is a significant difference between the two variances. The level of significance (α) is assumed to be 0.05 and the test is two-tailed because the null hypothesis may be rejected for the reason that either $s_1^2 > s_2^2$ or $s_1^2 < s_2^2$.

The F ratio is then calculated with the larger of the two variances defined as the numerator:

$$F = \frac{s_1^2}{s_2^2} = \frac{44.9}{0.40} = 112.25$$

The critical value of the F distribution that relates to the experimental design may be obtained by consultating the table of critical values of the F distribution (Appendix 7). This study is a two-tailed design in which α is 0.05 and the numbers of degrees of freedom associated with the numerator and denominator are both 11 (=12 – 1). Accordingly, the critical value of the F statistic is 3.47 ($F_{\alpha = 0.05, \text{two-tailed, num } df = 11, \text{ denom} df = 11}$). As the calculated F statistic was 112.25, the null hypothesis is rejected, i.e. the variances of the two groups are dissimilar.

It is therefore more appropriate to use a non-parametric method, namely the Mann–Whitney U test, to evaluate differences in the two sets of data.

(vi) Perform the statistical analysis

This is done in a stepwise fashion.

Step 1
The collective data from the two groups are pooled into one group, arranged numerically and ranked. The smallest value is assigned a rank of 1. In situations where there are tied values (identical values), an average rank is assigned. For example, in Table 8.9 there are two cases of the value 5.6 μg/mL. Each value must be given an identical rank and therefore the two values share the average of the third and fourth ranks, i.e. each value is ranked at 3.5. Similarly there are three identical cases of 5.8 μg/mL that have been initially assigned ranks 7, 8 and 9. These

Table 8.9 Numerical ranking of data presented in Table 8.8. Numbers in bold refer to data derived from the new drug treatment group

Numerical arrangement of data from treatments 1 and 2 (μg/mL)	Rank order of data from treatments 1 and 2
4.8	1
5.1	2
5.6	3.5
5.6	3.5
5.7	5.5
5.7	5.5
5.8	8
5.8	8
5.8	8
5.9	10
6	11
6.9	12
7.1	13
7.8	14
7.9	15
8.4	16
8.5	17
9.4	18
9.6	19
13.7	20
17.5	21
19.6	22
21	23
26.9	24

three values must share the same rank and accordingly an average of the three ranks is used for this purpose (8).

Step 2
The data (and the assigned ranks) are repartitioned into their original treatment groups. This is shown in Table 8.10. Next, the sums of the ranks for each treatment group are calculated. These values are required for the calculation of the Mann–Whitney U statistic.

Step 3 Calculation of the Mann–Whitney U statistic
The reader will remember that there are two forms of the Mann–Whitney U equation. The smaller calculated value of U should be used to interpret the statistical outcome of the analysis, so each U statistic needs to be calculated.

Table 8.10 Assignment of ranks to the data associated with the two treatment groups in Example 8.7

Established formulation		New formulation	
C_{max} (μg/mL)	Overall rank	C_{max} (μg/mL)	Overall rank
4.8	1	5.7	5.5
5.1	2	7.8	14
5.6	3.5	7.9	15
5.6	3.5	8.4	16
5.7	5.5	8.5	17
5.8	8	9.4	18
5.8	8	9.6	19
5.8	8	13.7	20
5.9	10	17.5	21
6.0	11	19.6	22
6.9	12	21.0	23
7.1	13	26.9	24
Sum of ranks	85.5	Sum of ranks	214.5

- Using N_1 (corresponding to the established formulation):

$$U = (N_1 N_2) + \frac{N_1(N_1 + 1))}{2} - R_1$$

$$= (12 \times 12) + \frac{12(12 + 1)}{2} - 85.5 = 136.5$$

- Using N_2 (corresponding to the new formulation):

$$U = (N_1 N_2) + \frac{N_2(N_2 + 1))}{2} - R_2$$

$$= (12 \times 12) + \frac{12(12 + 1)}{2} - 214.5 = 7.5$$

Step 4   Interpretation of the Mann–Whitney U statistic
The critical values of the Mann–Whitney U statistic are shown in Appendix 8. The table refers to the critical values of the statistic at a defined level of significance, i.e. for $\alpha = 0.05$ for a two-tailed test or $\alpha = 0.10$ for a one-tailed test. Furthermore, interpretation of the critical statistic requires knowledge of the size of each sample. The numerator (N_2) denotes the size of the larger sample group and N_1 denotes the size of the smaller group. In this current example the sample sizes are identical and therefore this factor is not relevant to the outcome of the

analysis, but it should be remembered when the sizes differ. From Appendix 8 it may be observed that when both N_1 and N_2 are equal to 12 and the level of significance is 0.05, the critical value of the Mann–Whitney U statistic for a two-tailed experimental design is 37. When the calculated (smaller) value of U is equal to or less than the critical value, the null hypothesis is rejected and the alternative hypothesis is accepted. Therefore, in Example 8.7 the alternative hypothesis is accepted, i.e. there is a significant difference between the pharmacokinetic properties (C_{max} in this case) of the two formulations. Furthermore, it may be concluded that micronisation of the therapeutic agent significantly increased the resultant maximum concentration of drug in the plasma of human volunteers.

8.2.2.2 Use of the Mann–Whitney U test for the analysis of large data sets

The largest value of N_2 that is included in the table of critical values of the Mann–Whitney U statistic is 20. An obvious question to ask is, 'What table is used to define the critical value when the sample size of the larger group exceeds this value?'. Under these circumstances it is assumed that the sampling distribution of the Mann–Whitney U statistic approximates to the normal distribution and therefore the standardised normal distribution may be employed to interpret the outcome of the statistical analysis. Under these circumstances the z value is calculated as before, i.e. the difference between the test value (the Mann–Whitney U statistic) and the mean is divided by the standard deviation:

$$z = \frac{U - (N_1 N_2/2)}{\sqrt{(N_1 \times N_2)(N_1 + N_2 + 1)/12}}$$

where U is the calculated Mann–Whitney U statistic (the smaller of the two possible calculated values), N_1 is the sample size of the smaller group and N_2 is the size of the larger group.

Following calculation of the z statistic, the statistical outcome is determined using the standardised normal distribution in conjunction with the parameters associated with the experimental design (number of tails, level of significance). The use of the Mann–Whitney U test for the determination of the similarity (or difference) between two treatment groups of large sample size is demonstrated in Example 8.8.

EXAMPLE 8.8 *Adherence of microorganisms to epithelial cells is thought to represent the initial stage of infection. A laboratory has developed a new drug (X), which it believes will demonstrate an ability* *to interfere with microbial adherence to epithelia. An* in vitro *experiment has been designed to investigate this hypothesis. In this, buccal epithelial cells were collected from a pool of donors and divided into two groups. One group was treated with the new drug and the other with sterile water, and then both groups were challenged with a fixed number of bacteria. Perform the appropriate statistical analysis to examine whether drug X exhibited a significant anti-adherent effect in the above experiment.*

Using a similar protocol to previous examples, the design criteria for the experiment should be defined.

(i) State the null hypothesis

The null hypothesis states that there is no difference between the mean number of adherent bacteria to epithelial cells that have been treated with either sterile water or the therapeutic agent (X).

> H_0: There is no difference between the abilities of either sterile water or drug X to reduce microbial attachment to epithelial cells *in vitro.*

In other words, drug X does not possess a significant microbial anti-adherence property in comparison to the experimental control (sterile water).

(ii) State the alternative hypothesis

The alternative hypothesis states that the adherence of bacteria to epithelial cells that have been treated with drug X is lower than to cells treated with sterile water.

> H_a: Drug X does possess a significant microbial anti-adherence property in comparison to the experimental control (sterile water).

(iii) State the level of significance (the rejection region)

In this example, it is assumed that the level of significance (α) is 0.05.

(iv) State the number of tails associated with the experimental design

This is an example of a one-tailed test because the study has been designed to identify whether bacterial adherence to epithelial cells treated with the therapeutic agent is less than to cells treated with sterile water. In this situation there is only one experimental outcome that is of interest to the investigator, and accordingly the experimental design is one-tailed.

The experiment is conducted and the numbers of bacteria (*Escherichia coli*) adherent to individual epithelial cells that had been previously treated with either sterile water or drug X are measured. The results are shown in Table 8.11.

(v)   *Select the statistical analytical method*

As outlined in the previous example, there are several questions that must be answered concerning both the experimental design and the statistical model to ensure that the most appropriate statistical test is chosen:

- First, two sets of data (treatments) are under comparison. These treatments are not related to each other, as each group of the epithelial cells received only one treatment. Consequently, a two-independent-samples statistical test should be used to analyse the comparative properties of the two data sets.
- The second question is whether a parametric or non-parametric method should be employed. Once more, the descriptive statistics of each group should be calculated and considered (Table 8.12). The mean and median of

Table 8.11   Number of bacteria adherent to individual epithelial cells that have been pre-treated with either sterile water (control) or therapeutic agent (drug X)

Number adherent to cells treated with sterile water	Number adherent to cells treated with drug X
25	12
35	12
45	21
65	24
32	1
14	2
10	0
2	0
3	1
56	4
12	0
25	0
46	3
23	2
45	14
12	6
	0
	2
	5
	0
	1

Table 8.12 Descriptive statistics (mean, median, mode, variance and standard deviation) of the number of adherent bacteria per epithelial cell following treatment with either sterile water or drug X

Descriptive parameters	Number of bacteria adherent to cells treated with sterile water	Number of bacteria adherent to cells treated with drug X
Mean	28.1	5.2
Median	25.0	2.0
Mode	Not applicable	0.0
Variance	366.4	51.3
Standard deviation	19.1	7.2

the data associated with the sterile water treatment are relatively close, but this is not the case for the data associated with the drug-treated epithelial cells. This raises doubts concerning the normality of the populations from which the data were derived.

The homogeneity of variances is assessed using the F test. The null hypothesis for this test states that there is no difference between the variances of the two groups; the alternative hypothesis states that there is a significant difference between the two variances. The level of significance (α) is assumed to be 0.05 and the test is two-tailed because the null hypothesis may be rejected for the reason that $s_1^2 > s_2^2$ or $s_1^2 < s_2^2$.

The F ratio is then calculated with the larger of the two variances defined as the numerator:

$$F = \frac{s_1^2}{s_2^2} = \frac{366.4}{51.3} = 7.14$$

The critical value of the F distribution that relates to this study may be obtained from Appendix 7. This study is a two-tailed design in which α is 0.05 and the numbers of degrees of freedom associated with the numerator and denominator are 15 ($=16-1$) and 20 ($=21-1$), respectively. Accordingly, the critical value of the F statistic is 2.57 ($F_{\alpha = 0.05, \text{ two-tailed, num } df = 15, \text{ denom } df = 20}$). As the calculated F statistic was 7.14, the null hypothesis is rejected, i.e. the variances of the two groups will be assumed to be dissimilar.

We may conclude that the most suitable statistical method to compare the central tendency of the two sets of data is a two-independent-samples non-parametric method, i.e. the Mann–Whitney U test.

Table 8.13 Numerical ranking of data presented in Table 8.11. Numbers in bold refer to the number of bacteria adherent to epithelial cells that had been treated with sterile water

Numerical arrangement of data from sterile water and drug treatments	Rank order of data from sterile water and drug treatments
0	3.5
0	3.5
0	3.5
0	3.5
0	3.5
0	3.5
1	8.0
1	8.0
1	8.0
2	11.5
2	11.5
2	11.5
2	11.5
3	14.5
3	14.5
4	16.0
5	17.0
6	18.0
10	19.0
12	21.5
12	21.5
12	21.5
12	21.5
14	24.5
14	24.5
21	26.0
23	27.0
24	28.0
25	29.5
25	29.5
32	31.0
35	32.0
45	33.5
45	33.5
46	35.0
56	36.0
65	37.0

(vi) Perform the statistical analysis

Step 1
Pool the data from the two groups into one group, arrange in numerical order and designate an appropriate rank to each datum (Table 8.13). As before, it should be remembered that tied ranks share an average rank value.

Step 2
Repartition the data into their original treatment groups and sum the ranks for each treatment group (Table 8.14).

Step 3   Calculate the appropriate statistic
As the sample size of the larger group exceeds 20, the normal approximation may be used for the statistical comparison of the two distributions.

Table 8.14 Assignment of ranks to the data associated with the two treatment groups described in Example 8.8

Drug treatment		Sterile water treatment	
Number of adherent bacteria per epithelial cell	Overall rank	Number of adherent bacteria per epithelial cell	Overall rank
0	3.5	2	11.5
0	3.5	3	14.5
0	3.5	10	19.0
0	3.5	12	21.5
0	3.5	12	21.5
0	3.5	14	24.5
1	8.0	23	27.0
1	8.0	25	29.5
1	8.0	25	29.5
2	11.5	32	31.0
2	11.5	35	32.0
2	11.5	45	33.5
3	14.5	45	33.5
4	16.0	46	35.0
5	17.0	56	36.0
6	18.0	65	37.0
12	21.5		
12	21.5		
14	24.5		
21	26.0		
24	28.0		
Sum of ranks	266.5	Sum of ranks	436.5

Thus, using the smaller sum of ranks, z is calculated:

$$z = \frac{U - (N_1 N_2/2)}{\sqrt{(N_1 \times N_2)(N_1 + N_2 + 1)/12}}$$

$$= \frac{266.5 - ((16 \times 21)/2)}{\sqrt{(16 \times 21)(16 + 21 + 1)/12}} = \frac{(266.5 - 168)}{32.6} = 3.02$$

Step 4   Interpret the calculated statistic
The two primary conditions of the experimental design were a level of significance (α) 0.05 and a negative one-tailed outcome. On the basis of this information and the standardised normal distribution (Appendix 1), the regions of acceptance and rejection of the null hypothesis may be defined. The region of acceptance of the null hypothesis is $-\infty$ to $+1.65$ and the region of rejection of the null hypothesis >1.65. Returning to Example 8.8, it may be observed that the calculated z statistic is 3.02 and therefore the null hypothesis is rejected. The adherence of bacteria to epithelial cells that had been pre-treated with drug X was significantly lower than to epithelial cells that had been treated with sterile water.

8.2.2.3   Use of the Mann–Whitney U test for the analysis of small data sets

Occasionally research within the pharmaceutical and related sciences involves the collection of small numbers of data. Indeed, in many scientific journals it is common to read that the experiment was performed in triplicate, implying that each data set consisted of three sample values. Students often ask what type of statistical test should be employed for the analysis of two such data sets. As the reader may recall, one of the requisites for the use of parametric statistical methods, e.g. Student's t test, is that the sample size should be large (>6). Therefore, in situations in which the sample size is less than this value it is customary to use a non-parametric test. If the sample size is greater than 6 the use of parametric tests is valid, providing that the other criteria for the use of such tests have been satisfied. These criteria have been outlined in previous examples. The use of the Mann–Whitney U test for the comparison of two sets of data (of small sample size) is illustrated in the following example.

EXAMPLE 8.9   *There have been reports of fracture of ureteral stents in patients. This is particularly dangerous as the fractured portions of the stent may migrate into and damage the kidney, and must be removed by surgical intervention. Fracture of stents implies that there have been* *alterations in their mechanical properties. Therefore, a university department has decided to investigate whether the duration of implantation of ureteral stents* in vivo *affects their mechanical properties.*

(i) State the null hypothesis

A suitable null hypothesis for this study is that time of implantation does not effect the mechanical properties of ureteral stents

(ii) State the alternative hypothesis

Conversely, the alternative hypothesis states that time of implantation decreases the resistance to mechanical fracture, i.e. adversely affects the mechanical properties of ureteral stents

(iii) State the level of significance

In this example, it is assumed that the level of significance (α) is 0.05.

(iv) Select the number of tails

In this investigation the investigators wish to find out if there is a decrease in the mechanical properties of ureteral stents associated with increased times of implantation *in vivo*. Therefore, there is only one outcome that is relevant to the study, i.e. there is only one outcome that will lead to the rejection of the null hypothesis. This study is therefore an example of a one-tailed investigation.

(v) Collect the experimental data

In the investigation, 3 ureteral stents were removed from patients after implantation in patients for 4 weeks and another 4 stents were removed after implantation for 16 weeks. Because of the difficulty in obtaining excised ureteral stents, the numbers of samples within each group (period of implantation) were limited. After removal, the mechanical properties of each stent were characterised by tensile analysis. The percentage elongations at break for each stent (a measure of the maximum deformation a material can withstand prior to fracture) were recorded and are displayed in Table 8.15.

(vi) Select the statistical test

As previously explained, the sample sizes of the two groups in this study are small and, therefore, it is difficult to assume or estimate that the distributions from which the samples were derived are normal. Furthermore, there are two sets of data (treatment groups) in this study

Table 8.15 Effect of implantation *in vivo* on the percentage elongation at break of ureteral stents

% Elongation after 4 weeks implantation	% Elongation after 16 weeks implantation
96.9	97.9
99.9	99.6
101.8	104.6
	100.2

that are unrelated. As a result a non-parametric, two-independent-samples test should be employed (e.g. the Mann–Whitney U test).

(vii)   Calculate the Mann–Whitney U statistic

In the case of small samples, the calculation of the Mann–Whitney U statistic requires that the data should be numerically ranked, as before; however, no mathematical formula is required to derive the numerical value U. Consequently, the data should initially be ranked, remembering to retain knowledge of the origins of each datum (Table 8.16).

The Mann–Whitney U statistic is then calculated by assigning the number of values in one group that precede the second group. This may be illustrated with reference to the above example. Firstly, calculate the number of values of the 4-week group that precede the 16-week group:

- below the value of 97.9 (16 weeks) there is one value in the 4-week group (96.9)
- below the value of 99.6 (16 weeks) there is one value in the 4-week group (96.9)
- below the value of 100.2 (16 weeks) there are two values in the 4-week group (96.9 and 99.9)
- below the value of 104.6 (16 weeks) there are three values in the 4-week group (96.9, 99.9 and 101.8).

Table 8.16 Ranking of the experimental data described in Table 8.15

Numerical ranking of data on the % elongation of ureteral stents	Original sample group
96.9	4 weeks
97.9	16 weeks
99.6	16 weeks
99.9	4 weeks
100.2	16 weeks
101.8	4 weeks
104.6	16 weeks

The numbers of values are then added together to produce the Mann–Whitney U statistic. In the above case, the statistic is 7 $(1 + 1 + 2 + 3)$.

This statistic was calculated by counting the number of values in the 4-week group that preceded those in the 16-week group. Of course, a Mann–Whitney U statistic could have also been calculated by counting the number of values in the 16-week group that preceded those in the 4-week group:

- below the value of 96.9 (4 weeks) there are no values
- below the value of 99.9 (4 weeks) there are two values in the 16-week group (97.9 and 99.6)
- below the value of 101.8 (4 weeks) there are three values in the 16-week group (97.9, 99.6 and 100.2).

The numbers of values are then added together to produce the Mann–Whitney U statistic. In this case, the statistic is 5 $(2 + 3)$.

As in previous descriptions of the use of the Mann–Whitney U test, the lower calculated U value is employed to interpret the outcome of the statistical analysis. Therefore, in Example 8.9, the calculated Mann–Whitney U statistic is 5.

Instead of calculating the two possible values of the Mann–Whitney U statistic, as described above, there is a mathematical shortcut that may be employed to render this process less laborious. One Mann–Whitney U statistic is calculated using the process described above, and the second possible Mann–Whitney U statistic is then calculated using the following formula:

$$U = N_1 \times N_2 - U^*$$

where N_1 and N_2 are the numbers of data in each treatment group and U^* is the value of the Mann–Whitney U statistic that has previously been calculated.

In Example 8.9, the first Mann–Whitney U statistic was calculated as 7. The second possible value may be calculated using the above formula:

$$U = N_1 \times N_2 - U^*$$
$$= (3 \times 4) - 7$$
$$= 5$$

The value so obtained is in agreement with that obtained using the earlier method.

(viii) Interpret the calculated Mann–Whitney U statistic

The calculated Mann–Whitney U statistic may be interpreted using the appropriate tables (Appendix 9). For small sample sizes the tables are divided into a series of smaller tables, each relating to size of the larger group (N_2). In the current example, $N_2 = 4$. The probability of observing the calculated Mann–Whitney U statistic (5) when the sample size of the smaller group (N_1) is 3 (i.e. the conditions of the experiment) is then extracted from the statistical table. In the current example, the probability of observing the calculated Mann–Whitney U statistic (5) when N_1 and N_2 are 3 and 4, respectively, is 0.43. Under the conditions of the experiment, the selected level of significance is 0.05, i.e. calculated probability values that are either equal to or less than 0.05 will allow the null hypothesis to be rejected. As the calculated value (0.43) exceeded 0.05, we have no reason to reject the null hypothesis. Therefore, there is no evidence to suggest that time of implantation in patients significantly reduced the percentage elongation at break of ureteral stents.

In Examples 8.7, 8.8 and 8.9, the Mann–Whitney U test was applied for the comparison of two independent sets of data that were measured in a ratio scale. However, this test may also be employed for the comparison of two sets of data whose measurement has been performed using an ordinal scale. The mechanics of the test are identical to those described in the previous examples and are outlined in the next example.

EXAMPLE 8.10 *Percutaneous local anaesthesia (anaesthesia of the skin) is an effective option for patients who wish to receive pain-free injections or local surgery (e.g. removal of facial port wine stains). A research unit wishes to compare the percutaneous local anaesthetic properties of two formulations, a gel and a cream, each containing 4% w/w of a local anaesthetic. In this study, it is proposed that each formulation will be applied to the forearm of volunteers for at least 45 min, removed and the degree of anaesthesia determined using a needle prick test. The pain associated with this test is measured in an ordinal scale, with 1 reflecting no pain (total anaesthesia) and 4 reflecting no anaesthesia. Values of 2 and 3 represent intermediate degrees of anaesthesia (i.e. 2 > 3). Using an appropriate statistical method, determine whether the nature of the formulation will affect the percutaneous local anaesthesia.*

Once more, the parameters associated with the experimental design should be detailed before the study begins.

(i) State the null hypothesis

The null hypothesis states that there is no difference in the percutaneous local anaesthetic properties of the two formulations:

> H_0: the gel and cream formulations have similar percutaneous local anaesthetic properties

(ii) State the alternative hypothesis

The alternative hypothesis states that there is a difference in the percutaneous local anaesthetic properties of the two formulations of the two formulations:

> H_a: the gel and cream formulations have different percutaneous local anaesthetic properties.

(iii) State the level of significance (the rejection region)

In this example, it is assumed that the level of significance (α) is 0.05.

(iv) State the number of tails associated with the experimental design

Once more, this is an example of a two-tailed test in which the null hypothesis may be rejected for two reasons: the degree of percutaneous local anaesthesia associated with the gel may be either higher or lower than that associated with the cream.

(v) Select the statistical analytical method

In this experimental design, the comparative effects of two formulations are under examination. It is proposed that two independent groups of volunteers will be used and each group will receive only one formulation. Therefore, this is an example of two-independent-samples experimental design. Furthermore, the data that will be collected in the clinical study is ordinal in nature, thus rendering invalid the application of parametric statistical tests. As a result, the comparative percutaneous local anaesthetic effects of the two formulations will be examined using a Mann–Whitney U test.

(vi) Collect the experimental data

In this study each group of volunteers received one formulation. Following the period of application (45 min), the formulation was removed and the degree of anaesthesia at the site of application was assessed using the needle prick test. The results of this study are shown in Table 8.17.

Table 8.17 Degree of percutaneous local anaesthesia, recorded as a pain score, associated with two formulations (gel and cream) containing 4% w/w local anaesthetic

Gel formulation	Cream formulation
1	2
1	3
1	3
1	4
2	3
1	2
2	3
1	2
1	

(vii) Perform the statistical analysis

Step 1
Pool the data from the two groups into one group, arrange in numerical order and designate an appropriate rank to each datum (Table 8.18).

Table 8.18 Numerical ranking of data presented in Table 8.17. Numbers in bold denote the pain scores associated with the cream formulation

Numerical order	Rank order
1	4
1	4
1	4
1	4
1	4
1	4
1	4
2	10
2	10
2	10
2	10
2	10
3	14.5
3	14.5
3	14.5
3	14.5
4	17

Step 2

Repartition the data into their original treatment groups and combine the ranks for each treatment group (Table 8.19). When there are tied values the average rank is given to each value. For example, in Table 8.19 there are 7 recorded pain scores with a magnitude of 1. Therefore to calculate the average pain score, the seven ranks are summed and averaged:

$$\text{Average} = \frac{(1 + 2 + 3 + 4 + 5 + 6 + 7)}{7} = 4$$

Step 3   Calculate the appropriate statistic

The sample size of the larger group is less than 20 and therefore the use of the normal approximation is not appropriate for the statistical comparison of the two distributions. Thus the conventional equation for the calculation of the Mann–Whitney U statistic may be used. In this case, the smaller value should be used to interpret the statistical outcome of the analysis and accordingly, each U statistic should be calculated.

Using N_1 (corresponding to the cream formulation), as N_1 refers to the smaller sample group, the Mann–Whitney U statistic may be calculated:

$$U = (N_1 N_2) + \frac{N_1(N_1 + 1))}{2} - R_1$$

$$= (8 \times 9) + \frac{8(8 + 1)}{2} - 105 = 3.0$$

Using N_2 (corresponding to the gel formulation), as N_2 refers to

Table 8.19 Assignment of ranks to the pain scores associated with the two formulations described in Example 8.10

Gel formulation		Cream formulation	
Pain score	Overall rank	Pain score	Overall rank
1	4.0	2	10.0
1	4.0	2	10.0
1	4.0	2	10.0
1	4.0	3	14.5
1	4.0	3	14.5
1	4.0	3	14.5
1	4.0	3	14.5
2	10.0	4	17.0
2	10.0		
Sum of ranks	48.0	Sum of ranks	105.0

the larger sample group:

$$U = (N_1 N_2) + \frac{N_2(N_2 + 1))}{2} - R_2$$

$$= (8 \times 9) + \frac{9(9 + 1)}{2} - 48.0 = 69.0$$

$$U^* = N_1 \times N_2 - U = (8 \times 9) - 69 = 3$$

Step 4   Interpret the Mann–Whitney U statistic
The calculated (smaller) U statistic may be interpreted after consideration of the properties of the experimental design and the table of critical
values of the Mann–Whitney U statistic. The main experimental parameters that must be known to enable interpretation of the outcome of the
clinical study are:

- the level of significance (0.05)
- the number of tails in the experimental design (two)
- the sizes of each set of data ($N_1 = 8$, $N_2 = 9$).

The critical value of the Mann–Whitney U statistic related to this study
is therefore 15 (from Appendix 7). When the calculated (smaller) value
of U (3) is equal to or less than the critical value, the null hypothesis is
rejected and the alternative hypothesis is accepted. Therefore, in this
example, the null hypothesis is rejected and the alternative hypothesis
accepted. It may therefore be concluded that there is a significant difference in the percutaneous local anaesthetic properties of the gel and
cream formulations. Furthermore, on the basis of the data depicted in
Table 8.17, it may be stated that the local anaesthetic activity of the gel
formulation is significantly greater than that of the cream formulation.

8.2.3 χ^2 Analysis for two independent samples: contingency tables

In Chapter 7, the χ^2 test was introduced for the analysis of one-sample
data. In this situation, the technique was referred to as a goodness-of-fit
test, in which a statistical comparison is carried out between the
numbers of actual observations associated with an event and the
expected number of observations (as defined by the null hypothesis). If
the expected and actual numbers of observations are in agreement then
there is said to be no *correlation* between the variables under consideration, i.e. the variables are said to be independent of one another.

The reader will recall that the one-sample χ^2 test involved
analysing the relationship between the observed and expected frequencies within different categories of a particular variable. In a two-sample
χ^2 analysis there are again two variables under consideration, one of

which may have several categories, e.g. 2×2, 2×3, 2×4. The null hypothesis in χ^2 analysis states that there is no correlation between the frequencies associated with the rows and those recorded in the columns. For this reason, the χ^2 analysis is referred to as a *test of independence*. At this stage it is useful to point out that there are also higher orders of χ^2 analyses, e.g. 3×4, 4×4. An introduction to the mechanics and applications of the χ^2 analysis to these higher orders of experimental design is provided in Chapter 11. The mechanics of the χ^2 analysis, independent of whether it is a one- or two-sample test, involve calculation of the expected values associated with the null hypothesis within the experimental design and, with knowledge of the observed values, calculation of the χ^2 statistic. The χ^2 statistic is then interpreted after consultation with the χ^2 distribution (Appendix 3). Once more, the χ^2 test is employed when the data is nominal in nature, i.e. when it is recorded as frequencies in discrete categories. As before, the use and interpretation of the χ^2 test is most appropriately illustrated by the use of examples.

The smallest contingency table that may be generated experimentally consists of two independent variables, each containing two categories. Such a design is composed of two columns and two rows and is therefore called a 2×2 *design*. Within the basic structure of a 2×2 contingency table, different experimental designs that are employed that are dependent on the nature of data collection. The first of these is referred to as a *double dichotomy system*. In this, the total number of observations is fixed but not the number of observations in the rows and totals (i.e. associated with the variables). The statistical analysis examines whether the variables are independent. A second experimental design is referred to as a *binomial comparative trial* and differs from the previous type as the total associated with either the rows or the column is specified before the study is carried out. Finally, certain experimental conditions are enforced in which the rows and columns in the 2×2 table are fixed. If the data are randomly sampled, this allows conclusions to be drawn concerning the nature of the population from which the samples were derived. The next examples illustrate some of these types of experimental designs and the application of the χ^2 test for the statistical analysis of data collected and presented in the 2×2 format.

EXAMPLE 8.11 *A national Department of Health is concerned with the number of deaths due to heart disease in men aged 40–50 years. Therefore, a study has been commissioned to investigate if there is a relationship between hypertension in men and their residence in either the north or south of the country. As a statistician, you have been asked to design and execute this study. Using an appropriate statistical test,* *examine whether there is a relationship between hypertension and geographical location.*

As before, it is important to establish the criteria for the statistical model.

(i) State the null hypothesis

The null hypothesis in a χ^2 analysis states that the variables are independent and therefore lack correlation. For Example 8.11, a suitable null hypothesis is that there is no relationship between the geographical location of residence (the north or south of the country) and the incidence of hypertension.

(ii) State the alternative hypothesis

In the χ^2 test, the alternative hypothesis states that there is a relationship (correlation) between the two variables. Therefore, a suitable alternative hypothesis for the above example is that there is a relationship between the location of residence and the incidence of hypertension.

(iii) State the level of significance

In this example, it is assumed that the level of significance (α) is 0.05.

(iv) State the number of tails associated with the experimental design

The number of tails associated with a particular experimental design is a statement of the number of outcomes associated with rejection of the null hypothesis. In this example there are two ways in which the null hypothesis may be rejected: the incidence of hypertension in the north of the country may be greater than in the south or vice versa. The experimental design associated with Example 8.11 is therefore two-tailed.

In the investigation, the blood pressures of 151 male volunteers aged 40–50 years resident in the north of the country and 179 resident in the south were measured. This is an example of a double dichotomy experimental design as a random sample of 330 men were included in the study, with no defined categorisation, i.e. no further specification of the location of residence of the chosen subjects. Only volunteers who had been resident in the relevant locations for over 20 years were admitted into the investigation. The patients were categorised as having normal or high blood pressure, commensurate with their age. The results from the study are presented in Table 8.20.

Table 8.20 Observed incidences of normal and high blood pressure (BP) in male volunteers (40–50 years of age) resident in the north and south of a country

Location	Normal BP	High BP	Totals
North	106	45	151
South	131	48	179
Totals	237	93	330

(v) Select an appropriate statistical test

In this study two variables are under examination, location and blood pressure. In each of these variables there are two categories, i.e. north or south and normal or high blood pressure. Consequently this is an example of a 2×2 experimental design. In this situation, the observed frequencies are located within the individual cells and the table is commonly referred to as a *contingency table*. One further point to note is the nature of the data, which has been recorded as frequencies (incidences) and is accordingly nominal in nature. Therefore, given the described properties of the experimental design, validation or rejection of the null hypothesis is most appropriately performed using a 2×2 χ^2 analysis.

(vi) Compute the χ^2 statistic

The equation employed for calculation of the χ^2 statistic was introduced in section 7.2.1. Computation of the χ^2 statistic involves an initial calculation of the expected frequencies for each cell in the contingency table, as defined by the null hypothesis, i.e. whenever there is independence between each variable:

$$\chi^2 = \sum \frac{(O_f - E_f)^2}{E_f}$$

where O_f is the observed frequencies in each cell and E_f is the expected frequencies for each cell (as defined by the null hypothesis).

In the case of a 2×2 χ^2 analysis, it is necessary to modify the above equation to allow for the use of a continuous probability distribution (the χ^2 distribution) for the calculation of the probability associated with discrete data (frequencies). The equation for the calculation of the χ^2 statistic is modified to include a correction term, referred to as the Yates correction for continuity:

$$\chi^2 = \sum \frac{[(O_f - E_f) - 0.5]^2}{E_f}$$

When higher orders of experimental design are employed, e.g. contingency tables composed of 2×3 or 2×4 cells, etc., this modification is not required.

As in previous examples, calculation of the χ^2 statistic is performed in a stepwise fashion.

Step 1 Calculate the expected frequencies associated with each cell
The expected frequencies associated with each cell are calculated by multiplying the row total associated with cell by the column total associated with the cell and dividing by the total number of observations in the study. The expected frequencies for the four cells (Table 8.21) are therefore:

- Cell representing normal blood pressure and north location:

$$E_f = \frac{(237 \times 151)}{330} = 108.4$$

- Cell representing high blood pressure and north location:

$$E_f = \frac{(93 \times 151)}{330} = 42.6$$

- Cell representing normal blood pressure and south location:

$$E_f = \frac{(237 \times 179)}{330} = 128.6$$

- Cell representing high blood pressure and south location:

$$E_f = \frac{(93 \times 179)}{330} = 50.4$$

Step 2 Calculate the corrected χ^2 statistic
The χ^2 statistic is calculated by calculating and adding the ratios of the squared differences between the observed and expected frequencies for

Table 8.21 Expected incidences of normal and high blood pressure (BP) in male volunteers (40–50 years of age) resident in the north and south of a country, as defined by the null hypothesis

Location	Normal BP	High BP	Totals
North	108.4	42.6	151
South	128.6	50.4	179
Totals	237	93	330

each cell (corrected for continuity) and the expected frequencies:

$$\chi^2 = \sum \frac{[(106-108.4)-0.5]^2}{108.4} + \frac{[(45-42.6)-0.5]^2}{42.6}$$
$$+ \frac{[(131-128.6)-0.5]^2}{128.6} + \frac{[(48-50.4)-0.5]^2}{50.4}$$
$$= 0.36$$

(vii) Interpret the χ^2 statistic

As described in section 7.2.1, the calculated χ^2 statistic is interpreted by comparing this value to the critical χ^2 statistic that defines the regions of acceptance and rejection of the null hypothesis. The critical values of the χ^2 statistic associated with these regions may be identified if the level of significance, the number of tails in the experimental design and the number of degrees of freedom associated with the study are known. The level of significance was set as 0.05 and the experimental design was two-tailed. The number of degrees of freedom for a χ^2 analysis is calculated using the following formula:

$$df = (R-1)(C-1)$$

in which R and C denote respectively the number of rows and columns in the contingency table. As this is a 2×2 contingency table, the number of degrees of freedom associated with Example 8.11 is 1. Therefore, when the number of degrees of freedom is 1 and the level of significance is 0.05, the critical value of χ^2 is 3.84, as we can see from the critical values of the χ^2 distribution (Appendix 3). Accordingly, the region associated with acceptance of the null hypothesis is $\chi^2 < 3.84$ and the region associated with rejection of the null hypothesis is $\geqslant 3.84$. In Example 8.11 the calculated χ^2 statistic was 0.36 and, as this value is less than 3.84, it may be concluded that the two variables are independent. More specifically, there is no difference in the incidences of hypertension in male subjects living in either the north or south of this particular country.

In Example 8.11 calculation of the χ^2 statistic was quite laborious, but a shortcut formula has been developed that includes the continuity correction:

$$\chi^2 = \frac{N[(AD-BC)-(N/2)]^2}{[(A+B)(C+D)(A+C)(B+D)]}$$

Here the symbols A, B, C and D refer to designated cells in the contingency table, whereas N, as before, refers to the total number of

Table 8.22 Designation of cells in a 2 × 2 contingency table

Variable 2	Variable 1		Total
	Category 1	Category 2	
Category 1	A	B	A + B
Category 2	C	D	C + D
Total	A + C	B + D	N

observations (the sum of the frequencies in all four cells). The designations of cells are illustrated in Table 8.22.

The use of this equation for the calculation of the χ^2 statistic is explained in Example 8.12. This example is also an illustration of the mechanics of the χ^2 analysis when the experimental design is one-tailed.

EXAMPLE 8.12 *A pharmaceutical company has developed two new anxiolytic drugs for the prevention of panic attacks in susceptible individuals. The company wishes to identify whether one of these drugs (Y) possesses superior anxiolytic properties to the other (X) as drug Y is more expensive to manufacture. A clinical trial has therefore been designed in which patients who suffer anxiety attacks are given a single dose of either drug X or drug Y and the incidence of anxiety attacks recorded for each patient over a 12 h period. More specifically, patients were asked whether (or not) they had experienced at least one anxiety attack over the 12 h period. In the study, it was decided that 135 and 186 patients should receive drugs X and Y respectively. The results of the outcome of the clinical trial are shown in Table 8.23.*

Once more, the experimental parameters must be defined.

(i) State the null hypothesis

A suitable null hypothesis for this clinical study is that there is no correlation (no dependency) between the two variables. Alternatively this may be stated as

H_0: there is no difference in the anxiolytic properties of drug X and drug Y

(ii) State the alternative hypothesis

The alternative hypothesis for this study states that there is a correlation between the two variables, i.e. the observed frequencies associated with the variables are dependent on each other. More specifically:

H_a: the incidence of anxiety attacks is lower in patients who received drug Y rather than drug X

(iii)   State the level of significance

In this example, it is assumed that the level of significance (α) is 0.05.

(iv)   State the number of tails associated with the experimental design

In this study the null hypothesis will be rejected only if the efficacy of drug Y is greater than that of drug X. Accordingly, there is only one outcome that will allow rejection of the null hypothesis, so this is an example of a one-tailed experimental design.

(v)   Compute the χ^2 statistic

This is an example of a binomial comparative design because the number of subjects entered into a particular classification was fixed before the start of the study. As this is a 2×2 contingency table, the χ^2 statistic may be calculated using the shortcut formula, as described above. With respect to this equation, the symbols A, B, C and D refer to the cells defined as drug X/no anxiety, drug X/anxiety, drug Y/no anxiety and drug Y/anxiety, respectively.

Therefore:

$$\chi^2 = \frac{N[(AD \times BC) - N/2]^2}{[(A+B)(C+D)(A+C)(B+D)]}$$

$$= \frac{321[((106 \times 17) - (19 \times 169)) - 321/2]^2}{[(106+19)(169+17)(106+169)(19+17)]}$$

$$= 2.49$$

(vi)   Interpret the outcome of the statistical analysis

The outcome of the statistical analysis is dependent on whether the calculated χ^2 statistic lies within the regions of acceptance or rejection of

Table 8.23   Incidences of anxiety attacks in patients over a 12-h period after administration of a single dose of either drug X or drug Y

Therapeutic agent	Incidence of anxiety attacks		Totals
	None	At least 1	
Drug X	106	29	135
Drug Y	169	17	186
Totals	275	46	321

the null hypothesis. Therefore, the first step in interpreting the calculated statistic is to define the ranges of values of χ^2 that define the acceptance and rejection regions. In Example 8.11, the level of significance was set at 0.05, the study was one-tailed and there is 1 df [(2 – 1)(2 – 1)]. The critical values of χ^2 values are provided in Appendix 3, but these values refer to a two-tailed design. For a one-tailed test in which $\alpha = 0.05$ and there is 1 df, the critical value associated with a probability of 0.1 is used. Therefore, for all one-tailed designs the critical value is that associated with 2α. From the table of critical values of χ^2, we can see that the critical statistic is 2.71. Consequently, if the calculated χ^2 value is less than 2.71 the null hypothesis is accepted, but if the calculated value is equal to or exceeds 2.71, the null hypothesis is rejected. In Example 8.12 the calculated χ^2 statistic was 2.49 and therefore the null hypothesis is accepted, i.e. drug X and drug Y have similar anxiolytic properties so there is no clinical advantage in using drug Y (remembering that it is also more expensive!).

The previous examples have illustrated the use of the χ^2 test for the analysis of data that has been presented in a 2×2 contingency table. This is the most straightforward experimental design of contingency table, as only two categories are allowed for each variable. In clinical research it is frequently difficult to categorise a particular variable into only two categories and therefore, on many occasions, contingency tables are assembled in which a variable is expressed by more than two categories. The mechanics of performing the χ^2 analysis for these experimental designs (e.g. 2×3, 2×4, etc.) is identical to that for the 2×2 design. However, it may be of interest to the reader to work through the following example to gain a further insight into the operation of the test.

EXAMPLE 8.13 *Two transdermal formulations have been developed for the cessation of smoking, one containing 2 mg and the other 4 mg of a therapeutic agent. One of the side-effects of the therapeutic agent is headache. Therefore, as part of a phase III clinical trial, the sponsor company wishes to examine whether there is a correlation between the concentration of therapeutic agent and severity of headache. Using an appropriate statistical test, examine whether the concentration of therapeutic agent increased the incidence of headache.*

The parameters of the experimental design should first be detailed.

(i) State the null hypothesis

In the χ^2 test the null hypothesis assumes that there is no correlation between the two variables, i.e. concentration of therapeutic agent and severity of headache are independent (i.e. not related).

(ii)   State the alternative hypothesis

The alternative hypothesis, as before, adopts an opposite view to that stated in the null hypothesis. Therefore, a suitable alternative hypothesis is that there is a correlation (relationship) between increasing the concentration of therapeutic agent in the transdermal formulations and the increased severity of headache.

(iii)   State the level of significance

In this example, it is assumed that the level of significance (α) is 0.05.

(iv)   State the number of tails associated with the experimental design

This clinical study has been commissioned to find out if the increased dose of therapeutic agent is associated with increased severity of headache. Pharmacologically, it is highly unlikely that a reciprocal relationship exists between drug concentration and severity of side-effects and accordingly, increasing the amount of therapeutic agent in the dosage form either will or will not increase the severity of headache. It has already been stated in the null hypothesis that there will be no increase in the severity of headaches from increasing the concentration of therapeutic agent, whereas the alternative hypothesis has stated that increasing the concentration of therapeutic agent will increase the severity of headache. As there is only one path along which the null hypothesis may be rejected (and the alternative hypothesis accepted), this study is an example of a one-tailed design.

(v)   Collect the experimental data

In the clinical study, the transdermal formulation containing 2 mg therapeutic agent was administered to 295 patients, whereas the formulation containing the higher concentration of agent was administered to 296 patients. Over a period of 12 h after administration of each transdermal formulation, the patients were asked to record both whether or not they experienced headache and the severity of any headache. The results are shown in Table 8.24.

(vi)   Select an appropriate statistical test

This investigation is an example of a 2×3 contingency table, i.e. there are two variables (concentration of therapeutic agent and headache) each consisting of two categories (two concentrations and three stages of headache). The data is nominal in nature, consisting of recorded

Table 8.24 Observed incidences and severity of headache associated with transdermal administration of two formulations containing different concentrations of therapeutic agent (2 mg and 4 mg)

Concentration of therapeutic agent	Number of recorded observations (O_f)			Total
	No headache	Mild headache	Severe headache	
2 mg	182	75	38	295
4 mg	155	91	50	296
Total	337	166	88	591

frequencies in each category, and it is assumed that the two variables are independent of one another. On the basis of this information, the most appropriate test to confirm or reject the null hypothesis is a 2×3 χ^2 analysis.

(vii) Carry out the χ^2 test

The mechanism for execution of the χ^2 test for two-samples in a 2×3 design is identical to that for the 2×2 design. Therefore, the initial main step in this process is to calculate the expected frequencies within each category as predicted by the null hypothesis. These expected frequencies are calculated by multiplying the values of the row total and the column total that are associated with each observed frequency and dividing this value by the overall number of participants in the study. The calculations of each expected frequency associated with the data described in Table 8.24 are shown below.

- Expected frequency (E_f) of the cell representing the lower concentration of therapeutic agent and no headache:

$$E_f = \frac{(337 \times 295)}{591} = 168.2$$

- Expected frequency (E_f) of the cell representing the higher concentration of therapeutic agent and no headache:

$$E_f = \frac{(337 \times 296)}{591} = 168.8$$

- Expected frequency (E_f) of the cell representing the lower concentration of therapeutic agent and mild headache:

$$E_f = \frac{(166 \times 295)}{591} = 82.9$$

- Expected frequency (E_f) of the cell representing the higher concentration of therapeutic agent and mild headache:

$$E_f = \frac{(166 \times 296)}{591} = 83.1$$

- Expected frequency (E_f) of the cell representing the lower concentration of therapeutic agent and severe headache:

$$E_f = \frac{(88 \times 295)}{591} = 43.9$$

- Expected frequency (E_f) of the cell representing the higher concentration of therapeutic agent and severe headache:

$$E_f = \frac{(88 \times 296)}{591} = 44.1$$

These calculated expected values are summarised in Table 8.25.

After the expected frequencies have been computed, the χ^2 statistic is calculated:

$$\chi^2 = \sum \left(\frac{O_f - E_f}{E_f}\right)^2$$

$$= \sum \frac{(182.0 - 168.2)^2}{168.2} + \frac{(155.0 - 168.2)^2}{168.8} + \frac{(75.0 - 82.9)^2}{82.9}$$

$$+ \frac{(91.0 - 78.8)^2}{78.8} + \frac{(38.0 - 43.9)^2}{43.9} + \frac{(50.0 - 44.1)^2}{44.1}$$

$$= (1.13 + 1.03 + 0.75 + 1.89 + 0.79 + 0.79) = 6.38$$

Note that no correction term for continuity has been applied to the above calculation. As mentioned earlier, when the degrees of freedom of an experiment are greater than 1, the continuity correction is not required.

Table 8.25 Expected incidences of headache associated with transdermal administration of two formulations containing different concentrations of therapeutic agent (2 mg and 4 mg)

Concentration of therapeutic agent	Number of expected observations (E_f)			Total
	No headache	Mild headache	Severe headache	
2 mg	168.2	82.9	43.9	295
4 mg	168.8	83.1	44.1	296
Total	337	166	88	591

(vii) Interpret the outcome of the χ^2 test

The outcome of the statistical test is interpreted by comparing the calculated value of χ^2 to the critical value associated with the experimental design. The critical value is defined by three parameters: the chosen level of significance, the number of tails and the number of degrees of freedom associated with the design. In this example, the experimental design is one-tailed and has a defined level of significance (0.05). The number of degrees of freedom may be calculated as before using the following equation:

$$df = (R - 1)(C - 1) = (2 - 1)(3 - 1) = 2$$

With this information the critical values of the χ^2 statistic may be found from the table in Appendix 3, remembering that for a one-tailed analysis the probability value that must be entered into the table is 2α (0.1). In Example 8.13, the critical value of χ^2 is therefore 4.60. Accordingly, if the calculated value is less than 4.60 the null hypothesis is accepted, but if the calculated value is equal to or greater than this critical value the null hypothesis is rejected. Reverting to Example 8.13, the calculated value is 6.38 and the null hypothesis is rejected. Therefore, it may be concluded that the variables are not independent and indeed there is a measure of correlation between the severity of headache and the concentration of therapeutic agent. In other words, as the concentration of therapeutic agent is increased the severity of headaches also increased.

It is important to note that there are some restrictions/modifications concerning the use of the χ^2 test for 2×3 (and greater) contingency tables. In these, the expected frequency should be greater than 5 in the vast majority of the cells. If this is not the case, then categories should be combined to ensure that this requirement is met.

8.2.4 The Fisher exact probability test for two independent samples

The Fisher exact test is another statistical method that may be employed to analyse the relationship between variables within the 2×2 experimental design. For this reason, the test is related, albeit not mathematically, to the 2×2 χ^2 analysis. Before introducing the mechanics of the Fisher exact probability test, it is appropriate to consider the design and limitations of the χ^2 test for the analysis of data collected in a 2×2 experimental design. In the design of a 2×2 experiment and subsequent analysis of the data using the χ^2 test, it is common for the experimental design to be a *double dichotomy*, in which the sample size is fixed but the number of observations in the rows and columns are not set; a *binomial comparative design*, in which the total in the two categories of a variable are set; or, occasionally, a design in which there are fixed totals for the rows and columns. Typically, the χ^2 test is employed for the analysis of all of these experimental designs. Furthermore, as has been shown in the various examples in section 8.2.3, calculation of the χ^2 statistic requires application of the continuity correction. However, although the χ^2 test is a useful technique for the analysis of nominal or ordinal data that have been presented in the form of a contingency table, there are restrictions concerning its use. If the total sample size is less than 20, or if it is between 20 and 40 and the smallest expected frequency in one of the cells is less than 5, the χ^2 test cannot be employed. Under these circumstances, the *Fisher exact probability test* is used instead.

In general the Fisher exact probability test is used for the analysis of 2×2 contingency tables that have fixed column and row totals, but the test may also be used for the analysis of double dichotomy and binomial comparative trial designs. However, in these latter cases, the test assumes that the row and column totals are actually fixed and hence the 'exactness' of the test in these circumstances is questionable. To fully explain the mechanics of the Fisher exact probability test, it is useful to use a sample 2×2 contingency table (Table 8.26). The probability (P) of recording a particular set of observations may be calculated using the following equation:

$$P = \frac{(A+C)!(B+D)!(A+B)!(C+D)!}{N!A!B!C!D!}$$

The terms in the numerator are the numbers of observations that are associated with the individual rows and columns.

In the above equation the calculation of the probability value associated with the recorded frequencies in each cell involves the use of factorials (denoted by!). A factorial is the product of all positive integers from 1 up to and including a defined integral. For example, the factorial of the integer 5 (denoted as 5!) is:

$$5! = 5 \times 4 \times 3 \times 2 \times 1 = 120$$

Table 8.26 A 2×2 contingency table

Variable Y	Variable X		Total
	Category 1	Category 2	
Category 1	A	B	A + B
Category 2	C	D	C + D
Total	A + C	B + D	A + B + C + D = N

The denominator in the probability equation is the product of all the factorial values associated with the frequency in each cell and the factorial of the total number of observations.

The Fisher exact probability may be employed to calculate the probability of both one- and two-tailed experimental designs, as illustrated in the following examples.

EXAMPLE 8.14 *A formulation unit in a university department is involved in the design and formulation of novel bioadhesive tablets that adhere to the oral mucosa and, in so doing, form the platform for controlled drug delivery to the oral cavity. Because of the prolonged contact between such dosage forms and the mucosa, one problem that may arise is mucosal damage at the site of attachment. Therefore, a clinical study has been designed to compare the mucosal damaging properties of two tablet formulations, of which one contains a bioadhesive polymeric component and the other does not. In this study, each formulation is allowed to contact the mucosa between the upper lip and gingiva for 60 min, after which the tablet is removed and the site of attachment assessed for mucosal damage. Using an appropriate statistical method, examine whether the bioadhesive tablet has a greater propensity to induce mucosal damage at the site of attachment.*

As before, it is important to define the parameters associated with the experimental design before the study begins.

(i) State the null hypothesis

A suitable null hypothesis for this study is that the mucosal damaging property of the bioadhesive formulation is similar to that of the non-bioadhesive formulation.

(ii) State the alternative hypothesis

One of the aims of the investigation is to identify if the bioadhesive formulation produces greater mucosal damage than the non-bioadhesive formulation. Therefore, a suitable alternative hypothesis is that the bioadhesive formulation is more damaging to mucosa than the non-bioadhesive counterpart.

(iii) State the level of significance

In this example, it is assumed that the level of significance (α) is 0.05.

(iv) Define the number of tails in the experimental design

The number of tails of an experimental design is a measure of the number of outcomes that will result in the rejection of the null hypothesis. In this example, the null hypothesis will be rejected (and the alternative hypothesis accepted) if the bioadhesive formulation is more damaging to the oral mucosa than the non-bioadhesive formulation. The design of this experiment is therefore one-tailed.

(v) Collect the experimental data

As previously stated, in this study each formulation was placed adjacent to the mucosa under the upper lip and allowed to reside for 60 min. Each formulation was then removed and the site of attachment assessed for mucosal damage. The results from the study are shown in Table 8.27.

(vi) Select the most appropriate statistical test

There are several aspects of the experimental design that enable the rational selection of the most appropriate statistical test to analyse the comparative effects of the two formulations. The data presented in Table 8.27 are nominal in nature and the study has been structured as a 2×2 contingency table. Therefore, there are two statistical tests that may be employed to evaluate whether or not there is a correlation between the variables: the χ^2 analysis and the Fisher exact probability test. But which is more appropriate for the current set of data? To answer this question one must consider the limitations of the use of the χ^2 analysis for two-samples in a 2×2 design. Two major points that must be considered are the overall sample size and the expected frequencies in each cell, as defined by the null hypothesis. The sample size in this clinical study was 26, which although relatively small,

Table 8.27 Damage to the oral mucosa resulting from contact with a bioadhesive formulation and a non-bioadhesive formulation

Tablet formulation	Recorded frequencies		Total
	No mucosal damage	Mucosal damage	
Non-bioadhesive formulation	9	3	12
Bioadhesive formulation	2	12	14
Total	11	15	26

does not specifically prohibit the use of the χ^2 analysis. However, because of the low magnitude of the frequencies in some cells, we should anticipate that the expected values in the individual categories in this study will be small. This is a sufficiently serious concern to preclude the use of the χ^2 analysis. Therefore, the most appropriate statistical test for the analysis of data in Table 8.27 is the Fisher exact probability test.

(vii) Calculate the probability

In the χ^2 test, a χ^2 statistic is calculated after mathematical considera-tion of the collected data. The outcome of the statistical analysis (acceptance or rejection of the null hypothesis) is then determined by a comparison of the calculated statistic with the critical statistic, as defined by the parameters of the experimental design. Conversely, in the Fisher exact probability test the exact probability associated with a study is calculated. If the calculated probability is less than the defined level of significance, the null hypothesis is rejected in favour of the alternative hypothesis. In this respect the Fisher exact probability test is analogous to the binomial test. The probability of observing the frequencies stated in Table 8.27 is calculated using the appropriate equation:

$$P = \frac{(A+C)!(B+D)!(A+B)!(C+D)!}{N!A!B!C!D!}$$

Therefore, substituting the data presented in Example 8.14 into this equation:

$$P = \frac{(9+2)!(3+12)!(9+3)!(2+12)!}{(26!)(9!)(3!)(2!)(12!)}$$

$$= \frac{(11!)(15!)(12!)(14!)}{(26!)(9!)(3!)(2!)(12!)} = \frac{2.18 \times 10^{39}}{8.41 \times 10^{41}}$$

$$= 0.0026$$

The calculated probability value refers to the probability of observing the configuration of data described in Table 8.27, but the test is not yet complete. In the Fisher exact probability test, the probability of observing more extreme deviations from the null hypothesis within the same marginal totals (the totals associated with the rows and columns) must be calculated. Tables 8.28 and 8.29 represent the other more extreme deviations associated with the clinical study.

Table 8.28 More extreme deviation of data from the null hypothesis concerning damage to the oral mucosa resulting from contact with a bioadhesive formulation and a non-bioadhesive formulation

Tablet formulation	Recorded frequencies		Total
	No mucosal damage	Mucosal damage	
Non-bioadhesive formulation	10	2	12
Bioadhesive formulation	1	13	14
Total	11	12	26

Table 8.29 Most extreme deviation of data from the null hypothesis concerning damage to the oral mucosa resulting from contact with a bioadhesive formulation and a non-bioadhesive formulation

Tablet formulation	Recorded frequencies		Total
	No mucosal damage	Mucosal damage	
Non-bioadhesive formulation	11	1	12
Bioadhesive formulation	0	14	14
Total	11	12	26

The probability of observing the frequencies stated in Table 8.28 is calculated as previously described:

$$P = \frac{(10 + 1)!(2 + 13)!(10 + 2)!(1 + 13)!}{(26!)(10!)(2!)(1!)(13!)}$$

$$= \frac{(11!)(15!)(12!)(14!)}{(26!)(10!)(2!)(1!)(13!)} = \frac{2.18 \times 10^{39}}{1.82 \times 10^{43}}$$

$$= 0.000\ 12$$

The probability of observing the frequencies stated in Table 8.29 is also calculated as previously described:

$$P = \frac{(11 + 0)!(1 + 14)!(11 + 1)!(0 + 14)!}{(26!)(11!)(1!)(0!)(14!)}$$

$$= \frac{(11!)(15!)(12!)(14!)}{(26!)(11!)(1!)(0!)(14!)} = \frac{2.18 \times 10^{39}}{1.40 \times 10^{45}}$$

$$= 0.000\ 0016$$

To obtain the overall probability, the calculated values are summed:

$$P = 0.0026 + 0.00012 + 0.0000016 = 0.0027$$

(viii) Interpret the outcome of the statistical analysis

The calculated value for the probability of observing the configuration of data presented in Table 8.27, and the more extreme deviations from the null hypothesis (Tables 8.28 and 8.29), refers to the probability of the null hypothesis being accepted. In this example this probability has been calculated as 0.0027. As this value is less than 0.05, the chosen level of significance, the null hypothesis is rejected in favour of the alternative hypothesis. Therefore, it may be concluded that the incidence of mucosal damage to the oral mucosa associated with the bioadhesive formulation was significantly greater than for the non-bioadhesive formulation.

As previous defined, Example 8.14 is a case of a one-tailed experimental design in which the Fisher exact probability test was employed to discern whether the bioadhesive formulation possessed more damaging properties than the non-bioadhesive control formulation after application the oral mucosa. As with other statistical tests, the Fisher exact probability test may be used for two-tailed experimental designs. Under these circumstances, the probability associated with the first tail is calculated as described in Example 8.14 and the calculated probability is doubled to estimate the probability contained within both tails. It has been argued that this method is inaccurate as the second tail may be smaller in magnitude than the first tail, thus invalidating the use of the first tail for the estimation of the area (probability) encompassed within the second tail. However, for the purposes of this text, we will assume that the areas in the two tails are comparable. Interested readers should consult a more specialised text (e.g. Siegel, 1956, or Sokal and Rohlf, 1981) for an explanation of the calculation of the second tail in the Fisher exact probability test.

To further clarify the use of the Fisher exact probability test for the analysis of data that has been organised in a 2×2 contingency table, in Example 8.15 a two-tailed experimental design has been chosen.

EXAMPLE 8.15 *A formulation unit wishes to design drug-loaded bioadhesive films for application to the periodontal pocket for the treatment of periodontal disease. It has been specified that such products should remain within the periodontal pocket for at least 1 week after application, to ensure controlled release of drug within this environment. The unit has manufactured two formulations containing bioadhesive* *polymers that have been defined as highly bioadhesive in in vitro studies; however, no information is available about their performance (residence) within the periodontal pocket. You have been asked to design an appropriate study to examine the comparative retention of the formulations within the periodontal pocket.*

To address this question, a clinical study has been proposed in which samples of each formulation were inserted into the periodontal pockets of volunteers and, 1 week later, the pockets were inspected to identify whether or not the formulations had been retained within this environment.

The parameters associated with the proposed study are as follows:

(i) State the null hypothesis

The null hypothesis for this study states that the two formulations will exhibit similar retention characteristics within the periodontal pocket, i.e. there will be no difference in the number of samples retained in or detached from the periodontal pocket. As in the χ^2 test, the null hypothesis assumes that the variables (formulations and retention or detachment) are independent and exhibit no correlation.

(ii) State the alternative hypothesis

In this situation, the alternative hypothesis states that there is a difference in the *in vivo* bioadhesive properties of the two formulations, i.e. the two variables are dependent.

(iii) State the level of significance

In this example, it is assumed that the level of significance (α) is 0.05.

(iv) Define the number of tails in the experimental design

In this experimental design, the alternative hypothesis states that the two formulations will differ in their bioadhesive properties. No preset direction to this difference has been assumed. Therefore, the alternative hypothesis will be accepted (and the null hypothesis rejected) if the retention properties of formulation 1 are either better or worse than those of formulation 2. As there are two potential outcomes, this is an example of a two-tailed design.

(v) Collect the experimental data

In the clinical study, the number of samples of formulations 1 and 2 that were retained within or detached from the periodontal pockets of volunteers were recorded 1 week after application. The results from the study are shown in Table 8.30.

(vi) Select the most appropriate statistical test

The data in Table 8.30 are nominal in nature and are presented in the form of a 2×2 contingency table. As in Example 8.14, the sample size in this study is small ($N = 17$) and furthermore, both the observed and expected frequencies in some cells are small. As before, these factors preclude the use of the χ^2 test for the analysis of the data. Therefore, the most appropriate statistical test for the analysis of data in Table 8.30 is the Fisher exact probability test.

(vii) Calculate the probability

The probability of observing the frequencies stated in Table 8.30 is calculated using the following equation:

$$P = \frac{(A + C)!(B + D)!(A + B)!(C + D)!}{N!A!B!C!D!}$$

Substituting the data presented in Table 8.30 into this equation,

$$P = \frac{(5 + 9)!(2 + 1)!(5 + 2)!(9 + 1)!}{(17!)(5!)(2!)(9!)!(1!)}$$

$$= \frac{(14!)(3!)(7!)(10!)}{(17!)(5!)(2!)(9!)(1!)} = \frac{9.57 \times 10^{21}}{3.10 \times 10^{22}}$$

$$= 0.309$$

Therefore, the probability of observing the data set described in Table 8.30 is 0.309 (30.9%). The next step in the test involves calculating the probability of observing more extreme deviations from the null hypothesis within the same marginal totals (the totals associated with the rows and columns). Table 8.31 represents the most extreme

Table 8.30 Effects of bioadhesive formulation on retention within or detachment from the periodontal pocket 1 week after insertion

Film formulation	Recorded frequencies		Total
	No. of films retained	No. of films detached	
Formulation 1	5	2	7
Formulation 2	9	1	10
Total	14	3	17

Table 8.31 Most extreme deviation of data from the null hypothesis concerning the effects of bioadhesive formulation composition on retention within or detachment from the periodontal pocket 1 week after insertion

Film formulation	Recorded frequencies		Total
	No. of films retained	No. of films detached	
Formulation 1	4	3	7
Formulation 2	10	0	10
Total	14	3	17

deviation associated with the clinical study. The probability of observing the frequencies stated in Table 8.31 is calculated as previously described:

$$P = \frac{(4+10)!(3+0)!(4+3)!(10+0)!}{(17!)(4!)(3!)(10!)(0!)}$$

$$= \frac{(14!)(3!)(7!)(10!)}{(17!)(4!)(3!)(10!)(0!)} = \frac{9.57 \times 10^{21}}{1.86 \times 10^{23}}$$

$$= 0.051$$

To obtain the overall probability, the calculated values are summed:

$$P = 0.309 + 0.051 = 0.36$$

(viii) Interpret the outcome of the statistical analysis

To interpret the outcome of the statistical analysis, the parameters associated with the experimental design should be fully considered. In this example, the level of significance has been determined as 0.05 and the experimental design is two-tailed. The Fisher exact probability test directly calculates the probability associated with a set of data (and the more extreme possible data sets), so statistical tables are not required to interpret the outcome of this test. Quite simply, if the calculated probability is less than 0.05, the null hypothesis is rejected, whereas if the calculated probability exceeds this value, the null hypothesis is accepted. The probability that has been calculated using the equations above refers to the probability associated with a one-tailed outcome. To translate this into a two-tailed outcome, the calculated probability value is doubled, under the assumption that the areas within the two tails are equivalent. Therefore, the probability associated with the clinical study in Example 8.14 is:

$$P = (0.36 \times 2) = 0.72$$

As this value is greater than 0.05, it may be concluded that the null hypothesis is accepted, i.e. there is no clinical difference in the two formulations with respect to their comparative residences within the periodontal pocket 1 week after implantation.

8.3 Conclusions

This chapter has described both the basic principles concerning statistical hypothesis testing of data composed of two samples and, more specifically, examples of the most common statistical tests that are employed to assess the similarity or difference between such sets of data. In particular, two distinct categories of statistical tests have been described, namely parametric and non-parametric methods, along with experimental situations that warrant the use of these categories of tests.

In the selection of the most appropriate statistical method for the analysis of two independent sets of data, the statistical analyst should ask several important questions:

- *What is the nature of measurement of the sets of data?* The parametric tests described in this chapter, the z test and the t test, may only be used if the data has been measured on, at least, an interval scale.
- *Are the populations from which the two sets of data have been sampled normally distributed?* This question cannot be answered definitively, but where possible the characteristics of the data set should be identified by the use of simple descriptive statistical data (mean, median, mode, etc.). As before, it is assumed that the statistical properties of each data set are good estimates of the population statistics. Theoretically, parametric tests should only be employed for the comparison of data sets that have been derived (sampled) from normally distributed populations, but in practice such tests may be used for data sets that deviate from this theoretical goal.
- *Are the variances of the sets of data similar?* One requirement concerning the use of parametric tests for the statistical comparison of two sets of unrelated data is homogeneity of variances. In this chapter the use and interpretation of a simple statistical test, the F ratio, for the statistical comparison of two variances have been described. Before using a parametric test, the analyst must be assured of the similarity of the variances of the two sets of data. Once more, the t test is valid even when there are departures from this assumption, but as the deviation becomes increasingly large, erroneous outcomes may result from the inappropriate use of parametric tests.

Despite the restrictions on the use of parametric tests for the analysis of two independent sets of data, it should be remembered that parametric tests are the most powerful statistical tests whenever the experimental design lends itself to this type of analysis. Therefore, parametric tests should be used whenever possible.

The choice of the most appropriate parametric test for the comparison of two independent sets of data is more straightforward, as the choice is simply whether to use the t test or the z test. The z test is used when the sample size is large (> 100, in which the standard deviation of the sample is assumed to be equivalent to the population standard deviation) or, alternatively, there is prior knowledge of the population standard deviation, e.g. as derived from production batch records. The calculated z statistic is interpreted using the standardised normal distribution. Conversely, the two-independent-samples t test is applied for the comparison of sets of data that are small in number. In pharmaceutical research, the t test is used more extensively than the z test as pharmaceutical experiments are generally replicated in relatively small numbers. In the calculation of the test statistic, the pooled standard deviation (the weighted standard deviation of the two groups) is derived from the data and, once more, is assumed to be good estimation of the pooled population standard deviation. In addition to the general restrictions on the use of parametric tests, one further restriction concerning the use of the Student's t test involves sample size. It is accepted that if the sample sizes of the two groups are small (<6), then the t test should not be applied. On the basis of such a restricted sample size, it is difficult to assume that population from which the data have been sampled is normally distributed. Finally, the calculated t statistic is interpreted using the t distribution.

When parametric tests are inapplicable, for some or all of the reasons specified above, non-parametric methods are applied to the analysis and comparison of two independently sampled sets of data. In this chapter the mechanics and applications of three such methods have been described: the Mann–Whitney U test, χ^2 analysis and the Fisher exact probability test. Each test has a unique function in the analysis and comparison of two independent sets of data.

- *The Mann–Whitney U test* is employed for the comparison of two sets of independently sampled data that have been measured on ordinal, interval or ratio scales. The method that is employed for the interpretation of the calculated Mann–Whitney U statistic is dependent on the size of the data sets. When the size of the larger data set is ⩽8, the exact probability of observing the U statistic may be determined from the appropriate Mann–Whitney U statistic table. When the size of the larger sample ranges between 9 and 20, the significance of the calculated U statistic is derived from the table which lists the critical values of U in the Mann–Whitney U test. When the size of the larger sample exceeds 20, it is assumed that the sampling distribution of the Mann–Whitney U statistic is normally distributed. Thus, the z statistic that is associated with the data sets may be calculated and the significance of this value interpreted using the standardised normal distribution.

- *The χ^2 test* is employed for the analysis of data that has been both collected in the form of a contingency table and measured in a nominal or ordinal scale. In this method, a χ^2 statistic is calculated and, as is the case for the z and t statistics, the probability associated with this statistic is determined by referring to the χ^2 probability distribution. The design of these contingency tables is flexible, but there are restrictions concerning the applicability of the χ^2 analysis for the analysis of two sets of independently collected data. For example, the expected frequency should be greater than 5 in the vast majority of cells for higher contingency tables, in which the degrees of freedom for the analysis are greater than 1. The use of the χ^2 analysis for 2×2 contingency tables is more restrictive and requires that a correction for continuity is applied to the calculation of the χ^2 statistic, that the total sample size should exceed 20 and that the expected frequencies in all cells are greater than 5.
- *The Fisher exact probability test* is employed for the comparison of two sets of data that have been arranged in a 2×2 contingency table and measured in either nominal or ordinal scales. It is used for those situations in which the χ^2 test is inappropriate, most notably whenever the combined sample size is less than 20 and the expected frequency in at least one cell is low (<5). Unlike the χ^2 test, the Fisher exact probability test does not calculate a critical statistic but rather generates an exact probability of observing the recorded data (and other more extreme cases). Therefore probability tables are not required for the interpretation of the Fisher exact probability test.

References

Siegel S. (1956). *Nonparametric Statistics for the Behavioural Sciences*. New York: McGraw-Hill.

Sokal R R, Rolf F J (1981). *Biometry*, 2nd edition. New York: W H Freeman.

9

Statistical hypothesis testing for two related samples

In the previous chapter the use of statistical methods for the comparison of data from two independent samples was described. The experimental design associated with such comparisons is commonplace in the pharmaceutical and related sciences, and, indeed, the associated statistical tests are relatively straightforward. However, in certain circumstances, the implementation of this type of statistical experimental design may be restricted. One of the major problems associated with two independent samples experimental designs is biological or patient variability. As a result of such variability, the variance associated with each set of data is increased and, accordingly, larger differences between mean samples are required to reject the null hypothesis. In clinical or animal research such variability may be sufficient to increase the (type II) error associated with the statistical measurement. Therefore, in this situation, the null hypothesis may be accepted when in fact it is false. One method by which the variability may be reduced is to increase the number of animals or patients in the study, but this has cost implications, particularly when human volunteers are involved. One way of addressing this problem is to employ a *matched-pairs* experimental design in which each subject is employed as his or her own control (Figure 9.1). There are several steps within this design. Only one group of patients is recruited into the study and, as a result, the total number of patients required to ensure appropriate statistical power may be only half that required for designs with two independent samples. The pool of volunteers receives the first treatment and the appropriate biological measurement is performed. There is then a washout period to ensure that treatment A has been sufficiently eliminated from each patient, hence reducing any interference with the biological properties of treatment B. After this washout period (the duration of which depends on the biological half-life of the therapeutic agent in question), treatment B is administered to each volunteer and, once more, the associated biological response is recorded. At this stage, statistical comparisons of the two sets of data associated with treatments A and B may be carried out using the appropriate parametric or non-parametric methods.

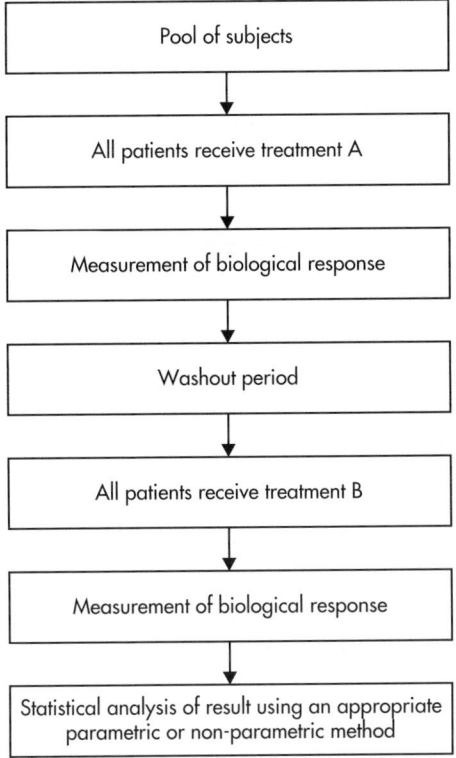

```
┌─────────────────────────────────────┐
│           Pool of subjects          │
└─────────────────────────────────────┘
                   │
                   ▼
┌─────────────────────────────────────┐
│     All patients receive treatment A│
└─────────────────────────────────────┘
                   │
                   ▼
┌─────────────────────────────────────┐
│   Measurement of biological response │
└─────────────────────────────────────┘
                   │
                   ▼
┌─────────────────────────────────────┐
│           Washout period            │
└─────────────────────────────────────┘
                   │
                   ▼
┌─────────────────────────────────────┐
│     All patients receive treatment B│
└─────────────────────────────────────┘
                   │
                   ▼
┌─────────────────────────────────────┐
│   Measurement of biological response │
└─────────────────────────────────────┘
                   │
                   ▼
┌─────────────────────────────────────┐
│ Statistical analysis of result using an appropriate │
│    parametric or non-parametric method │
└─────────────────────────────────────┘
```

Figure 9.1 Diagramatic representation of a matched-pairs experimental design.

In the above design each patient receives each treatment and, accordingly, it is possible to use each patient as his or her own biological control. The biological variation associated with intersubject differences is therefore less important because, in the case of interval or ratio data it is the differences between the effects of each treatment for each patient that will be analysed in the statistical analysis. Although two patients may differ by a substantial amount in their individual biological responses to particular treatments, the variability of the differences between treatments will be minimised. As previously stated, the analysis of data derived from a matched-pairs design may be performed using either parametric or non-parametric methods. In this chapter, the design and mechanics of one parametric method – the *paired-samples t test* – and two non-parametric methods – the *Wilcoxon signed-ranks test* and the *McNemar test* – will be explained, again with the aid of pharmaceutical examples. These examples will further illustrate the usefulness and applicability of matched-pairs experimental designs to the pharmaceutical and related sciences.

9.1 A parametric statistical test for two matched samples: the paired *t* test

9.1.1 Introduction and mechanics of the paired *t* test

The paired *t* test is a parametric statistical method that is similar in operation and interpretation to the one-sample *t* test. The one-sample *t* test examines the significance of the difference between a set of data and a fixed value, whereas the paired test examines the significance of the mean of the differences between the pairs of data and a fixed value, determined from the null hypothesis. The assumptions of the statistical model associated with the paired *t* test are similar to those that have been described for both the one-sample and two-independent-samples *t* tests. At the risk of becoming repetitive, it is still useful to consider these assumptions as, if the conditions of the experimental model are consistent with the assumptions of the paired *t* test, then that test is the most powerful method by which the results may be analysed. Therefore, it is assumed that:

- the data have been measured on an interval or ratio scale
- the two sets of data have been sampled from populations that are normally distributed
- the populations from which the two sets of data have been samples have similar variances
- the means and standard deviations of the two sets of sample data are good estimates of the central tendency and variability of the populations from which the data were sampled.

In addition, the paired *t* test requires that two further assumptions are valid:

- As the test is a paired test, the number of data sets in each treatment group must be equal.
- The calculation of the paired *t* statistic initially involves computation of the mean (and standard deviation) of the differences between each individual pair of data. Therefore, the test assumes that the calculated differences in means is derived from a normally distributed population of differences of means.

The calculation of the *t* statistic employs an equation that is related to that described for a one-sample *t* test:

$$t_{(df, \alpha)} = \frac{(\delta_m - \delta_{H_0})}{SE_{\text{difference}}} = \frac{(\delta_m - \delta_{H_0})}{s_{\text{difference}}/\sqrt{N}}$$

where $t_{(df, \alpha)}$ is the calculated t statistic under the conditions of the experimental design (i.e. number of degrees of freedom, number of tails and level of significance); δ_m is the observed (calculated) mean of the differences between the pairs of data; δ_{H_0} is the theoretical mean of the differences between the pairs of data, as defined by the null hypothesis; $s_{difference}$ is the observed (calculated) standard deviation of the differences between the pairs of data; and N is the number of pairs of data.

The mechanics and use of the paired t test are highlighted in the following examples.

EXAMPLE 9.1   *A company has designed a tablet formulation containing a natural product that has been reported to promote weight loss. To allow this claim to be included in the product literature, the company has been asked to substantiate this claim by carrying out a clinical trial. Therefore, the company has recruited 10 obese adult male volunteers and recorded their initial weights. Each volunteer was then asked to take one tablet twice daily for a 1-month period, following which their individual weights were recorded. The results of the clinical study are presented in Table 9.1. Using an appropriate statistical test, conclude whether or not the natural product was clinically successful.*

Before the start of the clinical study, the parameters of the experimental design are defined.

(i) State the null hypothesis

As before, the null hypothesis states that the formulation will have no effect on weight loss in the obese volunteers. Accordingly, there will be

Table 9.1 Effects of a tablet formulation containing a natural product on weight loss of 10 obese male volunteers

Patient number	Weight (kg) before start of clinical trial	Weight (kg) 4 weeks after after start of clinical trial
1	140	131
2	125	121
3	154	150
4	121	121
5	115	108
6	156	151
7	150	150
8	154	153
9	130	124
10	106	100

no difference in the weights of the volunteers before and after the clinical trial.

H_0: weights of patients at the start of the trial = weight of patients at the end of the trial

or in other words

H_0: weights of patients at the start of the trial – weight of patients at the end of the trial = 0.

In terms of the equation for computing the t statistic, the term μ_{H_0} refers to the difference as specified by the null hypothesis. On many occasions, and indeed unless specified in the experimental design, the term μ_{H_0} is equal to 0, denoting that no difference between the two treatments is expected under the terms of the null hypothesis.

(ii) State the alternative hypothesis

In this example the alternative hypothesis states that the formulation will have a significant effect on weight loss in the obese volunteers, i.e. the product will significantly reduce the weights of the volunteers:

H_a: weights of patients at the start of the trial > weight of patients at the end of the trial

(iii) State the level of significance

In this example, it is assumed that the level of significance (α) is 0.05.

(iv) State the number of tails in the experimental design

The number of tails of a particular experimental design reflects the number of ways in which the null hypothesis can be rejected. In Example 9.1, we are interested only in whether the formulation containing the natural product reduces the weight of volunteers. As there is only one outcome that will give rise to a rejection of the null hypothesis, this is an example of a one-tailed design.

(v) Select the most appropriate statistical test

After collection of the experimental data, the first choice that confronts the analyst is whether to use a parametric or non-parametric statistical test. One should always examine the applicability of parametric tests first because, if the conditions for their use are satisfied, they have greater power than their non-parametric counterparts. In particular, for statistical tests involving matched pairs of data, the major concern is whether or not the distribution of differences of means has been derived from a population of distributions of means that is normally distributed. This may seem quite complicated, but to make it easier to comprehend, the reader should imagine a situation in which the clinical study described in Table 9.1 is performed using not just 10 volunteers but a large number (a population). The difference in weight between the beginning and end of the trial for each volunteer is calculated and plotted as a frequency distribution. It is the normality of this distribution that validates the use of the two-sample paired t test. In the current example, we have only employed 10 volunteers and therefore we have to assume that the population is normally distributed before commissioning the use of a paired t test. However, a measure of confidence may be obtained by examining the mean and median of the differences in weight of the 10 volunteers. These are calculated as 4.2 kg (mean) and 4.5 kg (median), respectively. As these values are similar, we will assume that the weight differences are normally distributed and use a parametric test. The reader will by now be aware that a two-paired-samples t test is an appropriate statistical test for Example 9.1, but it is worthwhile reflecting on the nature of the experimental design described in this example. In particular, the reasons why a two-independent-samples t test cannot be employed in this situation should be highlighted. In Example 9.1, each patient acts as their own control, i.e. the weight difference associated with each volunteer is used in the statistical analysis. As may be observed from Table 9.1 the volunteers recruited into the study had a wide range of initial weights (106–156 kg) and because of this large range, it was more efficient to use each person as their own control. To employ a two-independent-samples t test the experimental design would have been modified:

- A larger number of patients would have been required (possibly two groups of 10 volunteers).
- Both groups would have been weighed at the start of the study and one group would have received the formulation containing the natural product whereas the other group would have received a placebo treatment (i.e. an identical formulation that was devoid of therapeutic agent). After 4 weeks, both groups of volunteers would have been reweighed and the weight of the two groups statistically compared.

Although this approach has the advantage of more rapid completion time, one major flaw is the intra-group variability of weights. Because the calculation of the t statistic utilises the standard error of the difference in means as the denominator, the difference in the observed means of the two groups will have to be greater to allow the null hypothesis to be rejected. Therefore, the reader should always examine whether the two treatment groups are linked (matched) in any fashion.

Assuming that the differences in the matched pairs are normally distributed, and in light of the paired nature of the data, the most appropriate statistical method to analyse the data sets described in Example 9.1 is the two-paired-samples *t* test.

(vi) Perform the statistical analysis

Execution of the paired *t* test is performed in a number of separate steps, as described below.

Step 1 Calculate the differences in the two data sets
The differences in the two data sets and the mean and standard deviation of these differences are calculated and compiled in tabular form (Table 9.2). In the calculation of the mean and standard deviation of the difference between the two treatments (start and end of the clinical trial in this example) the signs (positive or negative) of all values must be taken into consideration.

Step 2 Calculate the t statistic
The *t* statistic is calculated using the following equation:

$$t_{(df, a)} = \frac{(\delta_m - \delta_{H_0})}{s_{\text{difference}}/\sqrt{N}}$$

Table 9.2 Effects of a tablet formulation containing a natural product on weight loss of 10 obese male volunteers

Patient number	Weight (kg) before start of clinical trial	Weight (kg) 4 weeks after start of clinical trial	Difference (weight start – weight end)
1	140	131	9
2	125	121	4
3	154	150	4
4	121	121	0
5	115	108	7
6	156	151	5
7	150	150	0
8	154	153	1
9	130	124	6
10	106	100	6
		Mean difference	4.20
		Standard deviation of the difference	3.05

For Example 9.1, δ_m is the calculated mean of the differences between the groups (4.20 kg); δ_{H_0} is the hypothetical difference between the two groups, as defined by the null hypothesis (0); $s_{difference}$ is the calculated standard deviation of the differences between the groups (3.08 kg); and N is the number of pairs of volunteers in the study (10). Therefore:

$$t_{(df,\,\alpha)} = \frac{(\delta_m - \delta_{H_0})}{s_{difference}/\sqrt{N}} = \frac{(4.20 - 0)}{3.08/\sqrt{10}} = \frac{4.20}{0.97} = 4.33$$

(vii) Interpret the calculated statistic

The interpretation of the calculated t statistic is identical to that described for the t test with one sample or two independent samples. Accordingly, the calculated statistic is interpreted by initially identifying the critical value of t that defines the regions of acceptance and rejection of the null hypothesis. The important experimental parameters that define this value are,

- $\alpha = 0.05$
- one-tailed experimental design
- 9 df (In a paired t test the number of degrees of freedom is calculated by subtracting 1 from the total number of pairs of data; $10 - 1 = 9$.)

On the basis of this information the critical t value is 1.83 (9 df, $\alpha = 0.05$, one-tailed). Therefore, as this is a one-tailed test, if the calculated value of the t statistic is less than 1.83 the null hypothesis is accepted, but if the calculated value ≥ 1.83, the null hypothesis is rejected. Consequently, as the calculated value exceeded the critical value, the null hypothesis is rejected. Therefore, it may be concluded that the formulation containing the natural product promoted weight loss in a clinical study.

The previous example was an illustration of the mechanics of the one-tailed paired t test in which each of the individual differences between the paired data was always positive. The following example illustrates the mechanics of the test in a two-tailed design in which there are negative paired differences.

EXAMPLE 9.2   *A clinical testing facility has been asked to design and perform a study to compare the diuretic properties of two loop diuretics. As the manager of this facility, you have designed a paired-samples study in which a group of patients received an intravenous dose of diuretic A, the urine of each patient was collected over a defined period (6 h) and the volume of urine recorded. After a washout period of 2 weeks, the same volunteers received an intravenous dose of the second* diuretic (B), and the urine was collected and measured as before. The results of the study are shown in Table 9.3. Using an appropriate statistical test, determine whether the two therapeutic agents differ in their diuretic properties.

Before beginning the clinical studies, the experimental parameters should be clearly defined.

(i) State the null hypothesis

In this clinical study the null hypothesis states that there is no difference in the clinical efficacy (diuresis) of the two therapeutic agents:

> H_0: volume of urine generated after administration of therapeutic agent A = volume of urine generated after administration of therapeutic agent B

or in other words

> H_0: volume of urine generated after administration of therapeutic agent A − volume of urine generated after administration of therapeutic agent B = 0

(ii) State the alternative hypothesis

A suitable alternative hypothesis for this study is that there is a difference in the diuretic properties of the two formulations. Accordingly,

Table 9.3 Effects of intravenous administration of loop diuretics A and B on the total volume of urine collected over a 6-h period after injection

Patient number	Volume of urine collected (L)	
	Loop diuretic A	Loop diuretic B
01001	3.5	4.0
01002	4.0	4.2
01003	4.6	4.9
01004	7.1	5.6
01005	3.1	5.1
01006	5.5	5.0
01007	6.8	5.7
01008	5.1	7.1
01009	5.6	6.2
01001	3.8	5.2
01011	4.8	6.3
01012	6.9	6.4

H_a: diuretic property of therapeutic agent A ≠ diuretic property of therapeutic agent B

(iii) State the level of significance

In this example, it is assumed that the level of significance (a) is 0.05.

(iv) State the number of tails in the experimental design

In this example, there are two possible outcomes that will result in the rejection of the null hypothesis: the volume of urine produced after the administration of therapeutic agent A (and hence the diuretic properties) may be either greater or less than the volume of urine produced after administration of therapeutic agent B. Because there are two possible outcomes, the experimental design of Example 9.2 is two-tailed.

(v) Select the most appropriate statistical test

In the clinical study the comparative effects of two therapeutic agents are under investigation, so this is an example of a two-sample experimental design. More specifically, the two treatments are inextricably linked because of the paired nature of the design, i.e. each patient received each therapeutic agent and therefore acted as their own control. Accordingly, the statistical method used to examine the outcome of this clinical study should be a two-paired-samples test. The final piece of the jigsaw is whether a parametric or a non-parametric test should be used. Once more, the normality of the distribution of differences of the diuretic effects of each agent in each patient should be examined. The mean and median of this distribution are 0.41 L and 0.40 L, respectively, and because these two values are so similar, we will assume that the distribution of differences from which the data were sampled is normal.

Consequently, the most appropriate statistical test to examine whether there is or is not a difference in the diuretic properties of therapeutic agent A and therapeutic agent B is a two-paired-samples t test.

(vi) Perform the statistical analysis

We can calculate the t statistic in a stepwise fashion, as described for Example 9.1.

Step 1   Calculate the differences in the two data sets
The differences in the two data sets and the mean and standard deviation of these differences are calculated and compiled in tabular form (Table 9.4).

Table 9.4 Effects of intravenous administration of loop diuretics A and B on the total volume of urine collected over a 6-h period after injection

Patient number	Volume of urine collected (L)		Difference (B–A) (L)
	Loop diuretic A	Loop diuretic B	
01001	3.5	4.0	+0.5
01002	4.0	4.2	+0.2
01003	4.6	4.9	+0.3
01004	7.1	5.6	−1.5
01005	3.1	5.1	+2.0
01006	5.5	5.0	−0.5
01007	6.8	5.7	−1.1
01008	5.1	7.1	+2.0
01009	5.6	6.2	+0.6
01001	3.8	5.2	+1.4
01011	4.8	6.3	+1.5
01012	6.9	6.4	−0.5
		Mean difference (L)	0.41
		Standard deviation of the difference (L)	1.16

Step 2   Calculate the t statistic
To calculate the *t* statistic, the following information is required:

- the calculated mean of the differences between the groups (δ_m), i.e. 0.41 L
- the hypothetical difference between the two groups (δ_{H_0}), i.e. 0.0 L, as defined by the null hypothesis
- the calculated standard deviation of the differences between the groups ($s_{\text{difference}}$), i.e. 1.16 L
- the number of pairs of volunteers in the study (N), i.e. 12.

Therefore:

$$t_{(df,\alpha)} = \frac{(\delta_m - \delta_{H_0})}{s_{\text{difference}}/\sqrt{N}} = \frac{(0.41 - 0)}{1.16/\sqrt{12}} = \frac{0.41}{0.33} = 1.24$$

(vii)   Interpret the calculated statistic

The important experimental parameters that define the critical value of the *t* statistic are

- $\alpha = 0.05$
- two-tailed experimental design
- 11 *df* ($N - 1 = 12 - 1 = 11$)

On the basis of this information the critical t value is 2.20 (11 df, $\alpha = 0.05$, two-tailed). Therefore, calculated values that fall within the range $-2.20 < t < +2.20$ will result in acceptance of the null hypothesis. Conversely, values of t that are either $\geqslant +2.20$ or $\leqslant -2.20$ allow the null hypothesis to be rejected. The calculated value (+1.24) lies within the region denoting acceptance of the null hypothesis and accordingly it may be concluded that there was no clinical difference in the diuretic properties of the two therapeutic agents.

Further examples of the mechanics of the paired t test are provided below.

EXAMPLE 9.3 *A company currently manufactures parenteral suspensions by dispersing the therapeutic agent in the aqueous vehicle (containing surfactants, etc.) and reducing the particle size of the therapeutic agent by passing the formulation through a ball mill. The company is not satisfied by the efficiency of this process. It has been suggested that the process of particle size reduction should be improved to generate a product containing particles of lower average diameter; specifically, an alternative process should be examined in which the particle size of the therapeutic agent is reduced in the solid state using a jet microniser before incorporation into the aqueous vehicle. To examine this suggestion, eight batches of the therapeutic agent have been used to manufacture the parenteral formulation. Each batch was subdivided into two lots, one of which was jet micronised prior to formulation whereas the other was incorporated into the product and ball milled. Following manufacture the average particle size of each formulation was examined using an electrical zone impedance method (Coulter counter). The results are presented in Table 9.5. Examine whether there is a difference in the*

Table 9.5 Effects of two methods of particle size reduction (jet micronisation and ball milling) on the particle size of a therapeutic agent in a parenteral suspension formulation

Batch of therapeutic agent	Average particle size (μm)	
	Jet microniser	Ball mill
SL-0006	12.0	17.0
SL-9910	9.5	21.5
SL-9858	12.0	21.2
SL-0052	6.4	18.2
SL-9901	6.5	23.0
SL-0018	11.2	27.5
SL-9988	16.1	25.5
SL-0001	8.9	12.7

particle size of the therapeutic agent after particle size reduction by the two techniques.

To resolve this problem, the experimental parameters should be initially defined.

(i) State the null hypothesis

A suitable null hypothesis for this study is there is no difference in the particle size of the therapeutic agent following size reduction either by jet micronisation or by ball milling:

H_0: particle size following jet micronisation = particle size following ball milling

i.e.

H_0: particle size following jet micronisation – particle size following ball milling = 0

(ii) State the alternative hypothesis

The alternative hypothesis in this example is that the size of the particles of the therapeutic agent are dissimilar following size reduction by either jet micronisation or ball milling:

H_a: particle size following jet micronisation ≠ particle size following ball milling

i.e.

H_a: particle size following jet micronisation – particle size following ball milling ≠ 0

(iii) State the level of significance

In this example, it is assumed that the level of significance (α) is 0.05.

(iv) State the number of tails associated with the experimental design

In this example the alternative hypothesis states that the particle size of the therapeutic agent is dependent on the nature of the method used to reduce particle size. The nature of this difference is not specified and, accordingly, may result from the particles produced by jet micronisation being either larger or smaller than the particles produced by ball milling. Therefore, as a result of the two possible outcomes that will lead to rejection of the null hypothesis, this study is two-tailed.

(v) Select the most appropriate statistical test

This experiment is an example of a paired (matched) samples design in which eight batches of therapeutic agent have undergone particle size reduction both by jet milling and by micronisation. This is a good example of the application of this experimental design. Frequently, unless specified by the purchaser, the particle size distribution of different batches of a particular active ingredient or excipient may vary considerably. Therefore, the use of a paired-samples design minimises the effects of batch-to-batch differences on the inherent variability in the experiment, and hence on the statistical analysis. Before deciding on the most appropriate statistical method, one must consider whether a parametric or non-parametric technique should be used. To clarify this question, the descriptive statistics of the differences between the two sets of data should be examined. The mean and median of the sample of the differences are 10.5 μm and 10.6 μm, respectively. As these values are similar in magnitude, we will assume that the distribution of differences from which the data were sampled is approximately normal. The most appropriate statistical method to test the null hypothesis of Example 9.3 is therefore a two-paired-samples t test.

(vi) Perform the statistical analysis

Calculation of the t statistic may be performed in a stepwise fashion, as follows.

Table 9.6 Effects of two methods of particle size reduction (jet micronisation and ball milling) on the particle size of a therapeutic agent in a parenteral suspension formulation

Batch of therapeutic agent	Average particle size (μm)		Difference in particle size (ball mill – jet microniser)
	Jet microniser	Ball mill	
SL-0006	12.0	17.0	5.0
SL-9910	9.5	21.5	12.0
SL-9858	12.0	21.2	9.2
SL-0052	6.4	18.2	11.8
SL-9901	6.5	23.0	16.5
SL-0018	11.2	27.5	16.3
SL-9988	16.1	25.5	9.4
SL-0001	8.9	12.7	3.8
		Mean difference (μm)	10.5
		Standard deviation of the difference (μm)	4.7

Step 1 Calculate the differences in the two data sets

The differences in the two data sets and the mean and standard deviation of these differences are calculated and compiled in tabular form (Table 9.6)

Step 2 Calculate the t statistic

As before, the *t* statistic is calculated using the following equation:

$$t_{(df, a)} = \frac{(\delta_m - \delta_{H_0})}{s_{\text{difference}}/\sqrt{N}}$$

In Example 9.3, $\delta_m = 10.5 \ \mu m$, $\delta_{H_0} = 0.0 \ \mu m$, $s_{\text{difference}} = 4.7 \ \mu m$ and $N = 8$, so

$$t_{(df, a)} = \frac{(\delta_m - \delta_{H_0})}{s_{\text{difference}}/\sqrt{N}} = \frac{(10.50 - 0)}{4.7/\sqrt{8}} = \frac{10.5}{1.7} = 6.18$$

(vii) Interpret the calculated statistic

The first step in the interpretation involves identification of the critical *t* statistic, i.e. the region of acceptance and rejection of the null hypothesis. In this experiment, the following parameters are required to facilitate this process:

- $a = 0.05$
- two-tailed outcome
- 7 *df* (number of pairs – 1).

With this information in mind, the critical *t* value is 2.36 (Appendix 2). Consequently, the region of acceptance of the null hypothesis is $-2.36 < t_{\text{calculated}} < +2.36$, whereas the region of rejection of the null hypothesis is $t_{\text{calculated}} \geqslant +2.36$ or, alternatively, $t_{\text{calculated}} \leqslant -2.36$. The value of *t* calculated from the above equation is 6.18. As this calculated value exceeds the upper critical value, the null hypothesis is rejected. Therefore, it may be concluded that the method of particle size reduction does significantly affect the particle size of the finished product. In the above example, the average particle size of the product manufactured by jet micronisation of the active ingredient was significantly smaller than that prepared by ball milling.

It is extremely important to point out that in two-paired-sample *t* tests the null hypothesis may reflect the difference in the two groups that is important or relevant to the study. Therefore, it is not a prerequisite for this statistical method that the difference between the two treatment groups should be zero. This scenario is highlighted in the next example.

EXAMPLE 9.4   *The pharmaceutical company described in Example 9.3 wishes to examine whether jet micronisation can reduce the particle size of a parenteral product by 10 μm in comparison to the ball milled product, as this size reduction would represent a significant improvement in the physical stability of the formulation. Using the data given in Table 9.5, test this hypothesis using an appropriate statistical method.*

(i)   State the null hypothesis

A suitable revised null hypothesis is:

> H_0: average particle size after jet micronisation is up to 10 μm less than that after ball milling

or

> H_0: particle size after jet micronisation – particle size after ball milling = 10 μm

(ii)   State the alternative hypothesis

The revised alternative hypothesis is:

> H_a: average particle size after jet micronisation process is smaller than that after ball mill process by 10 μm or more

(iii)   State the level of significance

In this example, it is assumed that the level of significance (α) is 0.05.

(iv)   State the number of tails associated with the experimental design

This study has been designed to investigate whether the jet micronisation process may be used to produce particles that are at least 10 μm smaller than those produced by ball milling. The company is not interested in whether jet micronisation produces particles that are larger than those produced by ball milling. Subsequently, as there is only one experimental outcome that is of interest, and hence only one way in which the null hypothesis may be rejected, this is an example of a one-tailed experimental design.

(v)   Select the most appropriate statistical method

The data described in Table 9.5 will be analysed using a two-paired-samples *t* test. The rationale for this choice has been outlined previously.

(vi)   Perform the statistical analysis

Calculation of the *t* statistic may be performed in a stepwise fashion, as before.

Step 1   Calculate the differences in the two data sets

The differences in the two data sets and the mean and standard deviation of these differences have been calculated previously and are summarised in Table 9.6.

Step 2   Calculate the t statistic

The t statistic is calculated using the following equation:

$$t_{(df, \alpha)} = \frac{(\delta_m - \delta_{H_0})}{s_{\text{difference}}/\sqrt{N}}$$

In this current example, $\delta_m = 10.5 \, \mu m$, $\delta_{H_0} = 10.0 \, \mu m$, $s_{\text{difference}} = 4.7 \, \mu m$, and $N = 8$, so

$$t_{(df, \alpha)} = \frac{(\delta_m - \delta_{H_0})}{s_{\text{difference}}/\sqrt{N}} = \frac{(10.5 - 10.0)}{4.7/\sqrt{8}} = \frac{0.5}{1.7} = 0.29$$

(vii)   Interpret the calculated statistic

Although the data used to address the problem stated in Example 9.4 was derived from a previous example, it is incorrect to believe that the experimental conditions in Examples 9.3 and 9.4 are identical. The experimental parameters associated with the current example that are required to enable identification of the critical value of t are as follows:

- $\alpha = 0.05$
- *one*-tailed experimental design
- *7 df*

By referring to the table of the critical values of the t statistic (Appendix 2), the critical t value may be identified as 1.89. Therefore, the region of acceptance of the null hypothesis is $t_{\text{calculated}} < +1.89$, whereas the region of rejection of the null hypothesis is $t_{\text{calculated}} \geqslant +1.89$. From the data provided, the calculated value of t is 0.29 and, from the defined regions of acceptance and rejection of the null hypothesis, it may be concluded that jet micronisation does not lower the particle size of a product by more than 10 μm, when compared to the ball milling.

9.1.2   Sample size and power in two-paired-samples t tests

Previously in this chapter an analogy was drawn between the operations of the one-sample and two-paired-samples t test. It may therefore be unsurprising to read that the calculations of the sample size, power and indeed minimum detectable difference for one-sample and two-paired-samples t tests are similar. As before, calculation of these terms requires prior knowledge of the following parameters:

- the chosen level of significance (α)
- the standard deviation of the differences in individual paired samples (s)
- the probability of committing a type II error (β) (see Chapter 5)
- the difference between the mean of the individual differences and a hypothetical value that is presumed to be clinically or experimentally important (δ).

In this section, calculation of these various parameters of a paired-samples experimental design will be explained with the use of pharmaceutical examples.

EXAMPLE 9.5 *The clinical trials department of the pharmaceutical company described in Example 9.3 has calculated that a difference in particle size of 5 μm between the products produced by the two micronisation methods would be clinically relevant. Calculate the probability of detecting a difference in particle size of 5 μm between the two particle size reduction methods.*

The problem posed in this example may be addressed by calculating the power of the study. The power of a two-paired-samples test is calculated in an analogous manner to that for a one-sample test using the following equation:

$$t_{\beta(df)} = \frac{\delta}{\sqrt{s^2_{difference}/N}} - t_{\alpha(df)}$$

in which δ is the mean difference between the individual pairs of data that is thought to offer a practical difference; $s^2_{difference}$ is the variance of the difference between the individual pairs of data; N is the number of pairs of data; $t_{\alpha(df)}$ is the t value commensurate with the stated level of significance (α), number of tails and the number of degrees of freedom; and $t_{\alpha(df)}$ is the t value associated with committing a type II error at the defined number of degrees of freedom in a one-tailed scenario.

For the current example, the various terms in the above equation are $\delta = 5$ μm (as specified by the clinical trials department), $s^2_{difference} = (4.7)^2$, $N = 8$ and $t_{\alpha(df)}$ is 2.36 ($\alpha = 0.05$ and $df = 7$), as derived from the table of the critical values of the t statistic (Appendix 2). The t statistic associated with committing a β error may be calculated by inserting these data into the equation:

$$t_{\beta(df)} = \frac{5.0}{\sqrt{(4.7)^2/8}} - 2.36 = 0.65$$

The calculated value of $t_{\beta(df)}$ may be converted into the probability associated with committing a type II error under the conditions of the experiment (one-tailed design with 7 df). As the probabilities associated with the t statistic are not fully tabulated for 7 df, we are unable to interpret the calculated t value into an exact probability. Therefore, as before, it will be assumed that the calculated t value approximates to a z value and, as a result, the standardised normal distribution may be used to interpret the probability associated with the calculated value. Consulting the standardised normal distribution (Appendix 1) shows that a value of 0.65 is associated with a probability of 0.26. The power of the test is calculated by subtracting the calculated probability from 1, i.e.

$$power = (1 - \beta) = (1.00 - 0.26) = 0.74$$

Therefore, we may conclude that there is a 74% chance that a particle size difference of 5 μm will be observed between the two particle size reduction methods.

Two useful parameters were introduced in Chapter 7 provide a greater insight into experimental design and, indeed, are required to ensure that the experimental design has been optimised. They are the estimations of the sample size and the minimum detectable difference. The use and calculation of these parameters are explained in the following example.

EXAMPLE 9.6 *A pharmaceutical company develops and manufactures generic dosage forms. The most recent product that has been developed is a generic intranasal peptide spray that has been designed to provide bioequivalence (similar pharmacokinetic properties) to the proprietary brand. A basic knowledge of the pharmacokinetic responses of the generic and proprietary dosage forms has been gained from a pilot two-paired-samples clinical study. This has provided sufficient evidence to the generic company that the two dosage forms may be bioequivalent. You have been asked to design a larger bioequivalence study for the purpose of product registration and have decided, on the basis of cost and lower variability, to use a two-paired-samples design. How many volunteers should be recruited into the study?*

This is a classical example of the need for a well-planned experiment. Recruitment of too many volunteers will be costly to the company that is sponsoring the study, but if the number of volunteers is too small, the outcome of the study may be unclear because its power will be inadequate. Assuming that the differences in data from the two treatment groups are normally distributed, the number of volunteers required may be calculated with knowledge of the following parameters:

- The level of significance ($\alpha = 0.05$).
- An estimation of the variability of the differences between the two treatment groups. The standard deviation has been acquired from the information

generated within the pilot study and is 2.09 ng mL^{-1} h. This data refers to the area under the curve, a key pharmacokinetic property.

- The probability of committing a type II error (β). Remembering that the power of the study is $1 - \beta$, we wish to establish a study with a 90% power of detecting a difference between the two treatments of a defined value. Therefore, the β error will be set at 0.1.

- The difference (δ) between the two treatments that is accepted to be experimentally valid. The pharmaceutical company has been informed that if the areas under the curves of the two products differ by more than 10%, then they are deemed to be non-bioequivalent. Based on the data generated within the pilot study, this value of 10% may be assumed to represent 1.85 ng mL^{-1} h.

The process for calculating the sample size required for the study is iterative and has been described in Chapter 7. The equation used to calculate sample size is

$$N = \left(\frac{s}{\delta}\right)^2 (t_{\alpha(df)} + t_{\beta(df)})^2$$

In the current example, the values to be inserted into the right-hand side of the equation are $s = 2.09$ ng mL^{-1} h and $\delta = 1.85$ ng mL^{-1} h. Let us initially assume that 20 volunteers will be required for the clinical study as this will allow estimation of both $t_{\alpha(df)}$ and $t_{\beta(df)}$. Therefore $t_{\alpha(df)}$ is equal to $t_{(0.05, 19\ df,\ \text{two-tailed test})}$, i.e. 2.09. Similarly, $t_{\beta(df)}$ is equal to $t_{(0.10, 19\ df,\ \text{one-tailed test})}$, i.e. 1.33. Therefore, the estimated number of volunteers that are required for the clinical study is

$$N = \left(\frac{s}{\delta}\right)^2 \times (t_{\alpha(df)} + t_{\beta(df)})^2 = \left(\frac{2.09}{1.85}\right)^2 \times (2.09 + 1.33)^2 = 15.0$$

The next stage of the iterative process involves repeating the above calculation but this time using 15 as an estimated sample size. Accordingly, $t_{\alpha(df)} = t_{(0.05, 14\ df,\ \text{two-tailed test})}$, i.e. 2.14, and $t_{\beta(df)} = t_{(0.10, 14\ df,\ \text{one-tailed test})}$, i.e. 1.35. The improved estimation of the required sample size is

$$N = \left(\frac{s}{\delta}\right)^2 (t_{\alpha(df)} + t_{\beta(df)})^2 = \left(\frac{2.09}{1.85}\right)^2 (2.14 + 1.35)^2 = 15.6$$

Both calculations agree, so we can conclude that at least 15 volunteers should be included in the clinical study.

Another frequently asked question concerning experimental design is the minimum detectable difference, i.e. the smallest difference that may be observed between the mean difference and the null hypothesis. To explain this calculation, the data given in Example 9.6 will be used again.

EXAMPLE 9.7   *Using the data in Example 9.6, calculate the minimum detectable difference between the two treatments in terms of the area under the curve that may be identified in 90% of all volunteers.*

The equation that is employed to calculate minimum detectable difference is (symbol notation as described previously):

$$\delta = \left(\sqrt{\frac{s^2}{N}} \right) \times (t_{\alpha(df)} + t_{\beta(df)})$$

The statement *'may be identified in 90% of all volunteers'* is an important component of this analysis, as it defines the power of the study. Therefore, if the power of the study is 0.90, the probability associated with a β (type II) error is 0.1.

For the purpose of this calculation, assume the following values for the parameters described on the right-hand side of the equation: $s = 1.85$ ng mL^{-1} h, $N = 20$, $t_{\alpha(df)} = 2.09$ ($\alpha = 0.05$, 19 df, two-tailed) and $t_{\beta(df)} = 1.33$ ($\beta = 0.10$, 19 df, one-tailed). Substituting these terms into the equation above produces

$$\delta = \left(\sqrt{\frac{s^2}{N}} \right) \times (t_{\alpha(df)} + t_{\beta(df)})$$

$$= \left(\sqrt{\frac{1.85^2}{20}} \right) \times (2.09 + 1.33) = 1.40 \text{ ng mL}^{-1} \text{ h}^{-1}$$

Therefore, the minimum detectable difference associated with a 90% power is 1.40 ng mL^{-1} h^{-1}

9.2   Non-parametric hypothesis testing for two paired samples

By this stage, the reader will appreciate that for every parametric experimental design there is a non-parametric counterpart. The rationale for the use of non-parametric statistical tests for two paired samples is identical to that described in Chapter 8 for the non-parametric analysis of two independent samples. To further reinforce the dichotomy between parametric and non-parametric methods for the analysis of paired samples, remember that the experimental situations favouring the use of non-parametric tests are as follows:

- the distribution from which the differences in the two data sets have been sampled may be asymmetrical in nature
- the data may have been measured in a nominal or ordinal scale
- the variances of the populations (estimated by the variances of the samples) may be heterogeneous

Under these circumstances, or indeed if there is any reason to suggest that the experimental requirements of parametric statistical tests are invalid, a non-parametric statistical method must be used to analyse the difference between paired samples. Once the necessity of using a non-parametric method has been decided, the next question is the specific choice of method. Several non-parametric methods are used to examine differences between paired sets of data, but their operation depends on the nature of the measured data. In this chapter the mechanics and applications of two exemplar methods – *McNemar's test* and *Wilcoxon's signed-rank test* – will be described with the aid of pharmaceutical examples.

9.2.1 McNemar's test

McNemar's test is a statistical method that examines the differences between two paired samples in which the data has been collected in a 2×2 design and is nominal in nature. At first sight the presentation of data resembles a conventional contingency table. However, in a contingency table the null hypothesis in the statistical design assumes that there is no correlation between the rows and columns, i.e. the rows and columns are independent. In a two-paired-samples design, however, there is a relationship between the rows and columns as a result of the paired basis of the sampling process. It is helpful at this stage to illustrate the nature of the two-paired samples design relevant to analysis using McNemar's test, and the mechanics of the test.

In this type of analysis each patient or volunteer acts as their own control and, as before will be exposed to both treatments. Traditionally, this type of experimental design is employed to evaluate the response of the volunteers both before and after a particular treatment. Alternatively, this design may be employed to compare the effects of two treatments on the biological response of a group of volunteers. Example 9.8 illustrates a typical 2×2 paired-samples design.

EXAMPLE 9.8 *A packaging company has developed a new type of blister packaging for drugs that are used for the treatment of rheumatoid arthritis. However, before implementing a process to manufacture this new packaging, the company wishes to examine the acceptability of this system to patients. A group of volunteers with severe rheumatoid arthritis have been asked to comment on whether they like or dislike the design of a new type of blister packaging. After a 4-week period in which the patients were allowed to become accustomed to the new packaging, they were questioned again about its acceptability. The results are shown in Table 9.7. Using an appropriate statistical test,*

Table 9.7   Acceptability of a new type of blister packaging to patients with rheumatoid arthritis, initially and after 4 weeks of usage

Initial response	Response after 4 weeks	
	Acceptable	Unacceptable
Acceptable	13	6
Unacceptable	11	8

examine whether the new blister pack is more acceptable to patients with rheumatoid arthritis after a 4-week period of use.

As before, the parameters associated with the experimental design are initially defined.

(i)   State the null hypothesis

In this study the null hypothesis states that the acceptability of the packaging after the 4-week period is the same as that recorded at the beginning of the study.

(ii)   State the alternative hypothesis

The alternative hypothesis states that the acceptability of the packaging to the patients increases after the 4-week period during which the patients were allowed to become accustomed to the new presentation.

(iii)   State the level of significance

In this example, it is assumed that the level of significance (α) is 0.05.

(iv)   State the number of tails associated with the experimental design

In this study the null hypothesis will be rejected if the acceptability of the packaging increases after the 4-week period. As this is the only outcome of interest to the sponsor company, this is a one-tailed statistical analysis.

(v)   Select the most appropriate statistical method

This is an example of a data set that should be analysed using McNemar's test, but it is important that the exact reasons for this selection are clear to the reader. The important characteristics of the data set described in Table 9.7 are as follows:

- the data are paired, i.e. the same pool of volunteers are being used to evaluate the acceptability before and after the period of usage
- the data have been measured on a nominal scale

Therefore a non-parametric two-paired-samples statistical test (McNemar's test) must be employed to address the validity of the null hypothesis.

(vi) Perform the statistical analysis

Before carrying out the test, it is important to provide the reader with some background. In the 2×2 table (Table 9.7), two distinct profiles may be observed. The first involves the number of patients whose opinions have not been altered over the period of the study, i.e. those patients who found the packaging material to be either acceptable or unacceptable both at the start and at the end of the clinical study. For the purpose of this explanation, these responses have been denoted as cells A and D, respectively (Table 9.8).

Cells A and D represent data sets in which there have been no changes and are therefore referred to as *tied data*. These data sets are not employed in the statistical analysis. Conversely, data sets B and C represent changes in the responses of the volunteers over the course of the study. Cell B represents those patients who categorised the new packaging as acceptable at the start of the study but reversed their opinion after the 4-week trial period. The opposite is true for the patients described in cell C. These volunteers described the packaging as unacceptable to begin with, but their opinions had changed after the trial period. The values recorded in cells B and C are employed for the calculation because these observations are associated with a change in response. For this reason, McNemar's test is often referred to as *McNemar's test of significance of changes*.

Before the mathematical calculation of the test statistic, the null hypothesis and alternative hypotheses should be stated in terms of the frequency of observations in each cell. The null hypothesis stated that the trial period will not change the acceptability of the new packaging system and therefore the probabilities of recording values in cell B and cell C will be equal. Conversely, the alternative hypothesis for this one-tailed example states that the probability in cell C exceeds that of cell B.

Table 9.8 Acceptability of a new type of blister packaging to patients with rheumatoid arthritis, initially and after 4 weeks of usage

Initial response	Response after 4 weeks	
	Acceptable	Unacceptable
Acceptable	Cell A	Cell B
Unacceptable	Cell C	Cell D

McNemar's test is in effect a goodness-of-fit test in which the observed frequencies are compared to the expected frequencies, as defined by the null hypothesis. It may therefore be unsurprising to the reader that the calculated statistic in McNemar's test is the χ^2 statistic. The expected frequencies (E_f) of cells B and C, as defined by the null hypothesis are calculated as follows:

$$E_f = \left(\frac{B+C}{2}\right)$$

where B and C are the recorded frequencies associated with cells B and C, respectively.

The χ^2 statistic is calculated, as described previously (Chapters 7 and 8), but as only cells B and C are relevant, the calculation is performed only using these cells. Accordingly:

$$\chi^2 = \frac{(O_B - E_B)^2}{E_B} + \frac{(O_C - E_C)^2}{E_C}$$

where O_B and O_C are the observed frequencies in cells B and C, respectively, and E_B and E_C are the expected frequencies in cells B and C, respectively (as defined by the null hypothesis).

The χ^2 statistic may be rewritten as

$$\chi^2 = \frac{(O_B - ((B+C)/2))^2}{((B+C)/2)} + \frac{(O_C - ((B+C)/2))^2}{((B+C)/2)} = \frac{(B-C)^2}{(B+C)}$$

This test employs the χ^2 statistic for the interpretation of the validity of the null hypothesis. The number of degrees of freedom associated with the McNemar test is 1 (i.e. $(R-1)(C-1)$). In earlier chapters it was explained how the accuracy of the method may be improved by introducing a continuity correction into the above equation. This is necessary because the χ^2 distribution (a continuous distribution) is being employed to estimate a discrete distribution. With this in mind, the equation that is employed to calculate the χ^2 statistic within the McNemar test is

$$\chi^2 = \frac{(B-C)^2}{(B+C)} = \frac{[(B-C)-1]^2}{(B+C)}$$

To illustrate the calculation of the χ^2 statistic and the subsequent interpretation, we now return to the data presented in Example 9.8.

(vii) Calculate the χ^2 statistic

Using the above equation, the χ^2 statistic for 1 *df* may be calculated. As we are interested in the difference between cell C and cell B (as defined by the alternative hypothesis), the χ^2 statistic will be calculated by subtracting the frequency in cell B from that in cell C:

$$\chi^2 = \frac{[(C-B)-1]^2}{(B+C)} = \frac{[(11-6)-1]^2}{(11+6)} = \frac{16}{17} = 0.94$$

(viii) Interpret the calculated statistic

The initial step in the interpretation of the calculated χ^2 statistic involves the definition of the critical region. From the conditions of the experimental design (1 *df*, one-tailed, $\alpha = 0.05$) the critical value of χ^2 may be found from Appendix 3 as 2.71 (remembering that the probabilities illustrated in this table refer to two-tailed outcomes and therefore must be doubled to generate the probabilities associated with one-tailed designs. For this reason the χ^2 statistic associated with 0.1 is selected).

   In the current study, the critical region associated with the null hypothesis is $\chi^2 < 2.71$, whereas the alternative hypothesis is defined as $\chi^2 \geqslant 2.71$. As the calculated value is less than 2.71 the null hypothesis is accepted and therefore, it may be concluded that the acceptability of the new packaging system was not increased at the end of the 4-week trial period.

   To further consolidate the mechanics and application of McNemar's test, the reader should consider the following example.

EXAMPLE 9.9   *As part of a PhD programme, a scientist wishes to examine the comparative percutaneous local anaesthetic properties of two prototype formulations. It has been decided that a paired-samples study should be performed to reduce both the cost and variability of the study. In this, 40 volunteers have been recruited and (at different times) the formulations were applied to the right forearm of each volunteer for 30 min. The formulation was then removed and the degree of anaesthesia of the site tested by the needle prick test. The volunteers were asked to record whether pain was associated with this process. The results are shown in Table 9.9. Is there a clinical difference in the percutaneous local anaesthetic properties of the two products?*

Table 9.9 Comparative percutaneous local anaesthetic properties of two prototype formulations

Formulation B	Formulation A	
	Anaesthesia	No anaesthesia
Anaesthesia	8 (cell A)	6 (cell B)
No anaesthesia	15 (cell C)	11 (cell D)

As before, we define the parameters associated with the experimental design before the start of the clinical study.

(i) State the null hypothesis

In this example, the null hypothesis is that there is no clinical difference in the percutaneous local anaesthetic properties of the two formulations:

> H_0: probability associated with cell B = probability associated with cell C

(ii) State the alternative hypothesis

A suitable alternative hypothesis for this example is that there is a clinical difference in the percutaneous local anaesthetic properties of the two formulations:

> H_a: probability associated with cell B ≠ probability associated with cell C

(iii) State the level of significance

In this example, it is assumed that the level of significance (α) is 0.05.

(iv) State the number of tails associated with the experimental design

The null hypothesis may be rejected for two reasons: the clinical efficacy of formulation A may be either greater or less than that of formulation B. As there are two outcomes that will result in a rejection of the null hypothesis, this is a two-tailed experimental design.

(v) State the most appropriate statistical test

The experimental design is a paired design in which nominal data has been collected. Therefore, a non-parametric two-paired-samples design (McNemar's test) is the most appropriate statistical method for this clinical scenario.

(vi) Calculate the χ^2 statistic

In the calculation of the χ^2 statistic it is good practice to initially identify the cells that will be included in the calculation. From Table 9.9 it may be observed that cells A and D are tied, whereas cells B and C reflect differences between the two formulations. Therefore, cells B and C should be used in the calculation, as follows:

$$\chi^2 = \frac{[(15-6)-1]^2}{(15+6)} = \frac{[(15-6)-1]^2}{(11+6)} = \frac{64}{21} = 3.05$$

(vii) Interpret the calculated χ^2 statistic

The critical χ^2 statistic relating to this example may be determined from the table of the critical values of the χ^2 distribution (Appendix 3). Under the conditions of this study (1 *df*, two-tailed design, $\alpha = 0.05$) the critical χ^2 statistic is 3.84. Therefore, if the calculated value of the χ^2 statistic is equal to or exceeds this critical value, the null hypothesis is rejected. Conversely, if the calculated value is less than 3.84, the null hypothesis is accepted. As the calculated value of the χ^2 statistic is 3.05, the null hypothesis is accepted and it may be concluded that there was no clinical difference in the percutaneous local anaesthetic properties of the two formulations.

One final point about the use of the McNemar test concerns those cases in which the expected frequencies are small (i.e. less than 5). In these cases it is recommended that the binomial test should be employed for the analysis of the data sets, allowing x to be the smaller of the two observed frequencies (either B or C) and N to be the total number of observations in these two cells (B + C).

9.2.2 Wilcoxon's signed-rank test

Wilcoxon's signed-rank test is the non-parametric equivalent of the paired t test. It is used in situations in which the data have been measured using an ordinal, interval or ratio scale and, importantly, whenever the assumptions of the t test cannot be assured. Conversely, the Wilcoxon's signed-rank test may be used to analyse two-paired-samples data that are parametric in nature. Unfortunately, in the latter situation, the power associated with the use of the non-parametric test is approximately 95% of the power of the parametric comparator. For this reason, the analyst should not indiscriminately use the Wilcoxon's signed-rank test for the analysis of two-paired-sample data. This is a similar situation to that described for the use of the Mann–Whitney U test for the analysis of parametric independent data.

The mechanics of Wilcoxon's signed-rank test are similar to the paired t test in so far as both tests involve the initial calculation of the differences between pairs of data. As would be expected, the non-parametric test does not employ arithmetic manipulations (as these are invalid) but ranks the differences between the pairs in ascending order (initially ignoring the sign). The sign of the difference (+ or −) is re-assigned to the individual ranks and the positive and negative ranks are segregated. These individual ranks are used in the calculation of the associated statistic and hence the interpretation of the statistical outcome. The calculation of the test statistic associated with the

Wilcoxon signed-rank test depends on whether the sample size is small or large. To ensure complete understanding of the technique, the following examples have been designed to cover all aspects of this analytical test.

EXAMPLE 9.10 *Two therapeutic agents have been developed for the treatment of hypertension. Before setting up an extensive clinical trial the sponsor company has requested that the comparative effects of the two therapeutic agents (A and B) on diastolic blood pressure should be examined in a small pilot study. Design an appropriate methodology for the comparative assessment of the anti-hypertensive effects of the two agents and, in addition, statistically compare the effects of the two therapeutic agents using the results collected in the designed clinical study.*

Before starting the clinical study it is necessary to define the parameters of the experimental design.

(i) State the null hypothesis

In this study it will be assumed that the null hypothesis represents no difference between the anti-hypertensive effects of the two formulations. Therefore, the null hypothesis states that the diastolic blood pressure of the volunteers will be statistically similar after administration of either therapeutic agent (A or B):

H_0: diastolic blood pressure after administration of therapeutic agent A = diastolic blood pressure after administration of therapeutic agent B

(ii) State the alternative hypothesis

The alternative hypothesis states that there will be a difference in the anti-hypertensive properties of the two therapeutic agents:

H_a: diastolic blood pressure after administration of therapeutic agent A ≠ diastolic blood pressure after administration of therapeutic agent B

(iii) State the level of significance

In this example, it is assumed that the level of significance (α) is 0.05.

(iv) State the number of tails associated with the experimental design

The alternative hypothesis has stated that there will be a difference in the clinical efficacies of the two therapeutic agents but has not defined the nature of the difference. Therefore, the alternative hypothesis may be accepted because the anti-hypertensive property of therapeutic agent A is either greater or less than that of therapeutic agent B. As there are two possible outcomes associated with the rejection of the null hypothesis (and hence acceptance of the alternative hypothesis), the experimental design is two-tailed.

(v) Collect the experimental data

The statistical analyst has decided that a two-paired-samples experimental design should be employed, and for this purpose 10 volunteers who currently suffer from hypertension have been recruited into the study. On day 1 each volunteer received a single dose of a tablet formulation containing therapeutic agent A and the diastolic blood pressure was measured over the course of the next 8 h. After a washout period of 2 weeks, the volunteers received an identical tablet formulation containing therapeutic agent B and the blood pressure was measured as before. The results of the clinical study are shown in Table 9.10.

(vi) Select the most appropriate statistical test

The study has been designed as a two-paired-samples experimental design in which the data has been measured on a ratio scale. The data has not been collected and presented in the form of a contingency table, so McNemar's test cannot be used. There are two possible tests for the analysis of two-paired sample data that have been measured on a ratio scale, the paired t test and the Wilcoxon signed-rank test. Therefore, to

Table 9.10 Effects of a single dose of either therapeutic agent A or therapeutic agent B on the diastolic blood pressure of 10 male volunteers (45–55 years old). The data refer to measurements of blood pressure 2 h after administration of each agent.

Patient number	Diastolic blood pressure (mmHg) after administration	
	Therapeutic agent A	Therapeutic agent B
1	129	100
2	100	95
3	132	116
4	124	129
5	113	119
6	99	99
7	105	101
8	108	98
9	118	119
10	128	107

complete the selection process, the suitability of the above data sets for analysis using the parametric test must be investigated. The assumptions of the paired t test have been described in a previous section of this chapter. Accordingly, the normality of the distribution of differences between the two sets of data should be investigated by calculating and comparing the mean and median of the distribution (Table 9.11), which in this case are 7.30 and 4.50 mmHg, respectively. The difference between the mean and the median is sufficient to raise doubts about the validity of the parametric statistical method for the comparison of the two sets of data. Therefore, the most appropriate statistical method is the Wilcoxon signed-rank test.

(vii) Perform the statistical calculation

The statistic associated with the Wilcoxon signed-rank test may be easily calculated in a stepwise fashion, as described below.

Step 1   Calculate the difference between the pairs of data (Table 9.11)

mean difference (A–B) = 7.30 mmHg

median difference (A–B) = 4.50 mmHg

Step 2   Rank the differences, disregarding sign
Two points should be highlighted before carrying out this step.

Table 9.11   Differences between the effects of a single dose of either therapeutic agent A or therapeutic agent B on the diastolic blood pressure of 10 male volunteers (45–55 years old). The data refer to measurements of blood pressure 2 hours after administration of each agent

Patient number	Diastolic blood pressure after administration (mmHg)		Difference (A–B) (mmHg)
	Therapeutic agent A	Therapeutic agent B	
1	129	100	+29
2	100	95	+05
3	132	116	+16
4	124	129	−05
5	113	119	−06
6	99	99	0
7	105	101	+04
8	108	98	+10
9	118	119	−01
10	128	107	+21

- If there are values that share the same ranking, the assigned ranking should be calculated as the average of all the possible ranks. In Table 9.12 there are two differences of 5.0 mmHg. As these values are numerically identical they must possess the same ranking. Therefore, instead of assigning one value a rank of 3 and the other a rank of 4, both are ranked as 3.5. This technique was illustrated in Chapter 8 for the Mann–Whitney U test.
- Pairs of observation whose difference are zero are not included in the statistical analysis.

The individual differences are assigned a rank value, as shown in Table 9.12.

Step 3   Reallocate the signs (positive or negative) to the ranks and then segregate and individually sum the positive ranks and the negative ranks. The result is shown in Table 9.13

Table 9.12   Ranking of the differences between the effects of therapeutic agents A and B on the diastolic blood pressure of volunteers (data derived from Table 9.11)

Patient number	Change in diastolic blood pressure (mmHg) after administration of agent A or B	Assigned rank
1	+29	9.0
2	+05	3.5
3	+16	7.0
4	−05	3.5
5	−06	5.0
6	0	Not used in the analysis
7	+04	2.0
8	+10	6.0
9	−01	1.0
10	+21	8.0

Table 9.13   Positive and negative ranks associated with the data presented in Table 9.12

Positive ranks	Negative ranks
9.0	3.5
3.5	5.0
7.0	1.0
2.0	
6.0	
8.0	
Sum of positive ranks = 35.5	Sum of negative ranks = 9.5

(viii) *Interpret the statistical outcome based on the individual ranks*

The outcome of the statistical analysis is interpreted by consideration of the smaller sum of ranks, which in the present example is 9.5, in conjunction with the table of critical values of the smaller sum of ranks in the Wilcoxon signed-rank test (Appendix 10). Using this table and with knowledge of the relevant parameters relating to the experimental design (two-tailed design, $\alpha = 0.05$, number of untied ranks = 9), the critical value of the smaller sum of ranks (denoted by T) is 5. As in other statistical tests, the outcome of the statistical analysis is interpreted using this critical value. In the Wilcoxon signed-rank test, if the smaller sum of ranks is less than or equal to the critical value, then the null hypothesis is rejected and the alternative hypothesis is accepted. Conversely, if the calculated smaller sum of ranks (T) is greater than the critical value the null hypothesis is accepted. In the current example the calculated value of T (9.5) is greater than the critical value (5) and accordingly, the null hypothesis is accepted. Therefore, it may be concluded that there was no clinical difference in the anti-hypertensive properties of the two therapeutic agents.

Example 9.10 described a study involving a small number of pairs of volunteers. Unfortunately the table of critical values of the smaller sum of ranks in the Wilcoxon signed-rank test may not be used to interpret the outcome of the statistical analysis if the number of untied ranks is large. Under these circumstances it has been shown that if a series of studies were performed and the sum of the smaller ranks calculated, the distribution of these summed ranks would be more or less normally distributed with a mean of 0 and a standard deviation of ± 1. Therefore, in a similar fashion to the strategy employed for the Mann–Whitney U test, a z value may be calculated and employed for the interpretation of the outcome of the Wilcoxon signed-rank test. The equation that describes the relationship between the smaller sum of ranks (T), the mean (μ) and standard deviation (σ) is

$$z = \frac{T - \mu}{\sigma}$$

In terms of the Wilcoxon signed-rank test, μ and σ are calculated using the following equations:

$$\mu = \frac{N(N + 1)}{4}$$

$$\sigma = \sqrt{\frac{N(N + 1)(2N + 1)}{24}}$$

The equation that describes the z statistic may therefore be rewritten as

$$z = \frac{T - [N(N+1)/4]}{\sqrt{N(N+1)(2N+1)/24}}$$

Using the above equations, the Wilcoxon signed-rank test may be computed in terms of the z statistic and the outcome of the statistical analysis interpreted using the standardised normal distribution. An example of the mechanics and application of the Wilcoxon signed-rank test when the sample size is large is shown in Example 9.11.

EXAMPLE 9.11 *A weight control programme that has been developed by healthcare company A is claimed to significantly decrease the proportion of body fat over the first week of the programme. Company B, which also offers a weight control programme, is anxious about the efficacy of this competitor's programme and has commissioned a clinical study to investigate Company A's claim concerning the reduction in body fat over the first week of the programme. Therefore, a two-paired-samples study has been designed in which the body fat content of 30 female volunteers was initially measured using an electrical impedance method. Then the volunteers participated in Company A's new regimen for a 1-week period, at the end of which their fat content was measured once more. The results from the clinical trial are shown in Table 9.14. Do the results from the clinical study substantiate or invalidate Company A's claims for the efficacy of their weight control programme?*

This question may be resolved in the following fashion.

(i) State the null hypothesis

The null hypothesis for this example states that Company A's weight control programme does not significantly lower the proportion of body fat after 1 week of therapy.

> H_0: proportion of body fat at the start of the study = proportion of body fat after 1 week of therapy

or alternatively:

> H_0: proportion of body fat at the start of the study – proportion of body fat after 1 week of therapy = 0

(ii) State the alternative hypothesis

The aim of the investigation is to examine whether Company A's weight control programme significantly lowers the proportion of body fat. Therefore, the alternative hypothesis states that the weight control

Table 9.14 Effect of a weight control programme on the proportion of body fat in female volunteers. All measurements were taken before treatment and 1 week later

Patient number	Proportion of body fat (%)	
	Before treatment	After 1 week of treatment
1	25.3	23.8
2	38.2	30.2
3	31.6	32.2
4	24.8	22.6
5	36.5	28.6
6	19.8	18.2
7	18.4	18.9
8	36.9	29.5
9	39.4	33.5
10	35.2	32.5
11	19.2	22.5
12	19.6	19.1
13	24.5	22.1
14	28.4	26.8
15	30.0	27.1
16	38.9	31.5
17	35.2	33.9
18	39.2	34.6
19	19.9	21.0
20	37.9	36.5
21	32.7	32.7
22	28.8	28.7
23	22.5	22.1
24	22.6	21.4
25	28.9	26.9
26	30.4	29.2
27	19.6	19.6
28	22.5	22.8
29	25.4	26.0
30	29.6	25.8

programme significantly lowers the proportion of body fat in the female volunteers:

H_a: proportion of body fat at the start of the study > proportion of body fat after 1 week of therapy

or alternatively

H_a: proportion of body fat at the start of the study – proportion of body fat after 1 week of therapy > 0

(iii) State the level of significance

In this example, it is assumed that the level of significance (α) is 0.05.

(iv) State the number of tails in the experimental design

As previously stated, the main interest in this clinical trial is whether company A's weight control programme significantly lowers the proportion of body fat after 1 week of therapy. Company B, who have sponsored the study, are not concerned whether the new weight control programme is equivalent, or indeed inferior to other programmes. Their mission is to refute the claim of their competitor, company A. As there is only one outcome that will result in rejection of the null hypothesis, the experimental design is one-tailed.

(v) Select the most appropriate statistical test

The clinical study has been designed in a paired fashion, so a two-paired-samples statistical method should be used for the analysis of the data. The two tests that may be employed for the analysis of two-paired-samples data that have been measured on a ratio scale are the paired *t* test and the Wilcoxon signed-rank test. As one test is parametric and the other non-parametric, one method to selectively differentiate these tests is to assess the normality of the distribution of the differences of the pairs of data. The mean and median of the distribution of differences are 2.05% and 1.45%, respectively. Once more, the difference between the mean and median is sufficient to raise doubts about the validity of using a parametric statistical method to compare the two sets of data. Therefore, the most appropriate statistical method is the Wilcoxon signed-rank test. Furthermore, as the number of untied pairs of data exceeds 25, the analysis of the data may be performed using the normal approximation, i.e. the z statistic.

(vi) Perform the statistical calculation

Step 1   Calculate the difference between the pairs of data (Table 9.15)

   mean difference (before–after) = 2.05%
   median difference (before–after) = 1.45%

Step 2   Rank the differences, disregarding sign (Table 9.16)

Step 3   Reallocate the signs (positive or negative) to the ranks and then segregate and individually sum the positive ranks and the negative ranks (Table 9.17)

Table 9.15 Differences in the proportion of body fat of human female volunteers before and 1 week after the commencement of a weight control programme

Patient number	Proportion of body fat (%)		Difference (before – after)
	Before treatment	After 1 week of treatment	
1	25.3	23.8	1.5
2	38.2	30.2	8.0
3	31.6	32.2	−0.6
4	24.8	22.6	2.2
5	36.5	28.6	7.9
6	19.8	18.2	1.6
7	18.4	18.9	−0.5
8	36.9	29.5	7.4
9	39.4	33.5	5.9
10	35.2	32.5	2.7
11	19.2	22.5	−3.3
12	19.6	19.1	0.5
13	24.5	22.1	2.4
14	28.4	26.8	1.6
15	30.0	27.1	2.9
16	38.9	31.5	7.4
17	35.2	33.9	1.3
18	39.2	34.6	4.6
19	19.9	21.0	−1.1
20	37.9	36.5	1.4
21	32.7	32.7	0.0
22	28.8	28.7	0.1
23	22.5	22.1	0.4
24	22.6	21.4	1.2
25	28.9	26.9	2.0
26	30.4	29.2	1.2
27	19.6	19.6	0.0
28	22.5	22.8	−0.3
29	25.4	26.0	−0.6
30	29.6	25.8	3.8

(viii) Calculate the z statistic

The equation that may be employed to calculate the z statistic associated with the Wilcoxon signed-rank test has been previously defined as

$$z = \frac{T - [N(N+1)/4]}{\sqrt{N(N+1)(2N+1)/24}}$$

Table 9.16 Ranking of the differences in the proportion of body fat of female volunteers before and 1 week after the start of a weight control programme (data derived from Table 9.15). Figures in bold indicate negative differences

Patient number	Difference in body fat (before – after 1 week of treatment)	Assigned rank
21	0	Not used in the analysis
27	0	Not used in the analysis
22	0.1	1.0
28	**0.3**	**2.0**
23	0.4	3.0
7	**0.5**	**4.5**
12	0.5	4.5
3	**0.6**	**6.5**
29	**0.6**	**6.5**
19	**1.1**	**8.0**
24	1.2	9.5
26	1.2	9.5
17	1.3	11.0
20	1.4	12.0
1	1.5	13.0
6	1.6	14.5
14	1.6	14.5
25	2.0	16.0
4	2.2	17.0
13	2.4	18.0
10	2.7	19.0
15	2.9	20.0
11	**3.3**	**21.0**
30	3.8	22.0
18	4.6	23.0
9	5.9	24.0
8	7.4	25.5
16	7.4	25.5
5	7.9	27.0
2	8	28.0

For the current example, T denotes the sum of the smaller ranks ($T = 48.5$) and N denotes the number of untied pairs of data, i.e. data sets whose difference was not equal to zero ($N = 28$). Entering this information into the above equation allows the z statistic to be computed:

$$z = \frac{T - [N(N+1)/4]}{\sqrt{N(N+1)(2N+1)/24}} = \frac{48.5 - [28(28+1)/4]}{\sqrt{28(28+1)((2 \times 28)+1)/24}}$$

$$= \frac{-154.5}{43.9} = -3.52$$

Table 9.17 Positive and negative ranks associated with the data presented in Table 9.15

Positive ranks	Negative ranks
1.0	2.0
3.0	4.5
4.5	6.5
9.5	6.5
9.5	8.0
11.0	21.0
12.0	
13.0	
14.5	
14.5	
16.0	
17.0	
18.0	
19.0	
20.0	
22.0	
23.0	
24.0	
25.5	
25.5	
27.0	
28.0	
Sum of positive ranks = 357.5	Sum of negative ranks = 48.5

This study was a one-tailed design with a chosen level of significance of 0.05. The critical z statistic for this design may be obtained from the standardised normal distribution (Appendix 1) as -1.65. Subsequently, the null hypothesis will be accepted if the calculated z value is greater than -1.65 and rejected if the calculated z value is equal to or less than this value. The calculated z value (-3.52) lies within the region of rejection of the null hypothesis and therefore it may be concluded that Company A's weight control programme significantly lowered the proportion of body fat in human female volunteers after a 1 week treatment period.

9.3 Conclusions

This chapter has described the mechanics and applications of parametric and non-parametric statistical tests that are used to compare two samples in a paired experimental design. In this a group of volunteers, for example, is exposed to two treatments, or alternatively, a set of samples may be analysed by two methods. The paired-sample experimental design is a powerful method that allows each sample or patient to act as their own control and, as a result, is often employed whenever the intersubject or intersample variability is expected to be large or, under certain circumstances, when there are limitations on the cost of the study. This type of design should not be confused with a two-independent-samples experimental design, as in the latter the two samples are exposed to independent treatments. If a two-independent-samples statistical method, e.g. an unpaired t test, is used to examine data that has been collected in a paired design, the probability of committing a type II error is increased and may lead to an erroneous outcome (i.e. acceptance of the null hypothesis when the null hypothesis should be rejected). It is therefore important that the reader should understand the format of the two-paired-samples design, and also the most appropriate statistical test that may be employed to determine the differences or similarity between the data sets.

Once the reader has recognised that the data has been collected in a two-paired-samples experimental design, the next challenge is the choice of a parametric or non-parametric test for the comparison of the two data sets. First the nature of the data – i.e. nominal, ordinal, interval or ratio – should be examined. If the data is nominal in nature, an appropriate statistical method for the analysis of this type of data is the McNemar test. In this test, a χ^2 statistic is calculated and interpreted using the table of critical values of the χ^2 distribution. There is no parametric test that may be applied to this type of data. Assuming that the data has been measured on an interval or ratio scale, the data may be examined using either a parametric test (the two-paired-samples t test) or a non-parametric test (Wilcoxon signed-rank test). Which test to use depends on whether the conditions of the experiment comply with the requirements of the parametric test. In particular, the nature of the distribution of differences between the pairs of data should be examined. If there is insufficient evidence to conclude that this distribution is normally distributed, then the Wilcoxon signed-rank test should be used. Conversely, if the distribution is normally distributed, the parametric two-paired-samples t test must be used. Indiscriminate use of the Wilcoxon signed-rank test in situations that require the application of the paired t test will increase the chance of coming to an erroneous conclusion. As before, a t statistic is calculated in the two-paired-sample t test and this is statistically interpreted using the t distribution. In the case of the Wilcoxon signed-rank test the differences in the pairs of data are ranked and segregated into two categories (positive and negative ranks) and the smaller rank is used as the critical (T) statistic. If the number of untied samples is small, the significance of the calculated smaller sum of ranks (T) may be interpreted from the table containing the critical values of the smaller sum of ranks in the Wilcoxon signed-rank test. If the sample size is large (i.e. number of untied ranks $\geqslant 25$), it may be assumed that the distribution of values of T is normally distributed. Under these circumstances the smaller sum of ranks is used in the calculation of a z statistic, the significance of which is discerned from the standardised normal distribution. Finally, if the data has been measured on an ordinal scale, Wilcoxon's signed-rank test should be employed for the statistical analysis of paired data.

10

Parametric hypothesis testing for multiple samples

In Chapters 8 and 9 the theory and applications of techniques that may be used for the statistical comparison of two sets of data were described. The comparison of two sets of data, either paired or unpaired, is a common procedure in the pharmaceutical and related sciences, as the reader will by now have realised. However, in another type of experimental design common in scientific research more than two sets of data are collected and require simultaneous comparisons. Under these circumstances a multiple comparison test is employed. In this chapter, the mechanics and applications of multiple comparison statistical procedures, namely the *analysis of variance (ANOVA)* will be explained. As in the previous chapters, several pharmaceutical examples of these techniques will be provided to assist in their understanding.

10.1 One-way analysis of variance

Analysis of variance is a parametric statistical technique that has found extensive applications in scientific research, mainly because of its flexibility. Importantly, this method may be employed to analyse both paired and independent data and may also be used to simultaneously compare a large number of variables. The mechanics of the technique are more complex than those of the other parametric methods that have been described in previous chapters, but the reader should not be deterred by this. ANOVA is an extremely powerful technique and, once understood, it is invaluable in the execution and analysis of scientific research. To ensure understanding of this method, special attention will be paid to the theory of the technique, including the rationale for its use, before its applications of the technique are considered.

10.1.1 Introduction to ANOVA

Consider a clinical situation in which the comparative effects of three drugs on the concentration of cholesterol in the plasma of human volunteers are under investigation. In this study patients were recruited and divided into three independent groups and each group received one drug. A schematic representation of the experimental design is shown in Table 10.1. Applying the logic described in Chapter 8, the reader might examine for differences in the clinical performances of the three drugs by making the following statistical comparisons using a two-independent-samples t test:

- comparison of the means of group A and group B
- comparison of the means of group A and group C
- comparisons of the means of group B and group C

Although this may seem to be appropriate at first glance, it is unfortunately an incorrect method of examining for differences between the three treatment groups. When a single t test is used to compare the means of two sets of data, the level of significance (i.e. the probability of rejecting the null hypothesis when it is in fact true) is arbitrarily set (usually at 0.05). Therefore, in an individual analysis, e.g. in the comparison of the means of groups A and B, the probability of making a type I error is 0.05. Alternatively, it may be stated that the probability of accepting the null hypothesis in a two-sample t test when it is indeed true is 0.95. If the t test is applied to the experimental design in Table 10.1, then three separate analyses are required to test the null hypothesis that there is no difference between the means of the three treatments. Under these circumstances, the probability of accepting all null hypotheses $(\bar{X}_A = \bar{X}_B, \bar{X}_A = \bar{X}_C, \bar{X}_B = \bar{X}_C)$ is 0.86 (i.e. $0.95 \times 0.95 \times 0.95$). Conversely, the probability of committing a type I error for at

Table 10.1 Exemplar experimental design associated with the analysis of variance in which the effects of three therapeutic agents on blood cholesterol concentrations in patients has been examined

Plasma cholesterol concentration		
Drug A	Drug B	Drug C
Group 1 volunteer 1	Group 2 volunteer 1	Group 3 volunteer 1
Group 1 volunteer 2	Group 2 volunteer 2	Group 3 volunteer 2
Group 1 volunteer 3	Group 2 volunteer 3	Group 3 volunteer 3
Group 1 volunteer 4	Group 2 volunteer 4	Group 3 volunteer 4
Group 1 volunteer 5	Group 2 volunteer 5	Group 3 volunteer 5
Group 1 volunteer 6	Group 2 volunteer 6	Group 3 volunteer 6
Group 1 volunteer 7	Group 2 volunteer 7	Group 3 volunteer 7
Mean $= \bar{X}_A$	Mean $= \bar{X}_B$	Mean $= \bar{X}_C$
Variance $= \sigma_A^2$	Variance $= \sigma_B^2$	Variance $= \sigma_C^2$
Overall treatment mean $= \frac{1}{3}(\bar{X}_A + \bar{X}_B + \bar{X}_C)$		

least one null hypothesis is 0.14 (1.00 – 0.86). This problem is further complicated when more than three treatments are under comparison: as the number of treatment groups is increased the probability of committing a type I error is increased. This has serious consequences in terms of the conclusions that are associated with the statistical tests. As the probability of committing a type I error is increased, there is a greater probability that the null hypothesis will be rejected and, accordingly, a significance difference will be recorded between two treatments that in fact does not exist.

Because of the increased risk associated with the use of a series of *t* tests for executing multiple comparisons, a parametric statistical procedure, ANOVA, is recommended for the simultaneous comparison of more than two sets of data. As this method is a parametric statistical technique, its use is valid whenever the conditions of the experimental design conform to the assumptions of the test. These assumptions are similar to those described for other parametric statistical methods:

- The data must be measured on an interval or ratio scale. ANOVA may not be used to compare data that have been collected using nominal or ordinal scales.
- The populations from which the samples have been derived must possess similar variances. As before, this is referred to as *homogeneity of variance* and is statistically examined using the *F* test.
- The populations from which the samples have been derived must be normally distributed.
- The observations must be independent of each other. As in the *t* test, it is assumed that the selection of one sample associated with a particular group does not directly influence the selection of subsequent samples.

The reader will recognise these assumptions from the previous chapters. Furthermore, like the *t* test, ANOVA may be used to analyse data in which there are moderate deviations from the above assumptions. However, as the deviations become more marked, the use of ANOVA is invalidated.

10.1.2 Underlying mechanism of ANOVA

The mathematics that are required to perform ANOVA are relatively straightforward, but before the test can be carried out effectively it is important to understand the rationale of the calculations used. In ANOVA, the variances of each set of data are compared, from which conclusions concerning the similarity or dissimilarity of sample means may be formulated. To clarify this alternative approach, it is important to provide the reader with an insight into the mechanism behind the analysis of more than two sets of data using ANOVA.

In ANOVA, the variance of the data collected in a study, e.g. the cholesterol study described in Table 10.1, is effectively segregated into two major sources:

- Variability may occur due to differences in the responses of each patient within individual treatment groups. In Table 10.1, this variance corresponds to the *intragroup* variance, i.e. the variability between the seven individual volunteers in any of the three groups.
- The second source of variation is that which exists *between treatments*, which in Table 10.1 refers to the variability that exists between the three separate mean values.

In ANOVA, these two variances, termed respectively the *mean square error* and the *mean square between groups*, are calculated and compared. Alternative names for these terms are the *mean square within groups* and the *mean square treatment*.

To fully understand the mechanics of the ANOVA test it is important to comprehend the methods by which each of these mean squares is calculated. The mean square within groups is effectively the mean of the variability of the three groups. Therefore, in Table 10.1, the mean square error is calculated as follows:

$$MS_{error} = \left(\frac{\sigma_A^2 + \sigma_B^2 + \sigma_C^2}{3} \right)$$

Remember that one of the assumptions of ANOVA is homogeneity of variances and therefore, the above calculation is one measure of the population variance. If the sample sizes in the treatment groups are not equal, then the mean square error is calculated by pooling the variances, weighting each variance as a function of the number of degrees of freedom as described for the two-independent-samples *t* test.

The mean square treatment is a measure of the intergroup variability. This variability may be visualised as the variability of each treatment mean around the overall mean of the three treatments. In other words, the mean square treatment is the variance of the individual treatment means. If we assume that there are no differences between the three treatment groups, then it may be concluded either that the three samples in Table 10.1 have been sampled from a common population, or alternatively, that the three samples have been derived from three identical populations. The mean square treatment may be employed to obtain a second estimate of the common population from which the three treatment groups have been sampled, as described under the null hypothesis. For this purpose it should be remembered that, according to the central limit theorem, the variance of means sampled from a common population is equal to the variance of the population divided by the sample size, i.e. $s^2 = \sigma^2/N$ or alternatively $\sigma^2 = s^2 \times N$. Therefore, it may be observed that both the mean square error and the mean square treatment provide independent estimates of the variance of the population from which the individual sets of data have been sampled. The mean square error has been calculated without any reference to a null hypothesis, whereas the mean square treatment is computed on the basis that the null hypothesis is accepted, i.e. there is no difference between the treatment groups, or alternatively, the three samples have been derived from a single population. The fundamental basis of ANOVA involves the mathematical comparison (i.e. the ratio) of these two estimates. If the two estimates are in agreement, the null hypothesis is accepted, whereas if the two estimates differ, the null hypothesis is rejected in favour of the alternative hypothesis. The astute reader may at this point ask how large the difference between samples has to be in order to be considered significant. As in previous problems, the significance (or lack of significance) of differences between sample means is determined by calculating the ratio of the mean squares treatment to the mean squares error (termed the F statistic) and interpreting the significance of this ratio by reference to the F distribution:

$$F_{calculated} = \frac{MS_{treatment}}{MS_{error}} = \frac{\sigma^2_{treatment}}{\sigma^2_{error}}$$

If it is assumed that the sets of data have been sampled from a single population (as defined in the null hypothesis), then the two estimates of the population variance will be equal and hence, according to the above equation, the F ratio will be equal to unity. In effect, it is unlikely that the two estimates will be exactly equal and this reflects the variability of the magnitudes of means derived from any single population. However, the degree of this departure from normality is relatively small.

If the null hypothesis is false, then sample means will differ for two reasons:

- The treatments may be sufficiently different to be considered as being sampled from different populations. This is commonly referred to as a *treatment effect*, which in Table 10.1 reflects clinical differences in the cholesterol-lowering properties of the three drugs.
- Differences in the magnitude of sample means may also be a result of natural variability, akin to that described for the mean square error.

As the magnitude of the calculated F ratio departs from unity, it becomes more probable that the null hypothesis will be rejected. As in all statistical methods a critical value of F is defined before the collection of data, and if the calculated value of F is equal to or exceeds the critical value the null hypothesis is rejected in favour of the alternative hypothesis. Conversely, if the calculated value of F is less than the critical value, the null hypothesis is accepted. The F distribution therefore assigns a probability to the likelihood of observing a particular calculated F statistic under the conditions of the experimental design, and in this respect it is no different from other probability distributions.

10.1.3 Performing the ANOVA test

ANOVA is an extremely powerful and versatile test, so it is no surprise to discover that many different types of experimental design may be examined using this technique. The experimental model described in Table 10.1 is referred to as a *one-way* (or one-factor) *fixed-model ANOVA*. There are two key terms in this description that require clarification:

- The term *one-way* refers to the number of factors in the experimental model. At first glance the reader may be tempted to conclude that, because there are three treatments, there are three factors and, as a result, this should be a three-way design. This is a common misapprehension among students encountering this technique for the first time. The factor in Table 10.1 refers not to the number of treatments but to the general category that is under investigation, which in this example is the concentration of cholesterol in the plasma of human volunteers. The three treatments are therefore sub-categories of this single category (factor).
- In ANOVA the models may be either fixed or random in design. In the fixed model, the treatment groups have been selected to examine whether the defined treatments (drugs in Table 10.1) differ. The *fixed-model ANOVA* is frequently referred to as a model I ANOVA. Conversely, the *random model* refers to the situation in which the inclusion of different treatment groups has occurred at random, with no predetermined inferences.

As in previous chapters, the use and applications of the ANOVA will be highlighted with the use of pharmaceutical examples. To ensure that the reader understands the technique, the first examples will explain the mechanics of a simple one-way ANOVA. After this, the calculations associated with a more advanced ANOVA, referred to as a two-way ANOVA, will be described.

EXAMPLE 10.1 *Four new benzimidazole drugs (coded as A, B, C and D) are under assessment for their ability to eliminate intestinal worms. In a clinical evaluation, 28 cattle were subdivided into four groups, inoculated with larvae and each group treated with a single dose of a benzimidazole. Table 10.2 shows the counts of adult worms in each*

Table 10.2 Effects of administration of a single dose of four benzimidazoles on the number of adult worms in cattle

Drug A	Drug B	Drug C	Drug D
229	378	199	358
238	289	165	304
330	400	100	340
208	286	145	451
201	298	198	384
262	350	225	351
287	365	204	316

animal, 8 days after treatment. Using an appropriate statistical method, determine whether there is a difference in the clinical performance of the four drug treatments.

As in all previous examples, the parameters associated with the experimental design should be clarified before the study begins.

(i) State the null hypothesis

In the analysis of variance the null hypothesis assumes that there is no difference in the clinical efficacies of the four treatment groups, i.e. the means of the treatment groups are identical. In light of this, the null hypothesis may be stated as:

$$H_0: \bar{X}_A = \bar{X}_B = \bar{X}_C = \bar{X}_D$$

(ii) State the alternative hypothesis

In all examples described to date the alternative hypothesis has adopted an opposite outcome to the null hypothesis, and this is also the situation for the analysis of variance. Accordingly, in this example the alternative hypothesis states that there is a clinical difference between the clinical efficacies of the four drugs. In other words, the mean numbers of adult worms in each animal following treatment with the four drugs are not equal:

$$H_a: \bar{X}_A \neq \bar{X}_B \neq \bar{X}_C \neq \bar{X}_D$$

(iii) State the level of significance

In this example, it is assumed that the level of significance (α) is 0.05.

(iv) State the number of tails associated with the experimental design

In the examples discussed in Chapters 7 and 8, identification of the number of tails associated with an experimental design is an important process in the definition of the parameters associated with the experimental design. In ANOVA all experimental designs are two-tailed, so this decision is straightforward!

(v) Select the most appropriate statistical test

In Table 10.2, it may be observed that this is a one-factor analysis in which there are four sub-categories are present. The single factor may be referred to as the drug class (benzimidazole) and the four different types of drug in this class constitute the four sub-categories. As the study has been designed to examine the comparative effects of the four drugs on the number of adult worms in cattle, this is an example of a multiple comparison test. Consequently, for reasons explained in section 10.1.1, examination of the differences in the four drug treatments by a series of two-sample tests is invalid and therefore we must employ a statistical test that has the capacity to examine the differences or similarities between all four treatments simultaneously.

As in previous scenarios, there are both parametric and non-parametric multiple comparison tests, the choice of which depends on the compatibility of the experimental design with the assumption of the parametric test. The main assumptions associated with the use of a parametric multiple comparisons test (ANOVA) are that the populations from which the sets of data have been sampled should be normally distributed and their variances similar (homogeneous) and, in addition, the data must be measured in at least an interval scale. Therefore, before selecting the most appropriate statistical test it is important to examine the suitability of the experimental design (and associated data) for statistical manipulation using ANOVA.

The first assumption concerning the use of parametric tests is that the populations from which the sets of data have been sampled must be normally distributed with similar variances. As before, an initial impression of normality may be gained by consideration of the means and medians of each data set (Table 10.3).

Table 10.3 Summary of the central tendency of the data for the effects of four benzimidazoles on the number of adult worms in cattle. The figures represent the number of adult worms in each animal after treatment

Measure of central tendency	Drug treatment			
	Drug A	Drug B	Drug C	Drug D
Mean	250.7	338.0	176.6	357.7
Median	238.0	350.0	198.0	351.0

As may be observed from Table 10.3, the means and medians of each group are similar and therefore we will assume that the populations from which the data have been sampled are normally distributed. The next problem that must be considered is the possible homogeneity of variances. In the case of two independent samples the ratio of the two variances was calculated and the probability of the calculated ratio was abstracted from the F distribution to allow assessment of the homogeneity of variances of the two groups. In situations where there are three or more samples, there are defined tests that may be employed to compare the variances of each group, e.g. *Bartlett's test*. Unfortunately, the efficiencies of these tests are severely compromised when the data departs from normality. Because of this problem and also because the ANOVA test can operate when there is moderate heterogeneity of variances, many authors do not examine for homogeneity of variances before carrying out this test. However, in this chapter, the use of two inextricably related tests, the F *ratio* and the F_{max} test, for determining the homogeneity of variances before use of the one-way ANOVA is described. Unlike Bartlett's test, these tests consider the similarity or difference in variances in two treatments associated with the minimum and maximum variances.

The two F tests are related, indeed the F_{max} test is special variant of the F ratio. The mechanics and use of the F ratio were described in Chapter 8, and the reader may recall that this test can be used to compare the ratio of the variances of two groups when the numbers of samples in each group are either equal or unequal. The F_{max} test, which also examines the ratio between two variances, is employed when the numbers of samples in the treatment groups are identical. In the F_{max} test, the ratio of the largest variance to the smallest variance is calculated and the significance of this ratio, in terms of either the acceptance or rejection of the null hypothesis, is determined using the table of the critical values of the F_{max} test (Appendix 11). In Example 10.1, the variances associated with the four drugs (A, B, C and D) are 2109.91, 2170.33, 1842.29 and 2396.24, respectively. Before calculating the F_{max} statistic, the conditions associated with this analysis should be defined. Therefore, the null hypothesis states that there is no difference in the variances of the two treatments and the alternative hypothesis states that there is a difference. The level of significance is chosen as 0.05. The F_{max} statistic is calculated as follows:

$$F_{max} = \frac{s^2_{maximum}}{s^2_{minimum}} = \frac{2396.24}{1842.29} = 1.30$$

The critical F_{max} statistic may be derived from Appendix 11 with knowledge of the number of degrees of freedom (the number of observations in each treatment − 1), the total number of treatments (4, in this case) and the chosen level of significance ($\alpha = 0.05$). Therefore, the critical F_{max} statistic for Example 10.1 is 10.40 (6 df, 4 treatments, $\alpha = 0.05$). The null hypothesis is accepted if the calculated F_{max} statistic is less than the critical F_{max} statistic. Conversely, the null hypothesis is rejected if the calculated F_{max} statistic is equal to or is greater than the critical value. In Example 10.1 $F_{max\ calculated}$ (1.30) < $F_{max\ critical}$ (10.40) and accordingly, the null hypothesis is accepted, i.e. the variances described in Example 10.1 are homogeneous.

The nature of the data type is an important point that influences the final choice of statistical method. In Table 10.2 it may be observed that the data have been measured on a ratio scale, namely the number of adult worms in each animal. The parameters that influence the choice of statistical method for the comparison of the clinical effects of drugs A, B, C and D are as follows:

- It may be assumed that the populations from which each group of data has been sampled are normally distributed.
- It may be assumed that the variances of the populations from which each group of data has been sampled are similar (homogeneous).
- The data has been measured on at least an interval scale.

If these assumptions are satisfied, a parametric multiple comparisons method may be employed, i.e. ANOVA.

(vi) Perform the statistical test

The ANOVA method has been introduced as a method in which the variance associated with an experiment is partitioned into the mean square treatment and mean square error. The ratio of these is calculated and the probability associated with the calculated ratio is abstracted from the F distribution. This is an accurate description, but it is very concise and does not inform the reader of the mathematical functions that are required to generate the two mean square values. These mechanics of the ANOVA will therefore now be fully explained using the data presented in Example 10.1. In the experience of the author, the ANOVA is most easily performed in a stepwise fashion, as follows.

Step 1   Calculate the descriptive statistics associated with each treatment (sub-category)
The following descriptive statistics should be calculated and a new table (Table 10.4) generated to include these parameters:

- the sum of the values in each column ($\Sigma X_A, \Sigma X_B, \Sigma X_C, \Sigma X_D$)

Table 10.4 Effects of administration of a single dose of four benzimidazoles on the number of adult worms in cattle, showing the descriptive statistics that are used in the calculations associated with the one-way ANOVA. The figures represent the number of adult worms in each animal after treatment

Drug A	Drug B	Drug C	Drug D	Totals
229	378	199	358	
238	289	165	304	
330	400	100	340	
208	286	145	451	
201	298	198	384	
262	350	225	351	
287	365	204	316	
$\Sigma X_A = 1755.0$	$\Sigma X_B = 2366.0$	$\Sigma X_C = 1236.0$	$\Sigma X_D = 2504.0$	$\Sigma X = 7861.0$
$\Sigma X_A^2 = 452\,663.0$	$\Sigma X_B^2 = 812\,730.0$	$\Sigma X_C^2 = 229\,296.0$	$\Sigma X_D^2 = 910\,094.0$	$\Sigma X^2 = 2\,404\,783.0$
$\bar{X}_A = 250.7$	$\bar{X}_B = 338.0$	$\bar{X}_C = 176.6$	$\bar{X}_D = 357.7$	
$N_A = 7$	$N_B = 7$	$N_C = 7$	$N_D = 7$	$N = 28$

- the sum of the squares of values in each column ($\Sigma X_A^2, \Sigma X_B^2, \Sigma X_C^2, \Sigma X_D^2$), calculated by squaring each individual value in the treatment group and adding together all the squared values
- the mean of each column (treatment) ($\bar{X}_A, \bar{X}_B, \bar{X}_C, \bar{X}_D$)
- the number of observations in each treatment group (N_A, N_B, N_C, N_D).

Step 2   Calculate the total sum of squares
The term 'sum of squares' refers to the squared deviation between a datum point and the mean. The total sum of squares is therefore a measure of the squared deviation of all data points around the mean. In this fashion the data are assumed to represent a single large sample. The equation that is employed for the calculation of the total sum of squares is:

$$SS_{total} = \Sigma X^2 - \frac{(\Sigma X)^2}{N}$$

The term $(\Sigma X)^2/N$ is referred to as a *correction factor* and is employed in all computations in ANOVA.

Using the above equation the total sum of squares for Example 10.1 may be calculated:

$$
\begin{aligned}
\Sigma X^2 = {}& (229)^2 + (238)^2 + (330)^2 + (208)^2 + (201)^2 + (262)^2 + (287)^2 \\
& + (378)^2 + (289)^2 + (400)^2 + (286)^2 + (298)^2 + (350)^2 + (365)^2 \\
& + (199)^2 + (165)^2 + (100)^2 + (145)^2 + (198)^2 + (225)^2 + (204)^2 \\
& + (358)^2 + (304)^2 + (340)^2 + (451)^2 + (384)^2 + (351)^2 + (316)^2 \\
= {}& 2\,404\,873.0
\end{aligned}
$$

$$\frac{(\Sigma X)^2}{N} = \frac{(7861.0)^2}{28} = 2\,206\,975.75$$

Therefore, the total sum of squares is

$$SS_{total} = \Sigma X^2 - \frac{(\Sigma X)^2}{N} = 2\,404\,873.0 - 2\,206\,975.75 = 197\,897.25$$

Step 3   Calculate the sum of squares between treatments
The sum of squares between treatments is calculated using the following equation:

$$SS_{treatment} = \left(\frac{\Sigma X^2}{N}\right) - \frac{(\Sigma X)^2}{N}$$

In this computation the sum of data in each treatment group is squared and divided by the number of data, and all values are summed. As in the calculation of the total sum of squares, the correction term must be subtracted from the calculated value. Therefore, in the current example, the between-treatment sum of squares is:

$$SS_{treatment} = \left[\left(\frac{1755^2}{7}\right) + \left(\frac{2366^2}{7}\right) + \left(\frac{1236^2}{7}\right) + \left(\frac{2504^2}{7}\right)\right] - \frac{(7861.0)^2}{28}$$
$$= 146\,695.4$$

Step 4   Calculate the within-group sum of squares
The within-group sum of squares is calculated as the difference between the total sum of squares and the between-treatment sum of squares, i.e.:

$$SS_{error} = SS_{total} - SS_{treatment}$$

In Example 10.1, the within-group sum of squares is therefore:

$$197\,897.25 - 146\,695.4 = 51\,201.8$$

Step 5   Construct a summary table for the analysis of variance
The ANOVA table is basically a summary of the parameters that have been calculated above, and additionally a statement of the number of degrees of freedom associated with each source of variance. The total number of degrees of freedom for the experimental design is calculated by subtracting 1 from the total number of observations. In this example the total number of degrees of freedom is $N_{total} - 1 = 28 - 1 = 27$. The number of degrees of freedom associated with the between-treatments sum of squares is calculated by subtracting 1 from the total number of treatments, i.e. $4 - 1 = 3$. The number of degrees of freedom associated with the within-groups sum of squares is calculated by subtracting the number of degrees of freedom between treatments from the total number of degrees of freedom. These calculations

are summarised below:

- df_{total} = total number of observations − 1
- $df_{treatment}$ = total number of treatments − 1
- $df_{within} = df_{total} - df_{treatment}$.

Finally, the mean square is calculated by dividing the sum of squares for the treatment and error by the associated number of degrees of freedom.

With this information in mind, the ANOVA summary table is constructed (Table 10.5).

The reader will remember that the main basis of ANOVA is the independent calculation of the two components of the variance associated with the experiment. In the ANOVA table the F statistic is the ratio of these calculated variances, namely the ratio of the between-treatments mean square to the within-treatments (error) mean square.

Step 6   Define the critical F statistic
The critical F statistic is derived from the F distribution following consideration of the parameters of the experiment, namely the numbers of degrees of freedom associated with both the between-treatment mean squares and the within-groups mean squares and, additionally, the chosen level of significance. In this example, these parameters are as follows:

- level of significance $(\alpha) = 0.05$
- $df_{treatment} = 3$
- $df_{error} = 24$.

The degree of freedom in the numerator is the number of degrees of freedom associated with the treatment, whereas the degrees of freedom in the denominator is the df_{error}. Consequently, when $df_{treatment} = 3$, $df_{error} = 24$ and $\alpha = 0.05$, the critical value of the F statistic is 3.01 (Appendix 7). Interestingly, although the experimental design associated with ANOVA is always two-tailed, the rejection region is exclusively located in the upper part (right-hand side) of the distribution. Therefore, the number of tails in the experimental design is effectively one.

Table 10.5 Summary of the output of the analysis of variance concerning the effects of four benzimidazoles on the number of adult larvae in cattle

Source	Sum of squares	df	Mean square	F statistic
Between treatments (drug effects)	146 695.4	3	48 898.5	22.9
Within treatments (error)	51 201.8	24	2 133.4	
Total	197 897.2	27		

Step 7   Interpret the outcome of the statistical analysis
When the critical F statistic is known, the calculated F statistic may be compared to this value. Therefore, if the calculated value of F is equal to or greater than the critical value of F, the null hypothesis is rejected in favour of the alternative hypothesis. Conversely, if the calculated value of F is lower than the critical value, the null hypothesis is accepted. In Example 10.1, $F_{calculated}$ is greater than $F_{critical}$ and the null hypothesis is rejected in favour of the alternative hypothesis. We can therefore conclude that there is a difference in the clinical performance of the four benzimidazole drugs. As this is a multiple comparisons test, we cannot define the origin of the difference(s) at this point. To perform this, further statistical tests, known as *post-hoc tests*, must be employed, as described in a later section of this chapter.

   In the previous example, the experimental design was symmetrical in terms of equal numbers of observations in each group. However, it should be stressed that the numbers of samples in each group do not have to be equal to perform an ANOVA, although the ANOVA assumptions are less likely to be breached when the sample sizes are equal. The next example shows the ANOVA computations when the sample sizes are dissimilar.

EXAMPLE 10.2   *Three formulations of a controlled-release solid-dosage form containing salbutamol have been developed for the treatment of asthma. As the first stage of the development process, the pharmaceutical development laboratory has been asked to compare the release kinetics of the three formulations using the dissolution method described in the British Pharmacopoeia. The release kinetics of each formulation were experimentally determined and are presented in Table 10.6. Is there a difference between the release kinetics of the three formulations?*

Before the start of the experiment, the experimental parameters should be defined.

(i)   State the null hypothesis

In this experiment a suitable null hypothesis is that the mean rate of release of salbutamol form the three formulations is identical. Thus:

$$H_0: \ \mu_{formulation\ 1} = \mu_{formulation\ 2} = \mu_{formulation\ 3}$$

(ii)   State the alternative hypothesis

A suitable alternative hypothesis for this experiment is that the mean rate of release of salbutamol from the three formulations is not identical.

Table 10.6 The rates of release of salbutamol (mg/h) from three controlled release formulations

Formulation 1	Formulation 2	Formulation 3
4.21	3.69	5.00
5.23	3.99	6.55
4.01	4.25	6.02
6.00	4.08	6.11
5.25	5.22	4.88
6.41	2.99	4.29
4.52	5.66	6.00
4.18	4.25	5.45
6.05		5.04
4.66		

Remember, at this stage the alternative hypothesis cannot be stated in terms of the individual differences between the selected treatments. Thus:

$$H_a: \mu_{\text{formulation 1}} \neq \mu_{\text{formulation 2}} \neq \mu_{\text{formulation 3}}$$

(iii) State the level of significance

In this example, it is assumed that the level of significance (α) is 0.05.

(iv) State the number of tails associated with the experimental design

This is an example of a multiple hypothesis test, so the outcome is two-tailed.

(v) Select the most appropriate statistical test

The following points are determinants of the most appropriate statistical method for the experimental design described in Example 10.2.

- There are three treatments (formulations), so this is a case in which more than two means will be simultaneously compared and a multiple hypothesis test is required (either parametric or non-parametric).
- There is one factor in the experimental design (i.e. the formulation) of which there are three sub-categories (formulations 1, 2 and 3), so a one-way (single factor) multiple hypothesis test is required.
- To gain an insight into the normality of the populations from which the three treatments were sampled, the descriptive statistics of the three samples should be examined (Table 10.7). As may be observed, there is similarity between the mean and median of each data set and therefore, we will assume for the

Table 10.7 Summary of the central tendency of the data for the rates of release of salbutamol (mg/h) from three controlled-release formulations

Measure of central tendency	Formulation 1	Formulation 2	Formulation 3
Mean	5.05	4.23	5.48
Median	4.95	4.17	5.45

purposes of this analysis that the populations from which the data have been sampled are normally distributed.

- One of the assumptions of the ANOVA concerns homogeneity of variances of the various treatment groups and therefore this should be examined. In Example 10.2, the variances of formulations 1, 2 and 3 are 0.76, 0.70 and 0.54 mg^2/h^2, respectively. For the purpose of this analysis, we will assess the homogeneity of the variances of these groups. In Example 10.1, the F_{max} test was employed for this purpose. Although it is normally reserved for situations in which the numbers of observations in each group are identical, the homogeneity of variances in Example 10.2 may be evaluated using the F_{max} test. Therefore, to estimate the similarity of the variances of the data in Table 10.6, the F_{max} statistic associated with the largest (formulation 1) and smallest variances (formulation 3) may be calculated and interpreted using the table that describes the critical values of F_{max} (Appendix 11). The null hypothesis for this test assumes that there is no difference between the variances of these two formulations, whereas the alternative hypothesis assumes that the two variances are different. The level of significance has been defined as 0.05. The F ratio may be calculated as follows:

$$F_{max} = \frac{s^2_{maximum}}{s^2_{minimum}} = \frac{0.76}{0.54} = 1.41$$

The critical F_{max} statistic may be derived from Appendix 11, assuming that we know:

- the number of observations in each treatment. As there are 10 observations associated with treatment 1 and 9 associated with treatment 3, the smaller of these is employed in the analysis. Therefore, the number of degrees of freedom associated with this analysis is $N - 1 = 9 - 1 = 8$
- the chosen level of significance (0.05)
- the number of treatments in the multiple hypothesis test (3).

Therefore, the critical F_{max} statistic for Example 10.2 is 6.00. As the calculated F statistic (1.41) is less than the critical F statistic (6.00), the null hypothesis is accepted, i.e. the variances described in Example 10.2 may be assumed to be homogeneous.

Remember that ANOVA is relatively tolerant to departures in the assumptions both of the normality of populations and of the homogeneity of variances, and therefore the assumptions concerning these details in this current example are not excessive or potentially hazardous.

We can therefore conclude that the most appropriate statistical test for the analysis of Example 10.2 is a one-way ANOVA.

(vi) Perform the statistical test

Once more, to enhance understanding of this method, the ANOVA test is performed in a stepwise fashion.

Step 1 Calculate the descriptive statistics associated with each formulation (treatment) (Table 10.8)

Step 2 Calculate the total sum of squares
As stated in Example 10.1, the total sum of squares is calculated using the following formula:

$$SS_{total} = \Sigma X^2 - \frac{(\Sigma X)^2}{N}$$

Table 10.8 Comparative rates of release of salbutamol (mg/h) from three controlled-release formulations showing the terms that are used in the calculations associated with the ANOVA

Formulation 1	Formulation 2	Formulation 3	Totals
4.21	3.69	5.00	
5.23	3.99	6.55	
4.01	4.25	6.02	
6.00	4.08	6.11	
5.25	5.22	4.88	
6.41	2.99	4.29	
4.52	5.66	6.00	
4.18	4.25	5.45	
6.05		5.04	
4.66			
$\Sigma X_1 = 50.52$	$\Sigma X_2 = 34.13$	$\Sigma X_3 = 49.34$	$\Sigma X = 133.99$
$\Sigma X_1^2 = 262.03$	$\Sigma X_2^2 = 150.53$	$\Sigma X_3^2 = 274.80$	$\Sigma X^2 = 687.36$
$\bar{X}_1 = 5.05$	$\bar{X}_2 = 4.27$	$\bar{X}_3 = 5.49$	
$N_1 = 10$	$N_2 = 8$	$N_3 = 9$	$N = 27$

Accordingly, the total sum of squares in Example 10.2 is calculated as

$$\Sigma X^2 = (4.21)^2 + (5.23)^2 + (4.01)^2 + (6.00)^2 + (5.25)^2 + (6.41)^2$$
$$+ (4.52)^2 + (4.18)^2 + (6.05)^2 + (4.66)^2 + (3.69)^2$$
$$+ (3.99)^2 + (4.25)^2 + (4.08)^2 + (5.22)^2 + (2.99)^2$$
$$+ (5.66)^2 + (4.25)^2 + (5.00)^2 + (6.55)^2 + (6.02)^2$$
$$+ (6.11)^2 + (4.88)^2 + (4.29)^2 + (6.00)^2 + (5.45)^2 + (5.04)^2$$
$$= 687.36$$
$$\frac{(\Sigma X)^2}{N} = \frac{(133.99)^2}{27} = 664.94$$

Therefore, the total sum of squares is

$$SS_{total} = \Sigma X^2 - \frac{(\Sigma X)^2}{N} = 687.36 - 664.94 = 22.42$$

Step 3   Calculate the sum of squares between treatments
The sum of squares between treatments is calculated using the following equation:

$$SS_{treatment} = \left(\frac{\Sigma X^2}{N}\right) - \frac{(\Sigma X)^2}{N}$$

In the current example, the between treatment sum of squares is

$$SS_{treatment} = \left[\left(\frac{50.52^2}{10}\right) + \left(\frac{34.13^2}{8}\right) + \left(\frac{49.34^2}{9}\right)\right] - \frac{(133.99)^2}{27}$$
$$= 671.33 - 664.94 = 6.39$$

In the previous example the numbers of observations in each group were identical and therefore the denominators in the above calculation were identical. In this example, the numbers of observations in each group are different and, as a result, the denominators used in the equation have been modified to reflect these differences.

Step 4   Calculate the within-group sum of squares
The within-group sum of squares is calculated as the difference between the total sum of squares and the between-treatment sum of squares, i.e.

$$SS_{error} = SS_{total} - SS_{treatment}$$

In Example 10.2, the within-group (error) sum of squares is therefore

$$22.42 - 6.39 = 16.03$$

Step 5   Construct a summary table for the analysis of variance
The total number of degrees of freedom for the experimental design N_{total} is $27 - 1 = 26$, the number of degrees of freedom associated with the between-treatments sum of squares is $3 - 1 = 2$, and the number of degrees of freedom associated with the within-groups sum of squares is $26 - 2 = 24$. The mean square is calculated by dividing the sum of squares for the treatment and error by the associated number of degrees of freedom.

The summary table of the ANOVA is presented in Table 10.9.

Step 6   Define the critical F statistic
Definition of the critical F statistic for an ANOVA requires knowledge of the following parameters:

- the level of significance (i.e. 0.05, one-tailed interpretation of the F statistic)
- the number of degrees of freedom associated with the treatment (i.e. 2, the numerator in the table of the critical values of the F statistic)
- the number of degrees of freedom associated with the error (i.e. 24, the denominator in the table of the critical values of the F statistic).

The critical F statistic for Example 10.2 is therefore 3.40.

Step 7   Interpret the outcome of the statistical analysis
As in previous examples, the critical value of the F statistic is used to map the regions of acceptance and rejection of the null hypothesis. Therefore, if the calculated F value is less than the critical F value (3.04), the null hypothesis is accepted, whereas if the calculated statistic is equal to or greater then the critical F value, the null hypothesis is rejected in favour of the alternative hypothesis. In this example $F_{calculated} > F_{critical}$ and accordingly, the null hypothesis is rejected. Therefore, there is a significant difference between the rates of release of salbutamol from the three controlled-release formulations.

10.1.4   A-priori and *post-hoc* comparisons of treatments

In the discussion of ANOVA in the previous sections the null hypothesis was defined as a similarity between the means of the individual

Table 10.9 Summary of the output of the ANOVA for the comparative rates of release of salbutamol from three controlled-release formulations

Source	Sum of squares	df	Mean square	F statistic
Between treatments (formulation effects)	6.39	2	3.20	4.78
Within treatments (error)	16.03	24	0.67	
Total	22.42	26		

treatment groups and the alternative hypothesis as a difference between these means. Unfortunately, one of the problems of ANOVA is the nature of the rejection of the null hypothesis. For example, if an ANOVA has been performed to compare the means of three treatment groups and has recorded a rejection of the null hypothesis (Example 10.2), there may be several reasons for this outcome. In this case, the three means may be significantly different from one another, or alternatively two means may significantly differ. This cannot be discerned by ANOVA, so further statistical analyses are required to determine the origins of the rejection of the null hypothesis. These statistical tests are referred to as a-priori (planned) or *post-hoc* (unplanned) comparisons. These two terms refer to the nature of the decision to evaluate the individual treatments for their similarity or difference. An a-priori comparison is chosen before the collection of data and therefore no information about the differences in the means of the treatment groups is available. Conversely, *post-hoc* comparisons are performed after the computation of the means of each treatment group and the completion of the ANOVA. In this case, the analyst does have prior information about the relative differences between the treatment groups. As these two types of comparisons are distinct it will come as no surprise to the reader that the conditions for their use are different. Each comparison is discussed separately in the following sections.

10.1.4.1 A-priori (planned) comparisons

A-priori comparisons are referred to as planned comparisons because the statistical analyst generally has a predetermined comparison in mind before the experiment begins. This may involve a comparison between one product and a competitor in a multiple comparisons design, or between a control and a defined treatment. If such comparisons are premeditated then the chances of making a type I error are lower than when the comparisons are performed after the results have been received and analysed. To explain this detail, let us consider a multiple comparisons test in which there are four treatments. Typically the null hypothesis would state that there is no difference in the four means ($\bar{X}_1 = \bar{X}_2 = \bar{X}_3 = \bar{X}_4$) and for the purpose of this example, we can assume that after completion of the ANOVA the null hypothesis has been accepted. However, even under these conditions, it is possible that a difference exists between one set of means, but this difference has been masked in the outcome of the ANOVA as a result of the general similarities of the other treatments. This difference could have been between any of the following pairs:

- $\bar{X}_1$ and $\bar{X}_2$
- $\bar{X}_1$ and $\bar{X}_3$

- $\bar{X}1$ and $\bar{X}_4$
- $\bar{X}_2$ and $\bar{X}_3$
- $\bar{X}_2$ and $\bar{X}_4$
- $\bar{X}_3$ and $\bar{X}_4$

If the comparison had been planned before the experiment was carried out, the analyst would have a 1 in 6 probability of selecting the specific difference between the two treatments, i.e. the difference associated with a type I error. Conversely, in the *post-hoc* comparison, the means of the treatment groups are known and therefore it is straightforward to calculate the maximum difference between treatments and test for the significance of this difference. Under these circumstances the probability of observing a significant difference between groups is 1. Therefore, it is not unexpected that the *post-hoc* procedures that will be described in the following section usually have a restriction ensuring that the probability of making a type I error is maintained at the defined level.

One method that may be used to identify a-priori differences between treatments within a multiple comparisons experimental design is a two-independent-samples t test. In the introduction to multiple comparisons testing the reasons for avoiding the use of a series of t tests when more than two treatments were involved in the experimental design were identified. In particular it was shown that the probability of rejecting all null hypotheses was > 0.05 and therefore this approach was associated with a greater probability of making a type I error. However, the use of multiple t tests to perform a-priori comparisons is allowed, providing the pooled variance term of the t test is replaced with the mean square error that has been calculated in the ANOVA and the number of degrees of freedom associated with the t test is derived from the mean square error. In other words, the t test may be employed to perform planned (a-priori) multiple comparisons when the data has been analysed by a multiple hypothesis test (ANOVA). The use of the two-independent-samples t test for the planned comparison of data sets in a multiple hypothesis statistical design is shown in Example 10.3.

EXAMPLE 10.3 *A PhD student is concerned with the effects of solvent composition on the mechanical properties of polymer films, designed as tablet coatings. In particular, the graduate wishes to examine the comparative ultimate tensile strengths (UTS) of films that have been manufactured using a solvent evaporation process in conjunction with three different solvents (ethanol, dichloromethane and chloroform). From a consideration of the solubility parameters of the polymer and the solvents, and from previous work conducted in his laboratory, he believes that the UTS of the film cast from ethanol may be* *lower than for those cast from the other solvents. Consequently, six samples of the polymer were prepared by solvent evaporation, using these three solvents, and their UTS determined by tensile analysis. The results are shown in Table 10.10. Does solvent composition affect the ultimate tensile strength of the polymeric films?*

As the principles of the ANOVA test have been described in the previous examples, the description of ANOVA as applied to the data described in Example 10.3 is somewhat abridged here. As usual, the experimental parameters are defined before the experiment begins.

(i) State the null hypothesis

The UTS of films cast from the three solvents is identical:

$$H_0: \bar{X}_{\text{UTS ethanol}} = \bar{X}_{\text{UTS dichloromethane}} = \bar{X}_{\text{UTS chloroform}}$$

(ii) State the alternative hypothesis

The UTS of films cast from the three solvents is not identical:

$$H_a: \bar{X}_{\text{UTS ethanol}} \neq \bar{X}_{\text{UTS dichloromethane}} \neq \bar{X}_{\text{UTS chloroform}}$$

(iii) State the level of significance

In this example, it is assumed that the level of significance (α) is 0.05.

(iv) Select the most appropriate statistical test

The experimental data has been measured on a ratio scale, the mean and the median for each treatment are comparable and, in addition, the variances of three groups are similar $(F_{\text{max (calculated)}} = 1.53$, $F_{\text{max (critical)}} = 10.80)$. Therefore, we will assume that the experimental data conforms to the assumptions of the ANOVA.

Table 10.10 Effect of solvent composition on the ultimate tensile strength (MPa) of polymeric films produced by solvent evaporation from three solvents

Ethanol	Chloroform	Dichloromethane
230	248	245
245	235	257
231	257	265
240	256	248
255	261	251
234	244	261

(v) Perform the statistical test

Step 1   Calculate the descriptive statistics associated with each film (treatment) (Table 10.11)

Step 2   Calculate the total sum of squares

$$SS_{total} = \Sigma X^2 - \frac{(\Sigma X)^2}{N}$$

Therefore the total sum of squares in Example 10.2 is

$$SS_{total} = 1\,108\,563.0 - \frac{(4463)^2}{18} = 1986.9$$

Step 3   Calculate the sum of squares between treatments

$$SS_{treatment} = \left(\frac{\Sigma X^2}{N}\right) - \frac{(\Sigma X)^2}{N}$$

$$= \left[\left(\frac{1435^2}{6}\right) + \left(\frac{1501^2}{6}\right) + \left(\frac{1527^2}{6}\right)\right] - \frac{(4463)^2}{18} = 749.8$$

Step 4   Calculate the within-group sum of squares

$$SS_{error} = SS_{total} - SS_{treatment}$$

$$= 1986.9 - 749.8$$

$$= 1237.1$$

Table 10.11   Effect of solvent composition on the ultimate tensile strength of films produced by solvent evaporation showing the terms that are used in the calculations associated with the ANOVA

Ethanol	Chloroform	Dichloromethane	Totals
230	248	245	
245	235	257	
231	257	265	
240	256	248	
255	261	251	
234	244	261	
$\Sigma X_1 = 1435.0$	$\Sigma X_2 = 1501.0$	$\Sigma X_3 = 1527.0$	$\Sigma X = 4463.0$
$\Sigma X_1^2 = 343\,667.0$	$\Sigma X_2^2 = 375\,971.0$	$\Sigma X_3^2 = 388\,925.0$	$\Sigma X^2 = 1\,108\,563.0$
$\overline{X}_1 = 239.2$	$\overline{X}_2 = 250.2$	$\overline{X}_3 = 254.5$	
$N_1 = 6$	$N_2 = 6$	$N_3 = 6$	$N = 18$

Step 5   Construct a summary table for the analysis of variance

- The total number of degrees of freedom for the experimental design N_{total} is $18 - 1 = 17$.
- The number of degrees of freedom associated with the between-treatments sum of squares is $3 - 1 = 2$.
- The number of degrees of freedom associated with the within-groups sum of squares is $17 - 2 = 15$.

The summary table of the ANOVA is shown in Table 10.12.

Step 6   Define the critical F statistic
In this study, $\alpha = 0.05$, the number of degrees of freedom associated with the treatment is 2 and the number of degrees of freedom associated with the error is 15. From Appendix 7, the critical F statistic is found to be 3.68.

Step 7   Interpret the outcome of the statistical analysis
The region of acceptance of the null hypothesis is $F_{calculated} < F_{critical}$ (i.e. 3.68). Conversely, the region of rejection of the null hypothesis is $F_{calculated} \geqslant F_{critical}$ (i.e. 3.68). Therefore, as $F_{calculated}$ (4.54) > $F_{critical}$ (3.68), we may conclude that solvent composition significantly affected the UTS of polymeric films produced by the solvent evaporation technique. Unfortunately, the nature of the difference between the treatments is unknown, but perhaps the UTS of films cast from ethanol is lower than those cast from the other two solvents. An a-priori comparison is necessary to examine whether these differences are indeed apparent.

Comparison of the ultimate tensile strengths of films cast from ethanol and dichloromethane
The UTS of films cast from ethanol and dichloromethane may be easily compared using a two-independent-samples t test in which the pooled variance and the number of degrees of freedom are derived from the mean square error term. As before, the parameters associated with the two-sample comparison should be stated.

Table 10.12 Summary of the output of the ANOVA for the effect of solvent composition on the ultimate tensile strength of polymer films

Source	Sum of squares	df	Mean square	F statistic
Between treatments (solvent effects)	749.8	2	374.9	4.54
Within treatments (error)	1237.2	15	82.5	
Total	1987.0	17		

(i) State the null hypothesis

The mean UTS of films cast from ethanol is identical to the mean UTS of films cast from dichloromethane:

$$H_0: \bar{X}_{\text{UTS ethanol}} = \bar{X}_{\text{UTS dichloromethane}}$$

(ii) State the alternative hypothesis

The mean UTS of films cast from ethanol is not identical to the mean UTS of films cast from dichloromethane.

$$H_a: \bar{X}_{\text{UTS ethanol}} \neq \bar{X}_{\text{UTS dichloromethane}}$$

(iii) State the level of significance

In this example, it is assumed that the level of significance (α) is 0.05.

(iv) State the number of tails associated with the experimental design

In a-priori tests it is common practice for the comparisons to be two-tailed.

(v) Calculate the t statistic

The t statistic is calculated using the following formula (Chapter 8):

$$t = \frac{\bar{X}_{\text{UTS dichloromethane}} - \bar{X}_{\text{UTS ethanol}}}{\sqrt{s^2((1/N_{\text{UTS dichloromethane}}) + (1/N_{\text{UTS ethanol}}))}}$$

where $\bar{X}_{\text{UTS dichloromethane}}$ and $\bar{X}_{\text{UTS ethanol}}$ are the means of the two treatments, s^2 is the pooled variance, i.e. the mean square error in the ANOVA, and $N_{\text{UTS dichloromethane}}$ and $N_{\text{UTS ethanol}}$ are the numbers of observations in the two treatment groups. Therefore:

$$t = \frac{250.2 - 239.2}{\sqrt{82.5((1/6) + (1/6))}} = \frac{11.00}{5.24} = 2.10$$

(vi) Interpretation of the outcome of the statistical analysis

The first stage of the interpretative process involves the identification of the critical t statistic from the t distribution (Appendix 2). To determine the t statistic the following parameters are required:

- the level of significance ($\alpha = 0.05$)
- the number of tails (two)
- the number of degrees of freedom, i.e. the number of degrees of freedom associated with the mean square error (15).

On the basis of this information, the critical t statistic is 2.13 (Appendix 2). Therefore, if the calculated t statistic is greater than -2.13 and less than $+2.13$, the null hypothesis is accepted whereas if $t_{\text{calculated}} \geqslant +2.13$ or $\leqslant -2.13$, the null hypothesis is rejected in favour of the alternative hypothesis. In this comparison the calculated value of t is 2.10 and therefore the null hypothesis is accepted. Consequently, there is no difference in the UTS of films cast by solvent evaporation from either ethanol or dichloromethane.

Although the outcome of this analysis may appear to be definite, the calculated t statistic is numerically close to the critical t statistic and therefore the decision to accept or reject the null hypothesis is marginal. Under these circumstances it might be appropriate to repeat the experiment and increase the sample size in each treatment group.

Comparison of the UTS of films cast from ethanol and chloroform

(i) State the null hypothesis

The mean UTS of films cast from ethanol is identical to the mean UTS of films cast from chloroform:

$$H_0: \bar{X}_{\text{UTS ethanol}} = \bar{X}_{\text{UTS chloroform}}$$

(ii) State the alternative hypothesis

The mean UTS of films cast from ethanol is not identical to the mean UTS of films cast from chloroform.

$$H_a: \bar{X}_{\text{UTS ethanol}} \neq \bar{X}_{\text{UTS chloroform}}$$

(iii) State the level of significance

In this example, it is assumed that the level of significance (α) is 0.05.

(iv) State the number of tails associated with the experimental design

The design is two-tailed.

(v) Calculate the t statistic

The t statistic is calculated as before:

$$t = \frac{\bar{X}_{\text{UTS chloroform}} - \bar{X}_{\text{UTS ethanol}}}{\sqrt{s^2((1/N_{\text{UTS chloroform}}) + (1/N_{\text{UTS ethanol}}))}}$$

Therefore

$$t = \frac{254.5 - 239.2}{\sqrt{82.5((1/6) + (1/6))}} = \frac{15.3}{5.24} = 2.92$$

(vi) Interpret the outcome of the statistical analysis

The experimental parameters, and hence the critical t statistic, are identical to those used in the previous analysis. Therefore the critical t statistic is again 2.13 (Appendix 2).

In this comparison the calculated t statistic is greater than the critical t statistic and therefore the null hypothesis is rejected. The UTS of polymer films cast from chloroform by solvent evaporation is significantly greater than that of films cast from ethanol.

10.1.4.2 Post-hoc (unplanned) comparisons

The second category of comparisons performed in association with ANOVA are *post-hoc* comparisons. The comparisons are unplanned and are performed after statistical examination of the data and, for this reason, *post-hoc* comparisons are quite distinct from a-priori comparisons. Several different types of *post-hoc* comparison are available to the statistical analyst, but a full description of each of these is outside of the scope of this text. This section describes the use and applications of the most popular *post-hoc* comparisons: Fisher's least significant difference, Tukey's HSD test and Dunnett's test. For a full description of alternative *post-hoc* comparison methods, the interested reader should consult a more advanced text such as Sokal and Rohlf (1981) or Dunn and Clarke (1987).

Fisher's least significant difference (LSD) test

This method is similar to the two-independent-samples t test that is employed for the a-priori comparison of two data sets. The basic formula for calculation of the least significant difference is a rearrangement of the equation that describes the t statistic and, furthermore, both the t test and Fisher's LSD test employ the mean square error as the estimate of the pooled variance. However, one important difference between the two tests concerns the validity of their use. Fisher's LSD may only be used when the F statistic associated with the ANOVA is significant, whereas this is not the case for the two-independent-samples t test.

Fisher's LSD (FLSD) is calculated as follows:

$$FLSD = t_{\text{critical}} \sqrt{s^2 \left(\frac{1}{N_A} + \frac{1}{N_B} \right)}$$

where N_A and N_B are the sizes of the two treatment groups, s^2 is the pooled variance, estimated using the mean square error term in the ANOVA, and t_{critical} is the critical t statistic associated with the experimental design.

The use of Fisher's LSD test for the post-hoc comparisons of treatments will now be illustrated using the data from Example 10.3. It should be remembered that post-hoc tests are unplanned and are therefore performed to determine the nature of the differences between treatments. In this particular example, Fisher's LSD test is appropriate as a significant F value was recorded in the ANOVA.

Step 1 State the null hypothesis
The null hypothesis states that the means of the three treatment groups are identical:

$$H_0: \bar{X}_{\text{UTS ethanol}} = \bar{X}_{\text{UTS chloroform}} = \bar{X}_{\text{UTS dichloromethane}}$$

Step 2 State the alternative hypothesis
The alternative hypothesis states that the means of the three treatment groups are not identical:

$$H_a: \bar{X}_{\text{UTS ethanol}} \neq \bar{X}_{\text{UTS chloroform}} \neq \bar{X}_{\text{UTS dichloromethane}}$$

Step 3 State the level of significance
In this example, it is assumed that the level of significance (α) is 0.05.

Step 4 State the number of tails associated with the experimental design
As in the case of a-priori tests, all post-hoc tests are two-tailed.

Step 5 Calculate the least significant difference

$$FLSD = t_{\text{critical}} \sqrt{s^2 \left(\frac{1}{N_A} + \frac{1}{N_B} \right)}$$

where N_A and N_B are the sizes of the two treatment groups and s^2 is the pooled variance, estimated using the mean square error term in the ANOVA. t_{critical} is the t statistic that is associated with the defined level of significance ($\alpha = 0.05$), a two-tailed outcome and the number of degrees of freedom associated with the mean square error in the ANOVA (i.e. 15). We already know that for this design $t_{\text{critical}} = 2.13$. Therefore:

$$FLSD = t_{\text{critical}} \sqrt{s^2 \left(\frac{1}{N_A} + \frac{1}{N_B} \right)} = 2.13 \sqrt{82.5 \left(\frac{1}{6} + \frac{1}{6} \right)} = 11.1$$

Fisher's LSD is a measure of the least difference between two treatment groups that is associated with the rejection of the null hypothesis and, in effect, it may be regarded as a critical statistic. Accordingly, the null hypothesis is accepted if the difference between the treatment means is less than the calculated Fisher's LSD. Conversely, the null hypothesis is rejected if the difference between the treatments is equal to, or greater than the calculated Fisher's LSD.

Step 6 Calculate the differences between the means of the treatments groups

$$\overline{X}_{\text{dichloromethane}} - \overline{X}_{\text{ethanol}} = 250 - 239.2 = 11.0$$
$$\overline{X}_{\text{chloroform}} - \overline{X}_{\text{ethanol}} = 254.5 - 239.2 = 15.3$$
$$\overline{X}_{\text{chloroform}} - \overline{X}_{\text{dichloromethane}} = 254.5 - 250.2 = 4.2$$

Step 7 Interpret the outcome of the analysis

- $\overline{X}_{\text{dichloromethane}} - \overline{X}_{\text{ethanol}} = 11.0$. As this is less than the calculated Fisher's LSD, the null hypothesis is accepted. There is no difference in the UTS of polymer films cast from either ethanol or dichloromethane. It should be recognised that this value is extremely close to the critical difference, and therefore it may be useful to repeat this experiment to verify this outcome.
- $\overline{X}_{\text{chloroform}} - \overline{X}_{\text{ethanol}} = 15.3$. As this is greater than the calculated Fisher's LSD, the null hypothesis is rejected. The UTS of polymer films cast from chloroform is significantly greater than those cast from ethanol.
- $\overline{X}_{\text{chloroform}} - \overline{X}_{\text{dichloromethane}} = 4.2$. As this is less than the calculated Fisher's LSD, the null hypothesis is accepted. There is no difference in the UTS of polymer films cast from either chloroform or dichloromethane.

In addition to the requirement for a significant F in the ANOVA, it has been proposed that Fisher's LSD test should only be employed in the case of three treatments. When the number of treatment groups exceeds three, the overall probability of making a type I error increases and, as a result, the test identifies significant differences between treatment groups that may not be valid.

Finally, the test may be performed when the numbers of observations in each treatment group are dissimilar, and indeed, this is a useful application of the test. Despite the problems associated with the use of Fisher's LSD test, this test is one of the most powerful *post-hoc* tests when the experimental conditions favour its use.

Tukey's honestly significant difference (HSD) test

Tukey's honestly significant difference (HSD) test is a *post-hoc* test that is used to compare treatments with identical sample sizes. Like the Fisher's LSD test, an ANOVA is initially performed and the test is employed to identify differences between the individual treatments. However, unlike the Fisher's LSD, Tukey's HSD test may be executed when a non-significant F statistic has been recorded in the ANOVA. Furthermore, Tukey's HSD test is considered to be a more prudent test than the Fisher's LSD test and, as a result, a greater difference between the treatment groups is required to reject the null hypothesis. For this reason, the Fisher's LSD test is more powerful, i.e. will record smaller differences as significant, when the experimental conditions favour the use of this test. On the other hand, Tukey's HSD test will maintain the overall probability of making a type I error at a defined value, one of the major concerns of the Fisher's LSD test.

Tukey's HSD test calculates a critical difference between the means of treatment groups. If the actual difference between two groups is equal to or exceeds this critical value, then, as before, the null hypothesis is rejected and it may be concluded that the difference between the two treatments is significant. The equation that is employed to calculate the HSD statistic is another variant of the equation that is used for the two-independent-samples t test. However, there is one major difference: Tukey's HSD does not use the critical value of t associated with the experimental parameters but instead uses a different statistic, the *studentised range statistic* (q). The equation that is used for calculation of Tukey's HSD is

$$HSD = q \sqrt{\frac{s^2}{N}}$$

where q is the studentised range statistic, N is the number of observations in either group (this will be identical for each group) and s^2 is an estimate of the pooled variance, derived from the mean square error in the ANOVA. The studentised range statistic is obtained from consultation with the table of the critical values of this statistic (Appendix 12). As may be observed, selection of this statistic for inclusion into the above equation requires knowledge of the following parameters:

- the number of degrees of freedom associated with the mean square error in the ANOVA
- the total number of means (treatment groups) in the experimental design.

The use of the Tukey's HSD test is illustrated in the following example.

EXAMPLE 10.4   *A pharmaceutical company specialises in the formulation and production of therapeutic aerosols. As part of the development process for a new aerosol containing a therapeutic peptide, four types of valve (manufactured by four different companies) are under consideration for use in the aerosol delivery system. One primary concern of the pharmaceutical company is the reproducibility of the aerosol in terms of the amount of drug dispensed per actuation. Therefore, in a laboratory experiment, 10 actuations were dispensed from the aerosol system in conjunction with each of the 4 valves and the mass of therapeutic peptide delivery per actuation quantified using the Lowry assay. The results are shown in Table 10.13. Using an*

Table 10.13 Effect of valve design on the mass (μg) of therapeutic peptide released per actuation from an aerosol system

Valve 1	Valve 2	Valve 3	Valve 4
1.51	1.50	2.01	1.65
1.26	1.12	2.54	1.23
1.64	1.25	2.32	1.54
1.97	1.49	2.15	1.42
1.20	1.69	2.26	1.35
1.54	1.89	2.44	1.64
1.45	1.58	2.32	1.62
1.77	1.25	2.01	1.74
1.67	1.22	2.00	1.55
1.85	1.24	1.94	1.29

appropriate statistical method, determine whether the valves differ in performance and, if so, determine the nature of the difference(s).

(i) State the null hypothesis

The mean masses of therapeutic peptide released per actuation from the four types of valves are identical:

$$H_0: \quad \overline{X}_{\text{peptide released from valve 1}} = \overline{X}_{\text{peptide released from valve 2}}$$
$$= \overline{X}_{\text{peptide released from valve 3}} = \overline{X}_{\text{peptide released from valve 4}}$$

(ii) State the alternative hypothesis

The mean masses of therapeutic peptide released per actuation from the four types of valves are not identical:

$$H_a: \quad \overline{X}_{\text{peptide released from valve 1}} \neq \overline{X}_{\text{peptide released from valve 2}}$$
$$\neq \overline{X}_{\text{peptide released from valve 3}} \neq \overline{X}_{\text{peptide released from valve 4}}$$

(iii) State the level of significance

In this example, it is assumed that the level of significance (α) is 0.05.

(iv) Select the most appropriate statistical test

The following features of the experimental design directly influence the choice of the most appropriate statistical test:

- The data has been measured on a ratio scale.
- The mean and median for each treatment are comparable, and accordingly, we may assume that the populations from which the data have been sampled are normally distributed.

- The variances of the four treatment groups are similar (0.060, 0.061, 0.043 and 0.029 μg^2 for valves 1, 2, 3 and 4, respectively). Application of the F_{max} test shows that the calculated F_{max} statistic (2.10) is less than the critical F_{max} statistic (6.31 for 9 df, 4 treatments, $\alpha = 0.05$) and therefore, the null hypothesis (no difference between the variances of the four treatment groups) is accepted.

On the basis of these characteristics, ANOVA is assumed to be the most appropriate statistical method for the analysis of the experimental data.

(vi) Perform the ANOVA

The mechanics of the ANOVA test have been detailed in the previous examples and therefore, on this occasion, the only output table of the ANOVA has been presented (Table 10.14). However, it would be worthwhile for the reader to calculate the various parameters described in this table to ensure that the mechanics of this test are fully understood.

(vi) Define the critical F statistic

The critical F statistic in this experiment is obtained from the table of the critical values of the F distribution (Appendix 7) and is the value that is associated with the following parameters:

- $\alpha = 0.05$
- 3 df associated with the treatments (numerator)
- 36 df associated with the error (denominator).

Therefore, the critical F statistic for Example 10.4 is 2.86.

(vii) Interpret the outcome of the statistical analysis

As in previous examples, when the calculated F statistic is less than the critical F statistic the null hypothesis is accepted. Conversely, the null hypothesis is rejected (and the alternative hypothesis accepted) if the calculated F statistic is equal to or greater than the critical F statistic. In this

Table 10.14 Summary of the output of the ANOVA for the effect of valve design on the mass of therapeutic peptide released per actuation from an aerosol system

Source	Sum of squares	df	Mean square	F statistic
Between treatments (valve effects)	3.76	3	1.25	25.82
Within treatments (error)	1.75	36	0.05	
Total	5.51	39		

example $F_{calculated}$ (25.82) $> F_{critical}$ (2.86) and therefore the alternative hypothesis is accepted, i.e. the valves differ in the mass of therapeutic peptide released per actuation.

(viii) Perform an appropriate post-hoc comparison

Before the experiment was carried our there was no reason to consider a comparison of individual pairs of valves. After the ANOVA, in which it was concluded that the valves differed in their performance, it was decided to perform individual comparisons of pairs of data to identify the nature of the differences. Under these circumstances *post-hoc* comparisons should be employed. However, as there are several different types of *post-hoc* test, it is necessary to consider the experimental conditions to enable selection of the most appropriate comparison. With respect to Example 10.4, the following points should be considered.

- There are more than three treatment groups. As mentioned previously, it is usually recommended that the Fisher's LSD should not be employed when the number of treatments exceeds three as there is an increased risk of making a type I error.
- The numbers of observations in each treatment group are identical.
- The calculated F statistic (Table 10.14) denoted a significant treatment effect.

Under these circumstances Tukey's HSD test may be applied to make individual comparisons of pairs of treatments. This test is readily performed in a stepwise fashion, as presented below.

Step 1   State the null hypothesis
The null hypothesis states that there is no difference between the means of the four treatment groups, i.e.:

$$H_0: \bar{X}_{\text{peptide released from valve 1}} = \bar{X}_{\text{peptide released from valve 2}}$$

$$\bar{X}_{\text{peptide released from valve 1}} = \bar{X}_{\text{peptide released from valve 3}}$$

$$\bar{X}_{\text{peptide released from valve 1}} = \bar{X}_{\text{peptide released from valve 4}}$$

$$\bar{X}_{\text{peptide released from valve 2}} = \bar{X}_{\text{peptide released from valve 3}}$$

$$\bar{X}_{\text{peptide released from valve 2}} = \bar{X}_{\text{peptide released from valve 4}}$$

$$\bar{X}_{\text{peptide released from valve 3}} = \bar{X}_{\text{peptide released from valve 4}}$$

Step 2   State the alternative hypothesis
The alternative hypothesis states that there are differences between the

means of the three treatment groups, i.e.:

$$H_a: \bar{X}_{\text{peptide released from valve 1}} \neq \bar{X}_{\text{peptide released from valve 2}}$$

$$\bar{X}_{\text{peptide released from valve 1}} \neq \bar{X}_{\text{peptide released from valve 3}}$$

$$\bar{X}_{\text{peptide released from valve 1}} \neq \bar{X}_{\text{peptide released from valve 4}}$$

$$\bar{X}_{\text{peptide released from valve 2}} \neq \bar{X}_{\text{peptide released from valve 3}}$$

$$\bar{X}_{\text{peptide released from valve 2}} \neq \bar{X}_{\text{peptide released from valve 4}}$$

$$\bar{X}_{\text{peptide released from valve 3}} \neq \bar{X}_{\text{peptide released from valve 4}}$$

Step 3   State the level of significance
In this example, it is assumed that the level of significance (α) is 0.05.

Step 4   State the number of tails associated with the experimental design
Like a-priori tests, all *post-hoc* tests are two-tailed.

Step 5   Calculate the HSD statistic

$$HSD = q \sqrt{\frac{s^2}{N}}$$

where q is the studentised range statistic that is associated with the defined level of significance ($\alpha = 0.05$), a two-tailed outcome and the number of degrees of freedom associated with the mean square error in the ANOVA (i.e. 36) and the number of treatment means in the design (i.e. 4). Under these circumstances, $q = 3.82$ (this value has been determined by interpolation as the value is not readily available in the table of the critical values of the studentised range statistic.) N is the size of either of the two treatment groups (i.e. 10) and s^2 is the pooled variance, estimated using the mean square error term in the ANOVA, so

$$HSD = q \sqrt{\frac{s^2}{N}} = 3.82 \sqrt{\frac{0.05}{10}} = 0.27$$

The HSD statistic is similar to the Fisher's LSD statistic in that both are measures of the least difference between two treatment groups that are associated with the rejection of the null hypothesis. Similarly, if the difference between the treatment means is less than the calculated HSD, the null hypothesis is accepted, whereas the null hypothesis is rejected if the difference between the treatments is equal to or greater than the calculated HSD statistic.

Step 6 Calculate the absolute differences between the means of the treatments

$$\overline{X}_{\text{peptide released from valve 1}} - \overline{X}_{\text{peptide released from valve 2}} = 0.16$$

$$\overline{X}_{\text{peptide released from valve 1}} - \overline{X}_{\text{peptide released from valve 3}} = 0.61$$

$$\overline{X}_{\text{peptide released from valve 1}} - \overline{X}_{\text{peptide released from valve 4}} = 0.08$$

$$\overline{X}_{\text{peptide released from valve 2}} - \overline{X}_{\text{peptide released from valve 3}} = 0.78$$

$$\overline{X}_{\text{peptide released from valve 2}} - \overline{X}_{\text{peptide released from valve 4}} = 0.08$$

$$\overline{X}_{\text{peptide released from valve 3}} - \overline{X}_{\text{peptide released from valve 4}} = 0.70$$

Step 7 Interpretation of the outcome of the analysis

- $\overline{X}_{\text{peptide released from valve 1}} - \overline{X}_{\text{peptide released from valve 2}} = 0.16$. As this is less than the critical HSD (0.27), the null hypothesis is accepted. There is no difference in the mass of therapeutic peptide released per actuation from aerosols containing valve 1 and valve 2.
- $\overline{X}_{\text{peptide released from valve 1}} - \overline{X}_{\text{peptide released from valve 3}} = 0.61$. As this is greater than the critical HSD, the null hypothesis is rejected. The mass of therapeutic peptide released per actuation from aerosols containing valve 3 is significantly greater than from aerosols containing valve 1.
- $\overline{X}_{\text{peptide released from valve 1}} - \overline{X}_{\text{peptide released from valve 4}} = 0.08$. As this is less than the critical HSD, the null hypothesis is accepted. There is no difference in the mass of therapeutic peptide released per actuation from aerosols containing valve 1 and valve 4.
- $\overline{X}_{\text{peptide released from valve 2}} - \overline{X}_{\text{peptide released from valve 3}} = 0.78$. As this is greater than the critical HSD, the null hypothesis is rejected. The mass of therapeutic peptide released per actuation from aerosols containing valve 3 is significantly greater than from aerosols containing valve 2.
- $\overline{X}_{\text{peptide released from valve 2}} - \overline{X}_{\text{peptide released from valve 4}} = 0.08$. As this is less than the critical HSD, the null hypothesis is accepted. There is no difference in the mass of therapeutic peptide released per actuation from aerosols containing valve 2 and valve 4.
- $\overline{X}_{\text{peptide released from valve 3}} - \overline{X}_{\text{peptide released from valve 4}} = 0.70$. As this is greater than the critical HSD, the null hypothesis is rejected. The mass of therapeutic peptide released per actuation from aerosols containing valve 3 is significantly greater than from aerosols containing valve 4.

Dunnett's test

The *post-hoc* tests described in this chapter are examples of tests that may be applied to many situations in the pharmaceutical context and have been employed extensively by the author. The reader may encounter several other *post-hoc* tests, including the Newman–Keuls test, the Duncan multiple range test, the Scheffé test, and the Bonferroni test, but these are not described in this book. I have restricted the description of *post-hoc* tests to the Fisher's LSD test, Tukey's HSD test and Dunnett's test. The last of these is used when the analyst wishes to compare the mean of a control group to the means of other groups. Importantly, the use of Dunnett's test for the comparison of treatment groups with a control group does not increase the chance of making a type I error and, furthermore, this test is considered to be one of the most powerful available.

The mechanics of the test involve the calculation of a critical statistic using the following formula:

$$\text{critical statistic} = t_d \sqrt{\frac{2 \times s^2}{N}}$$

where t_d is Dunnett's t statistic, s^2 is the pooled variance and, as before, is estimated using the mean square error from the ANOVA, and N is the number of observations in either the treatment or the control group (these are identical).

Dunnett's t statistic (t_d) may be obtained from the appropriate table of critical values. As may be observed, information about two experimental parameters is required to enable selection of the t_d statistic that relates to the conditions of the experiment. These are:

- the number of treatments (including the control)
- the number of degrees of freedom associated with the pooled variance, i.e. the mean square error in the ANOVA.

As before, acceptance or rejection of the null hypothesis depends on whether the difference between the means of the treatment and control groups is either equal to or greater than the critical statistic or, alternatively, is less than the critical statistic. In the former scenario the null hypothesis is rejected in favour of the alternative hypothesis and in the latter case the null hypothesis is accepted.

The use of ANOVA in conjunction with Dunnett's test is illustrated in the following example.

EXAMPLE 10.5 *A medical device company manufactures poly(vinyl chloride) catheters for intermittent catheterisation. One of the main requirements of these devices is high lubricity to ensure ease of insertion and removal from the urethra. The medical device company is aware that the lubricity of their catheter is sub-optimal and, as a result, has asked another company that possesses catheter-coating technologies to design and develop a hydrogel coating for their standard PVC intermittent catheter. Following a development period, the catheter coating* company has provided PVC catheter samples that have been coated with one or the other of two different types of hydrogel systems. The medical device company has decided to evaluate the lubricity of these coated catheters, measured as a coefficient of friction using an American Standards for Testing Materials method, and to compare the results to those of the uncoated PVC catheter. The results from this study are shown in Table 10.15. Using an appropriate statistical method, determine whether the catheters differ in their lubricities and, if so, determine the nature of the difference(s).

Once more, we begin the analytical procedure by defining the experimental parameters.

(i) State the null hypothesis

The coefficients of friction (CoF) of the three urinary catheters are identical:

$$H_0: \overline{X}_{\text{CoF uncoated catheter}} = \overline{X}_{\text{CoF coating A}} = \overline{X}_{\text{CoF coating B}}$$

(ii) State the alternative hypothesis

The coefficients of friction (CoF) of the three urinary catheters are not identical:

$$H_a: \overline{X}_{\text{CoF uncoated catheter}} \neq \overline{X}_{\text{CoF coating A}} \neq \overline{X}_{\text{CoF coating B}}$$

(iii) State the level of significance

In this example, it is assumed that the level of significance (α) is 0.05.

Table 10.15 Comparative lubricities (expressed as a coefficient of friction) of an uncoated PVC catheter and PVC catheters that have been coated with two hydrogel biomaterials

Uncoated	Coating A	Coating B
0.62	0.13	0.22
0.65	0.15	0.25
0.55	0.18	0.23
0.51	0.14	0.21
0.57	0.21	0.16
0.66	0.23	0.14
0.53	0.15	0.15
0.60	0.18	0.19

(iv) State the number of tails associated with the experimental design

There are two tails associated with this analysis.

(v) Select the most appropriate statistical test

The following features of the experimental design directly influence the choice of the most appropriate statistical test:

- The data has been measured on a ratio scale.
- The data are composed of one category, which is subdivided into three treatments.
- The mean and median for each treatment are comparable, i.e. 0.59 and 0.59 for the uncoated catheter, 0.17 and 0.17 for the catheter with coating A and 0.19 and 0.20 for the catheter with coating B. Therefore, it may be assumed that the populations from which the data have been sampled are normally distributed
- The variances of the four treatment groups are similar (0.003, 0.001 and 0.002, respectively). This has been concluded by application of the F_{max} test to the data. The calculated F_{max} for this analysis is 3.00 (0.003/0.001) and the critical F_{max} (associated with $8 - 1 = 7$ df, a chosen level of significance of 0.05 and three treatments) is 6.94. As the calculated F_{max} is less than the critical F_{max}, the null hypothesis is accepted.

On the basis of these characteristics, a one-way ANOVA is the most appropriate statistical method for the analysis of the experimental data.

(vi) Perform the ANOVA

As in the previous example, only the output of the ANOVA has been presented (Table 10.16). For the reader who still requires practice in the computations associated with the ANOVA, it may be useful to calculate the various sums-of-squares terms that are described in the table.

(vii) Define the critical F statistic

The critical F statistic in this experiment is obtained from the table of the critical values of the F distribution (Appendix 7) and is the value that is

Table 10.16 Summary of the output of the ANOVA for the comparative lubricities (expressed as a coefficient of friction) of an uncoated PVC catheter and PVC catheters that had been coated with two hydrogel biomaterials

Source	Sum of squares	df	Mean square	F statistic
Between treatments (catheter effects)	0.871	2	0.436	220.683
Within treatments (error)	0.041	21	0.002	
Total	0.912	23		

associated with the following parameters:

- $\alpha = 0.05$
- 2 *df* associated with the treatments (numerator)
- 21 *df* associated with the error (denominator)

Therefore, the critical F statistic is 3.47. The reader will once more observe that the critical F statistic in the ANOVA is interpreted as a one-tailed value.

(viii) Interpret the outcome of the statistical analysis

As the critical F statistic ($F_{critical}$) is 3.47, the null and alternative hypotheses may be redefined as follows:

$$H_0: F_{calculated} < F_{critical} \ (3.47)$$
$$H_a: F_{calculated} \geqslant F_{critical} \ (3.47)$$

As the calculated F statistic (220.68) is greater than the critical F statistic (3.47), the null hypothesis may be rejected in favour of the alternative hypothesis. Therefore, the coefficients of friction of the three urinary catheters are dissimilar. The ANOVA simply concludes whether the null hypothesis is accepted or rejected; it does not identify the origin of the difference(s). To clarify this position, a *post-hoc* test must be applied to the experimental data.

(ix) Perform an appropriate post-hoc comparison

To select the most appropriate *post-hoc* statistical test, it is necessary to re-examine the nature of the experimental design.

- There are three treatment groups.
- The numbers of observations in each treatment group are identical.
- The calculated F statistic denoted a significant treatment effect.
- The experimental design involves comparisons between two treatments (two hydrogel-coated catheters) and a control (uncoated catheter).

Under these circumstances, and particularly because of the final point, the most appropriate *post-hoc* test for the comparison of the lubricities of the control and treatment catheters is Dunnett's test. This test is readily performed in a stepwise fashion, as presented below.

Step 1 State the null hypothesis
The null hypothesis states that there is no difference between the mean coefficient of friction of the uncoated catheter (control) and the

hydrogel-coated catheters (treatments):

$$H_0: \overline{X}_{\text{CoF uncoated catheter}} = \overline{X}_{\text{CoF coating A}}$$

$$\overline{X}_{\text{CoF uncoated catheter}} = \overline{X}_{\text{CoF coating B}}$$

Step 2   State the alternative hypothesis
The alternative hypothesis states that there are differences between the mean coefficient of frictions of the uncoated catheter (control) and the hydrogel-coated catheters (treatments):

$$H_a: \overline{X}_{\text{CoF uncoated catheter}} \neq \overline{X}_{\text{CoF coating A}}$$

$$\overline{X}_{\text{CoF uncoated catheter}} \neq \overline{X}_{\text{CoF coating B}}$$

Step 3   State the level of significance
In this example, it is assumed that the level of significance (α) is 0.05.

Step 4   State the number of tails associated with the experimental design
As before, this is a two-tailed test (two outcomes will allow the alternative hypothesis to be accepted).

Step 5   Calculate the critical statistic

$$\text{critical statistic} = t_d \sqrt{\frac{2 \times s^2}{N}}$$

where t_d is Dunnett's t statistic. This may be extracted from Appendix 13 as the statistic associated with the number of means in the experimental design (3), a two-tailed *post-hoc* design and the number of degrees of freedom associated with the mean square error in the ANOVA (21). On the basis of these parameters, the critical statistic for Example 10.5 is 2.37. The reader will observe in Appendix 13 that a critical value of the Dunnett's statistic is not available for 21 *df* (error term) and therefore, this value must be interpolated from the t_d values for 20 and 24 *df*, i.e. 2.37. s^2 is estimated using the mean square error from the ANOVA (0.002), and N is the number of observations in either the treatment or control group (8). Therefore the critical statistic is

$$t_d \sqrt{\frac{2 \times s^2}{N}} = 2.37 \sqrt{\frac{2 \times 0.002}{8}} = 0.053$$

As for other *post-hoc* tests, this critical statistic is the value of the difference between means that defines whether the null hypothesis is accepted or rejected. If the difference between the control and treatment means is equal to or greater than the critical statistic, the alternative hypothesis is accepted, whereas if the calculated difference between the control and treatment mean is less than the critical value the null hypothesis is accepted.

Step 6   Calculate the differences between the means of the control and treatment groups

$$\overline{X}_{\text{CoF uncoated catheter}} - \overline{X}_{\text{CoF coating A}} = 0.586 - 0.171 = 0.415$$

$$\overline{X}_{\text{CoF uncoated catheter}} - \overline{X}_{\text{CoF coating B}} = 0.586 - 0.194 = 0.392$$

Step 7   Interpretation of the outcome of the analysis

- $\overline{X}_{\text{CoF uncoated catheter}} - \overline{X}_{\text{CoF coating A}} = 0.415$. As this is greater than the critical statistic, the null hypothesis is rejected. The coefficient of friction of the PVC catheter coated with hydrogel A is significantly less than that of the uncoated PVC catheter.
- $\overline{X}_{\text{CoF uncoated catheter}} - \overline{X}_{\text{CoF coating B}} = 0.392$. As this is greater than the critical statistic, the null hypothesis is again rejected. The coefficient of friction of the PVC catheter coated with hydrogel B is significantly less than that of the uncoated PVC catheter.

10.2   Two-way analysis of variance

The preceding sections have described the use and mechanics of one-way ANOVA, the most basic design of this type of analysis. In this, the effect of an independent (fixed) variable, consisting of more than two treatment groups, on a dependent variable may be statistically compared. However, in the pharmaceutical and related sciences, there are situations in which the investigator may wish to examine the effects of more than one independent variable on a defined dependent variable. Under the appropriate circumstances (which will be outlined in this section), this type of experimental design is frequently referred to as a *factorial design* and the method that is used to statistically examine the effects of the independent factors on the dependent variable is *multi-factor ANOVA*. If there are two independent factors, the ANOVA is referred to as a two-way ANOVA, if there are three independent factors, it is a three-way ANOVA, and so on. Each factor within the ANOVA may be composed of several treatments, referred to as *levels*, and it is the combination of factors and treatments that defines the nature of the ANOVA. Therefore, if one factor is composed of three sub-categories (levels) and a second factor is composed of two sub-categories, this is an example of a two-way (two-factor) ANOVA, or more specifically, a 3×2 ANOVA. In a second scenario, consider a study in which the effects of three factors on a dependent variable are under evaluation. The first factor is composed of two levels and the second and third factors consist of three and four levels, respectively. The data may be analysed by an ANOVA, which, in this case is referred to as a three-way ANOVA and more specifically, a $2 \times 3 \times 4$ ANOVA. In this section the mechanics and applications of a two-way ANOVA are described. Unfortunately, space considerations forbid the description of three-way and higher ANOVA in this text; for details of the procedures associated with these higher analyses, the interested reader should refer to a more specialised text such as Sokal and Rohlf (1981) or Dunn and Clark (1987).

10.2.1 Mechanics and applications of the two-way ANOVA

At this stage, the perceptive reader may have a clear picture in mind of the nature of a two-way ANOVA, but for those who are still unclear, the typical design of a two-way ANOVA is illustrated in the following example.

EXAMPLE 10.6 *A pharmaceutical scientist wishes to formulate a gel formulation for the treatment of a skin condition. It has been suggested that the formulation should contain 2% w/w metronidazole and two polymeric ingredients, hydroxyethylcellulose (HEC) and polyacrylic acid (PAA); however, at this point the scientist is unclear of the exact concentrations required or their effects on the rheological properties of the formulation. Therefore, the scientist has prepared a series of formulations that contain two concentrations of each polymeric component (and 2% w/w metronidazole) and measured their zero-shear viscosity (ZSV) by flow rheometry. The results obtained are shown in Table 10.17. Using an appropriate statistical method, comment on the effects of increasing concentrations of both hydroxyethylcellulose and polyacrylic acid on the zero shear viscosities of the gel formulations.*

This is a typical experimental design for a two-way ANOVA. The effects of two factors – the concentration of HEC and the concentration of PAA – on the rheological properties of various gel formulations are under investigation. These factors are *independent* (*categorical*) variables, whereas the measured parameter, i.e. the ZSV, is the *dependent* (*continuous*) variable, which, in this example, has been measured on a ratio scale. Within each category, there are two sub-categories (levels) and accordingly, this example is a 2×2 ANOVA. It is an example of a factorial design, as the effects of one factor have been examined at both levels of the other factor, i.e. the effects of concentration of PAA (1% and 3%) have been examined at both levels of the second factor, i.e. 3% and 5% HEC. For this reason, Example 10.6 represents a complete factorial analysis.

Table 10.17 The effects of concentration of hydroxyethylcellulose (HEC) and polyacrylic acid (PAA) on the zero-shear viscosity (ZSV) of gel systems containing metronidazole (2% w/w)

Concentration of polymeric component (% w/w)		ZSV (MPa s)
HEC	PAA	
3	1	1.9
3	1	2.3
3	1	2.0
3	1	2.1
3	1	2.0
3	3	4.3
3	3	4.7
3	3	4.8
3	3	4.7
3	3	4.8
5	1	8.7
5	1	9.0
5	1	8.8
5	1	9.1
5	1	9.0
5	3	18.5
5	3	18.5
5	3	18.2
5	3	18.3
5	3	18.2

In the two-way ANOVA, the effects of two main factors on the dependent variable are simultaneously examined. Students often question the need for such an elaborate test. The eager undergraduate often suggests bisecting this design and performing two separate analyses on the data. In this scenario, the effect of increasing the concentration of HEC on the ZSV would be analysed using a two-independent-samples t test, and then the effect of increasing the concentration of PAA would be examined using the same statistical test. In doing this, an important feature of the two-way ANOVA would be lost, namely the interaction effect. By simultaneously assessing the effects of the two factors on the dependent variable, the two-way ANOVA can provide information on the interdependency of the two factors, i.e. how one factor can influence the outcome of the other. In this example, an interaction would be observed when the presence of PAA enhances the rheological properties of HEC to an extent that is greater than a simple addition of the properties of the two individual polymeric components. The concept of interactions should not be foreign to pharmaceutical and medical scientists, as it is frequently encountered in drug usage. For example, consider the antimicrobial effects of sulfamethoxazole and trimethoprim. Both agents are antibacterial, but when they are co-administered their antibacterial effects are greater than would be expected by simply adding the individual effects of the two agents. In microbiological terms, this phenomenon is termed *synergy* and would be validated within a two-way ANOVA by examining the statistical interaction effect. The reader will also be aware of drug interactions that affect the pharmacological properties of therapeutic agents. In an ANOVA, these interactions would be characterised in the statistical interaction term. The ability to identify interactions between factors is a powerful statistical tool and validates the use of the multifactor analysis of variance techniques.

The computations employed in the two-way ANOVA are identical to those described for the one-way ANOVA, but as two factors are now under consideration, there are more calculations and, in addition, the interpretation is slightly more complex. In practice, the computations in the two-way ANOVA involve the compression of the two factors to form two one-factor designs and the analysis is performed as if these were two one-way analyses of variance. This may seem strange, as it was stated earlier that situations involving multiple hypothesis testing should not be broken down into individual analyses. The use of a one-way ANOVA to statistically compare three or more treatments effectively maintains the probability of making a type I error at the defined level, whereas the application of a series of independent-samples t tests increases this probability and, in so doing, increases the chances of rejecting the null hypothesis. However, the two-way ANOVA does not suffer from this problem and accordingly maintains the probability of committing a type I error at the defined level and additionally, minimises the likelihood of committing a type II error. Indeed, these reasons are identical to those stated for the selection of a one-way ANOVA for multiple hypothesis testing at the expense of performing a series of two-independent-samples t tests.

From the above explanation it is apparent that an important step in the process of performing a two-way ANOVA is the compression of the factors, as this allows the effects of the individual factors to be assessed. This process is illustrated in Tables 10.18 and 10.19 for the data described in Example 10.6. The data corresponding to two factors in Example 10.6 have been compressed into a single factor, in this case, the concentration of HEC. This has been done by grouping all data relating to 3% HEC and grouping all data relating to the higher

Table 10.18 Compression of the data presented in Table 10.17 in terms of a single factor, i.e. ZSV (MPa s) of formulations containing 3% and 5% w/w HEC

HEC 3% w/w	HEC 5% w/w
1.9	8.7
2.3	9.0
2.0	8.8
2.1	9.1
2.0	9.0
4.3	18.5
4.7	18.5
4.8	18.2
4.7	18.3
4.8	18.2
$\bar{X}_{HEC\,3\%} = 3.36$ MPa s	$\bar{X}_{HEC\,5\%} = 13.63$ MPa s
$s^2_{HEC\,3\%} = 1.95$ (MPa s)^2	$s^2_{HEC\,5\%} = 24.76$ (MPa s)^2
$N_{HEC\,3\%} = 10$	$N_{HEC\,5\%} = 10$

Table 10.19 Compression of the data presented in Table 10.17 in terms of a single factor, i.e. ZSV (MPa s) of formulations containing 1% and 3% w/w PAA

PAA 1% w/w	PAA 3% w/w
1.9	4.3
2.3	4.7
2.0	4.8
2.1	4.7
2.0	4.8
8.7	18.5
9.0	18.5
8.8	18.2
9.1	18.3
9.0	18.2
$\bar{X}_{PAA\,1\%} = 5.48$ MPa s	$\bar{X}_{PAA\,3\%} = 11.51$ MPa s
$s^2_{PAA\,1\%} = 13.13$ (MPa s)^2	$s^2_{PAA\,3\%} = 52.00$ (MPa s)^2
$N_{PAA\,1\%} = 10$	$N_{PAA\,3\%} = 10$

concentration of this polymer. Therefore, the groups pertaining to 3% and 5% HEC actually each contain two sub-categories, namely 1% and 3% PAA. This process has been repeated in terms of the second factor, i.e. concentration of PAA, as shown in Table 10.19.

The two-way ANOVA effectively treats the analysis as if there are two separate one-factor analyses using the data presented in Tables 10.18 and 10.19. However, before explaining the mechanics of the technique, it is necessary to define the limitations of the use of this type of analysis. The limitations of the two-way ANOVA are identical to those already described for both the independent-samples t test and the one-way ANOVA:

- The data must be measured in an interval or ratio scale and each observation must be independent.
- The populations from which the samples have been derived must possess similar variances.
- The populations from which the samples have been derived must be normally distributed, thereby permitting the use of the mean as a measure of central tendency.

Before analysing the effects of increasing concentrations of HEC and PAA on the viscosity of gel formulations, it is important to define the parameters of the experimental design, as specified in all previous examples.

(i) State the null hypothesis

In this example, we are concerned with the effects of two independent factors on the viscosity of the gel formulations. Therefore, unlike the two-sample and one-factor multiple hypothesis tests, there are two null hypotheses, one associated with each of the main factors. There is also a null hypothesis associated with the interaction term. In Example 10.6 the null hypotheses are as follows:

- *Effect of PAA (factor 1).* A suitable null hypothesis for this factor is that as the concentration of PAA is increased there will be no change in the ZSV of the gel formulations:

$$H_0: \bar{X}_{\text{ZSV PAA 1\%}} = \bar{X}_{\text{ZSV PAA 3\%}}$$

- *Effect of HEC (factor 2).* In a similar fashion, the null hypothesis for the second factor may be stated as:

$$H_0: \bar{X}_{\text{ZSV HEC 3\%}} = \bar{X}_{\text{ZSV HEC 5\%}}$$

- *Interaction term.* The null hypothesis for the interaction term may be defined as the absence of an interaction effect between the two primary factors on the ZSV of the gel formulations.

(ii) State the alternative hypotheses

As there are two null hypotheses, it is no surprise that there are two alternative hypotheses in two-factor multiple hypothesis tests, each relating to the individual factors:

- *Effect of PAA (factor 1).* An alternative hypothesis for factor 1, the effect of PAA, is

$$H_a: \bar{X}_{\text{ZSV PAA 1\%}} \neq \bar{X}_{\text{ZSV PAA 3\%}}$$

- *Concerning the effect of HEC (factor 2).* Similarly, the alternative hypothesis for the second factor is

$$H_a: \bar{X}_{\text{ZSV HEC 3\%}} \neq \bar{X}_{\text{ZSV HEC 5\%}}$$

- *Interaction term.* The alternative hypothesis for the interaction term may be defined as the presence of an interaction effect between the two primary factors on the ZSV of the gel formulations.

(iii) State the level of significance

In this example, it is assumed that the level of significance (α) is 0.05.

(iv) State the number of tails associated with the experimental design

As there are two ways in which each null hypothesis may be rejected, this is a two-tailed experimental design.

(v) Select the most appropriate statistical test

In this example, the objective is to examine the effects of two independent factors on a dependent variable. Therefore a multiple hypothesis test is required and, accordingly, all two-sample methods are inappropriate. The point that must be addressed concerns the use of a parametric or non-parametric multiple hypothesis test. To answer this, the suitability of data for manipulation and analysis using a parametric technique should be evaluated. As in Example 10.1, the following questions should be addressed:

- *What is the nature of the data?* The data described in Example 10.6 has been measured in a ratio scale, hence validating the use of parametric analyses.
- *Are the populations from which the data have been sampled normally distributed and do they possess similar variances?* To gain an insight into the normality of the distribution, it is useful to compare the mean and median of each sample, as shown in Table 10.20. From the table it may be observed that the mean and median for each individual sample are similar in magnitude, as indeed are the variances of the four samples. The latter conclusion has been reached using an F_{max} test, as previously described. As a result of these simi-

Table 10.20 Summary of the central tendency and variance of the data concerning the ZSV of polymeric gel formulations containing HEC and PAA

Measure of central tendency	HEC 3%/ PAA 1%	HEC 3%/ PAA 3%	HEC 5%/ PAA 1%	HEC 5%/ PAA 3%
Mean (MPa s)	2.06	4.67	8.91	18.35
Median (MPa s)	2.01	4.69	8.98	18.29
Variance (MPa s)^2	0.03	0.04	0.03	0.03

larities, and the ability of parametric tests to accommodate slight or moderate deviations from both normality and homogeneity of variances, it is assumed that the data are suitable for analysis using a parametric statistical method.

Therefore, we may conclude that the above data may be statistically compared using a parametric technique that allows the simultaneous comparison of the effects of two independent parameters on a dependent variable, the ZSV in this example. For these requirements, a two-way ANOVA is the most appropriate statistical technique.

(vi) Perform the statistical test

As stated in the introduction to the two-way ANOVA, the calculations involved in this technique are similar to those already described for the one-way ANOVA, but the introduction of a second factor entails more calculations. To reduce the chance of miscalculations, the author recommends that the arithmetic manipulations associated with the two-way ANOVA should be performed in a stepwise fashion, as detailed below.

Step 1   Calculate the descriptive statistics associated with each cell
As in the one-way ANOVA, the following descriptive statistics should be calculated and summarised in tabular form (Table 10.21):

- the sum of the values (ΣX) and the sum of the square of the values in each cell (ΣX^2)
- the mean of each cell ($\bar{X}$)
- the number of observations in each cell (N)
- ΣX, ΣX^2 and N after the first factor has been collapsed (condensed) (Table 10.18). (This information will be used to statistically evaluate the effect of this factor on the dependent variable.)
- ΣX, ΣX^2 and N after the second factor has been collapsed (Table 10.19). (This information will be used to statistically evaluate the effect of this factor on the dependent variable.)
- ΣX_{total}, ΣX^2_{total} and N are then calculated using all data.

Step 2   Calculate the total sum of squares
The total sum of squares is calculated as previously described using the formula

$$SS_{total} = \Sigma X^2 - \frac{(\Sigma X_{total})^2}{N}$$

Using the data and descriptive statistics presented in Table 10.21,

$$SS_{total} = \Sigma X^2 - \frac{(\Sigma X)^2}{N} = 2209.9 - \frac{(169.9)^2}{20} = 766.60$$

Table 10.21   Effects of increasing concentrations of PAA and HEC on the zero-shear viscosity of gel formulations, showing the descriptive statistics used in the calculations associated with the two-way ANOVA

Factor 1: Concentration of PAA (% w/w)	Factor 2: Concentration of HEC (% w/w)		
	HEC 3%	HEC 5%	
PAA 1%	1.9	8.7	
	2.3	9.0	
	2.0	8.8	
	2.1	9.1	
	2.0	9.0	
	$\Sigma X_{3\%/1\%} = 10.3$	$\Sigma X_{5\%/1\%} = 44.6$	$\Sigma X_{PAA\ 1\%} = 54.9$
	$\Sigma X^2_{3\%/1\%} = 21.3$	$\Sigma X^2_{5\%/1\%} = 397.9$	$\Sigma X^2_{PAA\ 1\%} = 419.2$
	$\bar{X}_{3\%/1\%} = 2.1$	$\bar{X}_{5\%/1\%} = 8.9$	$\bar{X}_{PAA\ 1\%} = 5.5$
	$N_{3\%/1\%} = 5$	$N_{5\%/1\%} = 5$	$N_{PAA\ 1\%} = 10$
PAA 3%	4.3	18.5	
	4.7	18.5	
	4.8	18.2	
	4.7	18.3	
	4.8	18.2	
	$\Sigma X_{3\%/3\%} = 23.3$	$\Sigma X_{5\%/3\%} = 91.7$	$\Sigma X_{PAA\ 3\%} = 115.0$
	$\Sigma X^2_{3\%/3\%} = 108.8$	$\Sigma X^2_{5\%/3\%} = 1681.9$	$\Sigma X^2_{PAA\ 3\%} = 1790.7$
	$\bar{X}_{3\%/3\%} = 4.7$	$\bar{X}_{5\%/3\%} = 18.3$	$\bar{X}_{PAA\ 3\%} = 11.5$
	$N_{3\%/3\%} = 5$	$N_{5\%/3\%} = 5$	$N_{PAA\ 3\%} = 10$
	$\Sigma X_{HEC\ 3\%} = 33.6$	$\Sigma X_{HEC\ 5\%} = 136.3$	$\Sigma X_{total} = 169.9$
	$\Sigma X^2_{HEC\ 3\%} = 130.1$	$\Sigma X^2_{HEC\ 5\%} = 2079.8$	$\Sigma X^2_{total} = 2209.9$
	$\bar{X}_{HEC\ 3\%} = 3.4$	$\bar{X}_{HEC\ 5\%} = 13.6$	$\bar{X}_{total} = 8.5$
	$N_{HEC\ 3\%} = 10$	$N_{HEC\ 5\%} = 10$	$N_{total} = 20$

Step 3   Calculate the sum of squares associated with factor 1, the concentration of PAA

The sum of squares associated with the first factor is calculated using the condensed data (and associated descriptive statistics) and is performed by initially adding together the ratio of the square of the individual *row* totals for each concentration of PAA and the associated number of observations. The correction term is then subtracted from this total. This may be expressed mathematically as:

$$SS_{factor\ 1} = \sum \frac{(X_{row})^2}{N_{row}} - \frac{(\Sigma X_{total})^2}{N},$$

i.e.

$$SS_{PAA} = \left[\frac{(X_{PAA\ 1\%})^2}{N_{PAA\ 1\%}} + \frac{(X_{PAA\ 3\%})^2}{N_{PAA\ 3\%}} \right] - \frac{(\Sigma X_{total})^2}{N}$$

Using the data described in Example 10.6,

$$SS_{PAA} = \left[\frac{(54.9)^2}{10} + \frac{(115.0)^2}{10} \right] - \frac{(169.9)^2}{20} = 180.60$$

Step 4 Calculate the sum of squares associated with factor 2, the concentration of HEC

The sum of squares that is associated with factor 2, the concentration of HEC, is calculated in an identical manner to that described in step 3, but in this case, the *column* totals are used in place of the row totals. The formula that is used for this purpose is therefore

$$SS_{factor\ 2} = \sum \frac{(X_{column})^2}{N_{column}} - \frac{(\Sigma X_{total})^2}{N} ,$$

i.e.

$$SS_{HEC} = \left[\frac{(X_{HEC\ 3\%})^2}{N_{HEC\ 5\%}} + \frac{(X_{HEC\ 5\%})^2}{N_{HEC\ 5\%}} \right] - \frac{(\Sigma X_{total})^2}{N}$$

Inserting the appropriate statistical parameters, the sum of squares is thus calculated:

$$SS_{HEC} = \left[\frac{(33.6)^2}{10} + \frac{(136.3)^2}{10} \right] - \frac{(169.9)^2}{20} = 527.36$$

Step 5 Calculate the sum of squares associated with the interaction between the two factors

One of the strengths of the two-way ANOVA is the ability to mathematically determine whether (or not) the two factors influence each other and in so doing unexpectedly influence the magnitude of the dependent variable. The interaction sum of squares is calculated using the following formula:

$$SS_{interaction} = SS_{between\ groups\ (BG)} - SS_{factor\ 1\ (PAA)} - SS_{factor\ 2\ (HEC)}$$

The *SS* terms associated with the primary factors have been previously calculated, but two unknowns remain in the above equation: the sum of squares associated with the interaction and the between-groups sum of squares. Therefore, to calculate the interaction sum of squares it is necessary to firstly compute the between-groups sum of squares. This term is calculated by subtracting the correction factor from the total sum of the squares of each cell total divided by the number of observations in each cell. Mathematically, this formula bears a striking resemblance to the equations that have been employed to calculate the sum of squares for each factor:

$$SS_{BG} = \sum \frac{(X_{cell})^2}{N_{cell}} - \frac{(\sum X_{total})^2}{N}$$

$$SS_{BG} = \left[\frac{(X_{HEC\,3\%/PAA\,1\%})^2}{N_{HEC\,3\%/PAA\,1\%}} + \frac{(X_{HEC\,3\%/PAA\,3\%})^2}{N_{HEC\,3\%/PAA\,3\%}} + \frac{(X_{HEC\,5\%/PAA\,1\%})^2}{N_{HEC\,5\%/PAA\,1\%}} \right.$$

$$\left. + \frac{(X_{HEC\,5\%/PAA\,3\%})^2}{N_{HEC\,5\%/PAA\,3\%}} \right] - \frac{(\sum X_{total})^2}{N}$$

For the data described in Example 10.6, the between-groups sum of squares is calculated as

$$SS_{BG} = \left[\frac{(10.3)^2}{5} + \frac{(23.3)^2}{5} + \frac{(44.6)^2}{5} + \frac{(91.7)^2}{5} \right] - \frac{(169.9)^2}{20} = 766.11$$

With knowledge of the between-groups sum of squares, the interaction sum of squares may now be calculated

$$SS_{interaction} = SS_{between\,groups\,(BG)} - SS_{factor\,1\,(PAA)} - SS_{factor\,2\,(HEC)}$$

$$= 766.11 - 527.36 - 180.60$$

$$= 58.15$$

Step 6 Calculation of the within-groups (error) sum of squares
The final sum of squares term that is required for the computation of the two-way ANOVA is the within-groups (error) term. The reader will remember that this parameter is used to define the intragroup error in the one-way ANOVA, and its role is in the two-way test identical. As before, this term, after division by the number of associated degrees of freedom, is used as the denominator in the calculation of the F ratios in the analysis of variance.

The within-groups sum of squares is calculated as follows:

$$SS_{within\,groups} = SS_{total} - SS_{between\,groups}$$

so for the current example:

$$SS_{within\,groups} = 766.60 - 766.11$$

$$= 0.45$$

Step 7 Construct a summary table for the analysis of variance
The summary table for the two-way ANOVA is compiled in the same fashion as for the one-way ANOVA. Therefore, the sum of squares for the two primary factors, the interaction and the error are described, in addition to their associated numbers of degrees of freedom. The mean squares are determined as the ratio of the sum of squares of each parameter to the number of degrees of freedom. Finally, the F ratios are calculated by dividing the mean square errors into the mean squares relating to each factor and the interaction.

Before the calculations can be finalised, the numbers of degrees of freedom associated with the factors and interactions must be determined. The total number of degrees of freedom for the experimental design is calculated by subtracting 1 from the total number of observations. Thus, the total number of degrees of freedom in Example 10.6 is $N_{total} - 1 = 20 - 1 = 19$. The number of degrees of freedom associated with sum of squares for factor 1 (concentration of PAA) is calculated by subtracting 1 from the total number of levels in this factor, i.e. $2 - 1 = 1$. Similarly, the number of degrees of freedom for factor 2 is calculated by subtracting one from the total number of level of this factor, i.e. $2 - 1 = 1$. The number of degrees of freedom associated with the interaction component is obtained by multiplying the number of degrees of freedom associated with factor 1 by the number of degrees of freedom associated with factor 2, i.e. $1 \times 1 = 1$. Finally, the number of degrees of freedom associated with the error sum of squares is calculated by subtracting the sum of the number of degrees of freedom for factors 1 and 2 and the interaction from the total number of degrees of freedom, i.e. $19 - (1 + 1 + 1) = 16$.

The summary table for the two-way ANOVA, employed to compare the effects of HEC and PAA on the ZSV of gel formulations, may now be assembled (Table 10.22).

Table 10.22 Summary of the output of the analysis of variance for the effects of increasing concentrations of PAA and HEC on the ZSV of gel formulations

Source	Sum of squares	df	Mean square	F statistic
Concentration of PAA (factor 1)	180.60	1	180.60	6 020.00
Concentration of HEC (factor 2)	527.36	1	527.36	17 578.67
Interaction ([PAA] × [HEC])	58.15	1	58.15	1 938.33
Within treatments (error)	0.45	16	0.03	
Total		19		

The F statistics associated with each primary factor and the inter-action are calculated as follows:

$$F_{\text{calculated HEC}} = \frac{MS_{\text{HEC}}}{MS_{\text{error}}} = \frac{527.36}{0.03} = 17\,578.67$$

$$F_{\text{calculated PAA}} = \frac{MS_{\text{PAA}}}{MS_{\text{error}}} = \frac{180.60}{0.03} = 6020.00$$

$$F_{\text{calculated interaction}} = \frac{MS_{\text{interaction}}}{MS_{\text{error}}} = \frac{58.15}{0.03} = 1938.33$$

Step 8   Define the critical F statistics for each factor and the interaction term

As before, an important step in the determination of the outcome of the two-way ANOVA is the identification of the critical F statistic. In the one-way ANOVA only one critical F statistic is necessary, but in higher orders of ANOVA, separate F statistics are used for each primary factor and each interaction. In a two-way ANOVA, three critical F statistics are required. Identification of these requires the following information:

- the level of significance (0.05)
- the number of degrees of freedom associated with the numerator, i.e. the factor or interaction under consideration
- the number of degrees of freedom associated with the error term in the ANOVA (16 in the above example).

For factor 1, the concentration of PAA, the number of associated degrees of freedom is 1 and therefore, from the critical values of the F statistic (Appendix 7), the critical F statistic$_{(\alpha = 0.05, 1, 16)}$ is defined as 4.49.

Similarly, the number of degrees of freedom associated with factor 2, the concentration of HEC (the numerator), is 1, $\alpha = 0.05$, $df = 16$ and, accordingly, from Appendix 7, the critical F statistic is 4.49.

Finally, the interaction term has one associated degree of freedom and, under the conditions of the ANOVA, the critical F statistic$_{(\alpha = 0.05, 1, 16)}$ is determined from Appendix 7 as 4.49.

Step 9   Interpret the outcome of the statistical analysis

In the ANOVA the critical F statistic defines the region of acceptance and rejection of the null hypothesis. Therefore, if the calculated value of F is equal to or greater than the critical value of F, the null hypothesis is rejected in favour of the alternative hypothesis. Conversely, if the calcu-lated value of F is lower than the critical value, the null hypothesis is accepted. In this current example, the calculated statistic for each factor and the interaction term is compared to the relevant critical F statistic in the following way:

- *Significance of factor 1, the concentration of PAA.* Here, $F_{calculated}$ (6020.00) > $F_{critical}$ (4.49) and accordingly, the null hypothesis is rejected. Therefore, increasing the concentration of PAA from 1% to 3% w/w significantly increased the ZSV of the gel formulations.

- *Significance of factor 2, the concentration of HEC.* Here, $F_{calculated}$ (17 578.67) > $F_{critical}$ (4.49) and as a result, the null hypothesis is rejected. Therefore, increasing the concentration of HEC from 3% to 5% w/w significantly increased the ZSV of the gel formulations.

- *Significance of the interaction term.* The calculated F statistic for the interaction term is 1938.33, which exceeds the value of the critical F statistic (4.49). Consequently, the null hypothesis is rejected and we may be conclude that a significant interaction exists between the combined effects of HEC and PAA on the ZSV of the gel formulations.

Step 10   General conclusions

From the outcomes of the two-way ANOVA, we may conclude that the ZSV of the gel formulations was increased by increasing the concentrations of either HEC or PAA. One interesting further conclusion derived from the ANOVA relates to the significant interaction effect. This is a potentially complex aspect of statistics, and it is outside the scope of this text to delve deeply into the theoretical aspects of statistical interactions. However, as the experimental design described in Example 10.6 is quite straightforward, the basic principles and interpretations of statistical interactions can be described using this example. This will allow an insight into the usefulness of the interaction term within the process of statistical design. The basic concept of an interaction was presented using the example of antimicrobial synergy associated with combined antimicrobial chemotherapy (sulfamethoxazole and trimethoprim). This is an excellent example as it illustrates the enhancement in the dependent variable (number of non-viable bacteria) that may be achieved by the combination of these two therapeutic agents. In this example, these agents may be considered as primary factors in the ANOVA. A statistical interaction is generated in the ANOVA when the observed effect of increasing, e.g., the concentration of each agent has a unexpectedly greater or lesser effect on the dependent variable, i.e. more or less than would be expected by simple addition of the effects of the individual factors. Alternatively, an interaction may be considered to occur when the effect of changing the various levels of one factor on the dependent variable is dependent on the level of the second factor. This is referred to as *non-parallelism*. The finding of a significant statistical interaction in the ANOVA is an important observation in statistical analysis, and indeed, in some cases, information about the presence of the interaction may be just as important to the analyst as that of the presence of significant primary effects. When a statistical interaction has been identified, it is the role of the analyst, in conjunction with the other people involved in the design of the experiment, to interpret the basis of the interaction, e.g. physicochemical, biochemical, pharmacological or physiological.

In Example 10.6 it has been shown that increasing the concentrations of HEC and PAA had a greater effect on the ZSV than would have been predicted. To interpret the interaction, it is important to understand the nature of the dependent variable, in this case viscosity, the resistance of a substance to deformation. If a formulation has high viscosity, a greater stress will be required to obtain a given rate of shear than in formulations that are of lower viscosity. In Example 10.6, increasing the concentrations of either HEC or PAA would be expected to increase the ZSV of the formulations as these polymers autoentangle in solution in a concentration-dependent fashion. These random entanglements serve to increase the resistance of the formulation to deformation, as predicted from gelation theory. However, the observed synergy between the two polymers in their combined effects on the ZSV is of direct interest, as this may not be directly predicted by gelation theory. A possible explanation for this may involve physical entanglement between the HEC and PAA, resulting in greater entanglement. Without knowledge of the rheological properties of polymeric systems, this explanation for the statistical interaction could not have been formulated. The role of the ANOVA is thus to identify the presence of an event that may not be predicted by the null hypothesis.

The term 'interaction' may be misleading to pharmaceutical scientists, biochemists and chemists, who frequently use the term to refer to a physical or chemical association between animals, chemicals, macromolecules, etc. Statistically, however, an interaction refers to the lack of independence between two or more factors. When the term interaction is used, scientists often assume that the interaction term in the ANOVA provides evidence of an actual association. This misunderstanding is generally a function of the types of examples that are used in pharmaceutical statistics. Example 10.6 is a typical example. There a *statistical* interaction was observed between the effects of HEC and PAA on the ZSV of gel formulations, which, coincidentally, was explained by a *chemical* interaction between these two polymers. The misunderstanding may be elucidated by consideration of a non-chemical example. For example, a clinical study may be designed to investigate the effects of age (three levels) and gender (two levels) on blood pressure. If a statistical interaction is observed in this study, it does not imply a physical association between the different factors but rather points the analyst to the different effects of age on the blood pressure of men and women.

One useful method of visualising a statistical interaction is to display the means for each cell graphically and examine the relationships between the two factors. Remember that the presence of an interaction may be visually estimated by comparing the slopes of such plots. If the lines run parallel to each other, this is evidence of additivity and not interaction. If, however, the slopes of the lines are dissimilar, i.e. non-parallel, a statistical interaction is present.

The cell data in Example 10.6 is plotted in graphical format in Figure 10.1 to illustrate the presence of the interaction between HEC and PAA. The concentration of HEC has been selected as the abscissa and the mean ZSV as the ordinate. Alternatively, the concentration of PAA could have been chosen as the abscissa as shown in Figure 10.2. The lower slope depicts the change in mean ZSV as the concentration of HEC is increased from 3% to 5% w/w in gel formulations that contain 1% w/w PAA. The upper slope represents the change in ZSV as the concentration of HEC is similarly increased in gel formulations containing 3% w/w PAA. It may be observed in Figure 10.1 that the slope of the line relating to the formulation containing 3% PAA is visually greater than the slope for formulations containing the lower concentration of this polymer. Therefore in formulations containing 3% w/w PAA, increasing the concentration of HEC from 3% to 5% w/w had a greater effect on the ZSV than in formulations containing 1% w/w PAA. This disparity is evidence of the presence of a statistical interaction.

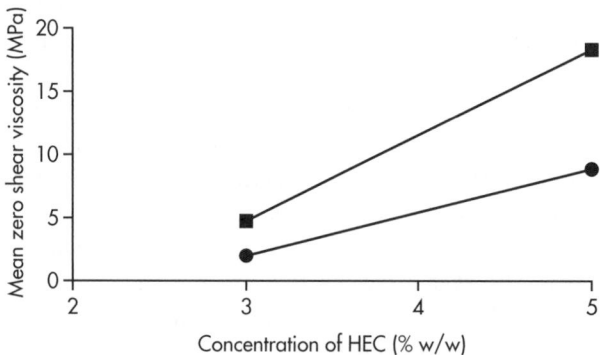

Figure 10.1 Effects of concentration of hydroxyethylcellulose (HEC) and polyacrylic acid (PAA) on the zero shear viscosity (ZSV) of gel formulations. Black circles and squares represent formulations that contained 1% w/w and 3% w/w of PAA, respectively.

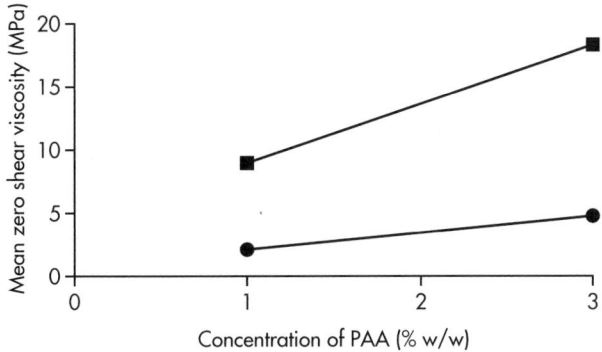

Figure 10.2 Effects of concentration of hydroxyethylcellulose (HEC) and polyacrylic acid (PAA) on the zero shear viscosity (ZSV) of gel formulations. Black circles and squares represent formulations that contained 3% w/w and 5% w/w of HEC, respectively.

As the reader will have appreciated by this stage, manual calculation of the two-way ANOVA is a laborious task, and such computations are now usually performed using a reliable computer statistical package, such as SPSS or StatView. It is nevertheless important that the reader gains an understanding of the mechanics of the higher ANOVAs, as this is necessary to ensure reliable interpretation of the output from the analysis.

The experimental design presented in Example 10.6 is the most straightforward design for the two-way ANOVA. There are of course more complex two-way designs and, as a general rule, as the complexities of these designs increase so does the difficulty of interpretating the outcome of the analysis. The following example illustrates the mechanics of a two-way design in which one of the factors is composed of more than two levels. It will be assumed that the data presented in this example is suitable for analysis using a two-way ANOVA. Nevertheless, it would be useful for the reader to confirm this assumption using the points of reference described in the previous example.

EXAMPLE 10.7   *A formulation scientist wishes to examine the effects of concentration of lubricant (magnesium stearate) and compression force on the time required for tablet disintegration. Tablets were formulated to incorporate either 0.5% or 1.0% w/w magnesium stearate and were manufactured by compression at 10, 15 or 20 tonnes in a pilot scale tablet press. The times required for disintegration of samples of 5 tablets that had been formulated using a defined concentration of magnesium stearate and compressed at a defined tonnage were examined according to the method described in the British Pharmacopoeia. The* *disintegration times of the various samples are shown in Table 10.23. Comment on the effects of concentration of lubricant and compression force on the disintegration time of the samples of tablets.*

The experimental design consists of the simultaneous examination of the effects of two independent factors (concentration of lubricant and compression force) on the disintegration time of tablets. This

Table 10.23 The effects of concentration of lubricant (magnesium stearate) and compression force on the disintegration times of tablets

Concentration of magnesium stearate (% w/w)	Compression force (tonne)	Disintegration time (min)
0.5	10	6.4
0.5	10	6.8
0.5	10	7.6
0.5	10	7.2
0.5	10	7.2
0.5	15	8.4
0.5	15	9.2
0.5	15	9.1
0.5	15	8.4
0.5	15	9.3
0.5	20	12.1
0.5	20	11.4
0.5	20	11.0
0.5	20	10.8
0.5	20	11.4
1.0	10	15.8
1.0	10	15.5
1.0	10	15.9
1.0	10	16.4
1.0	10	16.4
1.0	15	17.7
1.0	15	18.5
1.0	15	18.4
1.0	15	17.7
1.0	15	18.8
1.0	20	21.4
1.0	20	20.8
1.0	20	20.4
1.0	20	20.5
1.0	20	21.8

experiment is an example of a factorial design in which the data has been collected at all levels of each factor. For the sake of brevity, we will assume that the data is amenable to manipulation by a parametric technique (normally distributed, homogeneous variances, data measured on at least an interval scale, etc). As there are two independent factors, the most appropriate statistical (parametric) test is a two-way ANOVA and, accordingly, this will be employed to evaluate the effects of these factors on the dependent variable. The reader will observe that the design described in Example 10.7 possesses more levels in one of the factors (compression force) than in either of the factors in Example 10.6, and, as a result, the experimental design in the current example is more complex. A correct description of the design in Example 10.7 is a 3×2 factorial. Despite the greater intricacy associated with a 3×2 design, the calculations involved in the performance of the two-way ANOVA are identical to those employed for the 2×2 model.

As in previous examples, the following questions should be addressed.

(i) State the null hypothesis

This is a two-way ANOVA, so the validity of three null hypotheses (one for each factor and one for the interaction term) will be challenged:

- *Effect of magnesium stearate (factor 1).* A suitable null hypothesis for this factor is that increasing the concentration of magnesium stearate (MS) will not alter the disintegration time of the tablet samples:

$$H_0: \bar{X}_{\text{time MS } 0.5\%} = \bar{X}_{\text{time MS } 1.0\%}$$

- *Effect of compression force (factor 2).* Similarly, the null hypothesis for factor 2 may be stated as:

$$H_0: \bar{X}_{\text{time } 10\,t} = \bar{X}_{\text{time } 15\,t} = \bar{X}_{\text{time } 20\,t}$$

- *Interaction term.* The null hypothesis for the interaction term may be defined as the absence of an interaction effect between the two primary factors on the disintegration times of the tablets.

(ii) State the alternative hypotheses

As may be expected, there are alternative hypotheses for the two primary factors and the interaction term:

- *Effect of magnesium stearate (factor 1).* A suitable alternative hypothesis for this factor is that increasing the concentration of magnesium stearate will significantly alter the disintegration times of the tablet samples:

$$H_a: \bar{X}_{\text{time MS } 0.5\%} \neq \bar{X}_{\text{time MS } 1.0\%}$$

- *Effect of compression force (factor 2).* Similarly, the null hypothesis for factor 2 may be stated as:

$$H_a: \bar{X}_{\text{time 10 t}} \neq \bar{X}_{\text{time 15 t}} \neq \bar{X}_{\text{time 20 t}}$$

- *Interaction term.* Conversely, the alternative hypothesis for the interaction term may be defined as the presence of an interaction effect between the concentration of magnesium stearate and compression force on their effects of the disintegration times of tablet samples.

(iii) State the level of significance

In this example, it is assumed that the level of significance (α) is 0.05.

(iv) State the number of tails associated with the experimental design

As there are two ways in which each null hypothesis may be rejected, this is a two-tailed experimental design.

(v) Perform the statistical test

The calculations that are used in the two-way ANOVA will be performed in a stepwise fashion, as described in Example 10.6.

Step 1   Calculate the descriptive statistics associated with each cell
The data presented in Table 10.23 is expanded to include the descriptive statistics associated with each cell, namely the sum of each observation, the sum of the squares of each observation and the number of observations. The same procedure is then performed for the values associated with each row and column, after compressing each factor. These further considerations are shown in Table 10.24.

Step 2   Calculate the total sum of squares
The total sum of squares is calculated using the following formula:

$$SS_{\text{total}} = \sum X^2 - \frac{(\sum X_{\text{total}})^2}{N}$$

Using the information presented in Table 10.24,

$$SS_{\text{total}} = \sum X^2 - \frac{(\sum X)^2}{N} = 6431.37 - \frac{(412.30)^2}{30} = 764.99$$

Step 3   Calculate the sum of squares associated with factor 2, the compression force employed to manufacture the tablet samples
In Table 10.24, the effect of compression force on the disintegration times of the tablets is organised into columns. Condensation of the data in these columns allows the descriptive statistics for each column to be

Table 10.24 Effects of increasing concentration of magnesium stearate (MS) and compression force on the disintegration time of tablet samples, showing the descriptive statistics that are used in the calculations associated with the two-way ANOVA

Factor 1: Concentration of MS (% w/w)	Factor 2: Compression force			
	10 tonne	15 tonne	20 tonne	
MS 0.5% w/w	6.4	8.4	12.1	
	6.8	9.2	11.4	
	7.6	9.1	11.0	
	7.2	8.4	10.8	
	7.2	9.3	11.4	
	$\Sigma_{MS\,0.5\%/10t} = 35.20$	$\Sigma_{MS\,0.5\%/15t} = 44.40$	$\Sigma_{MS\,0.5\%/20t} = 56.70$	$\Sigma_{MS\,0.5\%} = 136.30$
	$\Sigma X^2_{MS\,0.5\%/10t} = 248.64$	$\Sigma X^2_{MS\,0.5\%/15t} = 395.06$	$\Sigma X^2_{MS\,0.5\%/20t} = 643.97$	$\Sigma X^2_{MS\,0.5\%} = 1287.67$
	$\bar{X}_{MS\,0.5\%/10t} = 7.04$	$\bar{X}_{MS\,0.5\%/10t} = 8.88$	$\bar{X}_{MS\,0.5\%/20t} = 11.34$	$\bar{X}_{MS\,0.5\%} = 9.09$
	$N_{MS\,0.5\%/10t} = 5$	$N_{MS\,0.5\%/15t} = 5$	$N_{MS\,0.5\%/20t} = 5$	$N_{MS\,0.5\%} = 15$
MS 1% w/w	15.8	17.7	21.4	
	15.5	18.5	20.8	
	15.9	18.4	20.4	
	16.4	17.7	20.5	
	16.4	18.8	21.8	
	$\Sigma_{MS\,1\%/10t} = 80.00$	$\Sigma_{MS\,1\%/15t} = 91.10$	$\Sigma_{MS\,1\%/20t} = 104.90$	$\Sigma_{MS\,1\%} = 276.00$
	$\Sigma X^2_{MS\,1\%/10t} = 1280.62$	$\Sigma X^2_{MS\,1\%/15t} = 1660.83$	$\Sigma X^2_{MS\,1\%/20t} = 2202.25$	$\Sigma X^2_{MS\,1\%} = 5143.70$
	$\bar{X}_{MS\,1\%/10t} = 16.00$	$\bar{X}_{MS\,1\%/15t} = 18.22$	$\bar{X}_{MS\,1\%/10t} = 20.98$	$\bar{X}_{MS\,1\%/} = 18.40$
	$N_{MS\,1\%/10t} = 5$	$N_{MS\,1\%/15t} = 5$	$N_{MS\,1\%/20t} = 5$	$N_{MS\,1\%} = 15$
	$\Sigma_{10t} = 115.20$	$\Sigma_{15t} = 135.5$	$\Sigma_{20t} = 161.60$	$\Sigma_{total} = 412.30$
	$\Sigma X^2_{10t} = 1529.26$	$\Sigma X^2_{15t} = 2055.89$	$\Sigma X^2_{20t} = 2846.22$	$\Sigma X^2_{total} = 6431.37$
	$\bar{X}_{10t} = 11.52$	$\bar{X}_{15t} = 13.55$	$\bar{X}_{20t} = 16.16$	$\bar{X}_{total} = 13.75$
	$N_{10t} = 10$	$N_{15t} = 10$	$N_{20t} = 10$	$N_{total} = 30$

calculated and this information is used to calculate the sum of squares associated with this factor:

$$SS_{factor\ 1} = \sum \frac{(X_{column})^2}{N_{column}} - \frac{(\sum X_{total})^2}{N},$$

i.e.

$$SS_{force} = \left[\frac{(X_{10t})^2}{N_{10t}} + \frac{(X_{15t})^2}{N_{15t}} + \frac{(X_{20t})^2}{N_{20t}}\right] - \frac{(\sum X_{total})^2}{N}$$

Using the data described in Table 10.24,

$$SS_{force} = \left[\frac{(115.20)^2}{10} + \frac{(135.5)^2}{10} + \frac{(161.60)^2}{10}\right] - \frac{(4121.30)^2}{30} = 108.21$$

Step 4 Calculate the sum of squares associated with factor 1, the concentration of magnesium stearate
In Table 10.24, the effect of concentration of magnesium stearate on the disintegration times of the tablets is organised into rows. Once more, the data in the rows is condensed, the associated descriptive statistics calculated, from which, the sum of squares for this parameter is calculated. The formula that is used for this purpose is

$$SS_{factor\ 1} = \sum \frac{(X_{row})^2}{N_{row}} - \frac{(\sum X_{total})^2}{N}$$

i.e.

$$SS_{MS} = \left[\frac{(X_{MS\ 0.5\%})^2}{N_{MS\ 0.5\%}} + \frac{(X_{MS\ 1\%})^2}{N_{MS\ 1\%}}\right] - \frac{(\sum X_{total})^2}{N}$$

Using the data presented in Table 10.24, the sum of squares for this factor is calculated:

$$SS_{MS} = \left[\frac{(136.30)^2}{15} + \frac{(276.00)^2}{15}\right] - \frac{(412.30)^2}{30} = 650.54$$

Step 5 Calculate the sum of squares associated with the interaction between the two factors
The reader will recall from Example 10.6 that the sum of squares associated with the interaction term is calculated in two parts. First, the

between-groups sum of squares is calculated:

$$SS_{BG} = \sum \frac{(X_{cell})^2}{N_{cell}} - \frac{(\sum X_{total})^2}{N}$$

$$= \left[\frac{(X_{MS\,0.5\%/10t})^2}{N_{MS\,0.5\%/10t}} + \frac{(X_{MS\,0.5\%/15t})^2}{N_{MS\,0.5\%/15t}} + \frac{(X_{MS\,0.5\%/20t})^2}{N_{MS\,0.5\%/20t}} + \frac{(X_{MS\,1\%/10t})^2}{N_{MS\,1\%/10t}} \right.$$

$$\left. + \frac{(X_{1\%\,MS/15t})^2}{N_{1\%\,MS/15t}} + \frac{(X_{1\%\,MS/20t})^2}{N_{1\%\,MS/20t}} \right] - \frac{(\sum X_{total})^2}{N}$$

The data from Table 10.24 is then inserted into the above equation:

$$SS_{BG} = \left[\frac{(35.20)^2}{5} + \frac{(44.40)^2}{5} + \frac{(56.70)^2}{5} + \frac{(80.00)^2}{5} \right.$$

$$\left. + \frac{(91.10)^2}{5} + \frac{(104.90)^2}{5} \right] - \frac{(412.30)^2}{30} = 759.32$$

With knowledge of the between-groups sum of squares, the interaction sum of squares may now be calculated:

$$SS_{interaction} = SS_{between\,groups\,(BG)} - SS_{factor\,2\,(force)} - SS_{factor\,1\,(MS)}$$
$$= 759.32 - 108.21 - 650.54$$
$$= 0.58$$

Step 6   Calculate the within-groups (error) sum of squares
The within-groups sum of squares is calculated by subtracting the between-groups sum of squares from the total sum of squares, i.e.

$$SS_{within\,groups} = SS_{total} - SS_{between\,groups}$$
$$= 764.99 - 759.32$$
$$= 5.67$$

Step 7   Construct a summary table for the analysis of variance
To enable computation of the mean squares associated with each primary factor and the interaction term, knowledge is required of the number of degrees of freedom associated with each of these parameters.

- The total number of degrees of freedom for the study is calculated by subtracting 1 from the total number of observations, i.e. $30 - 1 = 29$.
- The number of degrees of freedom associated with factor 2 (compression force) is calculated by subtracting 1 from the total number of levels in this factor, i.e. $3 - 1 = 2$.

- The number of degrees of freedom for factor 1 is similarly calculated by subtracting one from the total number of levels of this factor, i.e. $2 - 1 = 1$.
- The number of degrees of freedom associated with the interaction term is obtained by multiplying the number of degrees of freedom associated with the factor 1 by the number of degrees of freedom associated with factor 2, i.e. $2 \times 1 = 2$.
- The number of degrees of freedom associated with the error sum of squares is calculated by subtracting the sum of the number of degrees of freedom for factors 1 and 2 and the interaction from the total number of degrees of freedom, i.e. $29 - (2 + 1 + 2) = 24$.

With this information the summary table for the ANOVA corresponding to Example 10.7 may be formed (Table 10.25).

The F statistics associated with each primary factor and the interaction are calculated as shown below:

$$F_{\text{calculated force}} = \frac{MS_{\text{force}}}{MS_{\text{error}}} = \frac{54.10}{0.24} = 225.42$$

$$F_{\text{calculated MS}} = \frac{MS_{\text{MS}}}{MS_{\text{error}}} = \frac{650.54}{0.24} = 2710.58$$

$$F_{\text{calculated interaction}} = \frac{MS_{\text{interaction}}}{MS_{\text{error}}} = \frac{0.29}{0.24} = 1.21$$

Step 8   Define the critical F statistics for each factor and the interaction term

The comparisons of the calculated and critical F statistics for each primary factor and the interaction term form the basis of the interpretation of the outcome of the ANOVA. Therefore, the critical statistics for each these components must be defined and, as before, these are based on the level of significance ($\alpha = 0.05$), the number of degrees of freedom associated with the factor or interaction and the number of degrees of freedom associated with the error term in the ANOVA. The critical F

Table 10.25 Summary of the output of the analysis of variance concerning the effects of concentration of lubricant (MS) and compression force on tablet disintegration time

Source	Sum of squares	df	Mean square	F statistic
Compression force (factor 1)	108.21	2	54.10	225.42
Concentration of MS (factor 2)	650.54	1	650.54	2710.58
Interaction (force × [MS])	0.58	2	0.29	1.21
Within treatments (error)	5.67	24	0.24	
Total		29		

statistics for the effects of compression force, concentration of lubricant and the interaction between these terms will be addressed separately.

- *Factor 2, the compression force.* $\alpha = 0.05$, the number of degrees of freedom associated with factor one is 2 (i.e. $3 - 1$) and the number of degrees of freedom associated with the error term in the ANOVA is 24. From the table of the critical values of the F statistic (Appendix 7) the critical F statistic$_{(\alpha = 0.05, 2, 24)}$ is therefore 3.40.
- *Factor 1, the concentration of lubricant.* $\alpha = 0.05$, the number of degrees of freedom associated is 1 (i.e. $2 - 1$) and the number of degrees of freedom associated with the error term in the ANOVA is again 24. From the table of the critical values of the F statistic (Appendix 7) the critical F statistic$_{(\alpha = 0.05, 1, 24)}$ is therefore 4.26.
- *Interaction term.* $\alpha = 0.05$, the number of degrees of freedom is 2 (i.e. 2×1) and the number of degrees of freedom associated with the error term in the ANOVA is 24. From the table of the critical values of the F statistic (Appendix 7) the critical F statistic$_{(\alpha = 0.05, 2, 24)}$ is therefore 3.40.

Step 9   Interpret the outcome of the statistical analysis
The final part of the analysis is to compare the calculated F statistics with the critical F statistics, and accordingly accept or reject the null hypotheses defined at the start of the study. As there are three individual null (and alternative) hypotheses under consideration, each of these is considered individually.

- *Effects of compression force on tablet disintegration time.* $F_{calculated}$ (225.42) $> F_{critical}$ (3.40), so the null hypothesis is rejected. Therefore, increasing the tablet compression force over the range of values examined (from 10 tonnes to 15 tonnes to 20 tonnes) significantly increased tablet disintegration time.
- *Effects of concentration of lubricant on tablet disintegration time.* $F_{calculated}$ (2710.58) $> F_{critical}$ (4.26), so the null hypothesis is rejected. Thus, increasing the concentration of magnesium stearate from 0.5% to 1.0% w/w significantly increased the disintegration time of the tablets.
- *Significance of the interaction term.* The calculated F statistic for the interaction term is 1.23, which is less than the critical F statistic (3.40). Consequently, the null hypothesis is accepted, i.e. there is no interaction between the combined effects of compression force and concentration of magnesium stearate on performance of the tablets in terms of their disintegration times.

The effect of increasing compression force on the mean disintegration times of tablets containing either 0.5% or 1% w/w magnesium stearate is graphically presented in Figure 10.3. This graph shows that the disintegration times of the tablet formulations may be increased by increasing the compression force or by increasing the mass of lubricant

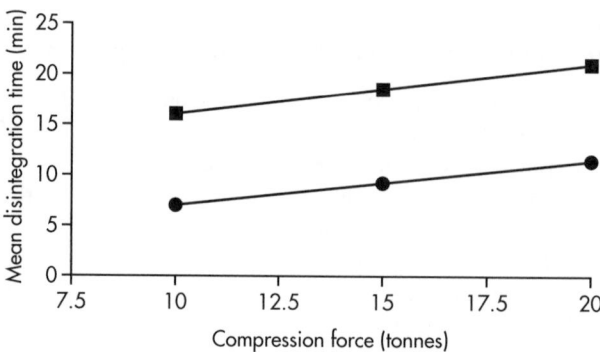

Figure 10.3 Effects of compression force and concentration of lubricant (magnesium stearate) on the mean disintegration times of tablets. Black circles represent formulations containing 0.5% magnesium stearate; black squares represent formulations containing 1.0% magnesium stearate.

in the formulation. The parallelism of the two slopes is evidence that the effects of these two parameters on the disintegration times of the tablets are independent of one another, an observation confirmed by the analysis of variance.

10.3 Repeated-measures ANOVA

Any discussion about the analysis of variance would be incomplete without a mention of a special type of experimental design, referred to as a *repeated-measures* or *split-plot* design. This type of design has been extensively used in certain areas of pharmaceutical research, e.g. clinical trials, and will be encountered by anyone embarking on a career in this field. As the title states, this experimental design is statistically examined using the ANOVA technique, hence the reason for including it in this chapter. To fully explain the theoretical basis of this technique is outside of the scope of this book, however, so the reader who wishes to explore this technique in more depth is advised to consult a more specialised text, e.g. Dunn and Clark (1987). The aim of this section is to introduce the repeated-measures experimental design and to illustrate the use of the ANOVA for the statistical comparison of data in such a design.

A logical starting point in the description of a repeated-measures design is the design associated with the one-way ANOVA. The reader will recall from section 10.1 that this is typically composed of more than two treatments, each containing a defined number of observations. In this the cells are independent of one another and accordingly the sampling of one observation does not affect the outcome of subsequent sampling. In a repeated-measures design, it is typical for the observations in each cell to be related to one another. A structure for this scenario is proposed in Example 10.8.

EXAMPLE 10.8 *A leading nutritionist has developed a new diet regimen to provide consistent and considerable weight loss over a 3-month period. To examine this claim, a company that markets a weight loss product has initiated a clinical trial. In this eight volunteers were recruited, weighed and introduced to the new diet regimen. The weights of the volunteers were recorded at defined intervals and are shown in Table 10.26. Using an appropriate statistical method examine whether or not the diet regimen provided consistent and considerable weight loss over the 3-month period, as specified by the nutritionist.*

At first glance the reader may be excused for feeling a degree of uncertainty about the nature of the experimental design. On one hand, the study would appear to be a two-factor multiple-comparisons test, in which the dependent variable is the weight of the patients and the two independent variables are the subjects and the time of inclusion within the diet regimen. This may erroneously allow the analyst to conclude that the most suitable statistical test for this problem is a two-way ANOVA (assuming that the data are suitable for analysis using a parametric method). However, the two factors (subjects and time) are not independent but are related in a paired fashion. Therefore, the weights of volunteers over the different times of inclusion on the diet regimen are obtained by performing multiple (repeated) measurements on each patient. The effect of time of inclusion on the diet regimen is effectively linked to each subject. This dependency therefore invalidates the use of the two-way ANOVA. Under these conditions, an ANOVA is

Table 10.26 The weights of eight patients monitored at the start and at different periods after the introduction of a new diet regimen

Volunteer	Weight (kg) after:			
	0 weeks	4 weeks	8 weeks	12 weeks
1	105	101	100	95
2	128	121	116	115
3	144	139	134	130
4	125	120	117	114
5	165	157	150	143
6	112	107	104	102
7	135	129	125	124
8	100	94	90	88

performed, but the calculations involved are modified to accommodate the relationship between the two factors. By using a common pool of subjects for the study (and not separate groups) the overall variability will be reduced. Significantly, the ANOVA that is applied to repeated-measures designs effectively removes the variability between volunteers from the measurement of error, thereby simplifying the effects of the primary factor (time of treatment in this example). The importance of this point should not be overlooked and can be illustrated by comparing the variability associated with the time of treatment and the volunteers. The variability associated with the time of treatment may be obtained by calculating the standard deviation associated with the totals in the columns, whereas the standard deviation associated with the row totals is a measure of the within-subjects variability. These calculations are shown in Table 10.27. As may be observed, the mean weight values associated with each time period are relatively similar, but the variabilities associated with each time period are large. Typically the average coefficient of variation for the four groups was about 0.17 (17%). However, the standard deviation associated with each subject (and hence the variability) is dramatically lower. Therefore, the variability associated with the treatment (time) may be primarily accredited to the inter-subject variability. Accordingly, the variability associated with each treatment group (due primarily to the within-subjects variability) may mask any true differences between the different times.

The problem of the inter-subject variability interfering with the statistical analysis and hence with the statistical outcome may be over-come by the use of a repeated-measures ANOVA. In this technique the inter-subject variability is effectively removed (partitioned), thus

Table 10.27 Summary of the descriptive statistics for the between-treatment (time) and within-subject data presented in Table 10.26

Columns in Table 10.26		Rows in Table 10.26	
Time (weeks)	Mean (±SD) weight (kg)	Subject	Mean (±SD) weight (kg)
0	126.75 ± 21.51	1	100.25 ± 4.11
4	121.00 ± 20.74	2	120.00 ± 8.94
8	117.00 ± 19.38	3	136.75 ± 6.07
12	113.88 ± 18.43	4	119.00 ± 4.69
		5	153.75 ± 9.43
		6	106.25 ± 4.35
		7	128.25 ± 4.99
		8	93.00 ± 5.29

reducing the error term (the denominator in the F ratio) and increasing the chances of rejecting the null hypothesis. The mechanics of the repeated-measures ANOVA, as applied to the data sets described in Example 10.8, are similar to those previously described for the two-way ANOVA. As before, the variability in the experimental design (calculated as a sum of squares) is subdivided into the between-subjects variability and the within-subjects variability. In the repeated-measures design, the within-subjects variability is further partitioned and accredited to either treatment (row) differences (time in Example 10.8) or alternatively, error. The degrees of freedom of each of these sums of squares may be calculated as follows:

- Total number of degrees of freedom = number of observations − 1.
- Between-subjects (rows) degrees of freedom = number of subjects (rows) − 1.
- Within-subjects degrees of freedom = number of subjects (rows) × (number of treatment groups − 1).
- Between-treatments (groups) degrees of freedom = number of treatments (groups) − 1.
- Error degrees of freedom (number of subjects/rows − 1) × (number of treatments/groups − 1).

With the above arguments in mind, we will analyse the clinical scenario described in Example 10.8 using a repeated-measures ANOVA. This example will be used to highlight the mechanics of this type of statistical analysis. As before, the critical statistical parameters associated with Example 10.8 will be defined before the collection of data.

(i) State the null hypothesis

The null hypothesis assumes that the diet regimen will not be successful:

$$H_0: \bar{X}_{\text{weight at 0 weeks}} = \bar{X}_{\text{weight at 4 weeks}} = \bar{X}_{\text{weight at 8 weeks}} = \bar{X}_{\text{weight at 12 weeks}}$$

(ii) State the alternative hypothesis

The alternative hypothesis states that there is a change in weight of the subjects as a function of time, i.e. the diet regiment is successful:

$$H_a: \bar{X}_{\text{weight at 0 weeks}} \neq \bar{X}_{\text{weight at 4 weeks}} \neq \bar{X}_{\text{weight at 8 weeks}} \neq \bar{X}_{\text{weight at 12 weeks}}$$

(iii) State the level of significance

In this example, it is assumed that the level of significance (α) is 0.05.

(iv) State the number of tails

As the null hypothesis may be rejected for two reasons, the test is two-tailed.

(v) Select the most appropriate statistical test

In the selection of the most appropriate statistical test, we will accept that the assumptions of parametric methods are valid, allowing the use of an appropriate parametric test. An examination of the experimental design shows that the effects of two factors on a dependent variable are under consideration, therefore suggesting that a conventional two-way ANOVA would be appropriate. However, upon further inspection, it may be observed that the two factors are dependent, with repeated measurements being performed on the same subjects. Therefore, under these conditions, the most appropriate statistical test is a repeated-measures ANOVA.

(vi) Perform the statistical test

As before, the mechanics of the repeated-measures ANOVA will be described in a stepwise fashion.

Step 1   Calculate the descriptive statistics
In Example 10.8, the descriptive statistics that are employed in the ANOVA are as follows:

- The sum of the squares of each observation (ΣX^2), which in this example is

$$\Sigma X^2 = (105^2 + 128^2 + 144^2 + \cdots + 102^2 + 124^2 + 88^2) = 470\ 163$$

- The sum of each individual value (ΣX), i.e.

$$\Sigma X = (105 + 128 + 144 + \cdots + 102 + 124 + 88) = 3829$$

- The correction term is calculated, as before, using the following formula:

$$CT = \frac{(\Sigma X_{total})^2}{N_{total}}$$

where N_{total} is the total number of observations.

Step 2   Calculate the total sum of squares (SS_{total})
The total sum of squares is calculated as before:

$$SS_{total} = \Sigma X^2 - CT$$

Inserting the data from Example 10.8, the total sum of squares is calculated as:

$$SS_{total} = \Sigma X^2 - \frac{(\Sigma X_{total})^2}{N} = 470\ 163 - \frac{(3829)^2}{32} = 11\ 999.22$$

Step 3   Calculate the between-subjects sum of squares (SS_{BS})
As in previous examples, the between-subjects (between-rows) sum of squares is calculated by subtracting the correction term from the ratio of

the sum of the squares of the row totals to the number of observations per row. Expressed mathematically, the between-subjects sum of squares is calculated as

$$SS_{BS} = \sum \frac{(X_{row})^2}{N_{row}} - \frac{(\sum X_{total})^2}{N_{total}}$$

$$= \begin{bmatrix} \dfrac{(X_{subject\ 1})^2}{N_{subject\ 1}} + \dfrac{(X_{subject\ 2})^2}{N_{subject\ 2}} + \dfrac{(X_{subject\ 3})^2}{N_{subject\ 3}} + \dfrac{(X_{subject\ 4})^2}{N_{subject\ 4}} \\[3mm] \dfrac{(X_{subject\ 5})^2}{N_{subject\ 5}} + \dfrac{(X_{subject\ 6})^2}{N_{subject\ 6}} + \dfrac{(X_{subject\ 7})^2}{N_{subject\ 7}} + \dfrac{(X_{subject\ 8})^2}{N_{subject\ 8}} \end{bmatrix}$$

Inserting the data from Example 10.8 (Table 10.26),

$$SS_{BS} =$$
$$\begin{bmatrix} \dfrac{(401)^2}{4} + \dfrac{(480)^2}{4} + \dfrac{(547)^2}{4} + \dfrac{(476)^2}{4} + \dfrac{(615)^2}{4} + \dfrac{(425)^2}{4} + \dfrac{(513)^2}{4} + \dfrac{(372)^2}{4} \end{bmatrix}$$
$$- \frac{(3829)^2}{32}$$

Alternatively, the above equation may be expressed as:

$$SS_{BS} = \left[\left(\frac{\begin{array}{c}401^2 + 480^2 + 547^2 + 476^2 \\ + 615^2 + 425^2 + 513^2 + 372^2 \end{array}}{4} \right) \right] - \frac{(3829)^2}{32}$$
$$= 11\ 183.50$$

Step 4 Calculate the between-groups sum of squares
The between-groups sum of squares is calculated in an analogous fashion to the between-columns sum of squares in previous examples. Once more, the descriptive statistics associated with each group (column) are used in the calculation of the overall between-groups (treatments) sum of squares ($SS_{treatment}$):

$$SS_{treatment} = \sum \frac{(X_{column})^2}{N_{column}} - \frac{(\sum X_{total})^2}{N_{total}}$$

$$= \begin{bmatrix} \dfrac{(X_{0\ weeks})^2}{N_{0\ weeks}} + \dfrac{(X_{4\ weeks})^2}{N_{4\ weeks}} + \dfrac{(X_{8\ weeks})^2}{N_{8\ weeks}} + \dfrac{(X_{12weeks})^2}{N_{12\ weeks}} \end{bmatrix}$$
$$- \frac{(\sum X_{total})^2}{N_{total}}$$

Using the data from Example 10.8,

$$SS_{treatment} = \left[\frac{(1014)^2}{8} + \frac{(968)^2}{8} + \frac{(936)^2}{8} + \frac{(911)^2}{8}\right] - \frac{(3829)^2}{32}$$

$$= 740.84$$

Step 5 Calculate the sum of squares associated with the error (SS_{error})
In the repeated-measures ANOVA, the sum of squares associated with the error is calculated as the difference between the total sum of squares and the sum of the between-subjects and between-groups sum of squares:

$$SS_{error} = SS_{total} - SS_{BS} - SS_{treatment}$$

$$= 11\ 999.22 - 11\ 183.50 - 740.84$$

$$= 74.88$$

Step 5 Construct a summary table for the ANOVA
The summary table for the repeated-measures ANOVA bears a striking resemblance to analogous tables in both the one- and two-way analyses of variance, but the repeated-measures ANOVA has two important distinguishing features.

- First, the main objective of the analysis is to partition the between-subjects variability from the error term and accordingly this is shown in the table as a separate sum-of-squares term. The between-subjects sum of squares is not involved in the calculation of an *F* ratio.
- Secondly, in Example 10.8, no replication of measurements was performed and therefore the error term is, in effect, the interaction term that is present in a conventional two-way ANOVA. The degrees of freedom for the error term are calculated by multiplying the between-subjects degrees of freedom by the treatment degrees of freedom (as is the case in the two-way ANOVA).

Bearing these differences in mind, the summary table for the ANOVA used to evaluate the efficacy of the diet regimen may be constructed as in Table 10.28.

Step 7 Identify the critical F statistic
The critical *F* statistic is the value in the table of the critical values of the *F* distribution that defines the regions of acceptance and rejection of the null hypothesis. As before, identification of this value requires knowledge of the chosen level of significance ($\alpha = 0.05$), the number of degrees of freedom associated with the treatment ($df = 3$) and the number of degrees of freedom associated with the error term ($df = 21$). From the table of the critical values of the *F* statistic (Appendix 7) the critical *F* statistic$_{(\alpha = 0.05, 3, 21)}$ is 3.07.

Table 10.28 Summary of the output of the analysis of variance for the weight loss of volunteers as a function of duration of time maintained on a novel diet regimen

Source	Sum of squares	df	Mean square	F statistic
Between subjects	11 183.50	7	1597.64	
Between treatments (time)	740.84	3	246.95	69.17
Error	74.88	21	3.57	
Total	11 999.22	31		

Step 8   Interpret the outcome of the statistical analysis
The final step in the statistical analysis of the efficacy of the novel diet regimen involves comparison of the magnitude of the calculated F statistic to the critical F statistic. The F statistic is calculated by dividing the mean square error into the between-treatments mean square:

$$F_{calculated} = \frac{MS_{treatment}}{MS_{error}} = \frac{246.95}{3.57} = 69.17$$

The null hypothesis is accepted if the calculated F statistic is less than the critical F statistic and rejected if the calculated F statistic is equal to or greater than this critical value. As the calculated F statistic (69.17) exceeds the critical F statistic (3.07), the null hypothesis is rejected in favour of the alternative hypothesis. Therefore, it may be concluded that the novel diet regimen did induce weight loss in the volunteers who had been recruited into the clinical study.

For the student who is still unclear about the need for a repeated-measures ANOVA, it is a useful exercise to repeat the statistical analysis using a one-way ANOVA. Under these circumstances, the statistical test does not acknowledge the variability associated with different volunteers. Therefore, in the analysis the independent factor is time, in which there are four categories (0, 4, 8 and 12 weeks). The table of data would now have a different appearance (Table 10.29).

Let us assume that the null hypothesis states that the weight of the patients remain constant over the 12-week period ($\overline{X}_{0\ weeks} = \overline{X}_{4\ weeks} = \overline{X}_{8\ weeks} = \overline{X}_{12\ weeks}$) and the alternative hypothesis states that duration within the diet regiment does influence the weight of the volunteers ($\overline{X}_{0\ weeks} \neq \overline{X}_{4\ weeks} \neq \overline{X}_{8\ weeks} \neq \overline{X}_{12\ weeks}$), the level of significance is 0.05 and that the data are amenable to analysis using a parametric technique. The null hypothesis may then be examined using a one-way ANOVA. The output from this test is displayed in Table 10.30. All calculations have been omitted, but is may be useful for the reader to work out these values using a calculator.

Table 10.29 Effect of duration within a novel diet regimen on the weight of volunteers after inclusion on a new diet regimen for different periods of time

Weight (kg) after:			
0 weeks	4 weeks	8 weeks	12 weeks
105	101	100	95
128	121	116	115
144	139	134	130
125	120	117	114
165	157	150	143
112	107	104	102
135	129	125	124
100	94	90	88

Table 10.30 Summary of the output of the ANOVA for the effect of duration of a diet regimen on the weight of volunteers

Source	Sum of squares	df	Mean square	F statistic
Between treatments (time effect)	740.84	3	246.95	0.61
Within treatments (error)	11 258.38	28	402.09	
Total	11 999.22	31		

Under the conditions of the experimental design (i.e. $\alpha = 0.05$, $df_{treatment} = 3$, $df_{error} = 28$) the critical F statistic is 2.95. As the calculated F statistic (0.61) is less than the critical F statistic, the null hypothesis is accepted and accordingly, it would have been concluded that the novel diet regimen was ineffective. This example serves to remind the reader that the incorrect choice of a statistical test may increase the probability of making a type II error. The ability of the repeated-measures design to separate the between-subjects variability is essential in the identification of a significant clinical effect.

10.4 Experimental design critertia of the ANOVA

Conducting pharmaceutical (and other) experiments may be expensive and time-consuming unless proper consideration is given to their design. The arguments concerning the need for the correct experimental design have been presented in Chapters 8 and 9. However, as there are at least three treatments (sample groups) in the ANOVA, there is a greater emphasis on the optimisation of experimental design in these situations.

As before, it is important to define the optimum design criteria. In this section, various aspects of experimental design will be discussed, namely, the power of the ANOVA, the sample size required to detect a specified difference between the means of treatment groups and finally, the minimum detectable difference between the means of samples or treatments. These topics will be fully discussed with the aid of pharmaceutical examples.

10.4.1 Power of the ANOVA and proposed sample size

The basic principles associated with the calculation of power in the ANOVA are similar to those already described for the t test, but in the case of the ANOVA a new statistic, ϕ (Greek phi), is calculated. The power is then interpreted from the tables of the critical values of the non-central F distribution (Appendix 14). It is not within the scope of this text to offer further explanations of this distribution. The reader need only remember that ϕ is used for calculating the power associated with the ANOVA. The power of the ANOVA may be calculated in a number of ways, depending on the information available to the analyst. These methods will be considered individually.

10.4.1.1 Determination of the power of an ANOVA after the completion of the analysis

In many situations an experiment will have been completed without any prior calculation of power. If the ANOVA has returned a rejection of the null hypothesis, the consequences of this are not dramatic. However, if the analysis has resulted in an acceptance of the null hypothesis, it is important to calculate the power associated with the study, as this will inform the analyst of the validity of the conclusion of the test. The reader will remember that if the null hypothesis is accepted where it is in fact false, a type II error has been made. Therefore, it is necessary to comment on the validity of accepting the null hypothesis.

The equation that is used to calculate ϕ is

$$\phi = \sqrt{\frac{(k-1)(MS_{treatment} - MS_{error})}{k \times MS_{error}}}$$

where k is the number of treatments (sample groups), $MS_{treatment}$ is the mean square associated with the treatment, as calculated in the ANOVA and MS_{error} is the mean square associated with the error, as calculated in the ANOVA.

To illustrate the power associated with an ANOVA, let us consider the following example.

EXAMPLE 10.9 *An engineering company specialises in the manufacture of pumps for the pharmaceutical industry. It has received a request to develop an efficient pump for the removal of a pseudoplastic gel from a manufacturing vat and, in response to this, has developed three potentially suitable types of pump. The company has decided to examine the time required to pump 10 kg of gel when each pump is operated at the maximum shear rate. The results of the experiment are summarised in Table 10.31. Using an appropriate statistical method, determine whether there is a difference in the performance of the three pumps.*

For the reasons presented in the previous examples (data measured on a ratio scale, assumed homogeneity of variances, similar means and medians for each treatment), an ANOVA has been used to compare the three sets of data. The reader should statistically evaluate the assumption of homogeneity of variances using the F_{max} test ($F_{max \, (calculated)} = 1.06$, $F_{max \, (critical)}$ 10.80, *outcome*: acceptance of null hypothesis, the variances are similar).

(i)   State the null hypothesis

There is no difference in the performances of the three pumps in terms of the times required to pump a 10-kg sample of gel:

$$H_0: \overline{X}_{pump \, 1} = \overline{X}_{pump \, 2} = \overline{X}_{pump \, 3}$$

(ii)   State the alternative hypothesis

There is a difference in the performances of the three pumps in terms of the times required to pump a 10-kg sample of gel:

$$H_a: \overline{X}_{pump \, 1} \neq \overline{X}_{pump \, 2} \neq \overline{X}_{pump \, 3}$$

Table 10.31 Times (s) required to pump 10-kg samples of a gel product using three different pumps

Pump 1	Pump 2	Pump 3
30.5	31.1	28.2
32.5	35.9	29.6
36.2	32.1	29.5
32.8	37.0	32.7
31.0	37.2	34.2
28.9	35.5	33.9
Mean: 32.0	Mean: 34.8	Mean: 31.3
Median: 31.8	Median: 35.7	Median: 31.2
Variance: 6.3	Variance: 6.7	Variance: 6.6

(iii) State the level of significance

In this example, it is assumed that the level of significance (a) is 0.05.

(iv) State the number of tails associated with the experimental outcome

There are two tails in the experimental design.

The summary table for the ANOVA is presented in Table 10.32. Under the conditions associated with the experimental design, i.e. $a = 0.05$, 2 df as the numerator, 15 df as the denominator, the critical statistic is defined as 3.68. Therefore, as the calculated F statistic (3.11) is less than the critical F statistic (3.68), the null hypothesis is accepted and, accordingly, it may be concluded that there is no difference in the performance of the three pumps in terms of the times required to pump 10 kg of gel.

Interestingly, although the calculated F statistic is less than the critical F statistic, the difference between these two values is not large. Indeed, if the level of significance (a) had been preset at 0.10 the critical F statistic associated with 2 and 15 df would have been 2.70 and, under these conditions, the null hypothesis would have been rejected in favour of the alternative hypothesis. Therefore, it is necessary to examine the above data sets to identify individual differences between the pumps. This is a situation in which a *post-hoc* test is required. Of the *post-hoc* tests that have been described in this text the most appropriate is Tukey's HSD test, as this may be employed when the calculated F statistic in the ANOVA is not significant. The experimental parameters associated with this *post-hoc* test are as follows:

Step 1   State the null hypothesis
The null hypothesis states that there is no difference between the means of the three treatment groups, i.e.

$$H_0: \overline{X}_{pump\ 1} = \overline{X}_{pump\ 2}$$

$$\overline{X}_{pump\ 1} = \overline{X}_{pump\ 3}$$

$$\overline{X}_{pump\ 2} = \overline{X}_{pump\ 3}$$

Table 10.32 Summary of the output of the ANOVA for the times required to pump 10-kg samples of a gel product using three different pumps

Source	Sum of squares	df	Mean square	F statistic
Between treatments (pump effects)	40.47	2	20.24	3.11
Within treatments (error)	97.52	15	6.50	
Total	93.13	17		

Step 2   State the alternative hypothesis
The alternative hypothesis states that there is/are differences between the means of the three treatment groups, i.e.

$$H_a: \overline{X}_{\text{pump 1}} \neq \overline{X}_{\text{pump 2}}$$
$$\overline{X}_{\text{pump 1}} \neq \overline{X}_{\text{pump 3}}$$
$$\overline{X}_{\text{pump 2}} \neq \overline{X}_{\text{pump 3}}$$

Step 3   State the level of significance and number of tails

$\alpha = 0.05$, two-tailed design.

Step 4   Calculate the HSD statistic

$$HSD = q \sqrt{\frac{s^2}{N}}$$

Here q is found from Appendix 12 under the conditions of the experiment, namely, 3 treatment groups, 15 *df* associated with the mean square error and $\alpha = 0.05$. Under these circumstances, $q = 3.67$. $N = 6$ is the size of either of the two treatment groups and $s^2 = 6.50$ is the pooled variance, estimated using the mean square error term in the ANOVA. Therefore

$$HSD = 3.67 \sqrt{\frac{6.50}{6}} = 3.82$$

Step 5   Calculate the absolute differences between the means of the treatment groups

$$\overline{X}_{\text{pump 1}} - \overline{X}_{\text{pump 2}} = -2.82 = 2.82$$
$$\overline{X}_{\text{pump 1}} - \overline{X}_{\text{pump 3}} = +0.63 = 0.63$$
$$\overline{X}_{\text{pump 2}} - \overline{X}_{\text{pump 3}} = +3.45 = 3.45$$

Step 6   Interpret the outcome of the analysis

- $\overline{X}_{\text{pump 1}} - \overline{X}_{\text{pump 2}} = 2.82$. As this is less than the critical HSD (3.82), the null hypothesis is accepted. There is no difference in the performances of pumps 1 and 2.
- $\overline{X}_{\text{pump 1}} - \overline{X}_{\text{pump 3}} = 0.63$. As this is less than the critical HSD (3.82), the null hypothesis is accepted. There is no difference in the performances of pumps 1 and 3.
- $\overline{X}_{\text{pump 2}} - \overline{X}_{\text{pump 3}} = 3.45$. As this is less than the critical HSD (3.82), the null hypothesis is accepted. There is no difference in the performances of pumps 2 and 3.

Therefore, in spite of the relative similarities of the critical and calculated F values in the ANOVA, no individual differences were identified in a *post-hoc* analysis.

Following the analysis of the data described in Example 10.9 with both an ANOVA and Tukey's HSD, it may be assumed that there were no differences between the performances of the pumps. However, before leaving this example, it is important to quantify the power of the study, as this will inform the analyst of the validity of the results obtained in the previous analyses.

The first step in this process involves the calculation of the ϕ value, using the equation given above:

$$\phi = \sqrt{\frac{(k-1)(MS_{treatment} - MS_{error})}{k \times MS_{error}}}$$

In this example, the number of treatment groups (k) is 3, $MS_{treatment}$ is 20.24 and MS_{error} is 6.50. Therefore:

$$\phi = \sqrt{\frac{(3-1)(20.24 - 6.50)}{(3 \times 6.50)}} = 1.19$$

The relevance of this calculated value may be determined by reference to Appendix 14, the table of critical values of the non-central F distribution. This table describes the probability of making a type II error. From this it may be observed that the probability of making a type II error requires knowledge of the calculated ϕ value (1.19), the stated α value (0.05), the number of degrees of freedom associated with the treatment (2) and the number of degrees of freedom associated with the error (15), both derived from the ANOVA associated with this example. From the table in Appendix 14, it may observed that the probability of making a type II (β) error is approximately 0.65. (The reader will have observed that the exact probability cannot be derived from the table and must be approximated.) With knowledge of the β error, the power may be calculated:

$$\text{power} = 1 - \beta$$
$$= 1.00 - 0.65$$
$$= 0.35$$

This is quite a low power. Expressed another way, it may be concluded that the probability of making a type II error is 0.65, i.e. the probability of accepting the null hypothesis (as we have concluded in this example) when the null hypothesis is actually false is 65%. In these terms, the conclusions derived from the ANOVA and Tukey's HSD may not be so definitive. This does not mean, however, that these conclusions are incorrect. In light of this knowledge it is appropriate to ask what measures may be initiated to improve the power of the study. This question may be answered with reference both to the equation that was described for the calculation of power and also to the table of critical values of the non-central F distribution (Appendix 14). As may be observed from Appendix 14, the probability of making a type II error decreases, and hence the power of the study increases, as ϕ increases. Therefore, to increase the power of the study, measures should be adopted to increase the value of ϕ. Referring to the previous equation, it may be observed that altering the following parameters will increase ϕ:

- decreasing the number of treatment groups (k)
- increasing the inter-treatment variability ($MS_{treatment}$).
- decreasing the within-treatment variability (MS_{error}).
- increasing the number of observations in the treatment groups (This is not directly apparent from the equation, but it will become apparent as the discussion of power is continued).

10.4.1.2 Determination of the power of an ANOVA before the collection of data

Frequently the analyst may wish to calculate the power of a study before collecting data. Power is a fundamental concern in the design of any experiment as it ensures that the experimental design is properly optimised and, as a result, the outcome of the analysis is not compromised by concerns over inadequate power. Therefore, where appropriate, the power should be determined before starting a study. The equation that may be employed to calculate ϕ (and hence the power of the study) is

$$\phi = \sqrt{\frac{N \Sigma(\overline{X} - \mu)^2}{k \times s^2}}$$

where N is the number of observations in a single treatment group (in this design, it is preferable that the sample sizes of each treatment group are identical); $(\overline{X} - \mu)^2$ is the square of the difference between the estimated mean of each treatment group and the mean of the estimated means of the treatment groups; k is the number of treatment groups; and s^2 is the estimated within-treatments variability (i.e. the error).

After calculating ϕ and with knowledge of the number of degrees of freedom associated with the treatments ($k - 1$) and the estimated within-group variability [$k(n - 1)$], the probability associated with a type II error, and hence the power of the study may be estimated. To illustrate the calculation of the power of a study, the scenario described in Example 10.9 will be used, but the wording of the scenario has been changed to highlight the differences in the information available to the analyst either before or after the collection of data.

EXAMPLE 10.10   *An engineering company specialises in the manufacture of pumps for the pharmaceutical industry. It has received a request to develop an efficient pump for the removal of a pseudoplastic gel from a manufacturing vat and has developed three potentially suitable types of pump. The company has estimated from previous pilot experiments that the mean times required to pump 10 kg of gel when each pump is operated at the maximum shear rate are 33.5, 36.0 and 32.6 s and the within-treatment (pump) variability is 6.0 s². The company is reluctant to begin a large trial of pump performance without prior knowledge of the power of the study. Therefore, as the statistical analyst you have been asked to calculate the power of the ANOVA pertaining to the experimental design.*

Referring to the previous equation, the following information is required for the calculation of ϕ:

- the number of treatment groups (k), i.e. 3
- the number of observations in each treatment group; for the purpose of this calculation, this value will be selected as 15
- the estimated mean of each group, i.e. 33.5 s for pump 1, 36.0 s for pump 2 and 32.6 s for pump 3
- the mean of the three estimated treatment means, i.e.

$$\left(\frac{33.5 + 36.0 + 32.6}{3} \right) = 34.03$$

- the estimated within-treatment variability, i.e. 6.0 s².

These parameters are then inserted into the equation to allow calculation of ϕ:

$$\phi = \sqrt{\frac{N \, \Sigma(\bar{X} - \mu)^2}{k \times s^2}}$$

$$= \sqrt{\frac{15 \times [(33.5 - 34.03)^2 + (36.0 - 34.03)^2 + (32.6 - 34.03)^2]}{3 \times 6.0}}$$

$$= 2.27$$

As before, the interpretation of this calculated value requires knowledge of the following parameters:

- the proposed level of significance, i.e. $\alpha = 0.05$
- the number of degrees of freedom associated with the treatments, i.e. $k - 1 = 3 - 1 = 2$

- the number of degrees of freedom associated with the error, i.e. $k (n - 1) = 3 \times (15 - 1) = 42$.

Under these conditions a ϕ value of 2.27 corresponds to a probability of committing a type II error of approximately 0.08 and, accordingly, the power of the ANOVA is approximately 0.92. This is a powerful study and would allow the analyst to have confidence of the output of the ANOVA.

It was stated earlier that the number of observations in each treatment group is a significant determinant of the power of the statistical analysis, and the reader should now understand this, from the equation described above. If in Example 10.10 we had arbitrarily selected 10 observations in each treatment group while retaining all other estimates, the power associated with the ANOVA could be calculated as

$$\phi = \sqrt{\frac{10 \times [(33.5 - 34.03)^2 + (36.0 - 34.03)^2 + (32.6 - 34.03)^2]}{3 \times 6.0}}$$

$$= 1.86$$

This equates to a probability of committing a type II error of approximately 0.21, or alternatively, a power of 0.79. Therefore, this example serves to illustrate the relationship between sample size and power. However, it should be remembered that as the sample size of each treatment group increases, the cost of the study would also increase. As a result, experimental design frequently involves a compromise between the sample size and power. Let us assume that in Example 10.10 that we wish to maintain the power of the study at 85%; the sample size that is associated with this value may be calculated by iteration. From the above calculations, it is known that sample sizes of 10 and 15 were associated with powers of approximately 0.79 and 0.92 and therefore, to establish a power of 0.85, the sample size must be intermediate between these values. Assuming that the sample size is 12 (and $\alpha = 0.05$), the calculation is repeated as above:

$$\phi = \sqrt{\frac{12 \times [(33.5 - 34.03)^2 + (36.0 - 34.03)^2 + (32.6 - 34.03)^2]}{3 \times 6.0}}$$

$$= 2.03$$

The numbers of degrees of freedom associated with the numerator and denominator are 2 and 33, respectively. Under these conditions, a ϕ value of 2.03 is associated with a probability of committing a type II error of 0.15, or alternatively, a power of approximately $(1 - 0.15) = 0.85$. Therefore, to establish a power of 0.85, a sample size of 12 is required in Example 10.10.

10.4.1.3 Calculation of the power of an ANOVA using the minimum detectable difference

Another method by which the power of an ANOVA may be estimated is by the use of a minimum detectable difference. In the previous method, two parameters were estimated, namely the means of each treatment group and the within-treatment variability. In this method, the within-treatment variability is once more estimated from a previous experiment and the minimum difference between two of the treatments that is expected to be of clinical (or non-clinical) relevance is defined. This difference represents the minimum difference between the largest and smallest means. As before, ϕ is mathematically calculated and the probability associated with this value determined from the table of the critical values of the non-central F distribution (Appendix 14). Under these circumstances, ϕ is calculated using the formula

$$\phi = \sqrt{\frac{N\delta^2}{2ks^2}}$$

where N is the number of observations in any group, δ is the minimum detectable difference that is expected to be important, k is the number of treatment groups and s^2 is the estimated variability. The use of this equation for the calculation of the power associated with an ANOVA is demonstrated in Example 10.11.

EXAMPLE 10.11 *The manufacture of steroid-containing polymeric rods for subcutaneous implantation involves dispersion of the therapeutic agent into the molten polymer and then extrusion of this polymer melt into a mould. The polymer used in this formulation is semi-crystalline. It is known that the degree of crystallisation of the polymer directly affects the clinical performance of the dosage form and that this property is affected by the rate at which the molten polymer is cooled in the extrusion process. Following the receipt of several complaints to the Committee on the Safety of Medicines, the company responsible for the manufacture of these dosage forms is concerned about the effects of cooling on the degree of crystallinity of the dosage forms and has decided to set up a study to investigate the relationship between cooling rate and crystallinity. In this study, 10 samples of the polymer will be produced using 5 cooling rates (2, 4, 6, 8 and 10 °C/min) and the percentage crystallinity of the formed dosage form characterised using differential scanning calorimetry. In a previous pilot study, the variability of the population was estimated as 5.6%, and it has been decided that the minimum detectable difference between the largest and smallest treatments that would constitute a potential clinical problem is 5%. As* *the statistical analyst you have been asked to calculate the power of the ANOVA that will be used to challenge the null hypothesis.*

The first step of this calculation involves computation and interpretation of ϕ:

$$\phi = \sqrt{\frac{N\delta^2}{2ks^2}}$$

where $N = 10$, $\delta = 5\%$, $k = 5$ and $s^2 = 5.6\%$. Therefore

$$\phi = \sqrt{\frac{10 \times 5^2}{2 \times 5 \times 5.6}} = 2.11$$

The interpretation of this calculated value requires knowledge of the level of significance ($\alpha = 0.05$), the number of degrees of freedom associated with the treatments ($k - 1 = 5 - 1 = 4$), the number of degrees of freedom associated with the error, i.e. $k (n - 1) = 5 \times 9 = 45$. The calculated ϕ value therefore corresponds to a probability of making a type II error of 0.05. Therefore, the power of the proposed study would be 0.95.

Once more, the power of the proposed analysis is high and, in light of the relationship between sample size and power, it would be typical (and expected) for the statistical analyst to recommend a smaller sample size. Although the power would thereby be reduced, the cost of the study to the parent company would be dramatically lower. Assuming that you have recommended that the size of each treatment should be 7, the calculated ϕ value would be

$$\phi = \sqrt{\frac{7 \times 5^2}{2 \times 5 \times 5.6}} = 1.77$$

The probability associated with making a type II error associated with this value (and $\alpha = 0.05$, $df_{\text{treatments}} = 4$ and $df_{\text{error}} = 30$) is approximately 0.14. Therefore, the power of the proposed study would be 0.86, an acceptable value for the hypothesis under investigation.

The reader should remember that this calculation may be transformed to enable the proposed sample size to be estimated before the start of the study. Under these conditions, the power of the study is defined at the beginning of the calculation, along with the estimates of variability and minimum detectable difference, and the sample size that corresponds to this specified value is estimated using an iterative process. Therefore, assume that in Example 10.11 that the power of the study has been defined as approximately 0.90 and the variability, level of significance and minimum detectable difference are as previously stated. From this information and using the previous equation, the sample size that provides this power value may be iterated.

Previously it was shown that samples sizes of 7 and 10 were associated with power levels of 0.86 and 0.95, respectively. Therefore, the sample size that is associated with a power of 0.90 must lie between these two values. First the suitability of a sample size of 8 will be examined:

$$\phi = \sqrt{\frac{8 \times 5^2}{2 \times 5 \times 5.6}} = 1.89$$

When $\alpha = 0.05$. $df_{treatments} = 4$ and $df_{error} = 35$, the probability of committing a type II error that is associated with a ϕ value of 1.89 is approximately 0.11 so the power of the proposed study is approximately 0.89.

Now let us examine the suitability of a larger sample size, i.e. 9:

$$\phi = \sqrt{\frac{9 \times 5^2}{2 \times 5 \times 5.6}} = 2.00$$

When $\alpha = 0.05$. $df_{treatments} = 4$ and $df_{error} = 40$, the probability of committing a type II error that is associated with a ϕ value of 2.00 is approximately 0.06 and the power of the proposed study is approximately 0.94.

It would therefore be appropriate to select a sample size of 8 in each treatment group to achieve a power in the ANOVA of approximately 0.90.

10.4.2 Estimation of the minimum detectable difference in the ANOVA

Another useful parameter that may be estimated before data collection begins is the minimum detectable difference. This is the smallest difference that may be detected under the conditions of the statistical analysis. It is particularly important to ensure that the ANOVA is capable of detecting differences between treatments that will be significant in terms of, e.g., clinical effect, stability, cost, and productivity. Otherwise an important aspect of the study may be masked.

The minimum detectable difference is calculated by rearranging the previous equation:

$$\phi = \sqrt{\frac{N\delta^2}{2ks^2}}$$

therefore $\quad \phi\sqrt{2ks^2} = \sqrt{N\delta^2}$

$$\delta = \frac{\phi\sqrt{2ks^2}}{\sqrt{N}}$$

The use of this equation is described in the next example.

EXAMPLE 10.12 *In a clinical study the effects of 3 drugs on the dias-tolic blood pressure of volunteers is under examination. In this study, 12 patients are allocated to each group and the patients in each group receive a single dose of one of the drugs. The comparative effects of the 3 drugs will be assessed using a one-way ANOVA. In a previous pilot study, the within-group variability was estimated as 10.1 mmHg². Assuming that the level of significance is 0.05 and the power of the pro-posed ANOVA is 0.80, estimate the minimum difference that may be detected between the drug treatments.*

To calculate the minimum detectable difference, the following parame-ters are inserted into the above equation: the number of treatments, $k = 3$; the estimated variability, $s^2 = 10.1$ mmHg²; the number of obser-vations in a treatment group, $N = 12$. ϕ is the value in the critical values of the non-central F distribution that corresponds to $\alpha = 0.05$, $df_{treatment} = 2$, $df_{error} = 33$ and a power of 0.8 (i.e. a 0.20 probability of committing a type II error), i.e. approximately 1.90. Therefore:

$$\delta = \frac{\phi\sqrt{2ks^2}}{\sqrt{N}} = \frac{1.90\sqrt{2 \times 3 \times 10.1}}{\sqrt{12}} = 4.27 \text{ mmHg}$$

The smallest difference between two treatment (drug) means that may be detected is thus 4.27 mmHg.

10.5 Conclusions

This chapter introduced the concept of simultaneously comparing three or more treatments and described examples of statistical methods by which this may be achieved. In light of the more complex natures and the greater number of statistical tests that may be used for this purpose, this chapter was restricted to only parametric methods, namely one-way and two-way analyses of variance (ANOVA). Before selecting these methods to resolve a statistical question, the analyst must be assured that both the nature of the data and the experimental design are appro-priate for statistical manipulation using this family of parametric tech-niques. The selection criteria for the ANOVA are identical to those previously described for parametric two-sample analyses. Therefore, the ANOVA may be used if the following are satified:

- the data has been measured on interval or ratio scales
- the populations from which the three or more sets of data have been sampled should be normally distributed

- the variances of the populations from which the three or more sets of data have been sampled should be similar in magnitude
- the number of observations in each treatment should be sufficiently large.

These assumptions may seem relatively inflexible yet, as in two-sample parametric tests, the ANOVA is sufficiently robust to tolerate moderate departures from the assumptions concerning homogeneity of treatment variances and normality of parent populations. However, the ANOVA assumes that the data have been measured in units that are amenable to arithmetic manipulations to gain information on the central tendency and dispersion of each data set, so the data must be measured on either interval or ratio scales. Similarly, if the number of observations in each treatment is too small, it is difficult to accurately estimate the means and variances of the parent populations using the sample data, thereby invalidating the use of the ANOVA. A similar situation exists concerning the use of the two-sample t test

The reader should be clear about the need for multiple-sample tests such as the ANOVA and, in particular, the problems associated with attempting to analyse such data sets using a series of two-independent-sample t tests. The strength of the ANOVA is that information about the effect of an independent variable on a particular outcome may be achieved while maintaining the probability of committing a type I error at a defined level. Unfortunately the same may not be said for the situation in which the ANOVA is substituted with a series of t tests. This approach dramatically increases the chance of committing a type I error, thereby leading to an unsubstantiated and erroneous rejection of the null hypothesis. Therefore, when it is required to statistically compare three or more treatments, a multiple-sample test such as ANOVA must be used.

In this chapter, the mechanics and applications of three types of ANOVA were described, with the aid of pharmaceutical examples: one-way ANOVA, the two-way ANOVA and repeated-measures one-way ANOVA. The appropriate test is selected according to the number of independent variables in the experimental design. Hence, in the one-way and two-way ANOVA there are one and two independent variables, respectively. In the one-way ANOVA with repeated measures, only one independent variable is present, but the nature of the design is different from that of the conventional one-way ANOVA because of the paired nature of the repeated-measures design. It is important that the reader appreciates the differences in these types of experimental designs.

The ANOVA is performed by calculating the F ratio associated with each independent variable and additionally, in the case of the two-way ANOVA, the F ratio associated with the interaction between the effects of the two primary variables. Following calculation of this ratio, the outcome of the statistical analysis is interpreted by comparing the calculated F ratio to the critical F statistic that is taken from the table of critical values of this statistic. To avoid erroneous interpretation of this outcome, the analyst must ensure that the critical F statistic is selected according to the properties of the experimental design. This requires knowledge of the numbers of degrees of freedom associated with the treatment (variable) and the error term and the level of significance.

One of the strengths of ANOVA is its ability to detect interactions between primary independent variables in two-way or higher experimental designs. The presence of a statistical interaction indicates that the effect of one variable on a particular response (the dependent variable) is dependent on the level (magnitude) of a second independent variable. When a statistical analysis has recorded a significant interaction effect, this often provides valuable information concerning the particular experiment or study. It is always worth considering the possible mechanisms of this statistical effect.

If the independent variable is composed of three or more sub-categories, a rejection of the null hypothesis implies that the variable has a significant effect on the magnitude of the dependent variable. However, it does not provide an insight into the differences between each individual sub-category with respect to this measured outcome. Therefore, to understand these individual differences (or lack of differences) it is necessary to perform either a-priori or *post-hoc* comparisons between individual treatments. Such tests employ the error term associated with the primary ANOVA, thereby increasing the likelihood of identifying individual differences between pairs of treatments. In this chapter several of these techniques were described, along with the rationale for their use. These tests are an important component of the process of statistical inference in multiple hypothesis tests.

References

Dunn O J, Clark V A (1987). *Applied Statistics: Analysis of Variance and Regression*, 2nd edition. New York: Wiley.
Scheffé H (1964). *The Analysis of Variance*. New York: Wiley.
Sokal R R, Rohlf F J (1981). *Biometry*, 2nd edition. New York: W H Freeman.

11

Non-parametric hypothesis testing for multiple samples

In the previous chapter, the mechanics and applications of methods that may be employed to simultaneously evaluate more than two hypotheses using parametric statistical tests were described. Through the course of Chapter 10 (and indeed Chapters 7, 8 and 9), the reader will have become aware of the implications of the use of parametric tests. In particular, this text has sought to highlight the applications and limitations of parametric statistical tests and the experimental situations that necessitate the use of such tests. In particular, it has been stated that the use of parametric tests is valid when:

- the samples (treatments) are derived from normally distributed populations
- the samples possess similar variances
- the data have been measured in at least an interval scale of measurement.

If these conditions cannot be assured, the analyst should turn to non-parametric methods of assessment. It should be remembered, however, that the use of many parametric tests may be valid in situations where there are moderate deviations from these assumptions, i.e. the data may not possess equal variances and the populations from which the data have been sample may deviate from normality. The nature of data measurement is an important determinant in the choice of statistical test. In parametric tests, the calculations, e.g. the mean and variance, require that the data is amenable to arithmetic manipulations and, accordingly, the data must be measured on either an interval or a ratio scale. If the data is nominal or ordinal, non-parametric tests must be employed to evaluate the validity of the null hypothesis.

In this chapter, three non-parametric multiple sample hypothesis tests are described: the χ^2 test, the Kruskal–Wallis test and Friedman's test. The conditions for the use these tests are specific, and again their mechanics and applications will be illustrated using pharmaceutical examples. When the data have been measured on at least an interval scale, the Kruskal–Wallis and Friedman's test are the non-parametric equivalent of the one-way and one-way repeated-measures/two-way analysis of variance and are therefore used when the assumptions of

ANOVA are invalid. It has proved impossible to combine parametric and non-parametric multiple-sample hypothesis tests into one chapter because of the amount of detail associated with these tests. However, otherwise the format of this chapter is similar to that of previous chapters.

11.1 χ^2 analysis for the comparison of three or more samples: higher contingency tables

The theory associated with the use of the χ^2 test for the comparison of more than two independent samples is an extension of that described for the one- and two-sample χ^2 tests. As before, in the χ^2 test the data is nominal in nature, i.e. the data is collected and presented as frequencies within discrete categories. In Chapter 8, the most straightforward experimental design that may be analysed using a χ^2 test was described, i.e. the 2×2 contingency table. When there are three or more independent groups, the complexity of these designs and their subsequent analysis is obviously increased. However, the reader should not be unduly concerned by this, as the mechanics of all χ^2 analyses are identical. In all cases, the expected numbers of observations in each cell (as defined by the null hypothesis) are compared to the recorded numbers of observation. The χ^2 statistic is calculated by summation of these individual comparisons and the outcome of the statistical analysis is interpreted by comparing the calculated χ^2 statistic to the critical χ^2 statistic. The experimental design and calculations associated with the χ^2 analysis when three or more columns or rows are present are shown in Example 11.1.

EXAMPLE 11.1 *A pharmaceutical company wishes to launch a new product on to the market but is unsure of the general public's preferred shape or type of solid dosage form. A market research company has been commissioned to examine whether there is a relationship between the acceptability of the shape or type of solid dosage form and patient age. To investigate this relationship, members of the public within three defined age groups (20–35 years, 36–50 years, 51–65 years) were asked to state their preference for a conventional round tablet, a caplet or a capsule. The results are recorded in Table 11.1. Using an appropriate statistical method, conclude whether or not there is a relationship between subject age and the preference for a particular shape of solid dosage form.*

As in previous examples, the criteria associated with the experimental design should be noted before the collection of data.

Table 11.1 Preference for different shapes of solid dosage forms stated by different age groups of respondents

Tablet shape	Age group (years)		
	20–35	36–50	51–65
Round	85	96	69
Caplet	80	85	64
Capsule	74	89	121

(i) State the null hypothesis

In the above example, the null hypothesis states that there is no relationship between the rows and columns, i.e. the variables are independent. Consequently, there is no relationship between subject age group and preference for a particular shape of solid dosage form.

(ii) State the alternative hypothesis

The alternative hypothesis adopts an opposing stance to the null hypothesis and therefore assumes that there is a correlation between subject age and preference for solid dosage form. Accordingly, the alternative hypothesis states that there is a relationship between subject age and solid dosage form.

(iii) State the level of significance

In this example, it will be assumed that the level of significance (α) is 0.05.

(iv) Select the most appropriate statistical test

Two basic variables are under consideration here: the shape or type of solid dosage form and the age group of respondents. More specifically, there are three discrete categories in each of these categories. The data housed within each cell is nominal in nature and the experimental design is a 3×3 contingency table. The validity of the null hypothesis may therefore be most appropriately examined using a χ^2 analysis.

(v) Compute the χ^2 statistic

The χ^2 statistic for higher contingency tables is calculated in an identical fashion to that described for 2×2 experimental designs: the χ^2 value for each cell is determined and these individual values are added together to generate an overall calculated χ^2 statistic. This value is then employed to determine the outcome of the statistical analysis. The χ^2 statistic is calculated using the following formula:

$$\chi^2 = \sum \frac{(O_f - E_f)^2}{E_f}$$

where O_f and E_f denote the observed and expected frequencies, respectively.

Using the above formula, the χ^2 test may be executed in a stepwise fashion.

Step 1   Calculate the expected frequencies associated with each cell
The expected frequencies are the frequencies associated with each cell as defined by the null hypothesis. The expected frequency for each cell is calculated individually by multiplying the row total associated with the cell by the column total associated with the cell and dividing the product by the total number of observations (respondents in this example). There are nine cells in Example 11.1 and the individual calculations of the expected frequency for each cell are shown below. It is good statistical practice to rewrite Table 11.1 to include the totals for each row and column (Table 11.2).

- *Cell representing 20–35 years age group and round tablets*

$$E_f = \frac{(column_{total} \times row_{total})}{observations_{total}} = \frac{(250 \times 239)}{763} = 78.3$$

- *Cell representing 36–50 years age group and round tablets*

$$E_f = \frac{(column_{total} \times row_{total})}{observations_{total}} = \frac{(270 \times 250)}{763} = 88.5$$

- *Cell representing 51–65 years age group and round tablets*

$$E_f = \frac{(column_{total} \times row_{total})}{observations_{total}} = \frac{(254 \times 250)}{763} = 83.2$$

Table 11.2 Preference for different shapes of solid dosage forms stated by different age groups of respondents, showing the row and column totals

Tablet shape	Age group (years)			Totals
	20–35	36–50	51–65	
Round	85	96	69	250
Caplet	80	85	64	229
Capsule	74	89	121	284
Totals	239	270	254	763

- Cell representing 20–35 years age group and caplets

$$E_f = \frac{(column_{total} \times row_{total})}{observations_{total}} = \frac{(239 \times 229)}{763} = 71.7$$

- Cell representing 36–50 years age group and caplets

$$E_f = \frac{(column_{total} \times row_{total})}{observations_{total}} = \frac{(270 \times 229)}{763} = 81.0$$

- Cell representing 51–65 years age group and caplets

$$E_f = \frac{(column_{total} \times row_{total})}{observations_{total}} = \frac{(254 \times 229)}{763} = 76.2$$

- Cell representing 20–35 years age group and capsules

$$E_f = \frac{(column_{total} \times row_{total})}{observations_{total}} = \frac{(239 \times 284)}{763} = 89.0$$

- Cell representing 36–50 years age group and capsules

$$E_f = \frac{(column_{total} \times row_{total})}{observations_{total}} = \frac{(270 \times 284)}{763} = 100.5$$

- Cell representing 51–65 years age group and capsules

$$E_f = \frac{(column_{total} \times row_{total})}{observations_{total}} = \frac{(254 \times 284)}{763} = 94.5$$

Step 2   *Calculate the χ^2 statistic*

$$\chi^2 = \sum \frac{(O_f - E_f)^2}{E_f}$$

$$= \left[\begin{array}{l} \dfrac{(85-78.3)^2}{78.3} + \dfrac{(96-88.5)^2}{88.5} + \dfrac{(69-83.2)^2}{83.2} \\[2ex] + \dfrac{(80-71.7)^2}{71.7} + \dfrac{(85-81.0)^2}{81.0} + \dfrac{(64-76.2)^2}{76.2} \\[2ex] + \dfrac{(74-89.0)^2}{89.0} + \dfrac{(89-100.5)^2}{100.5} + \dfrac{(121-94.5)^2}{94.5} \end{array} \right]$$

$$= [0.57 + 0.64 + 2.42 + 0.96 + 0.20 + 1.95 + 2.53 + 1.32 + 7.43]$$

$$= 18.02$$

(vi) Interpret the calculated χ^2 statistic

As in all statistical analyses, the validity of the null hypothesis is challenged by comparing the calculated statistic to the critical statistic, as defined by the null hypothesis. The value of the critical χ^2 statistic is dependent on the level of significance ($\alpha = 0.05$) and the number of degrees of freedom. The equation that is employed to calculate the number of degrees of freedom has been previously given in Chapter 8 as $df = (R - 1)(C - 1)$, where R and C denote the number of rows and columns, respectively.

Using this equation, we find that the number of degrees of freedom associated with Example 11.1 is $(3 - 1) \times (3 - 1) = 4$. From Appendix 3, the critical χ^2 statistic ($\chi^2_{(\alpha=0.05, 4df)}$) is 9.49. The null hypothesis is accepted when the calculated χ^2 statistic is less than the critical χ^2 statistic but rejected in preference to the alternative hypothesis when $\chi^2_{calculated} \geqslant \chi^2_{critical}$. In Example 11.1 $\chi^2_{calculated}$ (18.02) is greater than $\chi^2_{critical}$ (9.49) and, accordingly, the null hypothesis is rejected. It may therefore be concluded that there is a preference for a particular shape or type of solid dosage form among respondents in different age groups.

This conclusion highlights one of the problems associated with the χ^2 analysis of data that is composed of more than two rows and columns, i.e. we have identified that a significant relationship exists but there is no direct evidence of the nature of the preference. To gain a further insight into the nature of the relationship it is usual to examine the contribution of the χ^2 values of each individual cell to the overall χ^2 statistic and, in addition, to compare the sums of the χ^2 values of the individual factors. The individual χ^2 values associated with the data presented in Table 11.1 are shown in Table 11.3. As may be observed, the summed χ^2 values associated with the round tablet (3.63) and the caplet (3.11) are similar, but the value associated with the capsule is markedly greater (11.28). Furthermore, although there is a difference between the summed χ^2 values associated with the 20–35 years and 35–50 years age groups, the value associated with the 50–65 years group is markedly greater (11.80). We may therefore conclude that the major preference for shape or type of solid dosage form is associated with respondents in the 50–65 years age group. Furthermore, this older age group preferred

Table 11.3 χ^2 values associated with preferences for different shapes of solid dosage forms stated by different age groups of respondents

Tablet shape	χ^2 values associated with age group (years)			Totals
	20–35	36–50	51–65	
Round	0.57	0.64	2.42	3.63
Caplet	0.96	0.20	1.95	3.11
Capsule	2.53	1.32	7.43	11.28
Totals	4.06	2.16	11.80	18.02

the capsule to either the caplet or the conventional round tablet.

11.2 Kruskal–Wallis test

In section 10.2 the analysis of variance (ANOVA) was introduced as a statistical test to examine for differences between three or more samples. For this reason it is referred to as a *multiple hypothesis test*. This technique was shown to be more powerful than performing a series of two-sample tests to examine the validity of the individual null hypotheses. ANOVA is one of the most powerful statistical techniques available to the statistical analyst, but its use, like that of other parametric tests, is permitted only when the conditions of the experimental design are compatible with the assumptions of the test:

- The populations from which the data have been sampled are normally distributed.
- The populations from which the data have been sampled possess similar variances.
- The data must be measured on at least an interval scale, with an underlying continuous distribution.
- There must be a large number of recorded observations per sample group.

ANOVA is reasonably robust and, accordingly may be employed even when there are moderate departures from the assumptions of normality or equal variances. However, if the sample size is small, it is difficult to accurately predict the nature of the population and therefore ANOVA should not be used. Similarly, as ANOVA relies on arithmetic manipulations of the data sets to generate the mean and standard deviation of each sample, this technique may not be employed when the data is nominal or ordinal in nature. When the underlying assumptions of ANOVA have been violated, a non-parametric test that uses an identical design is employed. The non-parametric equivalent to one-way ANOVA is the *Kruskal–Wallis test*. In light of the importance of this technique, the underlying theory and the applications of this technique will be fully explained using pharmaceutical examples.

In the Kruskal–Wallis test, three or more independent groups of data are collected and the differences between these sets of data estimated. The mechanics of the test are similar to those of other related techniques, such as the Mann–Whitney U test, and involve ranking each individual datum. Using a defined formula, the sums of the ranks within each treatment are used to calculate a test statistic, which is, in turn, used to examine the validity of the null hypothesis. This process is described in the following example.

EXAMPLE 11.2 *Antibiotic-containing intramammary dosage forms are employed for the treatment and prophylaxis of infection in the udders of cattle. One issue in the development of these dosage forms for administration to dry (pregnant) cows is the milk withdrawal time, i.e. the period over which the first milk produced by the cows must be disposed of because it contains unacceptably high concentrations of antibiotic. Financially, farmers would prefer to use formulations that have as low a withdrawal time as possible as this ensures minimal wastage of milk. A research and development company has formulated an intramammary product for dry cows and wishes to investigate the milk withdrawal time of this product and compare this to three other commercially available products. All products contain the same concentration of a particular antibiotic. A clinical study has been arranged in which the four products are administered each to six individual cattle. The milk is then collected at regular intervals and the time required for the concentration of antibiotic in milk to fall below a defined limit measured. The results of the clinical trial are shown in Table 11.4. Using an appropriate statistical method, comment on the comparative milk withdrawal periods of the four intramammary products.*

Before data collection begins, the key points of the experimental design are documented.

(i) State the null hypothesis

Non-parametric tests do not use population parameters for the definition of the null and alternative hypotheses. Therefore, in light of this, a suitable null hypothesis for Example 11.2 is that there are no differences between the elimination times of the four products, i.e. all four products require the same milk withdrawal period.

Table 11.4 Milk withdrawal periods (h) associated with the single administration of four antibiotic-containing intramammary products

Product A	Product B	Product C	Product D
70	97	98	65
96	94	102	62
54	78	81	69
56	83	76	75
86	71	100	59
72	85	91	66

(ii) State the alternative hypothesis

A suitable alternative for the clinical study is that the four products do not require the same milk withdrawal period.

(iii) State the level of significance

In this example, it is assumed that the level of significance (α) is 0.05.

(iv) Select the most appropriate statistical test

In the experimental design, there is one independent variable, namely the antibiotic-containing intramammary formulations, of which there are four sub-categories under examination (products A, B, C and D). As the study has been designed to examine the comparative milk withdrawal periods of these four products, this is an example of a multiple comparison test. As described in section 10.2, it is improper to perform a series of two-sample comparisons and, therefore a statistical test should be used that will simultaneously examine the differences or similarities between all four treatments (products). The two most commonly used tests that are available to the statistical analyst are one-way ANOVA and the Kruskal–Wallis test. Which is the more appropriate here? To address this question, the data associated with each treatment must be thoroughly examined to identify whether the properties are compatible with the assumptions of ANOVA. In particular, the normality of the populations from which the samples have been derived, equivalence of variances of the parent populations, nature of the measured data and the number of observations per sample group must be considered. Each of these points should be examined individually.

To estimate the normality of the parent populations, it is useful to calculate and compare the means and medians of each data set. As stated previously, this is not a definitive measure of normality, but it is a useful estimation of this important property. The mean and median milk withdrawal times associated with the four products are shown in Table 11.5. The variance of each sample has also been included and will be discussed later. The means and medians of each group are, for the most part, similar and we will therefore assume that the populations from which the data have been sampled are normally distributed. A second important consideration is whether (or not) the samples possess similar variances. As previously discussed, there are statistical tests that will examine homogeneity or heterogeneity of variances (e.g. Bartlett's test), but there are limitations that often prohibit their use. However, visual inspection of the variances associated with the four treatments should raise suspicions about possible differences between the variances

Table 11.5 Summary of the descriptive statistics for the milk withdrawal times associated with the use of four dry-cow antibiotic-containing intramammary products

Measure of central tendency/variance	Product A	Product B	Product C	Product D
Mean (h)	72.3	84.7	91.3	66.0
Median (h)	71.0	84.0	94.5	65.5
Variance (h²)	271.1	94.7	115.1	31.2

of the products. Therefore, for the purpose of this example, it will be assumed that the variances of the four products are sufficiently dissimilar to compromise the use of the parametric ANOVA.

Summarising these concerns, we may conclude that the use of ANOVA would be inappropriate because of the possible dissimilarities of variances, so a non-parametric multiple-hypothesis test should be employed. As there is only one independent variable, the most appropriate statistical test to compare the milk withdrawal times associated with the use of the four products is the Kruskal–Wallis test.

(v) Perform the statistical test

The Kruskal–Wallis test may conveniently be executed in a stepwise fashion.

Step 1   Assign ranks to each observation
The Kruskal–Wallis test is a ranking test, so the first step is to pool all observations, ranking each individual observation and returning the ranks to the original treatment group. This process is shown in Table 11.6 for the data described in Table 11.4.

Table 11.6 Milk withdrawal times associated with the single administration of four antibiotic-containing intramammary products, illustrating the rank of individual observations

Product A		Product B		Product C		Product D	
Time (h)	Rank	Time (h)	Rank	Time (h)	Rank	Time (h)	Rank
70	8	97	21	98	22	65	5
96	20	94	19	102	23	62	4
54	1	78	13	81	14	69	7
56	2	83	15	76	12	75	11
86	17	71	9	100	24	59	3
72	10	85	16	91	18	66	6

Step 2   Calculate the sum of ranks associated with each treatment
This is performed by adding together each of the assigned ranks associated with a particular treatment. The sum of ranks (R) for each treatment is as follows:

$$\Sigma R_{\text{product A}} = (8 + 20 + 1 + 2 + 17 + 10) = 58$$
$$\Sigma R_{\text{product B}} = (21 + 19 + 13 + 15 + 9 + 16) = 93$$
$$\Sigma R_{\text{product C}} = (22 + 23 + 14 + 12 + 24 + 18) = 113$$
$$\Sigma R_{\text{product D}} = (5 + 4 + 7 + 11 + 3 + 6) = 36$$

Step 3   Calculate the between-groups sum of squares
The between-groups sum of squares (SS_{BG}) is calculated using the following equation:

$$SS_{BG} = \frac{(R_{\text{Product A}})^2}{N_{\text{Product A}}} + \frac{(R_{\text{Product B}})^2}{N_{\text{Product B}}} + \frac{(R_{\text{Product C}})^2}{N_{\text{Product C}}} + \frac{(R_{\text{Product D}})^2}{N_{\text{Product D}}}$$

where R is the sum of ranks associated with a particular treatment and N is the number of observations within a treatment group. The between-groups sum of squares in Example 11.2 is therefore:

$$SS_{BG} = \frac{(58)^2}{6} + \frac{(93)^2}{6} + \frac{(113)^2}{6} + \frac{(36)^2}{6} = 4346.3$$

Step 4   Calculate the Kruskal–Wallis statistic
The Kruskal–Wallis statistic (H) is calculated using the following formula:

$$H = \frac{12}{N(N+1)} \times SS_{BG} - 3(N+1)$$

where N is the total number of observations in the study and SS_{BG} is the between-groups sum of squares, as calculated in step 3. Inserting the relevant information into this equation allows calculation of the Kruskal–Wallis statistic:

$$H = \frac{12}{N(N+1)} \times SS_{BG} - 3(N+1)$$

$$= \frac{12}{24(24+1)} \times 4346.3 - 3(24+1) = 11.93$$

Step 5   Identify the critical Kruskal–Wallis statistic
As in other statistical techniques, comparing the calculated test statistic to the critical test statistic, i.e. the value that defines the regions of

acceptance and rejection of the null hypothesis, enables us to interpret the outcome of the experiment. When the experimental design is composed of no more than five treatment groups and the number of observations in each group is five or fewer, tables are available that depict the probability associated with the calculated H statistic. When the number of treatments or the number of observations in each group is more than five (as in Example 11.2), the sampling distribution of the Kruskal–Wallis statistic is approximated by the χ^2 distribution. Accordingly, in this scenario, the χ^2 distribution is used to identify the critical H statistic. To identify the critical value of H using the χ^2 distribution the following information is required:

- the number of degrees of freedom associated with the experimental design, obtained by subtracting 1 from the total number of treatment groups, i.e. $4 - 1 = 3$ in this example
- the level of significance (α), which in this design has been selected as 0.05.

The critical value of $H_{(\alpha = 0.05, 3\ df)}$ is therefore 7.81 (derived from Appendix 3).

Step 6   Interpret the outcome of the statistical analysis
The critical Kruskal–Wallis statistic provides information concerning the regions of acceptance and rejection of the null hypothesis. Accordingly, if the calculated Kruskal–Wallis statistic is less than the critical H statistic (7.81), the null hypothesis is accepted. Conversely, if $H_{\text{calculated}}$ is equal to or greater than H_{critical}, the null hypothesis is rejected in favour of the alternative hypothesis. In Example 11.2, the calculated Kruskal–Wallis statistic (11.93) is greater than the critical statistic (7.81) and, accordingly, the null hypothesis is rejected. Therefore, it may be concluded that the milk withdrawal periods associated with four intramammary products differ.

As in ANOVA, rejection of the null hypothesis can only be interpreted as a general difference in the comparative effects (milk withdrawal times in Example 11.2) of the four treatments. Unfortunately, information concerning the origins of the differences is not apparent. To identify the nature of the difference, one must perform non-parametric multiple comparison (*post-hoc*) tests in a similar fashion to that described for the ANOVA. The use of these tests is described in the next section.

Example 11.2 is a relatively uncomplicated example of the use of the Kruskal–Wallis test to simultaneously compare the similarities or differences between four populations. Two further experimental situations may occur that require clarification: the effects of unequal sample sizes, and the effects of ties on the calculation of the Kruskal–Wallis statistic. The effect of unequal sample sizes is addressed in the original equation that is employed for the calculation of the Kruskal–Wallis statistic. In this, the sum of squares between groups term (R) is determined with reference to the number of observations that are present in each column (treatment). The effect of ties is slightly more complex. The Kruskal–Wallis statistic is affected by the presence of tied values and, to compensate for this, the calculated statistic is divided by a correction factor (CF):

$$H_c = \frac{H}{CF}$$

where H_c is the corrected value of the Kruskal–Wallis statistic, H is the original (non-corrected) value of the Kruskal–Wallis statistic and CF is the correction factor. As before, each tied score is allocated a mean rank score, commensurate with the number of tied values. The correction factor is then calculated:

$$CF = 1 - \frac{\sum (t^3 - t)}{N^3 - N}$$

where t is the number of ties in a particular rank score, $\sum (t^3 - t)$ is the sum of all the individual values of $(t^3 - t)$ for each tied rank score and N is the total number of observations.

Further clarification of the use of the Kruskal–Wallis test in situations where the sample sizes are unequal or there are tied observations is presented in Example 11.3.

EXAMPLE 11.3 *The microbiological quality of water used in the production of a suspension for oral administration is a concern for the pharmaceutical industry. A pharmaceutical company uses three manufacturing suites for the manufacture of three different oral suspension formulations and has decided to examine and compare the total microbiological content of the water supply to the three suites. Samples of water entering each manufacturing vat were removed and the total number of bacteria enumerated using a seed plate technique. The results from these tests are shown in Table 11.7. Using an appropriate statistical method, comment on the comparative bacterial quality of the three water supplies.*

The important points that should be addressed before the study begins are as follows:

(i) State the null hypothesis

The null hypothesis for Example 11.3 states that there is no difference in the numbers of viable bacteria in the three water supplies.

Table 11.7 Total numbers of viable bacteria removed from the water supplies to three vats used in the manufacture of oral suspension preparations

Vat 1	Vat 2	Vat 3
1000	300	120
525	525	50
120	100	650
85	50	500
127	65	100
920	450	55
500	500	400
205	200	500
105		85
		120

(ii) State the alternative hypothesis

The alternative hypothesis states that the three supplies of water differ in their bacterial content.

(iii) State the level of significance

In this example, it is assumed that the level of significance (α) is 0.05.

(iv) Select the most appropriate statistical test

This study is an example of a multiple-sample hypothesis test as three treatments are under simultaneous comparison, and this invalidates the use of all two-sample statistical tests. On further inspection it may be observed that the situation warrants the use of a one-factor multiple-sample hypothesis test. The single factor in the study is the water supply, of which there are three sub-categories. With this information in mind, the reader should have narrowed down the choice of statistical test to either one-way ANOVA or the Kruskal–Wallis test. The next step involves an estimation of the suitability of the data for analysis using parametric ANOVA.

As before, the following points should be individually addressed:

- Have the data been measured on at least an interval scale?
- Is the number of observations in each sample greater than five?
- Are the populations from which the samples have been derived normally distributed?
- Do the populations from which the samples have been derived possess equal variances?

In this study, the data have been measured on a ratio scale and the sample size is sufficiently large to allow a parametric comparison. The normality of the parent populations may be estimated by comparing the mean and median for each treatment group (Table 11.8). The variances of the samples have been included in this table and their homogeneity is discussed later.

From Table 11.8, it may be observed that the mean and median values associated with manufacturing vats 1 and 3 are dissimilar, thereby raising doubts about the normality of the populations from which these observations have been sampled. Furthermore, there is concern about the possible heterogeneity of the variances of the three treatment groups. This raises serious doubts about the validity of ANOVA for analysis of the results of the study. Therefore, the most appropriate statistical method to examine the null hypothesis associated with Example 11.3 is the Kruskal–Wallis test.

(v) Perform the statistical test

The Kruskal–Wallis test is performed using the stepwise approach introduced in Example 11.2.

Step 1   Assign ranks to each observation
The data is pooled, ranked and returned to the original treatment groups, as shown in Table 11.9.

Step 2   Calculate the sum of ranks associated with each treatment
The sum of ranks (R) for each treatment is as follows:

$$\Sigma R_{vat\,1} = (27 + 23.5 + 11 + 5.5 + 13 + 26 + 20.5 + 15 + 9)$$
$$= 150.5$$
$$\Sigma R_{vat\,2} = (16 + 23.5 + 7.5 + 1.5 + 4 + 18 + 20.5 + 14)$$
$$= 105.0$$
$$\Sigma R_{vat\,3} = (11 + 1.5 + 25 + 20.5 + 7.5 + 3 + 17 + 20.5 + 5.5 + 11)$$
$$= 122.5$$

Table 11.8 Summary of the central tendency and variances of the data for the number of viable bacteria removed from water supplies to three vats used in the manufacture of oral suspension preparations

Measure of central tendency/variance	Vat 1	Vat 2	Vat 3
Mean	398.6	273.8	258.0
Median	205.0	250.0	120.0
Variance	129 151.3	39 333.9	52 045.6

Table 11.9 Numbers of viable bacteria removed from the water supplies to three vats used in the manufacture of three oral suspension preparations, illustrating the rank of each individual observation

Vat 1		Vat 2		Vat 3	
Number of viable bacteria	Rank	Number of viable bacteria	Rank	Number of viable bacteria	Rank
1000	27	300	16	120	11
525	23.5	525	23.5	50	1.5
120	11	100	7.5	650	25
85	5.5	50	1.5	500	20.5
127	13	65	4	100	7.5
920	26	450	18	55	3
500	20.5	500	20.5	400	17
205	15	200	14	500	20.5
105	9			85	5.5
				120	11

Step 3 *Calculate the between-groups sum of squares*
The between-groups sum of squares (SS_{BG}) is calculated as follows:

$$SS_{BG} = \frac{(R_{vat\ 1})^2}{N_{vat\ 1}} + \frac{(R_{vat\ 2})^2}{N_{vat\ 2}} + \frac{(R_{vat\ 3})^2}{N_{vat\ 3}}$$

Inserting the data from step 2, the between-groups sum of squares is therefore:

$$SS_{BG} = \frac{(150.5)^2}{9} + \frac{(105.0)^2}{8} + \frac{(122.5)^2}{10} = 5395.4$$

Note that the above calculation has considered the effects of different sample sizes by using the individual sample sizes as the denominators.

Step 4 *Calculate the uncorrected Kruskal–Wallis statistic*
With knowledge of the between-groups sum of squares, the Kruskal–Wallis statistic is computed:

$$H = \frac{12}{N(N + 1)} \times SS_{BG} - 3(N + 1)$$

$$= \frac{12}{27(27 + 1)} \times 5395.4 - 3(27 + 1) = 1.64$$

Step 5 *Calculate the correction factor*
There are tied ranks in Example 11.3. The Kruskal–Wallis statistic calculated in step 4 is therefore a biased estimate and the calculated statistic

must be corrected for the effect of ties. Mathematically, the correction factor was defined above as

$$CF = 1 - \frac{\sum (t^3 - t)}{N^3 - N}$$

where t is the number of ties in a particular rank score, $\sum (t^3 - t)$ is the sum of all the individual values of $(t^3 - t)$ for each tied rank score and N is the total number of observations. This equation may now be employed to calculate the correction factor for the effects of tied ranks in Example 11.3. To assist in this procedure, the tied ranks should be abstracted from Table 11.9, as follows:

1.5, 1.5

5.5, 5.5

7.5, 7.5

11, 11, 11

20.5, 20.5, 20.5, 20.5

23.5, 23.5

Bearing in mind that t is the number of ties in a particular rank score, the term $\sum(t^3 - t)$ is calculated:

$$\begin{aligned} \sum(t^3 - t) &= (2^3 - 2) + (2^3 - 2) + (2^3 - 2) \\ &\quad + (3^3 - 3) + (4^3 - 4) + (2^3 - 2) \\ &= (6) + (6) + (6) + (24) + (60) + (6) \\ &= 108 \end{aligned}$$

Using this information, the magnitude of the correction factor is determined:

$$CF = 1 - \frac{\sum (t^3 - t)}{N^3 - N} = 1 - \frac{108}{(27^3 - 27)} = 0.995$$

Step 6   Calculate the corrected Kruskal–Wallis statistic
The corrected Kruskal–Wallis statistic (H_c) is calculated as the ratio of the uncorrected statistic (H) to the correction factor, i.e.:

$$H_c = \frac{H}{CF} = \frac{1.64}{0.995} = 1.65$$

Although there are several tied values in Example 11.3, their overall effect is small. Only when there are a large number of ties does the correction factor appreciably affect the value of the uncorrected Kruskal–Wallis statistic. However, it is good statistical practice always to calculate the corrected Kruskal–Wallis statistic and to use this in interpreting the outcome of the statistical analysis.

Step 7   Identify the critical Kruskal–Wallis statistic
The reader will remember from the previous example that there are two possible tables from which the critical Kruskal–Wallis statistic may be determined: the critical values of the Kruskal–Wallis H distribution and the χ^2 distribution. To clarify the issue of which table to use, one must consider both the number of treatments and the number of observations per treatment. The table that describes the critical values of the Kruskal–Wallis H distribution is used when the number of observations in each treatment is small (usually less than five) or when the number of treatment groups is less than or equal to five. Conversely, the χ^2 distribution is employed to identify the critical test statistic when the number of observations in the treatment groups or the number of treatment groups exceeds five. In Example 11.3, there are only three treatment groups, but the number of observations in each group is sufficiently large to enable us to use the χ^2 distribution to determine the critical test statistic.

To identify the critical value of H using the χ^2 distribution, we need to know both the number of degrees of freedom associated with the experimental design and the level of significance. In this study there are 2 *df* (number of treatments – 1) and the level of significance is 0.05. Therefore the critical value of $H_{(\alpha = 0.05, 2\, df)}$ is 5.99.

Step 8   Interpret the outcome of the statistical analysis
As in all other tests, the critical statistic provides information on the regions of acceptance and rejection of the null hypothesis within the critical values of the χ^2 distribution. In Example 11.3, the calculated corrected Kruskal–Wallis statistic (1.65) is less than the critical statistic (5.99) and, accordingly, the null hypothesis is accepted. Therefore, it may be concluded that there is no difference in the bacterial content of the water supplies the three manufacturing vats.

One final experimental application of the Kruskal–Wallis test involves the analysis of data within a one-factor experimental design in which the number of observations in each treatment group is small. The mechanics of the test are identical to those described in Examples 11.2 and 11.3, but this time interpreting the outcome of the statistical analysis involves the use of the table of critical values of the Kruskal–Wallis H distribution. Furthermore, a characteristic trait of many published pharmaceutical studies using the one-factor design is the use of triplicate or quadruplicate measurements (replicates).

Example 11.4 typifies a statistical method that may be used to examine the validity of the null hypothesis in these situations. It should be stressed, however, that this is not the only test that may be applied under such experimental conditions.

EXAMPLE 11.4 *A clinical laboratory wishes to examine the elimination rate of an antimicrobial agent from the oral cavity following administration as a mouthwash. In particular, the laboratory is interested in the effect of concentration of antimicrobial agent on the elimination rate. Resources are limited, so the laboratory has decided to perform a clinical trial involving only 15 volunteers. The volunteers were divided into 4 groups and each group received a single administration of a mouthwash containing a defined concentration of antimicrobial agent. Saliva samples were collected for a period of 12 h after administration and the mass of antimicrobial agent present in the samples measured using high-performance liquid chromatography (HPLC). The elimination of the therapeutic agent was observed to follow first-order elimination kinetics, as shown in Table 11.10. Using an appropriate statistical method, determine whether or not the concentration of antimicrobial agent in the mouthwash formulations affected the elimination rate of the antimicrobial agent from the oral cavity.*

As before, the statistical nature of the study should be elucidated.

(i) State the null hypothesis

The null hypothesis for this study states that the elimination rate of the antimicrobial agent from the oral cavity is not dependent on the initial concentration of therapeutic agent administered as a mouthwash formulation. Alternatively, it may be stated that the elimination rate of the antimicrobial agent from the oral cavity will be similar for all four formulations.

Table 11.10 Effects of concentration of an antimicrobial agent on the subsequent elimination rate from the oral cavity after administration as a mouthwash

Formulation A (0.01% w/w)	Formulation B (0.05% w/w)	Formulation B (0.1% w/w)	Formulation C (0.5% w/w)
14.5	39.4	120.5	190.6
25.1	87.2	139.8	165.7
42.5	80.7	145.7	210.4
29.9	60.7	176.9	

Values in parentheses indicate the concentration of antimicrobial agent in the mouthwash formulations.

(ii) State the alternative hypothesis

A suitable alternative hypothesis for this study is that the elimination rate of the antimicrobial agent from the oral cavity is different for all four formulations, i.e. the elimination rate of the antimicrobial agent from the oral cavity is dependent on the initial concentration of the agent in the formulation.

(iii) State the level of significance

In this example, it is assumed that the level of significance (α) is 0.05.

(iv) Select the most appropriate statistical test

The selection of the most appropriate statistical test for the analysis of the data presented in Table 11.10 is relatively straightforward. This experimental design is another example of a one-factor multiple-sample analysis, in which there are four sub-categories within the single independent variable. Furthermore, the sample size in each of the treatment groups is relatively small, i.e. no more than four in all cases. In light of this it is difficult to assume that the populations from which the data have been sampled are normally distributed. Furthermore, owing to the small sample sizes, the sample variances may not provide reliable estimation of the population variances. Accordingly, it is difficult to satisfy two of the major assumptions of the ANOVA, i.e. the data have been sampled from normally distributed populations and that the variances of the parent populations are similar. Under these circumstances it is more appropriate (conservative) to statistically compare the effects of concentration on the elimination rate of an antimicrobial agent from the oral cavity following administration as a mouthwash using a non-parametric, one-factor multiple-sample hypothesis test, i.e. the Kruskal–Wallis test.

(v) Perform the statistical test

Step 1   Assign ranks to each observation
The data is pooled, ranked and returned to the original treatment groups, as shown in Table 11.11.

Step 2   Calculate the sum of ranks associated with each treatment
The sum of ranks (R) for each treatment is as follows:

$$\Sigma R_{\text{formulation A}} = (1 + 2 + 5 + 3) = 11$$
$$\Sigma R_{\text{formulation B}} = (4 + 8 + 7 + 6) = 25$$
$$\Sigma R_{\text{formulation C}} = (9 + 10 + 11 + 13) = 43$$
$$\Sigma R_{\text{formulation D}} = (14 + 12 + 15) = 41$$

Table 11.11 Effects of concentration of an antimicrobial agent on the subsequent elimination rate from the oral cavity after administration as a mouthwash, illustrating the rank of each individual observation

Formulation A (0.01% w/w)		Formulation B (0.05% w/w)		Formulation C (0.10% w/w)		Formulation D (0.50% w/w)	
Elimination rate (min^{-1})	Rank	Elimination (min^{-1})	Rank	Elimination rate (min^{-1})	Rank	Elimination rate (min^{-1})	Rank
14.5	1	39.4	4	120.5	9	190.6	14
25.1	2	87.2	8	139.8	10	165.7	12
42.5	5	80.7	7	145.7	11	210.4	15
29.9	3	60.7	6	176.9	13		

Step 3   Calculate the between-groups sum of squares
As before, the between-groups sum of squares (SS_{BG}) is determined using the following formula:

$$SS_{BG} = \frac{(R_{Formulation\ A})^2}{N_{Formulation\ A}} + \frac{(R_{Formulation\ B})^2}{N_{Formulation\ B}} + \frac{(R_{Formulation\ C})^2}{N_{Formulation\ C}} + \frac{(R_{Formulation\ D})^2}{N_{Formulation\ D}}$$

Inserting the data from step 2, the between-groups sum of squares is calculated as

$$SS_{BG} = \frac{(11)^2}{4} + \frac{(25)^2}{4} + \frac{(43)^2}{4} + \frac{(41)^2}{3} = 1209.1$$

Step 4   Calculate the Kruskal–Wallis statistic

$$H = \frac{12}{N(N+1)} \times SS_{BG} - 3(N+1)$$

$$= \frac{12}{15(15+1)} \times 1209.1 - 3(15+1) = 12.46$$

Step 5   Identify the critical Kruskal–Wallis statistic
In this example, there are four treatment groups with three or four observations in each. It is therefore more appropriate to use the table describing the critical values of the Kruskal–Wallis statistic to determine the critical test statistic. This table is shown in Appendix 15. To identify the critical value of H from this table requires knowledge both of the number of observations in each treatment (4, 4, 4 and 3) and the chosen level of significance (0.05). Given this information, the critical value of $H_{(\alpha = 0.05, 4, 4, 4, 3)}$ is therefore 7.14.

Step 6 Interpret the outcome of the statistical analysis
The critical statistic defines the regions of acceptance and rejection of the null hypothesis. If the calculated H statistic is less than the critical statistic, the null hypothesis is accepted, but if it is equal to or greater than the critical statistic, the alternative hypothesis is accepted. In Example 11.4, $H_{calculated}$ (12.46) > $H_{critical}$ (7.14) and, accordingly, the null hypothesis is rejected in favour of the alternative hypothesis. Therefore, it may be concluded the concentration of antimicrobial agent in a formulation affects its elimination from the oral cavity following administration as a mouthwash.

11.3 Friedman's test

Friedman's test is the non-parametric test that is employed for the analysis of data that have been collected in the form of a randomised block design or a one-factor repeated-measures design. In this respect the test may be considered to be the non-parametric equivalent of two-way ANOVA (without replication) or one-way repeated-measures ANOVA. As with the Kruskal–Wallis test, Friedman's test is employed to analyse such experimental designs when the data do not conform to the assumptions of ANOVA. For example, it may be improper to assume that the populations from which the data have been sampled are normally distributed, or that the variances of the populations possess similar variances. Furthermore, the data may be ordinal in nature. The basis hypothesis of Friedman's test is that the various treatments have been sampled either from the same population or from identical independent populations. In this respect, it is assumed that the ranks associated with each column are similar. A typical experimental design that may be analysed using Friedman's test is described in Example 11.5.

EXAMPLE 11.5 *A company that specialises in the research and development of novel drug delivery systems has developed an antibiotic-impregnated polymeric strip designed for attachment to the teeth, from which a therapeutic agent may be released into the oral cavity in a controlled fashion for the treatment of infective disorders of the superficial tissues. The company has designed a small clinical trial to examine the in vivo release properties of this system in which a polymeric strip is attached to the outer surface of a lower molar tooth of human volunteers. Saliva samples are collected from the patients at defined periods and the mass of therapeutic agent quantified using an appropriate analytical method. The results from the clinical study are shown in Table 11.12. The company wishes to claim that the release of drug into*

Table 11.12 Concentration (μg/mL) of therapeutic agent in saliva at defined time intervals after attachment of a drug-containing polymeric strip to the outer surface of a tooth

Patient number	Time after attachment			
	1 day	2 days	3 days	4 days
1	25.45	23.47	20.77	20.87
2	39.57	35.78	34.99	34.90
3	15.42	13.21	12.24	10.16
4	7.19	5.99	5.93	6.06
5	58.23	49.27	42.58	44.53
6	25.60	23.64	21.58	21.89

the oral cavity is constant over the first 4 days after attachment of the drug delivery system to the tooth. Using an appropriate statistical method, examine the validity of this claim.

The parameters associated with the experimental design are stated before data collection.

(i) State the null hypothesis

The null hypothesis for this study states that the concentration of therapeutic agent in saliva is constant for 4 days after attachment of the polymeric strips to the tooth surface of human volunteers

(ii) State the alternative hypothesis

A suitable alternative hypothesis for Example 11.5 is that the release of therapeutic agent from the polymeric strips is not constant for 4 days after attachment to the tooth surface of human volunteers, thereby invalidating the claim by the company.

(iii) State the level of significance

In this example, it is assumed that the level of significance (α) is 0.05.

(iv) Select the most appropriate statistical test

The experimental design described in Example 11.5 is recognisable as either a two-factor (independent variables) analysis without replication or, alternatively, a one-factor analysis with repeated measures. In the former, the two factors are the time of sampling (of which there are four sub-categories) and the patients (of which there are six sub-categories). In the latter design, the single factor is the time of sampling. The reader may recall that the repeated-measures one-factor analysis is, in effect, a paired experimental design. Therefore, in Example 11.5, each patient is acting as their own control, thereby reducing the overall error within the experiment. This is why the data described in Example 11.5 should not be analysed as a standard one-factor analysis, e.g. using a one-way ANOVA or the Kruskal–Wallis test. Therefore, two-way ANOVA or Friedman's test may be suitable methods to examine the validity of the null hypothesis. The choice of which of these two tests is more appropriate depends, as in previous examples, on whether the data conforms to the assumptions of parametric analysis. For the purpose of this section, we will assume that the requirements of the two way ANOVA are not met by the data described in Table 11.11 and, accordingly, the most appropriate statistical method to examine the validity of the null hypothesis is Friedman's test.

(v) Perform the statistical test

As previously stated, Friedman' test is another ranking test and therefore the reader should not be surprised to read that the first step in the execution of this test involves ranking the data. Unlike the Kruskal–Wallis test, the ranking procedure is performed across the rows and not down the columns. Therefore, the ranks for each treatment for

Table 11.13 Concentration (μg/mL) of therapeutic agent in saliva at defined time intervals after attachment of a drug-containing polymeric strip to the outer surface of a tooth, highlighting the ranks associated with each row

	Time after attachment			
Patient number	1 day	2 days	3 days	4 days
1	25.45	23.47	20.77	20.87
Rank for 1	4	3	1	2
2	39.57	35.78	34.99	34.90
Rank for 2	4	3	2	1
3	15.42	13.21	12.24	10.16
Rank for 3	4	3	2	1
4	7.19	5.99	5.93	6.06
Rank for 4	4	3	1	2
5	58.23	49.27	42.58	44.53
Rank for 5	4	3	1	2
6	25.60	23.64	21.58	21.89
Rank for 6	4	3	1	2
Sum of ranks (R)	24	18	8	10

each individual patient are recorded. The ranking process for Example 11.5 is shown in Table 11.13.

In Friedman's test the rank sums of the columns are used to calculate the test statistic (χ_r^2), using the following formula:

$$\chi_r^2 = \frac{12}{N_{rows}N_{columns}(N_{columns}+1)} \sum R^2 - 3N_{rows}(N_{columns}+1)$$

where N_{rows} and $N_{columns}$ denote the number of rows and columns, respectively, in the experimental design and $\sum R^2$ is the sum of the square of the individual ranks for each column. The Friedman test statistic may now be calculated, as follows:

$$\chi_r^2 = \left(\frac{12}{N_{rows}N_{columns}(N_{columns}+1)} \right)$$
$$\times (R^2_{1\,day} + R^2_{2\,days} + R^2_{3\,days} + R^2_{4\,days}) - 3N_{rows}(N_{columns}+1)$$

Inserting the data from Table 11.12 into the above equation gives

$$\chi_r^2 = \left(\frac{12}{6 \times 4(4+1)} \right) \times (24^2 + 18^2 + 8^2 + 10^2) - 3 \times 6(4+1) = 16.4$$

(vi) Identify the critical Friedman statistic

Once more an important stage in the process of statistical hypothesis testing is the identification of the critical test statistic. As in the Kruskal–Wallis test, identification of the test statistic associated with Friedman's test involves the use of one of two possible tables. A table may be used in which the critical values associated with the test statistic (χ_r^2) are defined for certain combinations of numbers of rows and columns. In particular, this table (Appendix 16) defines values of χ_r^2 when the number of columns and the number of rows are relatively small. Tables are available that provide critical values of χ_r^2 associated with higher variations of $N_{columns}$ and N_{rows}, but one can also define the critical value using the χ^2 distribution, as χ_r^2 is assumed to be distributed in a similar fashion to this distribution.

In Example 11.5, $N_{columns}$ and N_{rows} are 4 and 6, respectively, so the critical values of the χ_r^2 distribution will be used to determine the critical test statistic. This requires knowledge of the following experimental attributes:

- the level of significance, defined previously as 0.05
- the number of columns (4)
- the number of rows (6).

We can therefore see from the table in Appendix 16 that the critical test statistic is 7.60.

(vii) Interpret the statistical outcome

The null hypothesis is accepted or rejected by comparing the calculated test statistic to the abstracted critical test statistic. If the calculated test statistic is less than the critical test statistic, the null hypothesis is accepted. The calculated and critical test statistics are 16.4 and 7.60 and, accordingly, the null hypothesis is rejected in favour of the alternative hypothesis. Therefore, constant release of the therapeutic agent from the polymeric strips *in vivo* was not observed in this clinical study. Interestingly, if the sample size or the number of treatment groups is large enough for us to assume that Friedman's test statistic (χ_r^2) is distributed in a similar fashion to the χ^2 distribution, the outcome would be the same. In this case the critical χ^2 statistic is defined by the following parameters:

- the level of significance (0.05)
- the number of degrees of freedom (number of columns − 1 = 4 − 1 = 3).

On the basis of this information, the critical χ^2 statistic may be ascertained from Appendix 3 as 7.81 and, as the calculated statistic exceeded this value, the null hypothesis is rejected. The difference in the two test statistics may be attributed to the limitation of the assumption that, for the numbers of rows and columns, χ_r^2 is distributed in a similar fashion to the χ^2 distribution. It is obvious that larger samples are required to fulfil this assumption.

The next example provides the reader with a further description of the mechanics and application of Friedman's test.

EXAMPLE 11.6 *The owner of a chain of retail pharmacies wishes to compare the productivity of three locum pharmacists in a series of pharmacies within a particular city. Therefore, over the course of several weeks, the owner has assigned each pharmacist to work in different pharmacies on a defined day of the week and the number of prescription items dispensed by each pharmacist is recorded. The results of this study are shown in Table 11.14. The owner of the pharmacies believes that the productivities of the three pharmacists are different. Using an appropriate statistical method, examine the validity of this claim.*

The properties of the experimental design should be defined before the collection of data.

Table 11.14 The number of prescription items dispensed per day by three pharmacists in different pharmacies within a city

Location of pharmacy	Number of items dispensed		
	Pharmacist 1	Pharmacist 2	Pharmacist 3
North Street	108	108	115
West Street	76	84	85
High Street	157	164	168
Market Street	104	101	103

(i) State the null hypothesis

The null hypothesis for this study states that the productivities of the three pharmacists, defined as the number of prescription items dispensed per day, are similar.

(ii) State the alternative hypothesis

A suitable alternative hypothesis for this investigation states that the productivities of the three pharmacists are dissimilar, i.e. there are differences in the number of prescription items that the pharmacists dispense per day

(iii) State the level of significance

In this example, it is assumed that the level of significance (α) is 0.05.

(iv) Select the most appropriate statistical test

The experimental design described in Example 11.6 is an example of either a two-factor analysis without replication, in which the pharmacist and the pharmacy are the two independent variables, or alternatively, a one-factor analysis with replication, in which the repeated factor is the pharmacist. The two possible statistical methods that may be employed for the resolution of the posed problem are therefore either the one-way repeated-measures ANOVA or Friedman's test. The reader should have recognised that neither one-way ANOVA nor the Kruskal–Wallis test is suitable, because of the paired nature of the experimental design. The use of these methods would increase the experimental error, as a result of the large inter-pharmacy differences. Each pharmacy has an average number of prescription items dispensed in a working day, and this number will vary from one location to the other. A suitable statistical method should be able to accommodate this variability without adversely affecting the probability of making a type I error.

Returning to the choice of either parametric or non-parametric multiple-sample tests for the analysis of data presented in Table 11.14, it will be assumed that, because of the small number of observations recorded in the investigation, Friedman's test is more suitable. Under such circumstances it is difficult to assume normality and equal variances of the parent populations, and therefore the non-parametric test is a safer option.

(v) Perform the statistical test

Step 1 Rank the data across each treatment
The outcome of the ranking process for the data shown in Table 11.14 is shown in Table 11.15. There is one set of ties within the data set in this table. Unlike the Kruskal–Wallis test, no compensation for tied values is required in Friedman's test, so it is customary to replace the tied values with their average rank values. As may be observed from Table 11.15, the tied values were recorded along the row associated with the pharmacy in North Street (108 prescription items per day) and each of these values was replaced with an average rank (1.5).

Step 2 Calculate Friedman's test statistic

$$\chi_r^2 = \left(\frac{12}{N_{rows}N_{columns}(N_{columns}+1)}\right)$$
$$\times (R_{Pharmacist\,1}^2 + R_{Pharmacist\,2}^2 + R_{Pharmacist\,3}^2) - 3N_{rows}(N_{columns}+1)$$

Inserting the data from Table 11.15 into this equation,

$$\chi_r^2 = \left(\frac{12}{4 \times 3(3+1)}\right) \times (6.5^2 + 6.5^2 + 11^2) - 3 \times 4(3+1) = 3.38$$

Table 11.15 The number of prescription items dispensed by three pharmacists in different pharmacies within a city, highlighting the ranks associated with each row

Location of pharmacy	Number of items dispensed		
	Pharmacist 1	Pharmacist 2	Pharmacist 3
North Street	108	108	115
Rank for North Street	1.5	1.5	3
West Street	76	84	85
Rank for West Street	1	2	3
High Street	157	164	168
Rank for High Street	1	2	3
Market Street	104	101	103
Rank for Market Street	3	1	2
Sum of ranks (R)	6.5	6.5	11.0

(vi) Identify the critical Friedman statistic

The value of the critical test statistic may be abstracted directly from the table of the critical values of Friedman's χ_r^2 statistic (Appendix 16). Because of the small sample size (rows and columns), the value obtained from this table is more accurate than the value that may be derived from the table of the critical values of the χ^2 statistic. Therefore, it is important to employ the table that is more appropriate to the conditions of the experimental design in the identification of the critical test statistic. As before, the use of the table of the critical values of the χ_r^2 statistic requires knowledge only of the number of rows, number of columns and the level of significance (0.05). In Example 11.6, the numbers of rows and columns are 4 and 3, respectively, and therefore it may be observed from Appendix 16 that the critical χ_r^2 statistic is 6.50.

(vii) Interpret the statistical outcome

The outcome of the experimental scenario posed in Example 11.6 is interpreted, as before, by comparing the magnitude of the calculated χ_r^2 statistic to the critical χ_r^2 statistic found by reference to the table of critical values of this statistic. In (v) and (vi) above, the calculated and critical χ_r^2 statistics were determined as 3.38 and 6.50, respectively. As the calculated χ_r^2 statistic was lower than the critical χ_r^2 statistic, the null hypothesis is accepted. Therefore, there were no differences in the productivities of the three pharmacists in terms of the numbers of prescription items dispensed per day.

11.4   Non-parametric multiple comparison tests

Analogously to ANOVA, rejection of the null hypothesis using either the Kruskal–Wallis test or Friedman's test does not provide information concerning the origins of the proposed differences. Consequently, rejection of the null hypothesis informs the analyst that the three or more populations differ, but no conclusions may be drawn about the differences between individual pairs of populations. Therefore, as before, *post-hoc* statistical tests should be performed to analyse these individual differences. The use and applications of one test that is frequently used for the *post-hoc* analysis of data in which the null hypothesis has been rejected using either the Kruskal–Wallis or Friedman's tests are described here. This is the *Nemenyi test*, and its mechanics are similar to those of Tukey's HSD test. The subsequent examples explore the use of this multiple comparison test following initial analysis using either the Kruskal–Wallis and Friedman tests. The background to these examples has been addressed in earlier examples in this chapter.

EXAMPLE 11.7 *In Example 11.2 it was concluded, using the Kruskal–Wallis test, that the milk withdrawal periods for four intramammary products were significantly different. The sponsor of the clinical study is interested in determining the nature of the differences. Using a suitable* post-hoc *test, identify the nature of the differences between the individual pairs of treatments.*

The outcome of the primary analysis, the Kruskal–Wallis test, involved the rejection of the null hypothesis. Therefore, to interpret the nature of the differences between individual pairs of data, it is necessary to perform a suitable *post-hoc* test, i.e. Nemenyi's test. Note that after analysing a data set by a non-parametric multiple-sample test, one cannot use a parametric *post-hoc* test such as Tukey's HSD. In the author's experience, this is one of the errors most frequently committed by pharmacy students. The reader should remember that, in choosing a non-parametric multiple-sample test, the analyst has decided that the data do not fulfil the assumptions of the equivalent parametric test. If this is so for the primary analysis, it remains the case for the *post-hoc* test.

The non-parametric *post-hoc* test is performed using similar guidelines to previous parametric *post-hoc* tests. First, the experimental parameters should be clearly defined.

(i) State the null hypotheses

As there are four treatments, a total of six individual comparisons is possible:

- product A versus product B
- product A versus product C
- product A versus product D
- product B versus Product C
- product B versus Product D
- product C versus Product D.

Each of these individual comparisons has an associated null hypothesis. Consequently a generic null hypothesis may be established which states that there are no differences between the milk withdrawal periods of each pair of treatments.

(ii) State the alternative hypotheses

For each null hypothesis concerning the comparison of each individual pair of treatments, there is an accompanying alternative hypothesis. Once more a generic alternative hypothesis may stated: there are differences between the milk withdrawal periods of each pair of treatments.

(iii) State the level of significance

In this example, it is assumed that the level of significance (α) is 0.05.

(iv) Perform the individual post-hoc comparisons using Nemenyi's test

As Nemenyi's test is executed in a similar way to Tukey's HSD test, the reader may not be surprised to read that the equations used in both tests are generically similar. The calculated statistic derived using Tukey's test is obtained by dividing the difference between the means of the two treatment groups by the standard error of their difference. Similarly, in Nemenyi's test, the test statistic (q) is calculated by dividing the standard error into the difference between the rank sums of the two treatment groups. Mathematically, this is expressed as

$$q = \frac{(R_{\text{treatment 1}} - R_{\text{treatment 2}})}{SE}$$

The use of the Nemenyi test for the resolution of the problems described in Example 11.7 is outlined in a stepwise fashion below.

Step 1   Calculate the standard error
The standard error (SE) may be calculated using the following mathematical expression:

$$SE = \sqrt{\frac{N(NK)(NK + 1)}{12}}$$

where N is the number of observations in each treatment group (this equation assumes that the numbers of observations in each treatment group are identical) and K is the number of treatments. In Example 11.2 there were six observations in each group, so $N = 6$ and $K = 4$. Inserting this information into the above equation allows the standard error to be calculated:

$$SE = \sqrt{\frac{N(NK)(NK + 1)}{12}} = \sqrt{\frac{6(6 \times 4)(6 \times 4 + 1)}{12}} = \sqrt{300} = 17.32$$

Step 2   Calculate the differences between the rank sums of each pair of treatments

In Example 11.2 the rank sums of each treatment were as follows:

- product A   58
- product B   93
- product C   113
- product D   36

Step 3   Calculate the Nemenyi test statistic for each comparison

- *Comparison between products A and B*

$$q = \frac{(R_{\text{product A}} - R_{\text{product B}})}{SE} = \frac{(58 - 93)}{17.32} = 2.02$$

- *Comparison between products A and C*

$$q = \frac{(R_{\text{product A}} - R_{\text{product C}})}{SE} = \frac{(58 - 113)}{17.32} = 3.18$$

- *Comparison between products A and D*

$$q = \frac{(R_{\text{product A}} - R_{\text{product D}})}{SE} = \frac{(58 - 36)}{17.32} = 1.27$$

- *Comparison between products B and C*

$$q = \frac{(R_{\text{product B}} - R_{\text{product C}})}{SE} = \frac{(93 - 113)}{17.32} = 1.15$$

- *Comparison between products B and D*

$$q = \frac{(R_{\text{product B}} - R_{\text{product D}})}{SE} = \frac{(93 - 36)}{17.32} = 3.29$$

- *Comparison between products C and D*

$$q = \frac{(R_{\text{product C}} - R_{\text{product D}})}{SE} = \frac{(113 - 36)}{17.32} = 4.45$$

In all cases the sign of the calculated statistic has been removed.

Step 4   Identify the critical Nemenyi statistic

The critical test statistic is identified using the table of the critical values of the studentised range statistic (q). The reader will recall that this table was previously used to determine the critical test statistic for Tukey's *post-hoc* test. In Tukey's test, knowledge of three parameters was required to enable critical test statistic to be identified: the level of significance, the number of treatments (means) and the number of degrees of freedom associated with the within-groups term (denominator in the

F ratio). Similarly, in Nemenyi's test, the critical statistic is determined from the table of critical values of the studentised range statistic with knowledge of the level of significance, the number of treatments and the number of degrees of freedom, although the latter is not derived from the experiment design but is preset at infinity. The critical test statistic for the data presented in Example 11.7 may therefore be derived from Appendix 12 as 3.63 ($\alpha = 0.05$, 4 treatment groups, ∞ degrees of freedom).

Step 5   Interpret the outcome of the statistical analysis
Interpreting the outcome of the statistical analysis involves comparing the calculated statistic associated with each individual paired comparison (as performed in step 3) to the critical test statistic. As before, if the calculated statistic is less than the critical test statistic, the null hypothesis is accepted, whereas if the magnitude of the calculated statistic is equal to or greater than the critical test statistic, the null hypothesis is rejected in preference to the alternative hypothesis. Each of the individual comparisons is shown below, but it should be noted that to save time the analyst would normally examine the pair of treatments that offers the greatest calculated test statistic first for significance and then work backwards.

- *Comparison between products A and B*

  $q_{calculated}$ (2.02) < $q_{critical}$ (3.63)

  The null hypothesis is accepted and therefore it may be concluded that there is no difference in the milk withdrawal periods of products A and B.
- *Comparison between products A and C*

  $q_{calculated}$ (3.18) < $q_{critical}$ (3.63)

  The null hypothesis is accepted and therefore it may be concluded that there is no difference in the milk withdrawal periods of products A and C.
- *Comparison between products A and D*

  $q_{calculated}$ (1.27) < $q_{critical}$ (3.63)

  The null hypothesis is accepted and therefore it may be concluded that there is no difference in the milk withdrawal periods of products A and D.
- *Comparison between products B and C*

  $q_{calculated}$ (1.15) < $q_{critical}$ (3.63)

  The null hypothesis is accepted and therefore it may be concluded that there is no difference in the milk withdrawal periods of products B and C.
- *Comparison between products B and D*

  $q_{calculated}$ (3.29) < $q_{critical}$ (3.63)

The null hypothesis is accepted and therefore it may be concluded that there is no difference in the milk withdrawal periods of products B and D.
- *Comparison between products C and D*

$$q_{\text{calculated}}\ (4.45) > q_{\text{critical}}\ (3.63)$$

The null hypothesis is rejected and therefore it may be concluded that there is a significant difference in the milk withdrawal periods of products C and D. More specifically, based on the comparative rank scores of products C and D, it may be concluded that the milk withdrawal period of product D is significantly lower than that of product C.

In the previous example, the application of Nemenyi's test for the clarification of the basis of the rejection of the null hypothesis was described for a symmetrical experimental design, i.e. the numbers of observations in each treatment were identical. When the design is asymmetrical, i.e. the number of observations in each treatment is not identical, the equation that is used to determine the standard error is modified as follows:

$$SE = \sqrt{\frac{N(N+1)}{12}\left(\frac{1}{N_1} + \frac{1}{N_2}\right)}$$

where N is the total number of observations in the study and N_1 and N_2 are the numbers of observations in the two treatment groups that are under evaluation in the *post-hoc* analysis.

The calculation of the test statistic (Q) is also modified:

$$Q = \frac{(R_{\text{treatment 1}}/N_{\text{treatment 1}}) - (R_{\text{treatment 2}}/N_{\text{treatment 2}})}{SE}$$

$$= \frac{(R_{\text{treatment 1}}/N_{\text{treatment 1}}) - (R_{\text{treatment 2}}/N_{\text{treatment 2}})}{\sqrt{N(N+1)/12\ (1/N_1 + 1/N_2)}}$$

where Q is the test statistic (the critical values for this statistic are displayed in Appendix 17), $R_{\text{treatment 1}}$ and $R_{\text{treatment 2}}$ are the rank scores of the two treatments under comparison $N_{\text{treatment 1}}$ and $N_{\text{treatment 2}}$ are the numbers of observations in the two treatment groups. This is referred to as *Dunn's test*.

The use of the above equations is illustrated in the subsequent example.

EXAMPLE 11.8 *An analytical laboratory has been asked to analyse the concentration of drug in successive 10-mL aliquots of a suspension product, manufactured by three different pharmaceutical companies. Unfortunately, it is suspected that one of the products has been poorly formulated and will therefore provide an unreliable dose to patients.*

The laboratory has removed a series of aliquots of each product and quantified the mass of therapeutic agent present using a validated high-performance liquid chromatography (HPLC) method. The results of this investigation are shown in Table 11.16. Is there a difference in the drug content between the three different manufactured products? If so, determine the nature of the difference(s).

This problem will be addressed by initially defining the parameters associated with the experimental study.

(i) State the null hypothesis

In Example 11.8, the null hypothesis states that the drug content (per aliquot) of the three manufactured products is the same. In other words, the three populations from which the data have been sampled are similar or, alternatively, the three sets of sample data have been derived from one population.

(ii) State the alternative hypothesis

A suitable alternative hypothesis is that the drug content (per aliquot) of the three manufactured products is not the same.

(iii) State the level of significance

In this example, it is assumed that the level of significance (α) is 0.05.

(iv) Select the most appropriate statistical test

In the selection of the most appropriate test for the resolution of the problem, the first step involves interpretation of the general design of the study. In this example, three treatments will be compared and,

Table 11.16 Concentration of therapeutic agent (mg) in successive 10-mL aliquots of a suspension product manufactured by three different pharmaceutical companies

Product 1	Product 2	Product 3
115.5	113.5	120.6
121.2	114.9	135.4
118.5	118.4	145.2
116.9	119.6	110.5
115.4	114.8	125.8
117.0	116.1	135.2
117.8		128.5
		139.2
		119.5

accordingly, the statistical analysis must be a multiple-sample hypothesis test. Furthermore, this is a one-factor design: the single factor is the manufactured product, which is further subdivided into three categories (products 1, 2 and 3). With this information, the analyst is alerted to the potential suitability of either a parametric one-factor test (one-way ANOVA) or a non-parametric one-factor analysis (the Kruskal–Wallis test). To complete the selection of the most appropriate statistical test the analyst must initially examine the suitability of the measured data for analysis using the ANOVA. Therefore, the following points are addressed.

Are the populations from which the data have been sampled normally distributed?

One of the assumptions of ANOVA is that the parent populations are normally or pseudo-normally distributed. This question has been raised in several previous examples. The normality of a population may be rapidly estimated by comparing the descriptive statistics, namely the mean and median of each treatment. This information is presented in Table 11.17. Here the mean and median of each sample are comparable, suggesting that the distributions from which the data were derived are normally distributed.

Are the variances of the populations from which the data have been sampled similar in magnitude?

A second assumption of ANOVA is that the populations from which the data have been sampled have similar variances. The variances of each treatment are assumed to be representative of the variances of the parent populations and accordingly the variances of the three treatment groups are calculated and compared. The variances of the three populations are:

- product 1 $4.0 \ (\text{mg}/10 \ \text{mL})^2$
- product 2 $5.5 \ (\text{mg}/10 \ \text{mL})^2$
- product 3 $119.9 \ (\text{mg}/10 \ \text{mL})^2$.

Table 11.17 Summary of the central tendency of the data concerning the concentration of therapeutic agent (mg/10 mL) in successive aliquots of a suspension product manufactured by three pharmaceutical companies

Measure of central tendency	Product 1	Product 2	Product 3
Mean	117.5	116.2	128.9
Median	117.0	115.5	125.5

It is immediately apparent that the variance of product 3 vastly exceeds that of either product 1 or produce 2. However, the anxious statistician may wish to confirm this apparent disparity by applying the F_{max} test. Remembering that the F_{max} statistic is calculated as the ratio of the largest variance to the smallest variance, for this example it is

$$F_{max} = \frac{s^2_{largest}}{s^2_{smallest}} = \frac{s^2_{product\ 3}}{s^2_{product\ 1}} = \frac{119.9}{4.0} = 29.98$$

The critical F_{max} statistic may be derived from the table of the critical values of the F_{max} test. In this analysis, the level of significance is 0.05, the number of degrees of freedom is $N - 1$ (i.e. $7 - 1 = 6$) and the number of treatments in the experimental design is 3. When the two groups differ in the number of observations, the lower value may be employed in the determination of the critical F_{max} statistic, so the critical F_{max} statistic associated with these experimental parameters is 8.38. Finally, as the calculated value of F_{max} is greater than the critical value of F_{max}, it is assumed that the two variances are significantly different, thus violating one of the major assumptions of ANOVA.

What is the nature of measurement of the collected data?

One of the assumptions of ANOVA is that the data must be measured on at least an interval scale, whereas in the non-parametric equivalent, the Kruskal–Wallis test, the data may be ordinal, interval or ratio in nature. In this example, the data has been measured on a ratio scale, so either type of test is applicable.

What is the sample size of the treatments under comparison?

The accuracy of both the Kruskal–Wallis and ANOVA tests is influenced by small sample sizes, but the latter is particularly affected. Therefore, it is important to consider the sample size of each treatment before finally choosing the more appropriate test. As may be observed, the minimum sample size in the experimental design is six, so either type of test is applicable.

All of these factors influence the choice of the one-way ANOVA or the Kruskal–Wallis test for the statistical analysis of the data sets shown in Table 11.16. As there is a primary concern about the disparity of variances of the different populations, it is more appropriate to use the Kruskal–Wallis test to address the problem posed in Example 11.8. The interested reader may be comforted to know that the power efficiency of the Kruskal–Wallis test is about 95.5% of that of the ANOVA when the non-parametric test is employed in situations that are more appropriately addressed using ANOVA.

(v) Perform the statistical analysis

The Kruskal–Wallis test may be executed in a stepwise fashion.

Step 1   Assign ranks to each observation
All observations are pooled, ranked individually and the rank scores returned to their original treatment groups (Table 11.18).

Step 2   Calculate the sum of ranks associated with each treatment (product)
In this step, the individual rank scores in each column are added together.

$$\Sigma R_{\text{product } 1} = (6 + 16 + 12 + 8 + 5 + 9 + 10) = 66$$

$$\Sigma R_{\text{product } 2} = (2 + 4 + 11 + 14 + 3 + 7) = 41$$

$$\Sigma R_{\text{product } 3} = (15 + 20 + 22 + 1 + 17 + 19 + 18 + 21 + 13) = 146$$

Step 3   Calculate the between-groups sum of squares
The between-groups sum of squares (SS_{BG}) is determined using the following formula:

$$SS_{\text{BG}} = \frac{(R_{\text{product } 1})^2}{N_{\text{product } 1}} + \frac{(R_{\text{product } 2})^2}{N_{\text{product } 2}} + \frac{(R_{\text{product } 3})^2}{N_{\text{product } 3}}$$

Table 11.18 Mass (mg) of therapeutic agent in successive 10-mL aliquots of a suspension product manufactured by three different pharmaceutical companies, illustrating the rank score of each individual observation

Product 1		Product 2		Product 3	
Mass/ 10 mL	Rank	Mass/ 10 mL	Rank	Mass/ 10 mL	Rank
115.5	6	113.5	2	120.6	15
121.2	16	114.9	4	135.4	20
118.5	12	118.4	11	145.2	22
116.9	8	119.6	14	110.5	1
115.4	5	114.8	3	125.8	17
117.0	9	116.1	7	135.2	19
117.8	10			128.5	18
				139.2	21
				119.5	13
Rank total $(R_{\text{product } 1})$	66	Rank total $(R_{\text{product } 2})$	41	Rank total $(R_{\text{product } 3})$	146

For the data described in Table 11.18:

$$SS_{BG} = \frac{(66)^2}{7} + \frac{(41)^2}{6} + \frac{(146)^2}{9} = 3270.9$$

Step 4   Calculate the Kruskal–Wallis statistic
The Kruskal–Wallis statistic is calculated using the formula described in section 11.3:

$$H = \frac{12}{N(N+1)} \times SS_{BG} - 3(N+1)$$

$$= \frac{12}{22(22+1)} \times 3270.9 - 3(22+1) = 8.57$$

Step 5   Identify the critical Kruskal–Wallis statistic
In the experimental design described in this example, the number of treatments is three and the number of observations in each group is greater than five. We therefore assume that the distribution of the Kruskal–Wallis statistic is approximated by the χ^2 distribution. The critical statistic is abstracted from the table of critical values of the χ^2 statistic relevant to the following experimental parameters:

- $\alpha = 0.05$
- $df = 2$ (i.e. number of treatments – 1).

Therefore, under the above conditions, the critical test statistic ($H_{critical}$) is 5.99.

Step 6   Interpret the outcome of the statistical analysis
In this analysis the calculated value of the Kruskal–Wallis statistic (8.57) is greater than the critical test statistic (5.99), so the null hypothesis is rejected in favour of the alternative hypothesis. Therefore, it may be concluded that the three products differ in the concentration of therapeutic agent present in successive 10-mL aliquots.

The Kruskal–Wallis test has identified a generic difference between the three products with respect to the concentration of therapeutic agent present in a defined volume of product, but at this point no information is available about the nature of the difference. For example, is the concentration of therapeutic agent present in product 1 different from that in products 2 or 3, or is the concentration of therapeutic agent in product 2 different from that present in product 3? To answer these questions, one must employ a non-parametric *post-hoc* test. For this purpose the modified form of Nemenyi's test (Dunn's test) that accounts for differences in the number of observations in each treatment group will be used.

In total, three comparisons must be performed: product 1 versus product 2, product 2 versus product 3 and product 1 versus product 3. As before, the conditions of the statistical analysis should be outlined.

(i) State the null hypothesis

The null hypothesis in the series of *post-hoc* tests assumes that there are no differences between the various pairs of treatments. Accordingly, it may be assumed that the population distributions of products 1, 2 and 3 are similar or, alternatively that all three sets of data have been derived from a single population.

(ii) State the alternative hypothesis

The alternative hypothesis for each of the comparisons states that there are differences between each pair of treatments. Therefore, the concentration of therapeutic agent (per aliquot) in product 1 is different from that in either product 2 or 3 and similarly, there is a difference in concentration between products 2 and 3.

(iii) State the level of significance

In this example, it is assumed that the level of significance (α) is 0.05.

(iv) Perform the post-hoc analyses

In this example, three *post-hoc* analyses will be performed. These are individually described below. Once more, it should be noted that to save time the analyst would normally examine the pair of treatments that offer the greatest differences in mean rank scores first for significance, and then work backwards.

Compare products 1 and 2

Step 1   Calculate the standard error

$$SE = \sqrt{\frac{N(N+1)}{12}\left(\frac{1}{N_1}+\frac{1}{N_2}\right)} = \sqrt{\frac{22(22+1)}{12}\left(\frac{1}{7}+\frac{1}{6}\right)} = 3.61$$

Step 2   Calculate the mean rank of each treatment ($\bar{R}$)
The mean rank is the ratio of the rank score of a treatment to the number of observations associated with that treatment, i.e. $\bar{R}_{treatment} =$

$R_{treatment}/N_{treatment}$. Therefore

$$\overline{R}_{product\ 1} = \frac{R_{product\ 1}}{N_{product\ 1}} = \frac{66}{7} = 9.43$$

$$\overline{R}_{product\ 2} = \frac{R_{product\ 2}}{N_{product\ 2}} = \frac{41}{6} = 6.83$$

Step 3   Calculate the test statistic (Q)
The information generated in steps 1 and 2 allows calculation of the test statistic.

$$Q = \frac{(R_{treatment\ 1}/N_{treatment\ 1}) - (R_{treatment\ 2}/N_{treatment\ 2})}{SE}$$

$$= \frac{9.43 - 6.83}{3.61} = 0.72$$

Step 4   Identify the critical test statistic
The critical test (Q) statistic may be derived using the table of critical values of Q, as presented in Appendix 17. As may be observed from this table, knowledge of two parameters is required to define the critical test statistic, namely, the level of significance (0.05) and the number of treatments in the experimental design (three, in this example). The critical value of Q ($\alpha = 0.05$, 3 treatments) is 2.39.

Step 5   Interpret the outcome of the post-hoc analysis

$$Q_{calculated}\ (0.72) < Q_{critical}\ (2.39)$$

The null hypothesis is accepted and therefore it may be concluded that there is no difference in the concentration of therapeutic product in successive 10-mL aliquots of products 1 and 2.

Compare products 1 and 3

Step 1   Calculate the standard error

$$SE = \sqrt{\frac{N(N+1)}{12}\left(\frac{1}{N_1} + \frac{1}{N_2}\right)} = \sqrt{\frac{22(22+1)}{12}\left(\frac{1}{7} + \frac{1}{9}\right)} = 3.27$$

Step 2   Calculate the mean rank of each treatment (R̄)

$$\overline{R}_{product\ 1} = \frac{R_{product\ 1}}{N_{product\ 1}} = \frac{66}{7} = 9.43$$

$$\overline{R}_{product\ 3} = \frac{R_{Product\ 3}}{N_{product\ 3}} = \frac{146}{9} = 16.22$$

Step 3   Calculate the test statistic (Q)

$$Q = \frac{(R_{\text{treatment 3}}/N_{\text{treatment 3}}) - (R_{\text{treatment 1}}/N_{\text{treatment 1}})}{SE}$$

$$= \frac{16.22 - 9.43}{3.61} = 1.88$$

Step 4   Identify the critical test statistic
As before, the critical value of Q ($\alpha = 0.05$, 3 treatments) is 2.39.

Step 5   Interpret the outcome of the post-hoc *analysis*

$$Q_{\text{calculated}}\,(1.88) < Q_{\text{critical}}\,(2.39)$$

The null hypothesis is accepted and therefore it may be concluded that there is no difference in the concentration of therapeutic product in successive 10-mL aliquots of products 1 and 3.

Compare products 2 and 3

Step 1   Calculate the standard error

$$SE = \sqrt{\frac{N(N+1)}{12}\left(\frac{1}{N_1}+\frac{1}{N_2}\right)} = \sqrt{\frac{22(22+1)}{12}\left(\frac{1}{6}+\frac{1}{9}\right)} = 3.42$$

Step 2   Calculate the mean rank of each treatment ($\bar{R}$)

$$\bar{R}_{\text{product 2}} = \frac{R_{\text{product 1}}}{N_{\text{product 1}}} = \frac{41}{6} = 6.83$$

$$\bar{R}_{\text{product 3}} = \frac{R_{\text{product 3}}}{N_{\text{product 3}}} = \frac{146}{9} = 16.22$$

Step 3   Calculate the test statistic (Q)

$$Q = \frac{(R_{\text{treatment 3}}/N_{\text{treatment 3}}) - (R_{\text{treatment 2}}/N_{\text{treatment 2}})}{SE}$$

$$= \frac{16.22 - 6.83}{3.42} = 2.75$$

Step 4   Identify the critical test statistic
As before, the critical value of Q ($\alpha = 0.05$, 3 treatments) is 2.39.

Step 5   Interpret the outcome of the post-hoc *analysis*

$$Q_{\text{calculated}}\,(2.75) > Q_{\text{critical}}\,(2.39)$$

The null hypothesis is rejected and therefore it may be concluded that products 2 and 3 differ in the concentration of therapeutic product present in successive 10-mL aliquots. In particular, the rank scores inform the analyst that product 3 contains a greater concentration of therapeutic agent than product 2.

One further consideration when performing a non-parametric *post-hoc* test is to ensure that the correction has been applied to overcome the bias associated with the presence of tied values. It may be recalled that a correction factor was calculated and used in the final calculation of the Kruskal–Wallis statistic. Similarly, when there are tied rank scores in an experimental design, Dunn's equation for the calculation of the standard error is further modified as follows:

$$SE = \sqrt{\left(\frac{N(N+1)}{12} - \frac{\sum t}{12(N-1)}\right)\left(\frac{1}{N_1} + \frac{1}{N_2}\right)}$$

where N is the total number of observations in the experimental design, N_1 and N_2 are the numbers of observations in the two treatment groups under comparison, and $\sum t$ has previously been defined as $\sum(t^3 - t)$. The test statistic is calculated as before by diving the standard error into the difference in mean rank sums between the two treatment groups under comparison. The use of this equation is illustrated in Example 11.9.

EXAMPLE 11.9 *The preparation of solid dosage forms that contain a low mass of drug presents many challenges to the pharmaceutical industry. If preparations are formulated or prepared incorrectly, the reproducibility of drug content per tablet will be poor, which, in light of the potent nature of the therapeutic agent, may have dramatic consequences for the patient. A pharmaceutical company is in the process of selecting an appropriate method for the formulation of a tablet that contains 105 µg of a therapeutic agent and has identified three potentially suitable manufacturing methods for this dosage form. In a pilot study, three batches of tablets have been produced using each of these methods and the drug content of representative samples from these batches measured using an appropriate analytical method. The results are shown in Table 11.19. Using an appropriate statistical method, determine whether or not the manufacturing method significantly affects drug content per tablet.*

The starting point of the analytical procedure involves the definition of the important statistical parameters.

Table 11.19 Mass of therapeutic agent (μg) in tablets manufactured by three different processes

Wet granulation	Dry granulation	Direct compression
94	92	109
95	104	111
105	105	112
104	96	106
109	97	108
102	108	102
90	104	104
81	80	105
101		

(i) State the null hypothesis

In Example 11.9, the null hypothesis states that the mass of therapeutic agent per tablet is similar for each manufacturing method, i.e. drug content is independent of the method of manufacture.

(ii) State the alternative hypothesis

The alternative hypothesis states that the selected manufacturing method does affect the drug content of the tablets. Therefore, the mass of drug per tablet will differ depending on the selected method of manufacture.

(iii) State the level of significance

In this example, it is assumed that the level of significance (α) is 0.05.

(iv) Select the most appropriate statistical test

The following points are important determinants in the selection of the most appropriate statistical test to challenge the null hypothesis associated with Example 11.9:

- The data have been measured on a ratio scale.
- The number of observations in each treatment group is sufficiently large to enable analysis with either parametric or non-parametric statistical methods.
- The experiment has been designed as a multiple-samples test in which three treatments are under comparison. The three treatments may be classified as a single factor, so the three treatments may be compared using a one-factor analysis. As a result, the use of two-independent-samples tests cannot be recommended and therefore the choice of statistical test has been narrowed down to either one-way ANOVA or the Kruskal–Wallis test.

- The variances of the data associated with the wet granulation, dry granulation and direct compression processes were 76.1, 83.6 and 12.1 μg^2, respectively. Homogeneity of variances may be statistically assessed using the F_{max} test. In this the null hypothesis states that the variances of the three populations are similar, whereas, the alternative hypothesis states that the variances are heterogeneous. Assuming a level of significance of 0.05, the F_{max} statistic may be calculated:

$$F_{max} = \frac{s^2_{maximum}}{s^2_{minimum}} = \frac{s^2_{dry}}{s^2_{direct}} = \frac{83.6}{12.1} = 6.91$$

  From Appendix 11 and, under the conditions of the experimental design ($a = 0.05$, number of treatments = 3, $df = 8 - 1 = 7$), the critical F_{max} value is 6.94. The similarity between the calculated and critical F_{max} statistics implies that the variances of the populations from which the sample data have originated may be dissimilar. This disparity raises concerns over the validity of a parametric test to examine the truth of the null hypothesis.
- Are the populations from which the data have been sampled normally distributed? To examine the nature of the populations, the mean and median of the treatments groups are computed and compared (Table 11.20). As may be observed, the mean and median of each individual group are similar and therefore, we will assume that the populations from which the data were sampled are normally distributed.

On the basis of the above information, it is recommended that a non-parametric multiple-samples test, i.e. the Kruskal–Wallis test, is employed to examine the validity of the null hypothesis.

(v) Perform the statistical analysis

This may be conducted in a stepwise fashion, as before.

Step 1   Assign ranks to each observation (Table 11-21)

Step 2   Calculate the sum of ranks associated with each treatment

$$\Sigma R_{wet\ granulation} = (5 + 6 + 17 + 13.5 + 22.5 + 10.5 + 3 + 2 + 9)$$
$$= 88.5$$

Table 11.20 Summary of the central tendency of the data for the mass of therapeutic agent (μg) in tablets manufactured by three different processes

Measure of central tendency	Wet granulation	Dry granulation	Direct compression
Mean	97.89	98.25	107.13
Median	101.00	100.5	107.00

Table 11.21 Mass of therapeutic agent in tablets manufactured by three different processes, illustrating the rank score of each individual observation

Wet granulation		Dry granulation		Direct compression	
Mass (μg)/ tablet	Rank	Mass (μg)/ tablet	Rank	Mass (μg)/ tablet	Rank
94	5	92	4	109	22.5
95	6	104	13.5	111	24
105	17	105	17	112	25
104	13.5	96	7	106	19
109	22.5	97	8	108	20.5
102	10.5	108	20.5	102	10.5
90	3	104	13.5	104	13.5
81	2	80	1	105	17
101	9				

$$\Sigma R_{\text{dry granulation}} = (4 + 13.5 + 17 + 7 + 8 + 20.5 + 13.5 + 1)$$
$$= 84.5$$
$$\Sigma R_{\text{direct compression}} = (22.5 + 24 + 25 + 19 + 20.5 + 10.5 + 13.5 + 17)$$
$$= 152.0$$

Step 3   Calculate the between-groups sum of squares

$$SS_{\text{BG}} = \frac{(R_{\text{wet graulation}})^2}{N_{\text{wet graulation}}} + \frac{(R_{\text{dry graulation}})^2}{N_{\text{dry graulation}}} + \frac{(R_{\text{direct compression}})^2}{N_{\text{direct compression}}}$$

Therefore

$$SS_{\text{BG}} = \frac{(88.5)^2}{9} + \frac{(84.5)^2}{8} + \frac{152.0^2}{8} = 4650.8$$

Step 4   Calculate the uncorrected Kruskal–Wallis statistic
With knowledge of the between-groups sum of squares, the Kruskal–Wallis statistic is calculated:

$$H = \frac{12}{N(N+1)} \times SS_{\text{BG}} - 3(N+1) = \frac{12}{25(25+1)} \times 4650.8 - 3(25+1)$$
$$= 7.86$$

Step 5   Calculate the correction factor
As in Example 11.3, there are tied ranks and, accordingly, the calculated Kruskal–Wallis statistic must be modified to compensate for this. The

tied ranks in Example 11.9 are as follows:

> 10.5, 10.5
>
> 13.5, 13.5, 13.5, 13.5
>
> 17.0, 17.0, 17.0
>
> 20.5, 20.5
>
> 22.5, 22.5

In the calculation of the correction factor to account for the presence of ties, the term $\Sigma(t^3 - t)$ is first calculated:

$$\Sigma(t^3 - t) = (2^3 - 2) + (4^3 - 4) + (3^3 - 3) + (2^3 - 2) + (2^3 - 2)$$
$$= 6 + 60 + 24 + 6 + 6$$
$$= 102$$

With this information in mind, the correction factor is computed:

$$CF = 1 - \frac{\sum(t^3 - t)}{N^3 - N} = 1 - \frac{102}{(25^3 - 25)} = 0.993$$

Step 6   Calculate the corrected Kruskal–Wallis statistic
The corrected Kruskal–Wallis statistic (H_c) is calculated as the ratio of the uncorrected statistic (H) to the correction factor, i.e.

$$H_c = \frac{H}{CF} = \frac{7.86}{0.993} = 7.92$$

Step 7   Identify the critical Kruskal–Wallis statistic
The experimental design employed in Example 11.9 consisted of three treatments in which there were more than five observations. Under these circumstances, it may be assumed that the sampling distribution of the Kruskal–Wallis statistic is approximated by the χ^2 distribution and hence, the latter distribution is used to identify the value of the critical test statistic. In this example, there are 2 *df* (number of treatments − 1) and the level of significance is 0.05. Therefore, from the table in Appendix 3, the critical value of $H_{(a = 0.05, 2 \, df)}$ is 5.99.

Step 8   Interpret the outcome of the statistical analysis
The regions of acceptance and rejection of the null hypothesis are defined by the critical test statistic. If the calculated test statistic is less than the critical test statistic, the null hypothesis is accepted, whereas if the calculated test statistic is equal to or greater than the critical statistic, the null hypothesis is rejected in favour of the alternative hypothesis. In this example, $H_{calculated}$ (7.92) > $H_{critical}$ (5.99) and so the null hypothesis

is rejected. It may therefore be concluded that there is a difference in the mass of therapeutic agent per tablet associated with the three different manufacturing methods.

This conclusion has provided general information about the effects of processing conditions on the quality of the finished formulations. However, the sponsor of the study would like to explore the nature of the differences between the three manufacturing methods. For this purpose a non-parametric *post-hoc* statistical test is required. (Remembered that a parametric *post-hoc* test should not be applied to resolve the above question, as we have previously established that the statistical model does not meet the assumptions of a parametric statistical test.)

(vi) Perform the post-hoc analyses

In this example, three *post-hoc* analyses are performed to illustrate the use and interpretation of the modified equation. Once more, it should be noted that the analyst would normally initially examine the significance of the pair of treatments that offer the greatest differences in mean rank scores and then work backwards.

Compare wet granulation and dry granulation

Step 1   Calculate the standard error

$$SE = \sqrt{\left(\frac{N(N+1)}{12} - \frac{\sum(t^3 - t)}{12(N-1)}\right)\left(\frac{1}{N_1} + \frac{1}{N_2}\right)}$$

$$= \sqrt{\left(\frac{25(25+1)}{12} - \frac{102}{12(25-1)}\right)\left(\frac{1}{9} + \frac{1}{8}\right)} = 3.59$$

Step 2   Calculate the mean rank of each treatment ($\bar{R}$)

$$\bar{R}_{\text{wet granulation}} = \frac{R_{\text{wet granulation}}}{N_{\text{wet granulation}}} = \frac{88.5}{9} = 9.83$$

$$\bar{R}_{\text{dry granulation}} = \frac{R_{\text{dry granulation}}}{N_{\text{dry granulation}}} = \frac{84.5}{8} = 10.56$$

Step 3   Calculate the test statistic (Q)
The information generated in steps 1 and 2 is employed in the calculation of the test statistic:

$$Q = \frac{(R_{\text{dry granulation}}/N_{\text{dry granulation}}) - (R_{\text{wet granulation}}/N_{\text{wet granulation}})}{SE}$$

$$= \frac{10.56 - 9.83}{3.59} = 0.20$$

Step 4   Identify of the critical test statistic
The critical test statistic is taken from the table of critical values of Q in Appendix 17, with knowledge of the level of significance (0.05) and the number of treatments in the experimental design (3 in Example 11.9). The critical value of Q ($\alpha = 0.05$, 3 treatments) is 2.39.

Step 5   Interpret the outcome of the post-hoc analysis

$$Q_{\text{calculated}} (0.20) < Q_{\text{critical}} (2.39)$$

The null hypothesis is accepted and therefore it may be concluded that there is no difference in the concentration of therapeutic product of tablets manufactured using either the wet or dry granulation processes.

Compare wet granulation and direct compression

Step 1   Calculate the standard error

$$SE = \sqrt{\left(\frac{N(N+1)}{12} - \frac{\sum (t^3 - t)}{12(N-1)} \right) \left(\frac{1}{N_1} + \frac{1}{N_2} \right)}$$

$$= \sqrt{\left(\frac{25(25+1)}{12} - \frac{102}{12(25-1)} \right) \left(\frac{1}{9} + \frac{1}{8} \right)} = 3.59$$

Step 2   Calculate the mean rank of each treatment ($\bar{R}$)

$$\bar{R}_{\text{wet granulation}} = \frac{R_{\text{wet granulation}}}{N_{\text{wet granulation}}} = \frac{88.5}{9} = 9.83$$

$$\bar{R}_{\text{direct compression}} = \frac{R_{\text{direct compression}}}{N_{\text{direct compression}}} = \frac{152.0}{8} = 19.00$$

Step 3   Calculate the test statistic (Q)

$$Q = \frac{(R_{\text{direct compression}}/N_{\text{direct compression}}) - (R_{\text{wet granulation}}/N_{\text{wet granulation}})}{SE}$$

$$= \frac{19.00 - 9.83}{3.59} = 2.55$$

Step 4   Identify of the critical test statistic
From Appendix 17, the critical value of Q ($\alpha = 0.05$, 3 treatments) is 2.39.

Step 5   Interpret of the outcome of the post-hoc analysis

$$Q_{\text{calculated}} (2.55) > Q_{\text{critical}} (2.39)$$

The null hypothesis is rejected and therefore we may conclude that concentration of therapeutic product per tablet is dependent on whether wet granulation or direct compression is employed to manufacture the dosage form. Reference to the rank scores allows the analyst to conclude that tablets produced by direct compression contained a greater mass of therapeutic agent than those produced by wet granulation.

Compare dry granulation and direct compression

Step 1   Calculate the standard error

$$SE = \sqrt{\left(\frac{N(N+1)}{12} - \frac{\sum(t^3 - t)}{12(N-1)}\right)\left(\frac{1}{N_1} + \frac{1}{N_2}\right)}$$

$$= \sqrt{\left(\frac{25(25+1)}{12} - \frac{102}{12(25-1)}\right)\left(\frac{1}{8} + \frac{1}{8}\right)} = 3.67$$

Step 2   Calculate the mean rank of each treatment (R̄)

$$\bar{R}_{\text{dry granulation}} = \frac{R_{\text{dry granulation}}}{N_{\text{dry granulation}}} = \frac{84.5}{8} = 10.56$$

$$\bar{R}_{\text{direct compression}} = \frac{R_{\text{direct compression}}}{N_{\text{direct compression}}} = \frac{152.0}{8} = 19.00$$

Step 3   Calculate the test statistic (Q)

$$Q = \frac{(R_{\text{direct compression}}/N_{\text{direct compression}}) - (R_{\text{dry granulation}}/N_{\text{dry granulation}})}{SE}$$

$$= \frac{19.00 - 10.56}{3.67} = 2.30$$

Step 4   Identify the critical test statistic
From Appendix 17, the critical value of Q ($\alpha = 0.05$, 3 treatments) is 2.39.

Step 5   Interpret the outcome of the post-hoc analysis

$$Q_{\text{calculated}} (2.30) < Q_{\text{critical}} (2.39)$$

The null hypothesis is accepted and therefore it may be concluded that there is no difference in the drug content per tablet when the dosage form is manufactured by either dry granulation or direct compression.

For the final example of the use of a non-parametric *post-hoc* test, the data described in Example 11.5 will be used again. This example examines the release of therapeutic agent from a drug-containing polymeric strip attached to the tooth surface of human volunteers. On the basis of the paired experimental design and the unsuitability of the data for analysis using a parametric method (i.e. repeated-measures one-way ANOVA), Friedman's test was selected as the most appropriate statistical test. After the application of this test, the null hypothesis was rejected in favour of the alternative hypothesis, and it may therefore be of interest to the sponsor of the study to examine the data further in order to identify the origins of this statistical outcome. The procedure is demonstrated in the following example.

EXAMPLE 11.10   *In Example 11.5 the release of therapeutic agent from polymeric strips into saliva following attachment to the teeth of human volunteers was examined as a function of time (1, 2, 3 and 4 days after application). After statistical analysis of the data collected in this study it was concluded that the release of therapeutic agent was not constant with respect to time. Unfortunately this outcome did not match the expectations of the company sponsoring the study. However, to guide future development of the product, you have been requested to provide further details concerning the release of therapeutic agent at the different sampling periods, and, in particular, the disparities between the concentration of drug in saliva at these periods. Define the most appropriate statistical method that may be used for this purpose and what differences existed concerning the concentration of drug in saliva at each sampling period.*

The experimental parameters should be detailed, as follows:

(i)   State the null hypotheses

There are four different sampling periods and, as a result there are six possible multiple comparison tests, each of which has an associated null (and indeed alternative) hypothesis. To simplify matters, a single null hypothesis will be established for the experiment. This may be stated as follows:

- H_0:   Concentration at day 1 = concentration at day 2
- H_0:   Concentration at day 1 = concentration at day 3
- H_0:   Concentration at day 1 = concentration at day 4
- H_0:   Concentration at day 2 = concentration at day 3
- H_0:   Concentration at day 2 = concentration at day 4
- H_0:   Concentration at day 3 = concentration at day 4

(ii)   State the alternative hypothesis

The alternative hypothesis for each set of comparisons states that there is a difference in the concentration of drug at each time period, i.e.:

- H_a: Concentration at day 1 ≠ concentration at day 2
- H_a: Concentration at day 1 ≠ concentration at day 3

- H_a: Concentration at day 1 ≠ concentration at day 4
- H_a: Concentration at day 2 ≠ concentration at day 3
- H_a: Concentration at day 2 ≠ concentration at day 4
- H_a: Concentration at day 3 ≠ concentration at day 4

(iii) State the level of significance

In this example, it is assumed that the level of significance (α) is 0.05.

(iv) Select the most appropriate statistical test

The question raised in Example 11.10 is a typical scenario that requires the application of a *post-hoc* statistical test. The parent analysis (Example 11.5) employed a non-parametric statistical method (Friedman's test) to address the validity of the null hypothesis and therefore, a non-parametric *post-hoc* analysis should be used to identify differences between individual pairs of treatments. Furthermore, the *post-hoc* test should be compatible with the initial (parent) analysis, i.e. Friedman's test. Under these conditions Nemenyi's test may be applied, but in this example we will calculate the critical difference between mean rank sums that defines acceptance or rejection of the null hypothesis and then compare this value to the calculated differences between the mean rank sums of each pair of treatments. In essence, this is a more direct approach than has been employed in previous examples.

Step 1 Define the critical difference in the mean rank scores
The critical difference (CD) is mathematically determined using the following equation:

$$CD = \sqrt{\left(\frac{k(k+1)}{6N}\right)\chi^2_{\text{critical}}}$$

where k is the number of treatments in the experimental design, $N = 6$ is the number of observations in each treatment group and χ^2_{critical} is the critical statistic associated with the experimental design. In this example, the number of observations in each group is sufficiently large to allow the use of the χ^2 distribution to estimate the critical Friedman's statistic. In this design, there are 4 treatments ($4 - 1 = 3$ df) and the level of significance is 0.05. Therefore the critical test statistic is 7.81.

The critical difference in the mean rank scores may then be calculated:

$$CD = \sqrt{\left(\frac{k(k+1)}{6N}\right)\chi^2_{\text{critical}}} = \sqrt{\left(\frac{4(4+1)}{6\times 6}\right)\times 7.81} = 2.08$$

Step 2   Calculate the mean rank score associated with each treatment
The mean rank score is the ratio of the rank sum of each treatment to
the number of observations associated with that treatment, i.e.

$$\overline{R}_{day\ 1} = \frac{R_{day\ 1}}{N_{day\ 1}} = \frac{24}{6} = 4.00$$

$$\overline{R}_{day\ 2} = \frac{R_{day\ 2}}{N_{day\ 2}} = \frac{18}{6} = 3.00$$

$$\overline{R}_{day\ 3} = \frac{R_{day\ 3}}{N_{day\ 3}} = \frac{8}{6} = 1.33$$

$$\overline{R}_{day\ 4} = \frac{R_{day\ 4}}{N_{day\ 4}} = \frac{10}{6} = 1.67$$

*Step 3   Calculate the differences between the mean rank scores of the
pairs of treatments*

$$\overline{R}_{day\ 1} - \overline{R}_{day\ 2} = 4.00 - 3.00 = 1.00$$
$$\overline{R}_{day\ 1} - \overline{R}_{day\ 3} = 4.00 - 1.33 = 2.67$$
$$\overline{R}_{day\ 1} - \overline{R}_{day\ 4} = 4.00 - 1.67 = 2.33$$
$$\overline{R}_{day\ 2} - \overline{R}_{day\ 3} = 3.00 - 1.33 = 1.67$$
$$\overline{R}_{day\ 2} - \overline{R}_{day\ 4} = 3.00 - 1.67 = 1.33$$
$$\overline{R}_{day\ 4} - \overline{R}_{day\ 3} = 1.67 - 1.33 = 0.34$$

Step 4   Interpret the outcome of each statistical comparison
As previously stated, this example involved six individual comparisons.
To ensure understanding of this statistical test, the outcome of the most
relevant comparisons will be considered independently. In all cases the
null hypothesis is accepted when the calculated difference between the
mean rank scores is less than the critical difference. Conversely, the
alternative hypothesis is accepted when the calculated difference
between the pairs of rank scores is either equal to or greater than the
critical difference. This will form the basis of the statistical outcome.

- *Comparison between day 1 and day 2*
  Calculated difference between mean rank scores (1.00) < CD (2.08)
  The null hypothesis is accepted and it may be concluded that the
  concentration of drug in saliva at day 1 is similar to that observed at day 2,
  i.e. constant drug release was observed over the 2-day period.
- *Comparison between day 1 and day 3*
  Calculated difference between mean rank scores (2.67) > CD (2.08)
  The null hypothesis is rejected and it may be concluded that the
  concentration of drug in saliva at day 1 is greater than that observed at day 3,
  i.e. constant drug release was not observed over the 3-day period.

- *Comparison between day 1 and day 4*
  Calculated difference between mean rank scores (2.33) > CD (2.08)
    The null hypothesis is rejected and it may be concluded that the concentration of drug in saliva at day 1 is greater than that observed at day 4, i.e. constant drug release was not observed over the 4-day period.
- *Comparison between day 2 and day 3*
  Calculated difference between mean rank scores (1.67) < CD (2.08)
    The null hypothesis is accepted and it may be concluded that the concentration of drug in saliva at day 2 is similar to that observed at day 3.

From these *post-hoc* tests, it may be concluded that a constant rate of drug release was obtained for the first 2 days after application, but the release rate altered after this period. The sponsor company may only claim for constant release over this initial period and not the 4-day period as originally proposed.

11.5 Conclusions

In this chapter, the theory and applications of several non-parametric techniques that may be employed to compare three of more treatments have been described with the aid of pharmaceutically relevant examples. These tests are used to examine the validity of the null hypothesis when the experimental design, and in particular the data collected within this design, do not conform to the assumptions of parametric statistical tests. Consequently, the tests described in this chapter are employed when

- the data has been measured in nominal, ordinal, interval or ratio scales and is composed of three of more treatment groups
- the populations from which the treatment data have been sampled are non-normally distributed
- the variances of the populations from which the treatment data have been sampled are dissimilar
- the sizes of the sample groups are unduly small.

Three non-parametric tests that may be employed for the comparison of three or more treatment groups were selected for discussion in this chapter: χ^2 analysis, the Kruskal–Wallis test and Friedman's test. The use of each of these tests is dictated by the nature of the experimental design.

The χ^2 test is employed whenever the data are nominal in nature, or are measured as discrete categories within an ordinal scale of measurement. The test involves the comparison of the observed values within a category to the values that would be expected according to the null hypothesis. The outcome of the statistical analysis (i.e. the magnitude of the calculated statistic) is interpreted using the χ^2 distribution.

The Kruskal–Wallis test is the non-parametric equivalent of one-way ANOVA and is applied to data that have been measured on either ordinal, interval or ratio scales. In this design the data are allocated to a single factor that is, in turn, divided into a series of sub-categories (treatments). The mechanics of the test involve ranking the data associated with each treatment and using these ranks in the calculation of a test statistic (H). of The relevance of the calculated Kruskal–Wallis statistic is interpreted either after consulting the χ^2 distribution or directly from the table of values of probabilities associated with the test statistic (H).

Friedman's test may be employed for the comparison of data that has been measured on at least an ordinal scale. It is the non-parametric equivalent of either repeated-measures one-way ANOVA or two-way ANOVA without replication. As in the Kruskal–Wallis test, the data are allocated rank scores and these scores are used to calculate a Kruskal–Wallis test statistic (χ_r^2). The calculated test statistic is interpreted by comparison with the critical statistic that has been derived either from the χ^2 distribution or, alternatively, directly from the table of values of probabilities associated with the test statistic.

Finally, in this chapter, the theory and applications of a non-parametric *post-hoc* test (Nemenyi's test with associated modifications) were described. The reader will recall from the previous chapter that in situations where the independent variable(s) is composed of three or more sub-categories, a rejection of the null hypothesis implies that the variable has a significant effect on the magnitude of the dependent variable. *Post-hoc* tests are employed to provide an insight into the differences between each individual sub-category with respect to this measured outcome.

12

Linear regression and correlation

The terms *regression* and *correlation* are frequently employed within the pharmaceutical and related sciences to describe the relationship that exists between variables. Unfortunately, these terms are often used interchangeably, which is a mistake. Identification and interpretation of the relationships that exist between two variables are important statistical processes, so it is important at the outset to define regression and correlation accurately. Both terms refer to the relationship between variables, but they differ in the nature of the variables.

- In simple *regression* involving two variables, it is assumed that one variable is dependent and the other independent
- Conversely, in the *correlation* of two variables both are assumed to be dependent variables.

Classical pharmaceutical examples of regression include the relationships that exist between concentration of a therapeutic agent in solution and the associated analytical response (e.g. absorbance in ultraviolet spectroscopy, fluorescence intensity in fluorescence spectroscopy, peak area in high-performance liquid chromatography) or alternatively, the rate of release of drug from an implantable drug delivery system and the degree of cross-linking of the polymer matrix. In both of these examples the response of one variable (analytical response or drug release) is dependent on the magnitude of the second, independent variable (concentration of therapeutic agent in solution or degree of polymer cross-linking). One cannot, however, conclude that the concentration of drug is dependent on the analytical response as other factors may influence this response, e.g. the presence of other components within the solution or the performance of the analytical equipment. Similarly, the degree of polymer cross-linking is not dependent on the on the rate of drug release but on other factors such as the chemistry of the polymer, the chemistry of the cross-linking agent, the conditions under which the cross-linking process is performed. These examples should serve to illustrate the relationship that exists between independent and dependent variables.

Conversely, when the response of one variable changes as a function of a second variable and there is no obvious interplay between the independent and dependent variables, correlation is employed to define the nature of the relationship between the two variables. For example, in a clinical study an inverse relationship may be observed between blood cholesterol levels and aerobic fitness, but it is wrong to conclude that everyone with high blood cholesterol is unfit.

Hopefully these examples will have illustrated the difference between the terms regression and correlation. The remainder of this chapter will describe the theory and applications of regression and correlation, as before using pharmaceutical examples to aid understanding of these topics.

12.1 Linear regression analysis

In the previous section simple regression was defined as the relationship between two variables, one independent and the other dependent. When a relationship exists, a scientist will wish to define it mathematically, as this will enable accurate predictions of the response of the dependent variable to a change in the magnitude of the independent variable. The simplest relationship between two variables is a linear (straight line) relationship. *Linear regression analysis* is a statistical technique that mathematically defines the nature of the linear relationship between an independent and a dependent variable. There are numerous applications of linear regression analysis in the pharmaceutical and related sciences, for example:

- *The construction of calibration curves in pharmaceutical analysis.* Here the relationship between the concentration of a therapeutic agent and a defined analytical response (e.g. absorbance, peak area) is determined. Knowledge of this relationship allows the pharmaceutical analyst to calculate the concentration of therapeutic agent in samples following measurement of the analytical response. The term *calibration curve* may seem misleading, as the relationship between the two variables is actually linear (although mathematicians would argue that a straight line is a type of curve).
- *The accuracy of an analytical method for the determination of a therapeutic agent within a defined matrix.* In the regulatory process for a pharmaceutical product, the accuracy of the analytical method that is designed to determine the concentration of the therapeutic agent, e.g. for the purposes of stability studies, must be quantified. A typical method of doing this involves spiking the 'blank' formulation with known masses of therapeutic agent and subsequently determining the mass of agent within the formulation using the analytical method. Under ideal circumstances, i.e. in the absence of error associated with the operator or analytical equipment or interference with the method by other formulation ingredients, the mass of drug as determined using the analytical method should be identical to the known mass of added drug. Regression may be employed to examine the validity of this

relationship.

- *Identification of a linear (i.e. a directly proportional) relationship between two physicochemical properties.* For example, it is known that the rate of shear of a Newtonian liquid is directly proportional to the shearing stress applied. Therefore, if the flow properties of a pharmaceutical system are suspected to be Newtonian, the relationship between the shearing stress and the rate of shear should be determined experimentally and the linearity of the relationship between these two parameters statistically defined.

12.1.1 Mathematical description of linearity

In linear regression the relationship between two variables is described in terms of a *line of best fit*. The reader has probably been doing this visually for many years, in school science experiments. Typically, a student will attempt to select the gradient so that the line contacts as many points as possible, or so that the distance and number of points above the selected line are equal to those below the line. This ad-hoc method may satisfy the needs of school science experiments, but it requires mathematical intervention to improve its accuracy. Therefore linear regression analysis has evolved as a statistical process to mathematically predict the linear nature of the relationship between two variables. To understand this process it is necessary to remind the reader of the mathematical description of a straight line:

$$y = a + bx$$

where y and x are the dependent and independent variables, respectively, b is the slope (gradient) of the line and a is the intercept of the line, i.e. the value of y when $x = 0$. (The equation of a straight line is sometimes stated as $y = mx + c$, in which m and c replace the terms b and a in the above equation.)

From this equation it may be observed that the relationship between two variables may be mathematically described from knowledge of two parameters – the slope and the intercept – and, accordingly, these fundamental parameters are calculated in linear regression.

Assuming that there is a linear relationship between two variables, the equation for a straight line may be employed to determine the exact relationship between them, as shown in the following example.

EXAMPLE 12.1 *One stage in the industrial manufacture of ben-zylpenicillin by fermentation involves extraction of the active agent from the fermentation liquor into an organic solvent. The viscosity of the chosen organic solvent partly controls the efficiency of this extraction stage, so it is customary to examine the viscosity of individual* *batches of solvent to ensure that it is within the specifications of the extraction process. The viscosity of a Newtonian liquid (η), of which the solvent is an example, may be defined as the ratio of the shearing stress (τ) to the rate of shear ($\dot{\gamma}$), i.e. $\eta = \tau/\dot{\gamma}$. The manufacturer has stated that the viscosity of a new batch of organic solvent is 0.1 Pa s. As a quality control scientist you have been asked to perform an independent measurement of viscosity. How can you do this?*

The definition of viscosity states that there is a directly proportional relationship between the shearing stress and rate of shear, so if the shearing stress and the rate of shear are plotted as the x and y variables, the resultant graph should be linear. Based on the manufacturer's measurement of viscosity the shearing stress may be predicted at different rates of shear, e.g.

$$\eta = \frac{\tau}{\dot{\gamma}}$$

therefore

$$\dot{\gamma} \times \eta = \tau$$

When the rate of shear is 20 s^{-1}, the theoretical shearing stress may be calculated as $0.1 \times 20 = 20$ Pa. The remaining calculations in this series are shown in Table 12.1.

With knowledge of the relationship between the two variables, an experiment may be designed to determine the viscosity of the organic solution. Using a rheometer, the sample is exposed to an increasing rate of shear (20, 40, 60, 80 and 100 s^{-1}) and the associated shearing stress measured. Representative results from this experiment are also shown in Table 12.1.

The theoretical relationship between the rate of shear and shearing stress is shown in Figure 12.1. As may be observed a line of best fit has been applied to the relationship that, in this example, passes through

Table 12.1 Effect of increasing rate of shear of a pharmaceutical formulation on the resultant shearing stress

Rate of shear (s^{-1})	Theoretical shearing stress (Pa)	Shearing stress obtained experimentally (Pa)
20	2	1.8
40	4	4.1
60	6	6.2
80	8	8.4
100	10	9.8

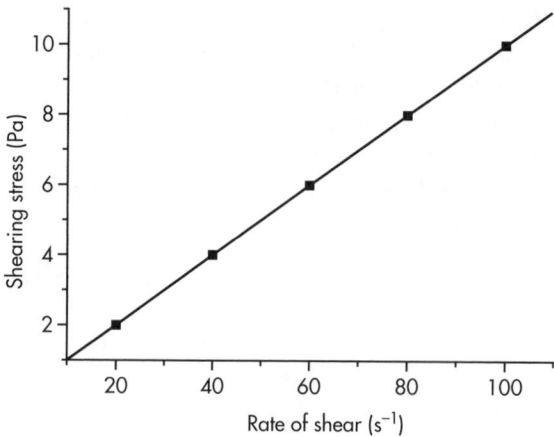

Figure 12.1 Theoretical relationship between the rate of shear of a pharmaceutical formulation and the application of shearing stresses of increasing magnitude.

the centre of each datum point. This is of course to be expected, as a theoretical relationship is definitive. Conversely, the relationship between these two variables, as determined experimentally, is shown in Figure 12.2. For comparison, the line of best fit for this set of data has been included. In contrast to Figure 12.1, the line of best fit in Figure 12.2 does not pass through each datum, but it is obvious to the eye that the line bisects the data, with the number of data and their distance above the line of best fit being similar to those below the line.

One obvious question concerns the disparity between the two sets of data and their associated lines of best fit. Despite the uncomplicated nature of the experimental procedure, the difference in the theoretical and experimental relationships between the rate of shear and shearing stress may be attributed to experimental error–operator error, small differences in the rheological properties of aliquots of the organic solvent, or machine variability. This example serves to highlight both the variability associated with any experimental procedure and, in addition, the difficulty of experimentally reproducing theoretical predictions.

The discussion so far has revolved around the visual differences between the lines of best fit of two sets of data. No details have yet been given of how these lines of best fit were generated. The visual method is not a responsible way of characterising the relationship between two variables (contrary to the beliefs of many students). In statistics a mathematical approach is adopted to define the linear relationship between two variables. In the absence of error, the relationship is definitive and the line of best fit passes through the central portion of each datum

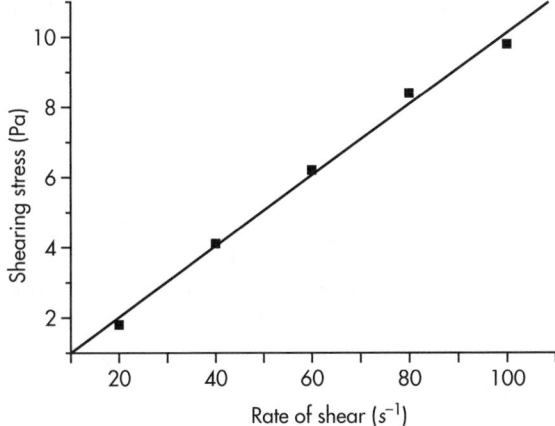

Figure 12.2 Experimental relationship between the rate of shear of a pharmaceutical formulation and the application of shearing stresses of increasing magnitude.

point (Figure 12.1). However, as this scenario is rarely seen experimentally, the line of best fit is mathematically defined as the line that minimises the difference between the each experimental datum point (y) and the equivalent point as defined by the line of best fit (Y). This concept is illustrated in Figure 12.3.

As previously described, the properties of a straight line are defined in terms of the slope, sometimes referred to as the *regression coefficient*, and the intercept of the line on the y axis, i.e. when the corresponding value on the x axis is 0. From early mathematical

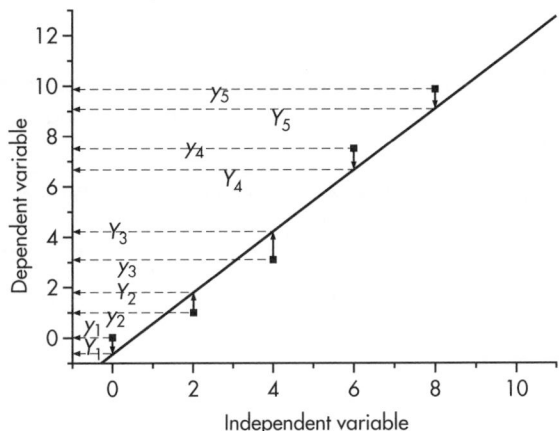

Figure 12.3 Relationship between an independent variable and a dependent variable as determined using linear regression analysis.

training the reader will recall that the slope is the gradient of the line. The slope (*b*) of a line of best fit is calculated by using the following equation:

$$b = \frac{N(\sum Xy) - (\sum X)(\sum y)}{N(\sum X^2) - (\sum X)^2}$$

where *N* is the number of pairs of data, $\sum X$ is the sum of all *X* values, $\sum y$ is the sum of all *y* values, $\sum X^2$ is the sum of the squares of all *X* values, $(\sum X)^2$ is the square of the sum of all *X* values and $\sum Xy$ is the sum of the product of each pair of values.

The use of this equation will be illustrated with reference to the data described in Table 12.1.

Theoretical shearing stress

The intercept and slope of the line of best fit relating to the relationship between the rate of shear of an organic solvent and the theoretical shearing stress required to maintain this rate of shear may be readily calculated in a simple stepwise fashion.

Step 1   Calculate the descriptive statistics associated with the regression
From the above equation the main parameters that are associated with the regression are $\sum y$, $\sum X^2$ and $(\sum X)^2$. Therefore, the first step in the calculation of a slope involves the calculation of these parameters. For convenience, these parameters are incorporated into the table of data, as shown in Table 12.2.

Step 2   Calculate the slope of the line of best fit
The slope of the line of best fit may now be calculated by inserting the

Table 12.2   Effect of increasing rate of shear of a pharmaceutical formulation on the resultant shearing stress, incorporating important parameters that are employed in linear regression analysis

Rate of shear (s⁻¹) (X)	Theoretical shearing stress (Pa) (y)	Product of X and y (Xy)
20	2	40
40	4	160
60	6	360
80	8	640
100	10	1000
$\sum X = 300$, $\bar{X} = 60$ $\sum X^2 = 22\,000$	$\sum y = 30$, $\bar{y} = 6$	$\sum Xy = 2200$

regression parameters into the appropriate equation:

$$b = \frac{N(\Sigma\, Xy) - (\Sigma\, X)(\Sigma\, y)}{N(\Sigma\, X^2) - (\Sigma\, X)^2} = \frac{(5 \times 2200) - (300)(30)}{(5 \times 22\,000) - (300)^2} = \frac{2000}{20\,000}$$

$$= 0.10 \text{ Pa s}$$

Therefore, the slope of the line (the viscosity in this example) is 0.1 Pa s. (Remember that the units of the calculated parameter must be included.)

Step 3 Calculate the intercept
Once the slope of the line has been calculated, finding the intercept is straightforward. Remembering that mathematically a straight line may be defined as $Y = a + bX$, the value of the intercept of the line of best fit may be calculated as follows:

$$a = \bar{y} - (b \times \bar{X})$$

where $\bar{Y}$ and $\bar{X}$ denote the mean of the Y and X values respectively. Therefore, the intercept of the line of best fit is:

$$a = \bar{y} - (b \times \bar{X})$$
$$= 6 - (0.1 \times 60)$$
$$= 0 \text{ Pa}$$

i.e. the line passes through the origin.

Experimentally measured shearing stress
The intercept and slope of the line of best fit for the experimentally observed shearing stress may be similarly be calculated in a stepwise fashion.

Step 1   Calculate the descriptive statistics associated with the regression
As before, the main parameters associated with the regression are calculated and incorporated into the original table of data (Table 12.3).

Step 2   Calculate the slope of the line of best fit
The slope of the line of best fit may now be calculated by inserting the regression parameters into the appropriate equation:

$$b = \frac{N(\Sigma\, Xy) - (\Sigma\, X)(\Sigma\, y)}{N(\Sigma\, X^2) - (\Sigma\, X)^2} = \frac{(5 \times 2234) - (300)(30.30)}{(5 \times 22000) - (300)^2} = \frac{2080}{20\,000}$$

$$= 0.104 \text{ Pa s}$$

Therefore, the slope of the line (the viscosity in this example) is 0.104 Pa s.

Step 3   Calculate the intercept
The intercept of the line of best fit is calculated as before, by rearranging

Table 12.3 Effect of increasing rate of shear of a pharmaceutical formulation on the resultant shearing stress, incorporating important parameters that are employed in linear regression analysis

Rate of shear (s⁻¹) (X)	Shearing stress obtained experimentally (Pa) (y)	Product of X and y (Xy)
20	1.8	36
40	4.1	164
60	6.2	372
80	8.4	672
100	9.8	990
$\Sigma X = 300$, $\bar{X} = 60$ $\Sigma X = 22\,000$	$\Sigma y = 30.30$, $\bar{y} = 6.06$	$\Sigma Xy = 2234$

the equation describing a straight line:

$$a = \bar{y} - (b \times \bar{X})$$
$$= 6.06 - (0.104 \times 69)$$
$$= -0.18 \text{ Pa}$$

The disparity between the theoretical calculations of the slope and intercept and their experimentally derived counterparts is due to statistical error, as discussed previously.

One further significant point about the mathematical description of linear relationships is the need for simultaneous expression of the slope and the intercept to achieve a comprehensive understanding of the properties of the relationship. Once these two parameters have been clearly defined, the mathematical description of the line is complete and all the properties of the relationship are known. Knowledge of the slope or the intercept alone does not identify the relationship between two variables. This problem is illustrated in Figures 12.4a and b. In these figures the mass of drug released *in vitro* from six different formulations of a solid dosage form has been plotted as a function of time. In Figure 12.4a, the rates of release of the drug from three selected formulations, as defined by their slopes, are different, yet the intercept on the y axis for each formulation is identical. Conversely, in Figure 12.4b, the rate of release of drug from the three selected formulations is identical (parallel slopes) but the values of the y intercept are disparate. Therefore, although there are similarities between the six formulations in terms of the relationship between the mass of drug released as a function of time, the relationship for each formulation is unique.

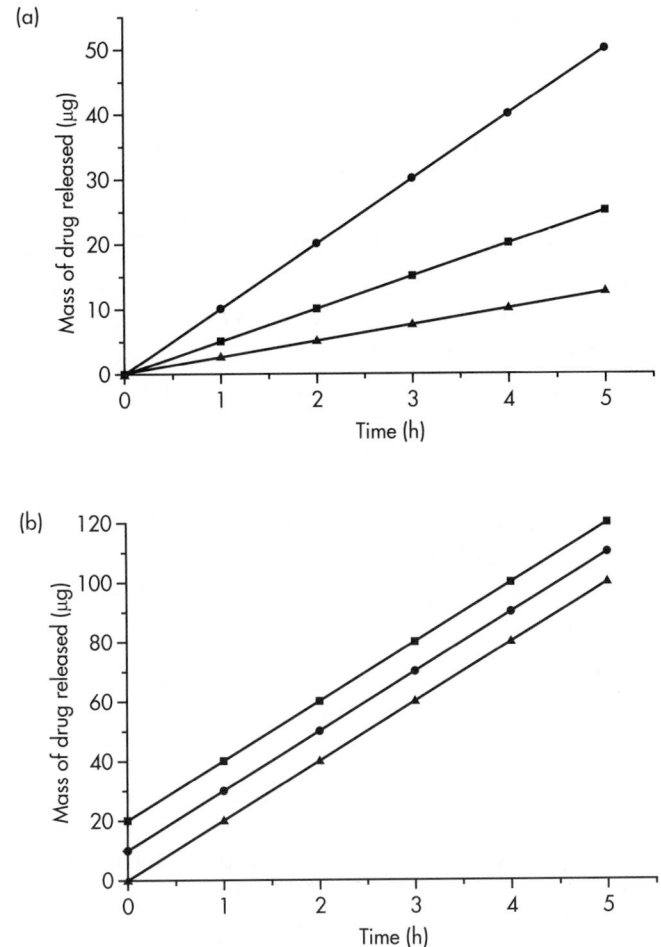

Figure 12.4 Mass of drug released in vitro as a function of time from six different formulations of a solid dosage form.

Accordingly, in linear regression analysis, both the slope and the *y* intercept should be calculated and expressed.

In all the examples that have been described so far, the application of linear regression to experimental or theoretical data has generated a positive slope. In many circumstances in the pharmaceutical and related sciences, the slope has as a negative value. This is not abnormal, and the analyst should consider the nature of the experiment before relegating the calculation to the waste bin. A negative slope simply refers to an inverse relationship between two variables, i.e. as the independent variable decreases the dependent variable increases. The process of linear regression for this type of response is identical to that shown earlier. However, to ensure clarity on this issue, the application of linear regression under these circumstances is illustrated in the following example.

EXAMPLE 12.2 *A company that specialises in the formulation of controlled-release drug delivery systems wishes to examine the diffusion of a therapeutic agent across a novel porous polymeric system, designed for use as a tablet coating. For this purpose, it has been decided to use a side-by-side diffusion apparatus in which the donor and receptor compartments are separated by a film of the novel polymer. The donor compartment contains a solution of known concentration of the therapeutic agent; the receptor compartment contains buffer at pH 7.4, but no drug. To examine the rate of diffusion of the drug from the donor compartment to the receptor compartment through the polymeric film (10 cm² surface area), samples of solution from the donor compartment are removed at defined periods and the mass of drug is quantified using a suitable analytical method. The results of the study are shown in Table 12.4. Using an appropriate statistical method, calculate the flux of the drug across the polymeric membrane.*

Theoretically, the diffusion of a therapeutic agent across a polymeric membrane is defined by the following equation:

$$\frac{dM}{dt} = \frac{DAkC_d}{h}$$

where D is the diffusion coefficient of the drug across the polymeric film, A is the surface area of the film exposed within the side-by-side diffusion cell, k is the membrane : buffer (donor) partition coefficient and h is the thickness of the polymeric film. All of the above terms are constant, so if the concentration of drug in the donor compartment (C_d)

Table 12.4 Concentration of drug in the donor compartment as a function of time in a side-by-side diffusion experiment designed to examine drug flux across a novel porous polymeric film

Time (h)	Mass of therapeutic agent in the donor compartment (mg)
1	248.7
2	246.6
3	244.9
4	243.4
5	242.1
6	241.9
7	240.1

remains constant (i.e. remains within 90% of the original concentration at the start of the experiment), the diffusion of drug across the membrane will be constant (linear). The flux (J) is defined as

$$J = \frac{1}{S} \times \frac{dM}{dt}$$

Therefore, the flux may be calculated experimentally by plotting the concentration of drug remaining in the donor compartment as a function of time, determining of the slope using linear regression analysis and dividing the calculated value of the slope by the surface area (S) of the membrane. In light of this, the relationship between the mass of drug in the donor compartment and time is established using linear regression analysis.

Step 1   Calculate the descriptive statistics associated with the regression
The main parameters associated with the regression are calculated and incorporated into the original table of data (Table 12.5).

Step 2   Calculate the slope of the line of best fit
The slope of the line of best fit may now be calculated by inserting the regression parameters into the following equation:

$$b = \frac{N(\Sigma\, Xy) - (\Sigma\, X)(\Sigma\, y)}{N(\Sigma\, X^2) - (\Sigma\, X)^2} = \frac{(7 \times 6759.60) - (28)(1703.0)}{(7 \times 140) - (28)^2}$$

$$= \frac{-366.8}{196} = -1.87 \text{ mg/h}$$

Table 12.5   Concentration of drug in the donor compartment as a function of time in a side-by-side diffusion experiment designed to examine drug flux across a novel porous polymeric film, incorporating important parameters that are employed in linear regression analysis

Time (h)	Mass of therapeutic agent in the donor compartment (mg)	Product of X and y
1	248.7	248.7
2	247.6	495.2
3	244.9	734.7
4	242.4	969.6
5	242.1	1210.5
6	240.2	1441.2
7	237.1	1659.7
$\Sigma X = 28$, $\bar{X} = 4$ $\Sigma X^2 = 140$	$\Sigma y = 1703.0$, $\bar{y} = 243.29$	$\Sigma Xy = 6759.6$

Therefore, the slope of the line is 1.87 mg/h. The minus sign indicates an overall decrease in concentration in the donor cell over the course of the experiment. To calculate the flux of the therapeutic agent across the novel porous polymeric film, it is necessary to divide the calculated rate of diffusion (slope) by the surface area of the polymeric film within the diffusion apparatus (10 cm^2). Therefore the flux of the therapeutic agent across the polymeric film is 0.187 mg h^{-1} cm^{-2}.

Step 3   Calculate the intercept
With the above knowledge the intercept is calculated as before:

$$a = \bar{y} - (b \times \bar{X})$$
$$= 243.29 - (-1.87 \times 4)$$
$$= 250.77 \text{ mg}$$

It is important that the sign associated with the slope is included in the above equation, otherwise the result will be incorrect.

A graphical representation of the line of best fit for the data set described in Example 12.2 (i.e. $b = -1.87$ mg/h, $a = 250.77$ mg) is shown in Figure 12.5.

12.1.2   Assumptions of linear regression analysis

At this stage the reader should have a basic understanding of the mechanism by which a line of best fit may be applied to a set of data. However, the application of linear regression analysis to experimentally derived data involves more than the definition of the slope and intercept

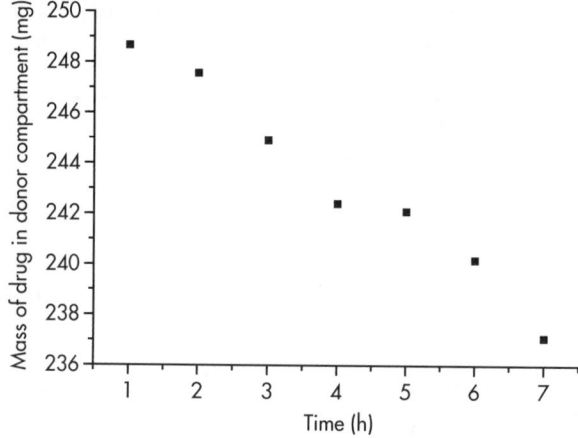

Figure 12.5   Rate of diffusion of a therapeutic agent across a novel porous polymeric film, assessed using a side-by-side diffusion apparatus.

of the line of best fit. Typically, the statistical analyst will wish to examine hypotheses concerning the regression or, in some cases, compute the confidence intervals associated with regression parameters. However, before this can be done, several assumptions concerning the regression process must be satisfied:

- For each value of x the corresponding y value has been sampled from a population that is normally distributed.
- Each of the populations from which the y values have been sampled must possess a similar variance. When this assumption is invalid, a process referred to as *weighted regression* is carried out to characterise the relationship between the two variables, but this technique is beyond the scope of this book.
- The y values have been randomly sampled from their populations and the sampling process is unbiased.
- There is no error associated with the measurement of each x value. The reader will appreciate that there is in fact error associated with the measurement of each x value, but as the extent of this is much less than that associated with the measurement of the corresponding y values, this is a relatively secure assumption.
- A linear relationship does in fact exist between the independent and dependent variables. This may seem nonsensical, but the author has encountered several cases in which students have attempted to perform a linear regression on two variables whose relationship is non-linear. An example of this is shown in Figure 12.6. This figure is a graphical representation of the release of a therapeutic agent from a heterogeneous polymer matrix plotted as a function of time. Linear regression analysis has been employed to generate a line of best fit to this data. As may be observed, the line of best fit does not adequately describe the mathematical relationship between the two variables and it is therefore erroneous to attempt to report a linear relationship. The

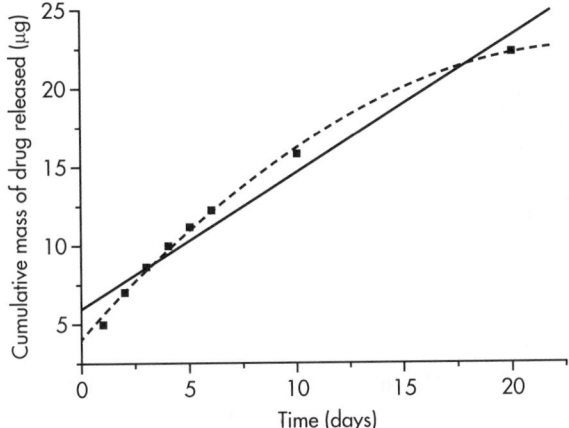

Figure 12.6 Relationship between cumulative mass of drug released from a polymeric matrix and time, as determined using an *in vitro* dissolution test.

true relationship (the cumulative mass of drug released is proportional to $t^{0.5}$) is presented as a dashed line.

One further comment concerning the application of linear regression relates to the general suitability of the data for statistical manipulation by this method. Two further potential problems associated with the use of linear regression are shown in Figure 12.7a and b. In Figure 12.7a the data is clustered into two sections of the graph with no available data to describe the intermediate region. Therefore, the analyst can not be certain that, following application of linear regression, the line

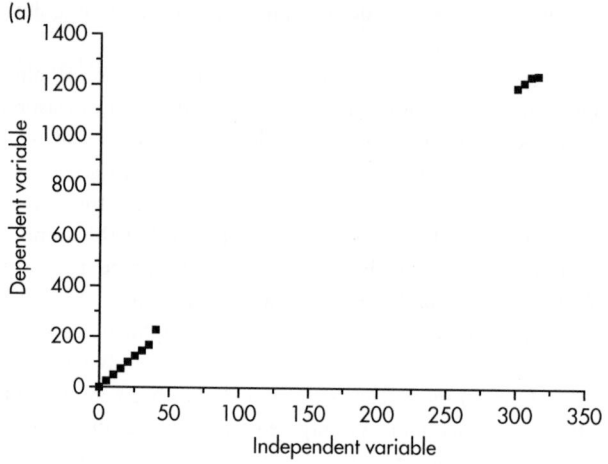

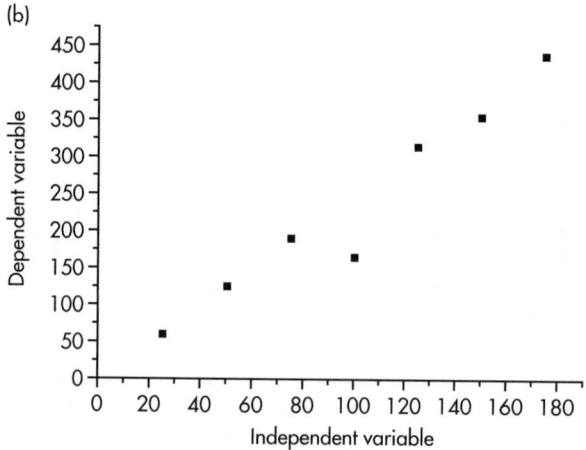

Figure 12.7 Experimental scenarios in which direct application of linear regression may be disadvantageous.

of best fit is suitable to describe this intermediate region, i.e. the section of the graph that is devoid of data. If a complete set of data had been collected, the relationship between the two variables might be found to be non-linear. In Figure 12.7b enough data has been collected to examine the relationship between the independent and dependent variables. However, calculation of line of best fit associated with the data is compromised by the presence of the datum corresponding to an x value of 100. In statistical terms this datum may represent an outlier and should be removed before carrying out the linear regression analysis.

12.1.3 Application of linear regression analysis to replicate measurements

In all the examples that have described so far in this chapter, a single measurement of the independent variable has been performed for each chosen x value. The reader will be aware of the need to perform replicate measurements of experimental data and accordingly, linear regression is most frequently performed on replicate measurements of the independent variable associated with each value of the independent variable. The mechanics of linear regression analysis for replicate measurements are identical to those described through the course of this chapter. However, to enhance the readers' understanding of this statistical technique, the following example describes the application of this technique in detail.

EXAMPLE 12.3 *Reservoir systems are dosage forms which have a coating applied to their external surface to control the subsequent release of therapeutic agent into body fluids. One way in which the release of the therapeutic agent from such systems may be modified is by altering the formulation of the coating system. In a laboratory study the rates of release of a therapeutic agent from tablets that have been coated to a defined thickness with a polymeric coating composed of different blends of two polymers (A and B) have been examined. The results are displayed in Table 12.6. Using an appropriate statistical method, examine the relationship between the composition of the polymeric coating and the subsequent rate of release of therapeutic agent.*

Step 1 Calculate the descriptive statistics associated with the regression
The main parameters associated with the regression are calculated and incorporated into the table of data (Table 12.7).

Table 12.6 Effects of the composition of a polymeric coating on the subsequent rate of release (μg/h) of a therapeutic agent from tablets *in vitro*

Proportion of A : B	Replicate 1	Replicate 2	Replicate 3	Replicate 4
0 : 100	124	136	129	121
20 : 80	151	155	162	154
40 : 60	170	179	180	175
60 : 40	202	209	211	215
80 : 20	230	235	225	224
100 : 0	265	274	260	257

Table 12.7 Effects of the composition of a polymeric coating on the subsequent rate of release of a therapeutic agent from tablets *in vitro*, incorporating important parameters that are employed in linear regression analysis

Proportion of A : B	Rate of release of therapeutic agent (μg/h)	Product of X and y
0	124	0
0	136	0
0	129	0
0	140	0
20	151	3 020
20	155	3 100
20	165	3 300
20	154	3 080
40	170	6 800
40	179	7 160
40	190	7 600
40	175	7 000
60	202	12 120
60	209	12 540
60	211	12 660
60	215	12 900
80	230	18 400
80	235	18 800
80	225	18 000
80	224	17 920
100	265	26 500
100	280	28 000
100	260	26 000
100	257	25 700
$\Sigma X = 1200$, $\bar{X} = 50$ $\Sigma X^2 = 88\ 000$	$\Sigma y = 4681$, $\bar{y} = 195.04$	$\Sigma Xy = 270\ 600$

Step 2 Calculate the slope of the line of best fit
The slope of the line of best fit may now be calculated by inserting the regression parameters into the appropriate equation, remembering that the number of pairs of data (N) is 24:

$$b = \frac{N(\Sigma\, Xy) - (\Sigma\, X)(\Sigma\, y)}{N(\Sigma\, X^2) - (\Sigma\, X)^2} = \frac{(24 \times 270\ 600) - (1200)(4681)}{(24 \times 88\ 000) - (1200)^2}$$

$$= \frac{877\ 200}{672\ 000} = 1.31\ \mu g/h$$

Step 3 Calculate the intercept
With the above knowledge the intercept is calculated as before:

$$a = \bar{y} - (b \times \overline{X})$$
$$= 195.04 - (1.31 \times 50)$$
$$= 129.54\ \mu g/h.$$

Step 4 Summary
The slope (b) and intercept (a) of the line of best fit, as determined by linear regression analysis, are 1.31 $\mu g/h$ and 129.54 $\mu g/h$, respectively. A graphical representation of the relationship between the rate of drug release and composition of the polymeric coating is shown in Figure 12.8.

12.1.4 Statistical methods for the assessment of the relationship between two variables

The examples that have been described in this chapter so far have considered experimental situations in which a series of measurements of a dependent variable have been made as a function of a defined independent variable. Analysis of the data by linear regression has enabled a description of the relationship between the two variables to be mathematically determined. In scientific experiments, this mathematical relationship may then be used to estimate the value of the dependent variable associated with an experimentally measured independent variable. For example, in pharmaceutical analysis a calibration curve is established in which the relationship between the dependent variable (concentration of drug in a defined matrix, e.g. buffer, formulation, biological tissue) and the independent variable (analytical response) is mathematically defined by linear regression. Subsequently, the concentration of drug in a matrix may be determined by measurement of the analytical response and, from the linear regression, calculation of the x value associated with this response.

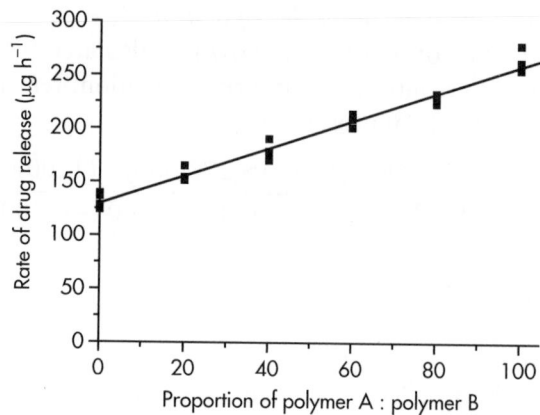

Figure 12.8 Effect of polymeric coating composition on the rate of release of a therapeutic agent from a tablet.

The above discussion hinges on the assumption that a linear rela-tionship actually exists between the two variables, i.e. the slope $(b) > 0$ or < 0. As in all statistical methods, it is assumed that the data collected in the sampling process are representative of the population(s) from which the data were extracted. If the sample data is not representative of the population, the linear relationship that has been identified by linear regression may be invalid. Consequently, it is important to examine the reliability of linear regression analysis and, in so doing, the statistical analyst may ascertain whether this result is indeed representative of the population from which the data have been sampled. The process by which this task is performed is similar to other statistical tests described in previous chapters. As before, the null and alternative hypotheses, the level of significance and the number of tails associated with the experi-mental design are defined. In linear regression analysis, it is assumed that the null hypothesis states that the slope is equal to zero, whereas the alternative hypothesis states that the slope is not equal to zero. The number of tails refers to the number of ways in which the null hypoth-esis may be rejected. There are two statistical tests that may be employed to determine the validity of the relationship between the two variables, as defined by the line of best fit, the analysis of variance and the two-independent-samples t test.

12.1.4.1 Analysis of variance and linear regression analysis

The application of the analysis of variance method to examine the validity of linear regression analysis is similar to that described in Chapter 10. Therefore, in this technique, the F ratio is calculated and is used to determine whether the null hypothesis should be accepted or rejected. If the null hypothesis is accepted, we may be conclude that there is no relationship between the two variables and therefore the line of best fit that has been calculated by linear regression is not representative of the relationship that exists in the population from which the sample data were derived. Conversely, if the null hypothesis is rejected, we conclude that the slope is not equal to zero and hence the relationship defined by linear regression analysis is accurate. The mechanics of the ANOVA involve the calculation of three sum-of-squares terms: the total sum of squares (SS_{total}), the regression sum of squares ($SS_{regression}$) and the residual sum of squares ($SS_{residual}$).

- *Total sum of squares (SS_{total})*. This is the sum of the squares of the differences between each y value as determined experimentally and that predicted from the linear regression analysis, and is calculated using the following formula:

$$SS_{total} = \Sigma(y - Y)^2 = \Sigma y^2 - \frac{(\Sigma y)^2}{n}$$

where y denotes the individual experimentally collected measurements of the dependent variable and n is the number of pairs of data that is collected experimentally. The total sum of squares is therefore a measure of the variability of the data from the predicted relationship.

- *Regression sum of squares ($SS_{regression}$)*. This is a measure of the variability between the individual experimentally determined y values and is calculated using the following equation:

$$SS_{regression} = \frac{[(\Sigma Xy) - (\Sigma X \Sigma y/n)]^2}{\Sigma X^2 - (\Sigma X)^2/n}$$

where X and y denote the individual measurements of the independent and dependent variables and n is the number of pairs of data that is collected experimentally.

- *Residual sum of squares ($SS_{residual}$)*. This is a measure of the variability of the data around the line of best fit that has been defined by linear regression. If all the data fall exactly on the calculated line of best fit, this would imply that the experiment has no associated error and, accordingly, the residual sum of squares is equal to zero. The residual sum of squares is calculated with knowledge of the total and regression sum of squares as follows:

$$SS_{residual} = SS_{total} - SS_{regression}$$

- *Calculation of the F ratio*. The F ratio is calculated in a similar fashion to that described in Chapter 10 and is the ratio of the regression mean squares to the residual mean squares, i.e.

$$F = \frac{MeanSquares_{regression}}{MeanSquares_{residual}}$$

Interpretation of the relevance of the calculated F ratio involves comparing the calculated F statistic (ratio) to the critical F statistic, which is obtained from the table of the critical values of the F distribution (Appendix 7) under the conditions of the experimental design.

The following examples illustrate the use of ANOVA in the process of linear regression.

EXAMPLE 12.4 *In Example 12.2 linear regression analysis was performed to evaluate the relationship between time and concentration of therapeutic agent in the donor compartment in a diffusion experiment. Using an appropriate statistical method, examine the validity of the calculated linear relationship between these two variables.*

The important descriptive statistics associated with this example, as depicted in Table 12.5, are $\Sigma X = 28$, $\Sigma y = 1703$, $(\Sigma Xy) = 6759.6$, $\Sigma X^2 = 140$, $\Sigma y^2 = 414\ 161.1$, slope $(b) = -1.87$ mg/h and intercept $(a) = 250.77$ mg.

The application of statistical methods within linear regression analysis will be treated in the same manner as all other statistical tests and, as a result, the experimental parameters are once more defined.

(i) State the null hypothesis

The null hypothesis for this example states that a linear relationship does not exist between time and the concentration of drug present in the donor solution:

H_0: $\beta = 0$, where β is the slope of the population.

(ii) State the alternative hypothesis

The alternative hypothesis for this example states that there is a (linear) relationship between time and the concentration of drug present in the donor solution:

H_a: $\beta \neq 0$

(iii) State the level of significance

In this example, it is assumed that the level of significance (α) is 0.05.

(iv) Perform the ANOVA

As in previous examples, the execution of the ANOVA associated with linear regression will be performed in a stepwise fashion to maintain clarity.

Step 1   Calculate the total sum of squares

$$SS_{total} = \Sigma\, y^2 - \frac{(\Sigma\, y)^2}{n} = 414\,416.1 - \frac{(1703)^2}{7} = 100.53$$

Step 2   Calculate the regression sum of squares

$$SS_{regression} = \frac{[(\Sigma\, Xy) - (\Sigma\, X\, \Sigma\, y/n)]^2}{\Sigma\, X^2 - ((\Sigma\, X)^2/n)} = \frac{[(6759.6) - (28 \times 1703)/7]^2}{140 - (28)^2/7}$$

$$= \frac{2745.76}{28} = 98.06$$

Step 3   Calculate the residual sum of squares

$$SS_{residual} = SS_{total} - SS_{regression} = 100.53 - 98.06 = 2.47$$

Step 4   Construct a summary table for the analysis of variance
The summary table for the ANOVA gathers all the relevant information that is required to calculate the F ratio (F statistic). $SS_{regression}$ and $SS_{residual}$ are transposed into their equivalent mean squares by dividing by the appropriate number of degrees of freedom. In this example the total number of degrees of freedom refers to the total number of pairs of data in the regression – 1, i.e. $7 - 1 = 6$. The number of degrees of freedom associated with the regression is always 1 in simple linear regression. The number of degrees of freedom associated with the residual sum of squares is calculated by subtracting the number of degrees of freedom associated with the regression from the total number of degrees of freedom.

With this information in mind, the ANOVA summary table is constructed (Table 12.8).

Step 5   Define the critical F statistic
The critical F statistic is derived from the F distribution after consideration of the parameters of the experiment, i.e. the numbers of degrees of freedom associated with both the regression and residuals

Table 12.8 Summary of the output of the analysis of variance for the linear regression of time and concentration of drug in the donor compartment in a diffusion experiment

Source	Sum of squares	df	Mean square	F statistic
Regression	98.06	1	98.06	200.12
Residual	2.47	5	0.49	
Total	100.53	6		

and, additionally, the chosen level of significance. In this example, these parameters are as follows:

- level of significance $(\alpha) = 0.05$
- $df_{\text{regression}} = 1$
- $df_{\text{residual}} = 5$

Under these experimental conditions the critical value of the F statistic is derived from the table of the critical values of the F distribution (Appendix 7) and is 6.61.

Step 6   Interpret the outcome of the statistical analysis
Compare the value of the critical F statistic to that of the calculated F statistic. If the critical F statistic is greater than the calculated statistic, the null hypothesis is accepted, whereas, if the calculated value is either equal to or greater than the critical value, the null hypothesis is rejected in favour of the alternative hypothesis. In this example, $F_{\text{calculated}} > F_{\text{critical}}$ and, accordingly, the null hypothesis is rejected, i.e. the slope of the line of best fit, generated by linear regression, is not equal to zero. Therefore, it may be concluded that the calculated linear relationship between time and concentration of drug in the donor cell of a diffusion cell is valid.

To illustrate a further example of the use of the ANOVA in conjunction with linear regression, the nature of the relationship between the composition of a tablet coating and the associated *in vitro* rate of release of a therapeutic agent, described in Example 12.3, is examined further in the next example.

EXAMPLE 12.5   *In Example 12.3, linear regression analysis was performed to examine the nature of the relationship between the polymer composition of a tablet coating and the subsequent rate of release of a therapeutic agent from the solid dosage form. Using an appropriate statistical method, examine the validity of the calculated linear relationship between these two variables.*

As before, the relevant descriptive statistics associated with the linear regression are stated: $\Sigma X = 1200$, $\Sigma y = 4681$, $\Sigma(Xy) = 270\,600$, $\Sigma X^2 = 88\,000$, $\Sigma y^2 = 961\,977$, slope $(b) = 1.31\ \mu g/h$, intercept $(a) = 129.54\ \mu g/h$.

Using a similar format to previous examples, the experimental parameters are defined.

(i)   State the null hypothesis

The null hypothesis for this example states that a linear relationship does not exist between polymer composition and the rate of release of therapeutic agent from the solid dosage form:

H_0: $\beta = 0$, where β is the slope of the population.

(ii) State the alternative hypothesis

The alternative hypothesis for this example states that there is a (linear) relationship between polymer composition and the rate of release of therapeutic agent from the solid dosage form:

H_a: $\beta \neq 0$

(iii) State the level of significance

In this example, it is assumed that the level of significance (α) is 0.05.

(iv) Perform the ANOVA

Step 1 Calculate the total sum of squares

$$SS_{total} = \Sigma y^2 - \frac{(\Sigma y)^2}{n} = 961977 - \frac{(4681)^2}{24} = 48986.96$$

Step 2 Calculate the regression sum of squares

$$SS_{regression} = \frac{[(\Sigma Xy) - \Sigma X \Sigma y/n]^2}{\Sigma X^2 - (\Sigma X)^2/n}$$

$$= \frac{[(270\,600) - (1200 \times 4681)/24]^2}{88\,000 - (1200)^2/24} = 47\,710.80$$

Step 3 Calculate the residual sum of squares

$$SS_{residual} = SS_{total} - SS_{regression}$$
$$= 48\,986.96 - 47\,710.8$$
$$= 1276.16$$

Step 4 Construct a summary table for the analysis of variance
The numbers of degrees of freedom (df) associated with the regression parameters are:

- df_{total} = number of observations − 1 = 24 − 1 = 23
- $df_{regression}$ = 1
- $df_{residual} = df_{total} - df_{regression}$ = 23 − 1 = 22

With this information, the mean sum of squares for each regression parameter is calculated and the ANOVA summary table constructed (Table 12.9).

Table 12.9 Summary of the output of the analysis of variance concerning the linear regression of tablet coating composition and subsequent rate of drug release

Source	Sum of squares	df	Mean square	F statistic
Regression	47 710.80	1	47 710.80	822.46
Residual	1 276.16	22	58.01	
Total	48 986.96	23		

Step 5   Define the critical F statistic
The critical F statistic is determined using Appendix 7, based on the following information concerning the statistical design:

- level of significance $(\alpha) = 0.05$
- $df_{\text{regression}} = 1$
- $df_{\text{residual}} = 22$

Under these experimental conditions the critical value of the F statistic is 4.30.

Step 6   Interpret the outcome of the statistical analysis
In this example, the calculated F statistic is greater than the critical F statistic, so the null hypothesis is rejected in favour of the alternative hypothesis. Therefore, it may be concluded that the linear relationship, defined using linear regression, is valid.

One of the primary assumptions of linear regression is of course that a linear relationship exists between two variables. An example in which a linear regression was an inappropriate method to describe such a relationship was illustrated earlier in this chapter in Figure 12.6. It is naive to imagine that all relationships are linear in nature, but this does not preclude the use of linear regression to examine the nature of the relationship. Under these circumstances, the non-linear relationship between the two variables is mathematically transformed into a linear relationship. The following example illustrates this principle.

EXAMPLE 12.6   *Controlled-release formulations for intravaginal administration may conveniently be prepared by mixing the therapeutic agent with polydimethylsiloxane and cross-linking this system within an appropriate mould. In a pharmaceutical company, a batch of intravaginal silicone rings (IVR) has been prepared using this technique and the release of drug from six samples examined using a modification of the USP dissolution method. The percentage of the original mass of drug released as a function of time was determined, and the results are shown in Table 12.10. Using an appropriate statistical method, examine the*

Table 12.10 Experimental examination of the release of a therapeutic agent from intravaginal silicone rings as a function of time. Release is expressed as the percentage of the original mass of drug released

Time (days)	% of original mass of drug released					
	IVR 1	IVR 2	IVR 3	IVR 4	IVR 5	IVR 6
0.5	14.16	14.24	14.01	14.36	14.14	14.1
1.0	20.56	20.15	21.39	19.64	19.99	20.14
2.0	28.61	28.04	28.46	28.19	27.99	28.54
3.0	33.99	34.60	34.76	34.79	34.50	34.49
4.0	39.61	39.10	41.12	40.64	40.9	39.91
5.0	44.51	43.99	44.96	45.10	44.51	44.71
6.0	49.68	49.61	51.01	50.43	50.13	49.91
7.0	53.16	53.05	52.69	53.04	52.61	52.99

relationship between the release of therapeutic agent from these systems and time.

The release of therapeutic agents from controlled-release systems may be conveniently described by the following generic equation (Peppas, 1985):

$$\frac{M_t}{M_\infty} = kt^n$$

where M_t/M_∞ is the fractional drug release, i.e. the percentage of the original mass of drug released as a function of time (t), k is the release rate, t is the time of release and n is the release exponent. Therefore, as the relationship between the mass of drug released and time is non-linear, the application of linear regression to this situation is invalid. However, the above equation may be mathematically manipulated to enable the application of linear regression analysis. Thus,

$$\frac{M_t}{M_\infty} = kt^n$$

$$\ln \frac{M_t}{M_\infty} = \ln k + n \ln t$$

From the above equation it may be predicted that there is a linear relationship between the natural logarithm of the fractional drug release and the natural logarithm of time, the intercept and slope being defined by the natural logarithm of the release rate and the release exponent, respectively. With this in mind, the data in Table 12.10 is transformed by application of natural logarithms to both the percentage drug released and time (Table 12.11).

Table 12.11 Logarithmic transformations of the data obtained from experimental examination of the release of a therapeutic agent from intravaginal silicone rings as a function of time

In [Time (days)]	In % of original mass of drug released					
	IVR 1	IVR 2	IVR 3	IVR 4	IVR 5	IVR 6
−0.69	2.65	2.66	2.64	2.66	2.65	2.65
0.0	3.02	3.00	3.06	2.98	3.00	3.00
0.69	3.35	3.33	3.35	3.34	3.33	3.35
1.10	3.53	3.54	3.55	3.55	3.54	3.54
1.39	3.68	3.67	3.72	3.70	3.71	3.69
1.61	3.80	3.78	3.81	3.81	3.80	3.80
1.79	3.91	3.90	3.93	3.92	3.91	3.91
1.95	3.97	3.97	3.96	3.97	3.96	3.97

The relationship between the natural logarithms of both the percentage drug release and time may now be found, combining the approaches that have been described previously.

Application of linear regression analysis

Step 1   Calculate the descriptive statistics associated with the regression
The main parameters associated with the linear regression procedure are calculated and presented as a table (Table 12.12).

Step 2   Calculate the slope of the line of best fit
The slope of the line of best fit may now be calculated by inserting the regression parameters into the appropriate equation. In this example the number of observations (N) is 48.

$$b = \frac{N(\Sigma Xy) - (\Sigma X)(\Sigma y)}{N(\Sigma X^2) - (\Sigma X)^2} = \frac{(48 \times 182.20) - (47.04)(167.52)}{(48 \times 82.16) - (47.04)^2}$$
$$= 0.50$$

Step 3   Calculation of the intercept
With the above knowledge the intercept may be calculated:

$$a = \bar{y} - (b \times \bar{X})$$
$$= 3.49 - (0.50 \times 0.98)$$
$$= 3.00$$

Remembering that the y axis is represented as a natural logarithm, the real value of the y intercept may be calculated by determining the

Table 12.12 Logarithmic transformations of the data obtained from experimental examination of the release of a therapeutic agent from intravaginal silicone rings as a function of time, incorporating important parameters that are employed in linear regression analysis

ln [Time (days)] (X)	ln % of original mass of drug released (y)	Product of X and y
−0.69	2.65	−1.83
−0.69	2.66	−1.84
−0.69	2.64	−1.82
−0.69	2.66	−1.84
−0.69	2.65	−1.83
−0.69	2.65	−1.83
0.00	3.02	0.00
0.00	3.00	0.00
0.00	3.06	0.00
0.00	2.98	0.00
0.00	3.00	0.00
0.00	3.00	0.00
0.69	3.35	2.31
0.69	3.33	2.30
0.69	3.35	2.31
0.69	3.34	2.30
0.69	3.33	2.30
0.69	3.35	2.31
1.10	3.53	3.88
1.10	3.54	3.89
1.10	3.55	3.91
1.10	3.55	3.91
1.10	3.54	3.89
1.10	3.54	3.89
1.39	3.68	5.12
1.39	3.67	5.10
1.39	3.72	5.17
1.39	3.70	5.14
1.39	3.71	5.16
1.39	3.69	5.13
1.61	3.80	6.12
1.61	3.78	6.09
1.61	3.81	6.13
1.61	3.81	6.13
1.61	3.80	6.12
1.61	3.80	6.12
1.79	3.91	7.00
1.79	3.90	6.98

continued

Table 12.12 *Continued*

In [Time (days)] (X)	In % of original mass of drug released (y)	Product of X and y
1.79	3.93	7.03
1.79	3.92	7.02
1.79	3.91	7.00
1.79	3.91	7.00
1.95	3.97	7.74
1.95	3.97	7.74
1.95	3.96	7.72
1.95	3.97	7.74
1.95	3.96	7.72
1.95	3.97	7.74
$\Sigma X = 47.04$, $\bar{X}0.98$ $\Sigma X^2 = 82.16$	$\Sigma y = 167.52$, $\bar{y} = 3.49$	$\Sigma Xy = 182.20$

antilogarithm of the calculated value:

$$y = e^{3.00} = 20.09\% \ \text{day}^{-0.5}$$

Step 4 Summary
The slope (*b*) and intercept (*a*) of the line of best fit, as determined by linear regression of the logarithmically transformed data are 0.50 and 20.09% day$^{-0.5}$, respectively. A graphical representation of the relationship between the natural logarithm of the percentage drug release and natural logarithm of time is shown in Figure 12.9. The release rate of the drug from the intravaginal ring is defined as the *y* intercept in the above regression and is of course a parameter that is of great interest to the formulation scientist. However, of similar importance is the use of regression analysis to determine the magnitude of the release exponent as this provides an insight into the mechanism of drug release from the formulation. From the regression analysis the slope of the line of best fit was identified as 0.50, a value that confirms diffusion as the predominant mechanism of drug release from these systems.

Having mathematically defined the relationship between the two variables in the form of a line of best fit, it is important to statistically examine the nature of the relationship using an appropriate statistical test. For the purpose of this example, ANOVA will be employed.

First, the relevant descriptive statistics are expressed: $\Sigma X = 47.04$, $\Sigma y = 167.52$, $\Sigma(Xy) = 182.20$, $\Sigma X^2 = 82.16$, $\Sigma y^2 = 593.6$.

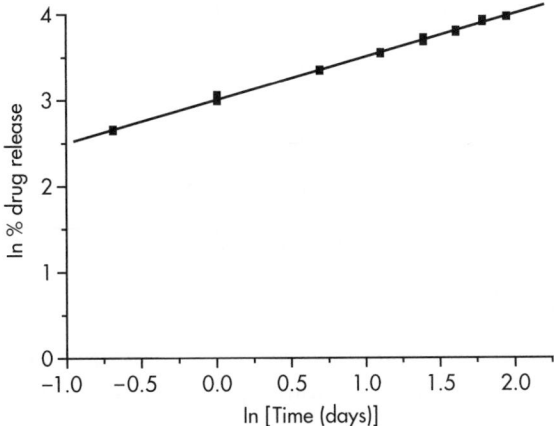

Figure 12.9 Release of a therapeutic agent from intravaginal silicone rings as a function of time.

(i) State the null hypothesis

The null hypothesis states that a linear relationship does not exist between the natural logarithm of the percentage of drug released and the natural logarithm of time:

$$H_0: \quad \beta = 0$$

(ii) State the alternative hypothesis

The alternative hypothesis states that a linear relationship does exist between the natural logarithm of the percentage of drug released and the natural logarithm of time:

$$H_a: \quad \beta \neq 0$$

(iii) State the level of significance

In this example, it is assumed that the level of significance (α) is 0.05.

(iv) Perform the ANOVA

Step 1   Calculate the total sum of squares

$$SS_{total} = \Sigma y^2 - \frac{(\Sigma y)^2}{n} = 593.67 - \frac{(167.52)^2}{48} = 9.03$$

Step 2 Calculate the regression sum of squares

$$SS_{regression} = \frac{[(\sum Xy) - \sum X \sum y/n]^2}{\sum X^2 - (\sum X)^2/n}$$

$$= \frac{[(182.20) - (47.04 \times 167.52)/48]^2}{82.16 - (47.04)^2/48} = 9.01$$

Step 3 Calculate the residual sum of squares

$$SS_{residual} = SS_{total} - SS_{regression} = 9.03 - 9.01 = 0.02$$

Step 4 Construct a summary table for the analysis of variance
The numbers of degrees of freedom (df) associated with the regression parameters are:

- df_{total} = number of observations $- 1 = 48 - 1 = 47$
- $df_{regression} = 1$
- $df_{residual} = df_{total} - df_{regression} = 47 - 1 = 46$

The mean sum of squares for each regression parameter is calculated and the ANOVA summary table is finalised (Table 12.13).

Step 5 Define the critical F statistic
The critical F statistic is determined using Appendix 7, on the basis of the following information about the statistical design:

- level of significance $(\alpha) = 0.05$
- $df_{regression} = 1$
- $df_{residuals} = 46$

Under these experimental conditions the critical value of the F statistic is 4.05.

Step 6 Interpret the outcome of the statistical analysis
In Example 12.6, $F_{calculated}$ (22 525) > $F_{critical}$ (4.05), so the null hypothesis is rejected in favour of the alternative hypothesis. Therefore, we may conclude that the linear relationship between the natural logarithms of the two variables, as defined by linear regression, is valid.

Table 12.13 Summary of the output of the analysis of variance for the linear regression of the natural logarithm of the percentage drug release and the natural logarithm of time

Source	Sum of squares	df	Mean square	F statistic
Regression	9.01	1	9.01	22 525
Residual	0.02	46	4×10^{-4}	
Total	9.03	47		

12.1.4.2 *t tests and linear regression analysis*

In the previous section, the use of ANOVA in conjunction with linear regression analysis for the examination (and validation) of the relationship between an independent variable and a dependent variable was detailed. The *t* test may also be used for this purpose, and has several advantages over the ANOVA technique. For example, in ANOVA the alternative hypothesis is stated as 'the slope of the line of best fit is not equal to zero', implying that rejection of the null hypothesis may be due to either a positive or a negative slope. The outcome is therefore two-tailed. There may be instances in which the analyst wishes to specify the nature of the rejection of the null hypothesis, i.e. $\beta < 0$ or $\beta > 0$. These are examples of one-tailed designs and they are analysed by the exclusive use of the *t* test. The reader will recall from Chapter 10 that the experimental design associated with ANOVA is always two-tailed. In addition, the *t* test is employed when the analyst wishes to compare a regression parameter to a defined value, other than zero. Under certain circumstances, it is more relevant to compare the slope or intercept to an experimentally or clinically relevant value. For example, an analyst may wish to compare the performance of two analytical methods for the analysis of a series of solutions. If the two methods are comparable, the slope of the linear regression would be expected to be 1 and therefore it is experimentally more relevant to base the null hypothesis on this expected slope. As before, the equation for the calculation of the *t* statistic is the ratio of the difference between an experimentally measured (b_{measured}) and hypothesised ($b_{\text{hypothesised}}$) parameter and the standard error of the said parameter (s_b). For example, if the parameter under investigation is the slope of the line of best fit, the formula for the *t* statistic is calculated using the following equation:

$$t = \frac{(b_{\text{measured}} - b_{\text{hypothesised}})}{s_b}$$

To illustrate the use of the *t* test for the examination of the relationship between two variables in conjunction with linear regression, the data presented in Examples 12.2 and 12.6 will be examined.

EXAMPLE 12.7 *In Example 12.2, linear regression analysis was performed to examine the nature of the relationship between time and the concentration of therapeutic agent within the donor cell in a diffusion experiment. Examine the validity of the calculated linear relationship between these two variables using the Student's t test.*

The execution of the Student's *t* test involves an initial definition of the parameters associated with the experimental design. The null and alternative hypotheses and the level of significance have been previously stated, as follows.

(i) State the null hypothesis

The null hypothesis for this example states that a linear relationship does not exist between time and the concentration of drug present in the donor solution:

H_0: $\beta = 0$, where β is the slope of the population.

(ii) State the alternative hypothesis

The alternative hypothesis for this example states that there is a (linear) relationship between time and the concentration of drug present in the donor solution:

H_a: $\beta \neq 0$

(iii) State the level of significance

In this example, it is assumed that the level of significance (α) is 0.05.

(iv) State the number of tails associated with the experimental design

In this example, the alternative hypothesis states that the magnitude of the slope is not equal to zero. Therefore, the null hypothesis may be rejected if the slope is either greater than or less than zero and accordingly, this study is an example of a two-tailed design.

(v) Perform the Student's t test

As the magnitude of the slope has been hypothesised to be zero, the t statistic associated with the regression analysis may be stated as

$$t = \frac{(b_{calculated} - 0)}{s_b}$$

The slope has previously been calculated by linear regression as 1.87 mg/h, so the only unknown value in the above equation is the standard error of the slope. This parameter is calculated using the following formula:

$$s_b = \sqrt{\frac{s_{y.X}^2}{\Sigma (X - \overline{X})^2}}$$

where $(X - \overline{X})^2$ is the square of the difference between each X value and the mean of all X values and $s_{y.X}^2$ is the variance of the dependent variable (y). If the line of best fit coincides with the experimentally recorded data, this value is small, whereas if the recorded and calculated responses are disparate, the variance of the dependent variable is large. This parameter is calculated as follows:

$$s_{y.X}^2 = \frac{\Sigma(y - \bar{y})^2 - b^2[\Sigma(X - \bar{X})^2]}{N - 2}$$

where y is an experimental measure of the dependent value, $\bar{y}$ is the mean of the dependent variable, X is the independent variable $\bar{X}$ is the mean of the independent variable and b is the slope, calculated using linear regression analysis. Therefore, the standard error of the slope is calculated by initially calculating the variance of the independent variable ($s_{y.X}^2$). The application of the Student's t test to the data described in Example 12.2 is performed in the stepwise fashion shown below.

An estimate of the variance of the dependent variable may also be obtained from the output of the ANOVA. In this, $s_{y.X}^2$ is equivalent to the residual mean squares (error) value (approximately 0.49 in this example).

Step 1   Calculate the relevant descriptive statistics
The important descriptive statistics that are required for the calculation of the t statistic are $\Sigma(y - \bar{y})^2$ and $\Sigma(X - \bar{X})^2$. The calculation of these two parameters is considered independently.

- *Calculation of $\Sigma(y - \bar{y})^2$*

$$\begin{aligned}\Sigma(y - \bar{y})^2 = {} & [(248.7 - 243.29)^2 + (247.6 - 243.29)^2 + (244.9 - 243.29)^2 \\ & + (242.4 - 243.29)^2 + (242.1 - 243.29)^2 + (240.2 - 243.29)^2 \\ & + (237.1 - 243.29)^2] = 100.51\end{aligned}$$

- *Calculation of $\Sigma(X - \bar{X})^2$*

$$\begin{aligned}\Sigma(X - \bar{X})^2 = {} & [(1 - 4)^2 + (2 - 4)^2 + (3 - 4)^2 + (4 - 4)^2 + (5 - 4)^2 \\ & + (6 - 4)^2 + (7 - 4)^2] = 28\end{aligned}$$

Step 2   Calculate the variance of the dependent variable

$$s_{y.X}^2 = \frac{\Sigma(y - \bar{y})^2 - b^2[\Sigma(X - \bar{X})^2]}{N - 2} = \frac{(100.51) - (1.87)^2(28)}{7 - 2} = 0.52$$

Step 3   Calculate the standard error of the slope

$$s_b = \sqrt{\frac{s_{y.X}^2}{\Sigma(X - \bar{X})^2}} = \sqrt{\frac{0.52}{28}} = 0.14$$

Step 4   Calculate the t statistic
From the previous equation,

$$t = \frac{(b_{calculated} - 0)}{s_b} = \frac{-1.87 - 0}{0.14} = -13.14$$

Step 5   Identify the critical t statistic
The critical t statistic for this statistical test may be obtained from the table of the critical values of the t distribution (Appendix 2), providing the relevant information is available, namely, the level of significance, the number of degrees of freedom and the number of tails associated with the experimental design. The level of significance has previously been established as 0.05 and the number of tails is 2. The number of degrees of freedom is determined by subtracting 2 from the total number of observations and, thus, in this example this value is 5 (7 – 2). The critical t statistic ($t_{\alpha = 0.05,5df,\text{two-tailed}}$) is therefore 2.57.

Step 6   Interpret the outcome of the statistical analysis
The critical t statistic defines the region of acceptance of the null hypothesis within the t distribution. Therefore, if the calculated t statistic falls within the region defined by $-2.57 < t < +2.57$, the null hypothesis is accepted. Conversely, if the calculated t statistic is equal to, or greater than $+2.57$, or less than or equal to -2.57, the null hypothesis is rejected in favour of the alternative hypothesis. In this example, $t_{calculated}$ (-13.14) is less than the lower boundary that defines the null hypothesis, so the null hypothesis is rejected.

We may therefore conclude that the linear relationship between time and the concentration of therapeutic agent in the donor cell that was defined by linear regression analysis is valid.

The reader is aware that the properties of the line of best fit, calculated using linear regression, are the slope and y intercept. In many pharmaceutical examples, it may be of interest to the analyst to compare the calculated value of the y intercept to a hypothesised value. Consider the scenario in Example 12.7 in which the initial mass of therapeutic agent in the donor cell was 251 mg. The analyst may wish to examine whether the calculated value of the y intercept is a good representation of the known value, i.e. the initial mass. Once more, this question may be statistically examined using the Student's t test. The equation that may be used for this purpose is identical to that described for the examination of the properties of the slope. Hence:

$$t = \frac{(a_{measured} - a_{hypothesised})}{s_a}$$

This equation will now be used to compare the calculated value of the y intercept to the actual value of this parameter.

(i) State the null hypothesis

The null hypothesis for this example states that the initial mass of drug in the donor solution as calculated using linear regression analysis ($mass_{LR}$) is similar to the known initial mass ($mass_{actual}$):

$$H_0: \quad mass_{LR} = mass_{actual}$$

(ii) State the alternative hypothesis

The alternative hypothesis for this example states that the initial concentration of drug in the donor solution as calculated using linear regression analysis ($mass_{LR}$) is dissimilar to the known initial concentration ($mass_{actual}$):

$$H_a: \quad mass_{LR} \neq mass_{actual}$$

(iii) State the level of significance

In this example, it is assumed that the level of significance (α) is 0.05.

(iv) State the number of tails associated with the experimental design

In this example there are two possible outcomes that may result in the rejection of the null hypothesis. The null hypothesis will be rejected if the calculated initial mass of drug in the donor solution is either less or more than the actual (hypothesised) value. This is therefore a two-tailed statistical design.

(v) Perform the Student's t test

As the actual (hypothesised) mass of drug in the donor solution is 251 mg, the t statistic may be defined as:

$$t = \frac{(a_{measured} - a_{hypothesised})}{s_a} = \frac{(250.77 - 251.00)}{s_a}$$

The y intercept has previously been calculated by linear regression as 250.77 mg. Calculation of the associated t statistic requires knowledge of the standard error of the y intercept (s_a). This parameter is calculated using the following formula:

$$s_a = \sqrt{s_{y.X}^2 \left[\frac{1}{N} + \frac{\overline{X}^2}{\Sigma(X - \overline{X})^2} \right]}$$

where $(X - \bar{X})^2$ is the square of the difference between each X value and the mean of all X values and $s_{y.X}^2$ is the variance of the dependent variable (y).

The statistical analysis is described in a stepwise fashion, as before.

Step 1   Calculate the relevant descriptive statistics
The important descriptive statistic that is required for the calculation of the t statistic is $\Sigma(X - \bar{X})^2$. This has been calculated in the previous section as 28.

Step 2   Calculate the variance of the dependent variable
This has been calculated in the previous section as 0.52.

Step 3   Calculate the standard error of the intercept

$$S_a = \sqrt{s_{y.X}^2 \left[\frac{1}{N} + \frac{\bar{X}^2}{\Sigma(X - \bar{X})^2}\right]} = \sqrt{0.52 \times \left[\frac{1}{7} + \frac{4^2}{(28)}\right]} = 0.61$$

Step 4   Calculate the t statistic
From the previous equation,

$$t = \frac{(a_{measured} - a_{hypothesised})}{S_a} = \frac{(250.77 - 251.00)}{0.61} = -0.38$$

(note: the initial mass of therapeutic agent added to the donor compartment was 251 mg).

Step 5   Identify the critical t statistic
The critical t statistic for this statistical test has been defined in the previous section. Therefore, the critical t statistic associated with 5 degrees of freedom ($N - 2$), a defined level of significance (0.05) and a two-tailed test is 2.57, as in the previous section.

Step 6   Interpret the outcome of the statistical analysis
As described previously, the region of acceptance of the null hypothesis within the t distribution is $-2.57 < t < +2.57$ whereas the regions of rejection of this hypothesis are either $t \geqslant +2.57$ or $t < -2.57$. In this example, $t_{calculated}$ (−0.38) lies within the region of acceptance of the null hypothesis and hence it may be concluded that the calculated mass of therapeutic agent in the donor solution and the actual value are statistically similar.

EXAMPLE 12.8   *An analytical division of a pharmaceutical company has developed an analytical method for the determination of therapeutic agent in a formulation. The next stage of the programme for implementation of this method into the company involves an assessment of the reproducibility of the method. Therefore, a series of formulations* *(devoid of drug) were spiked with known masses of therapeutic agent and the masses of therapeutic agent added to each formulation were quantified using the analytical method. Acceptability of the method is dependent on the ability to accurately determine the mass of drug added. The results for this study are shown in Table 12.14. Examine the relationship between the two variables using linear regression analysis and comment on the similarities/differences between the expected and measured regression parameters.*

Initially linear regression analysis should be performed to determine the mathematical relationship between the two variables.

Step 1   Calculate the descriptive statistics associated with the regression
The descriptive statistics involved in the calculation of the linear relationship between the variables are calculated and presented in tabular form (Table 12.15).

Step 2   Calculate the slope of the line of best fit
The slope of the line of best fit is obtained using the above data (remembering that $N = 20$):

$$b = \frac{N(\Sigma\, Xy) - (\Sigma\, X)(\Sigma\, y)}{N(\Sigma\, X^2) - (\Sigma\, X)^2} = \frac{(20 \times 2165.72) - (152.00)(161.02)}{(20 \times 2120.00) - (152.00)^2}$$

$$= \frac{18\,839.36}{19\,296.00} = 0.98$$

Step 3   Calculate the intercept
With the above knowledge the intercept is calculated as before:

$$a = \bar{y} - (b \times \bar{X})$$
$$= 8.05 - (0.98 \times 7.60)$$
$$= 0.60 \text{ mg}$$

Table 12.14   Quantification of the mass of therapeutic agent added to a formulation using an analytical method

Mass of drug added (mg)	Mass of drug determined using the analytical method (mg)			
	Sample 1	Sample 2	Sample 3	Sample 4
1	1.98	1.57	2.01	1.95
2	2.55	2.96	2.12	2.45
5	5.25	5.15	5.36	5.49
10	10.05	10.54	10.35	10.24
20	20.12	20.15	20.42	20.31

Table 12.15 Quantification of the mass of therapeutic agent added to a formulation using an analytical method, incorporating important parameters that are employed in linear regression analysis

Mass of drug added (mg)	Mass of drug determined using the analytical method (mg)	Product of X and y
1.00	1.98	1.98
1.00	1.57	1.57
1.00	2.01	2.01
1.00	1.95	1.95
2.00	2.55	5.10
2.00	2.96	5.92
2.00	2.12	4.24
2.00	2.45	4.90
5.00	5.25	26.25
5.00	5.15	25.75
5.00	5.36	26.80
5.00	5.49	27.45
10.00	10.05	100.50
10.00	10.54	105.40
10.00	10.35	103.50
10.00	10.24	102.40
20.00	20.12	402.40
20.00	20.15	403.00
20.00	20.42	408.40
20.00	20.31	406.20
$\Sigma X = 152.00$, $\bar{X} = 7.60$ $\Sigma X^2 = 2120.00$	$\Sigma y = 161.02$, $\bar{y} = 8.05$ $\Sigma y^2 = 2217.33$	$\Sigma Xy = 2165.72$

Step 4 Summary

The slope (b) and intercept (a) of the line of best fit, as determined by linear regression analysis are 0.98 and 0.60 mg, respectively. The slope of the line is dimensionless. A graphical representation of the relationship between these two variables is shown in Figure 12.10.

Once the regression parameters have been defined, the next stage is to evaluate their validity using either the ANOVA or t test procedures. For the purpose of this example, the former method will be employed.

(i) State the null hypothesis

The null hypothesis for this example states that a linear relationship

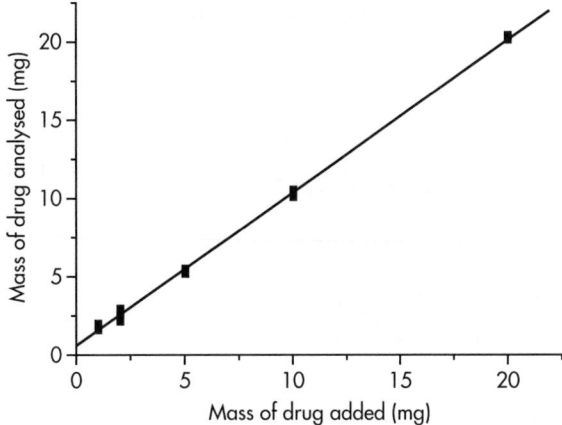

Figure 12.10 Relationship between the masses of drug added to samples of a blank formulation and those quantified in the samples using an analytical method.

does not exist between the masses of drug added to the formulations and the subsequent masses of drug quantified by an analytical method:

$$H_0: \quad \beta = 0$$

(ii) State the alternative hypothesis

The alternative hypothesis for this example states that there is a (linear) relationship between the masses of drug added to the formulations and the subsequent masses of drug quantified by an analytical method:

$$H_a: \quad \beta \neq 0$$

(iii) State the level of significance

In this example, it is assumed that the level of significance (α) is 0.05.

(iv) Perform the ANOVA

As in previous examples, the ANOVA will be performed in a series of steps.

Step 1   Calculate the total sum of squares

$$SS_{total} = \Sigma\, y^2 - \frac{(\Sigma\, y)^2}{n} = 2217.33 - \frac{(161.02)^2}{20} = 920.96$$

Step 2   Calculate the regression sum of squares

$$SS_{regression} = \frac{[(\Sigma\, Xy) - \Sigma\, X \Sigma\, y/n]^2}{\Sigma\, X^2 - (\Sigma\, X)^2/n}$$

$$= \frac{[2165.72 - (152.00 \times 161.02)/20]^2}{2120.00 - (152.00)^2/20} = 919.68$$

Step 3   Calculate the residual sum of squares

$$SS_{residual} = SS_{total} - SS_{regression}$$

$$= 920.96 - 919.68$$

$$= 1.28$$

Step 4 Construct a summary table for the analysis of variance (Table 12.16)
Initially, the numbers of degrees of freedom associated with each sum of squares is determined.

- total number of degrees of freedom $= N - 1 = 20 - 1 = 19$
- $df_{regression} = 1$
- $df_{residual} = 18$

Step 5   Define the critical F statistic
The critical F statistic is determined from Appendix 7 with knowledge of the following parameters:

- level of significance $(\alpha) = 0.05$
- $df_{regression} = 1$
- $df_{residual} = 18$

Under these experimental conditions the critical value of the F statistic is 4.41.

Step 6   Interpret the outcome of the statistical analysis
The null hypothesis is accepted if the calculated F statistic is less than the critical F statistic, whereas if the calculated statistic is equal to or greater than the critical F statistic the null hypothesis is rejected in favour of the

Table 12.16 Summary of the output of the analysis of variance for the linear regression of relationship between the masses of drug added to samples of a blank formulation and those quantified in the samples using an analytical method

Source	Sum of squares	df	Mean square	F statistic
Regression	919.68	1	919.68	13 138.29
Residual	1.28	18	0.07	
Total	920.96	19		

alternative hypothesis. In this example, $F_{\text{calculated}}(13\ 138.29) > F_{\text{critical}}$ (4.41), therefore the null hypothesis is rejected. The linear relationship between the two variables is assumed to be valid.

At this point, the linear relationship between the two variables has been confirmed. However, in this example, two further points are of interest to the statistical analyst:

- If the analytical method is reliable, the masses of drug quantified in the formulation should be similar to known masses of drug added. Therefore, the slope of the relationship should be equal to 1.
- If there is no interference with the analytical method by components of the formulation, the y intercept should be 0, i.e. if no drug is added the analytical method should not record a response.

These two scenarios represent hypotheses that may be addressed using the t test.

Statistical comparison of the calculated slope to the predicted slope

(i) State the null hypothesis

The null hypothesis states that the slope of the linear relationship between the masses of drug added to samples of a formulation and the masses quantified by the analytical method will be equal to 1:

$$H_0: \quad \beta = 1$$

(ii) State the alternative hypothesis

The alternative hypothesis states that the slope of the linear relationship between the masses of drug added to samples of a formulation and the masses quantified by the analytical method will not be equal to 1:

$$H_a: \quad \beta \neq 1$$

(iii) State the level of significance

In this example, it is assumed that the level of significance (α) is 0.05.

(iv) State the number of tails associated with the experimental design

In this example there are two routes by which the null hypothesis may be rejected in favour of the alternative hypothesis: the calculated slope may be either greater than or less than 1, so this is an example of a two-tailed study.

(v) Perform the Student's t test

This test will be executed using the information derived from the ANOVA.

Step 1   Determine the variance of the dependent variable
This may be calculated from first principles (see previous examples) or, alternatively, it may be assumed that the variance of the dependent variable is equal to the residual mean squares that was calculated in the ANOVA, i.e. 0.07.

Step 2   Calculate the standard error of the slope

$$s_b = \sqrt{\frac{s_{y.X}^2}{\Sigma(X - \overline{X})^2}} = \sqrt{\frac{0.07}{964.80}} = 0.009$$

Step 3   Calculate the t statistic

$$t = \frac{(b_{\text{calculated}} - b_{\text{hypothesised}})}{s_b} = \frac{0.98 - 1.00}{0.009} = -2.22$$

Step 4   Identify the critical t statistic
The critical t statistic is obtained from the table of the critical values the t distribution (Appendix 2) under the conditions of the experiment, namely:

- the level of significance (α) is 0.05
- $df = 18$ (20 – 2)

The critical t statistic ($t_{\alpha = 0.05, 18df, \text{two-tailed}}$) is therefore 2.10.

Step 5   Interpret the outcome of the statistical analysis
For the t distribution the regions of acceptance and rejection of the null hypothesis are as follows:

$$H_0: \quad -2.10 < t < +2.10$$
$$H_a: \quad t > +2.10 \text{ or } t < -2.10$$

In this example, $t_{\text{calculated}}$ (−2.22) is less than the lower boundary that defines the null hypothesis (−2.10) and, as a result, the null hypothesis is rejected.

We may therefore conclude that the results from the analytical method concerning the masses of drug in the formulation differ from the known masses within the formulations. However, as the reader will observe, the calculated t value is close to the boundary between H_0 and H_a (the critical t value), it would be appropriate to repeat the study and increase the sample size to ensure that this conclusion is valid.

Statistical comparison of the calculated intercept to the predicted intercept

(i) State the null hypothesis

The null hypothesis states that the intercept of the linear relationship between the masses of drug added to samples of a formulation and the masses quantified by the analytical method will be equal to 0:

$$H_0: \quad a_{\text{analytical method}} = 0$$

(ii) State the alternative hypothesis

The alternative hypothesis states that the intercept of the linear relationship between the masses of drug added to samples of a formulation and the masses quantified by the analytical method will not be equal to 0:

$$H_a: \quad a_{\text{analytical method}} \neq 0$$

(iii) State the level of significance

In this example, it is assumed that the level of significance (α) is 0.05.

(iv) State the number of tails associated with the experimental design

As in the previous calculation, the null hypothesis will be rejected if $a > 0$ or $a < 0$, so this is an example of a two-tailed outcome.

(v) Perform the Student's t test

Step 1 Calculate the variance of the dependent variable
This has been calculated in the previous section as 0.07.

Step 2 Calculate the standard error of the intercept

$$s_a = \sqrt{s_{y.x}^2 \left[\frac{1}{N} + \frac{\bar{X}^2}{\Sigma(X - \bar{X})^2} \right]} = \sqrt{0.07 \times \left[\frac{1}{20} + \frac{7.60^2}{964.8} \right]} = 0.088$$

Step 3 Calculate the t statistic

$$t = \frac{(a_{\text{measured}} - a_{\text{hypothesised}})}{s_a} = \frac{(0.60 - 0.00)}{0.088} = 6.82$$

Step 4 Identify the critical t statistic
The critical t statistic for this statistical test has been defined previously as $(t_{\alpha = 005, 18df, \text{two-tailed}}) = 2.10$.

Step 5 Interpret the outcome of the statistical analysis
In this example, the calculated t statistic (6.82) is larger than the critical t statistic (2.10) and accordingly the null hypothesis is rejected in favour of the alternative hypothesis. We may therefore conclude that the y intercept associated with the analytical method is significantly greater than 0. Once more this is an interesting and experimentally useful finding as it suggests that a component within the formulation has

interfered with the analytical method. This would account for the estimated mass of 0.60 mg of therapeutic agent in the formulation when in fact no drug was present. As a result, the analytical method may require some further development to overcome this problem.

12.1.5 Calculation of confidence intervals in linear regression analysis

In Chapter 6 the concept of confidence intervals was introduced as a measure of the reliability of a statistical parameter. In the pharmaceutical and related sciences, statistical hypotheses concerning population statistics are formulated and challenged using sample data. It is unacceptable to assume that the statistical information generated from samples will be identical to the corresponding population measurement, but it is important to obtain a measure of the quality of the estimation of the population parameter from the sample parameter. For this purpose confidence intervals are employed. As for other statistical parameters, the slope and intercept have been calculated using linear regression analysis based on sample data and are assumed to be good estimates of slope and intercept of the parent population. Accordingly, when the slope and intercept are recorded it is customary to cite the confidence intervals associated with these parameters in linear regression analysis. Calculation of the confidence intervals associated with the slope and y intercept is performed as in Chapter 6. The generic equation that is employed for the calculation of confidence interval is therefore

$$CI_{95\%} = \text{parameter} \pm (t)(SE_{\text{parameter}})$$

where the term 'parameter' refers to either the slope or the y intercept.

The use of this equation for the calculation of the 95% confidence intervals associated with the slope and intercept described in Example 12.8 is illustrated in Example 12.9.

EXAMPLE 12.9 *In the previous example, the slope and intercept of the linear relationship between the masses of drug added to samples of a formulation and the quantified masses of drug in the formulation, as determined using an analytical method, were determined. Calculate the 95% and 99% confidence limits for estimating the true values of the slope and intercept.*

95% Confidence intervals for the slope
The calculated values of the slope and the standard error of the slope, as determined in Example 12.8, are 0.98 and 0.009, respectively. The t statistic may be derived from the table of the critical values of the t statistic

(Appendix 2) on the basis of the following experimental parameters:

- $\alpha = 0.05$
- two-tailed experimental design
- 18 df

The critical t statistic ($t_{0.05,\text{two-tailed},18df}$) is therefore 2.10.

The slope, standard error of the slope and t statistic associated with the experimental design are then inserted into the generic equation to facilitate calculation of the 95% confidence intervals:

$$CI_{95\%} = \text{parameter} \pm (t)(SE_{\text{parameter}})$$
$$= 0.98 \pm (2.10 \times 0.009)$$
$$= 0.98 \pm 0.02$$

Therefore, we may conclude that there is a 95% chance that the true (population) value of the slope lies within the range 0.96–1.00.

99% Confidence intervals for the slope
This calculation is identical to the previous one, with the exception that the value of the critical t statistic differs. As before, the t statistic is determined from the table of the critical values of the t statistic (Appendix 2) on the basis of the following experimental parameters:

- $\alpha = 0.01$
- two-tailed experimental design
- 18 df

The critical t statistic ($t_{0.01,\text{two-tailed},18df}$) is therefore 2.88, so

$$CI_{95\%} = \text{parameter} \pm (t)(SE_{\text{parameter}})$$
$$= 0.98 \pm (2.88 \times 0.009)$$
$$= 0.98 \pm 0.03$$

We may therefore concluded that there is a 99% chance that the true (population) value of the slope lies within the range 0.95–1.01.

95% Confidence intervals for the intercept
The calculated values of the intercept and the standard error of the intercept (Example 12.8) are 0.60 mg and 0.088 mg, respectively. The critical t statistic ($t_{0.05,\text{two-tailed},18df}$) has been defined above as 2.10, so

$$CI_{95\%} = \text{parameter} \pm (t)(SE_{\text{parameter}})$$
$$= 0.60 \pm (2.10 \times 0.088)$$
$$= 0.60 \pm 0.18$$

Therefore, we may conclude that there is a 95% chance that the true (population) value of the intercept lies within the range 0.42–0.78 mg.

99% Confidence intervals for the intercept

The critical t statistic ($t_{0.01,\text{two-tailed},18df}$) has been defined above as 2.88, so

$$CI_{95\%} = \text{parameter} \pm (t)(SE_{\text{parameter}})$$
$$= 0.60 \pm (2.88 \times 0.088)$$
$$= 0.60 \pm 0.25$$

Therefore we may conclude that there is a 99% chance that the true (population) value of the intercept lies within the range 0.35–0.85 mg.

12.1.6 Prediction of the magnitude of dependent and independent variables using linear regression analysis

Linear regression analysis allows the relationship between an independent variable and a dependent variable to be determined mathematically. This relationship will have been examined by selecting a series of values to represent the independent variable, and determining the corresponding values of the dependent variable experimentally. It is not feasible to select every value of the independent variable for experimental examination, but the rational selection of a representative range of values allows the relationship to be securely defined. With knowledge of the mathematical relationship between two variables it is possible to predict the values of either the dependent or the independent variable. This is an extremely important application of linear regression and therefore the estimation of the dependent variable associated with a defined X value (independent variable) and estimation of the independent variable associated with a defined Y value (dependent variable) will be individually addressed, once more with the aid of pharmaceutical examples.

In both situations, estimation of the magnitude of the unknown variable is performed by rearrangement of the equation that relates the independent and dependent variables. As $Y = a + bX$, an unknown dependent variable may be estimated by inserting the known value of the independent variable and the slope and intercept (obtained from linear regression analysis). However, for the reasons described in Chapter 6 and in this section, it is unlikely that the calculated value of the dependent variable is identical to the corresponding population value. Therefore, whenever an estimation of the dependent variable at a defined independent variable is performed, the confidence intervals associated with the estimated value should be included.

12.1.6.1 Calculation of the confidence intervals for the estimated Y variable associated with a defined value of X

The confidence intervals for the estimated Y variable associated with a defined value of X are calculated using the following equation:

$$CI_{95\%} = Y_{estimate} \pm (t)(SE_{Y \, estimate})$$

Y is the calculated estimate of the dependent variable and $SE_{Y \, estimate}$ is the standard error of the estimated Y value. The standard error term in the above equation is calculated as follows:

$$s_{Y \, estimate} = \sqrt{s_{Y.X}^2 \left[\frac{1}{N} + \frac{(X - \bar{X})^2}{\Sigma(X - \bar{X})^2} \right]}$$

where $s_{Y.X}^2$ is the variance of the dependent variable, N is the number of observations, $(X - \bar{X})^2$ is the square of the difference between the defined value of the independent value and the mean of the independent variable, and $\Sigma(X - \bar{X})^2$ is the sum of the squares of the differences between each independent value and the mean of the independent variable.

Once the standard error of the Y estimate has been obtained, the confidence intervals may be easily calculated. To illustrate this procedure consider the following example.

EXAMPLE 12.10   *In Example 12.3 it was shown that a linear relationship existed between the ratio of two polymeric components in the coating of a solid dosage form and the subsequent rate of release of a therapeutic agent from the dosage form. The parameters associated with the regression were 1.31 µg/h (slope) and 129.54 µg/h (intercept).*

- Calculate the 95% confidence intervals for the true slope and intercept.
- Estimate the rate of drug release from a solid dosage form that has been coated with a 45 : 55 blend of the two polymers and, in addition, provide 95% confidence intervals for the true estimate.
- Estimate the rate of drug release from a solid dosage form that has been coated with a 90 : 10 blend of the two polymers and, in addition, provide 95% confidence intervals for the true estimate.

Calculate the 95% confidence intervals for the true slope and intercept
The 95% confidence intervals for the true slope are calculated as follows:

$$CI_{95\%} = slope \pm (t)(SE_{slope})$$

The t statistic may be derived from the table of the critical values of the t statistic (Appendix 2) on the basis of the following experimental parameters:

- $\alpha = 0.05$
- two-tailed experimental design
- 22 *df*

The critical t statistic $(t_{0.05,\text{two-tailed},22df})$ is therefore 2.07.

The standard error of the slope is calculated using the following equation, as previously documented, using the residual mean squares from the ANOVA (Table 12.9) as the estimate of $s^2_{y.x}$.

$$s_b = \sqrt{\frac{s^2_{Y.X}}{\Sigma(X-\overline{X})^2}} = \sqrt{\frac{58.01}{28\,000}} = 0.046$$

Therefore, the 95% confidence intervals are calculated:

$$CI_{95\%} = \text{slope} \pm (t)(SE_{\text{slope}})$$
$$= 1.31 \pm (2.07 \times 0.046)$$
$$= 1.31 \pm 0.10\,\mu g/h.$$

Consequently, there is a 95% chance that the true (population) value of the slope lies within the range 1.21–1.41 mg/h.

The 95% confidence intervals for the true intercept are calculated in a similar fashion:

$$CI_{95\%} = \text{slope} \pm (t)(SE_{\text{intercept}})$$

The critical t statistic $(t_{0.05,\text{two-tailed},22df})$ was previously defined above as 2.07. The standard error of the intercept (s_a) is calculated using the following equation, remembering that $s^2_{y.x}$ has been estimated from the residual means squares in the ANOVA:

$$s_a = \sqrt{s^2_{Y.X}\left[\frac{1}{N}+\frac{\overline{X}^2}{\Sigma(X-\overline{X})^2}\right]} = \sqrt{58.01\times\left[\frac{1}{24}+\frac{50^2}{28\,000}\right]} = 2.76$$

$$CI_{95\%} = \text{parameter} \pm (t)(SE_{\text{parameter}})$$
$$= 129.54 \pm (2.07 \times 2.76)$$
$$= 129.54 \pm 5.71\,\mu g/h.$$

Therefore, we may conclude that there is a 95% chance that the true (population) value of the intercept lies within the range 123.83–135.25 $\mu g/h$.

Drug release rate from a solid dosage form coated with a 45 : 55 polymeric blend

The release rate of the therapeutic agent may be obtained with reference to the regression equation. In this example, $a = 129.54\,\mu g/h$, $b = 1.31\,\mu g/h$ and the defined value of X is 45. With this information, Y may be calculated:

$$Y = 129.54 + (1.31 \times 45)$$
$$= 188.49\,\mu g/h.$$

Therefore, the estimated rate of release of therapeutic agent from a tablet that has been coated with a $45:55$ polymeric blend is $188.49\ \mu g/h$. However, it is unlikely that this value will be identical to the corresponding population value, so a measure of the reliability of the estimation must be expressed in terms of confidence intervals.

First, the standard error of the estimated Y value must be calculated:

$$s_{Y\,estimate} = \sqrt{s_{Y.X}^2\left[\frac{1}{N} + \frac{(X - \bar{X})^2}{\Sigma(X - \bar{X})^2}\right]}$$

$$= \sqrt{58.01 \times \left[\frac{1}{24} + \frac{(45 - 50)^2}{28\ 000}\right]} = 1.57$$

This, in turn, facilitates the calculation of the 95% confidence intervals:

$$CI_{95\%} = Y_{estimate} \pm (t)(SE_{estimate})$$

$$= 188.49 \pm (2.07 \times 1.57)$$

$$= 188.49 \pm 3.25\ \mu g/h.$$

The t statistic has been selected from the table of the critical values of the t distribution according to the parameters of the study, namely $\alpha = 0.05$, 22 df and a two-tailed outcome. Therefore, there is a 95% probability that the true value of the rate of release of therapeutic agent from a dosage form coated with a $45:55$ ratio of polymeric components A and B lies within the range $185.24–191.74\ \mu g/h$.

Drug release rate from a solid dosage form coated with a $90:10$ polymeric blend
The regression parameters are $a = 129.54\ \mu g/h$, $b = 1.31\ \mu g/h$ and $X = 90$, so

$$Y = 129.54 + (1.31 \times 90)$$

$$= 247.44\ \mu g/h.$$

Therefore, the estimated rate of release of therapeutic agent from a tablet that has been coated with a polymeric blend composed of a $90:10$ ratio of components A and B is $247.44\ \mu g/h$.

The confidence intervals associated with this estimated value are calculated by initially working out the standard error of the estimated value:

$$s_{Y\,estimate} = \sqrt{s_{Y.X}^2\left[\frac{1}{N} + \frac{(X - \bar{X})^2}{\Sigma(X - \bar{X})^2}\right]}$$

$$= \sqrt{58.01 \times \left[\frac{1}{24} + \frac{(90 - 50)^2}{28\ 000}\right]} = 2.39$$

This value is then used in the determination of the 95% confidence intervals:

$$CI_{95\%} = Y_{\text{estimate}} \pm (t)(SE_{\text{estimate}})$$
$$= 247.44 \pm (2.07 \times 2.39)$$
$$= 247.44 \pm 4.95 \ \mu g/h.$$

Therefore, there is a 95% probability that the true value of the rate of release of therapeutic agent from a dosage form coated with a 90 : 10 ratio of polymeric components A and B lies within the range 242.49–252.39 $\mu g/h$.

The reader will have observed that the sizes of the ranges of the confidence intervals for these two estimated Y values are different. The confidence intervals increase as the difference in the stated X value and the mean X value $(X - \bar{X})$ increases. Therefore, the size of the confidence intervals will be at a minimum (but not zero) when $X - \bar{X} = 0$.

12.1.6.2 Calculation of the confidence intervals for the estimated X variable associated with a defined Y value

Under certain circumstances an investigator may wish to predict the values of the independent (X) variable that are associated with a defined measurement of the dependent (Y) variable, a process that is referred to as *inverse prediction*. This process is performed by rearrangement of the line of best fit, as determined using linear regression analysis, $Y = a + bX$, as follows:

$$X = \frac{(Y - a)}{b}$$

After estimation of the X variable, it is appropriate to provide details of the confidence of this estimation, i.e. the confidence intervals. The equation that is used for this purpose is more complex that that used for the calculation of confidence intervals associated with the prediction of the Y variable. This is due, in part, to the asymmetrical distribution of confidence intervals around the estimated X variable. The confidence intervals associated with an estimated X value are calculated as follows:

$$CI_{95\%} = \bar{X} + \frac{b(y - \bar{Y})}{D} \pm K$$

where $\bar{X}$ is the mean of the X variable, $\bar{Y}$ is the mean of the Y variable, b is the slope of the regression and D and K are coefficients that are independently calculated as follows:

$$D = b^2 - ts_b^2$$

where b is the slope of the regression, t is the value of the critical t statistic under the conditions of the experiment, and s_b is the standard error of the slope.

$$K = \frac{t}{D} \sqrt{s_{Y.X}^2 \left[D\left(1 + \frac{1}{N}\right) + \frac{(y - \overline{Y})^2}{\Sigma X^2} \right]}$$

where $s_{y.X}^2$ is the variance of the dependent variable, D is the coefficient derived above, N is the number of observations, y is the defined value of the dependent variable, $\overline{Y}$ is the mean of the Y values, t is the value of the critical t statistic under the conditions of the experiment and ΣX^2 is the sum of the squares of all X values.

The confidence intervals associated with an estimated value of X are calculated by combining the previous three equations:

$$CI_{95\%} = \overline{X} + \frac{b(y - \overline{Y})}{(b^2 - ts_b^2)}$$

$$\pm \left(\frac{t}{(b^2 - ts_b^2)} \sqrt{s_{Y.X}^2 \left[(b^2 - ts_b^2)\left(1 + \frac{1}{N}\right) + \frac{(y - \overline{Y})^2}{\Sigma X^2} \right]} \right)$$

The reader will observe that the confidence intervals are symmetrical around the mathematical term

$$CI_{95\%} = \overline{X} + \frac{b(y - \overline{Y})}{D}$$

and not around the estimated value itself, i.e. $X = (Y - a)/b$.

The use of this equation for the inverse prediction of the X value and calculation of the associated confidence intervals is shown in the following example.

EXAMPLE 12.11 *The chemical stability of pharmaceutical suspension of a therapeutic agent is a typical example of pseudo-zero-order kinetics, in which the mass of undegraded drug decreases as a linear function of storage time, i.e. $C = C_0 - kt$ where C is the mass or concentration of (undegraded) drug at a defined time of sampling (t), C_0 is the original mass or concentration of drug and k is the rate of degradation. In a study, an investigator wishes to examine the chemical degradation of a pharmaceutical suspension containing a therapeutic agent. Consequently, three independent batches of the product were manufactured and samples of each batch were stored in their final packaging under defined environmental conditions (temperature and humidity). At defined intervals, samples were removed and the mass of undegraded drug was determined using a high-performance liquid chromatography*

(HPLC) assay to indicate stability. The results of the investigation are shown in Table 12.17.

- Using an appropriate statistical method, examine the linear relationship between the mass of undegraded drug and time of storage.
- In terms of chemical stability, the shelf-life of the product is defined as the time required for the concentration of therapeutic agent to degrade to 90% of the nominal original concentration within the sample. If the nominal mass of drug in the formulation is 100 mg, estimate the shelf-life of the product.

Linear relationship between mass of undegraded drug and storage time

Step 1   Calculate the descriptive statistics associated with the regression (Table 12.18)

Step 2   Calculate the slope of the line of best fit

$$b = \frac{N(\sum Xy) - (\sum X)(\sum y)}{N(\sum X^2) - (\sum X)^2}$$

$$= \frac{(21 \times 19\,633.8) - (216.0)(1989.3)}{(21 \times 3510.0) - (216.0)^2} = -0.64 \text{ mg/month}$$

The negative slope denotes that a reduction in the original concentration of drug has occurred over the period of storage.

Step 3   Calculate the intercept
The intercept is calculated using the above information:

$$a = \bar{y} - (b \times \bar{X})$$
$$= 94.73 - (-0.64 \times 10.29)$$
$$= 101.32 \text{ mg}$$

Table 12.17 Effect of storage on the stability of a therapeutic agent in a suspension formulation

Time of storage (months)	Mass of undegraded drug (mg) after storage		
	Batch 1	Batch 2	Batch 3
0	103.2	101.2	100.8
3	101.2	99.1	98.3
6	99.4	97.4	96.0
9	97.8	95.2	93.4
12	93.1	93.5	91.8
18	88.4	90.2	89.2
24	87.1	87.8	85.2

Table 12.18 Effect of storage on the stability of a therapeutic agent in a suspension formulation, incorporating important parameters that are used in linear regression analysis

Time of storage (months)	Mass of undegraded drug (mg) after storage	Product of X and y
0	103.2	0
0	101.2	0
0	100.8	0
3	101.2	303.6
3	99.1	297.3
3	98.3	294.9
6	99.4	596.4
6	97.4	584.4
6	96.0	576
9	97.8	880.2
9	95.2	856.8
9	93.4	840.6
12	93.1	1117.2
12	93.5	1122
12	91.8	1101.6
18	88.4	1591.2
18	90.2	1623.6
18	89.2	1605.6
24	87.1	2090.4
24	87.8	2107.2
24	85.2	2044.8
$\Sigma X = 216.0$, $\bar{X} = 10.29$ $\Sigma X^2 = 3510.0$	$\Sigma y = 1989.3$, $\bar{y} = 94.73$ $\Sigma y^2 = 189\,010.7$	$\Sigma Xy = 19\,633.8$

Step 4 Summary

The line of best fit that describes the relationship between the time of storage and the mass of undegraded drug is

$$y = 101.32 - 0.64X$$

The next stage of the analysis involves validation of the linearity of the relationship between the two variables, which, in this case will be performed in a stepwise fashion using ANOVA.

(i) State the null hypothesis

The null hypothesis for Example 12.11 states that a linear relationship does not exist between the time of storage and the mass of undegraded drug:

$$H_0: \quad \beta = 0$$

(ii) State the alternative hypothesis

The alternative hypothesis for Example 12.11 states that a linear relationship does exist between the time of storage and the mass of undegraded drug:

$$H_a : \beta \neq 0$$

(iii) State the level of significance

In this example, it is assumed that the level of significance (α) is 0.05.

(iv) Perform the ANOVA

As in previous examples, the ANOVA will be performed in a series of steps.

Step 1   *Calculate the total sum of squares*

$$SS_{total} = \Sigma y^2 - \frac{(\Sigma y)^2}{N} = 189\ 010.7 - \frac{(1989.3)^2}{21} = 567.15$$

Step 2   *Calculate the regression sum of squares*

$$SS_{regression} = \frac{[(\Sigma Xy) - \Sigma X \Sigma y/n]^2}{\Sigma X^2 - (\Sigma X)^2/n}$$

$$= \frac{[196\ 33.8 - (216.00 \times 1989.3)/21]^2}{3510.0 - (216.0)^2/21} = 531.62$$

Step 3   *Calculate the residual sum of squares*

$$SS_{residual} = SS_{total} - SS_{regression}$$

$$= 567.15 - 531.62$$

$$= 35.53$$

Step 4   *Construct a summary table for the analysis of variance (Table 12.19)*

Initially, the numbers of degrees of freedom associated with each sum of squares are determined.

- $df_{total} = N - 1 = 20$
- $df_{regression} = 1$
- $df_{residuals} = 19$

Step 5   *Define the critical F statistic*

The critical F statistic is determined from Appendix 7 with knowledge of

Table 12.19 Summary of the output of the analysis of variance concerning the linear regression of the relationship between the time of storage of a pharmaceutical suspension and the mass of undegraded drug

Source	Sum of squares	df	Mean square	F statistic
Regression	531.62	1	531.62	284.29
Residual	35.53	19	1.87	
Total	567.15	20		

the following parameters:

- $\alpha = 0.05$
- $df_{regression} = 1$
- $df_{residual} = 19$

Under these experimental conditions the critical value of the F statistic is 4.38.

Step 6   Interpretation of the outcome of the statistical analysis
As the calculated F statistic is greater than the critical F statistic, the null hypothesis is rejected. Therefore, the linear relationship between the two variables is valid.

Estimate the shelf-life of the product
The shelf-life of the product is regarded as the time taken for the concentration of therapeutic agent in the formulation to reduce to 90% of the nominal concentration. In this example, the shelf-life is therefore the time taken for the mass of drug in the container to reduce to 90 mg. As the mass of therapeutic agent is the dependent variable and time of storage is the independent variable in the linear regression analysis, inverse prediction is required to estimate the shelf-life.

Rearrangement of the linear regression equation allows the mean shelf-life to be calculated:

$$Y = 101.32 - 0.64X$$

Therefore, setting $y = 90$ mg (i.e. 90% of the nominal mass of therapeutic agent),

$$X = \frac{Y - 101.32}{-0.64} = \frac{90 - 101.32}{-0.64} = 17.69 \text{ months}$$

As before, it is unlikely that this estimated shelf-life is identical to the corresponding population value, so a measure of the reliability of the estimation must be expressed in terms of confidence intervals. The 95%

confidence intervals associated with the estimated value of the independent variable are calculated using the following equation:

$$CI_{95\%} = \bar{X} + \frac{b(y - \bar{Y})}{D} \pm K$$

As there are two unknown coefficients in this equation (D and K), these must be initially resolved.

- *Calculation of D*

$$D = b^2 - ts_b^2$$

  where b is the slope (-0.64 mg/month), t is the critical t statistic associated with the experimental design ($t_{19df,\text{two-tailed},\alpha = 0.05} = 2.09$) and s_b is the standard error of the slope, determined using the following equation:

$$s_b = \sqrt{\frac{s_{Y.X}^2}{\Sigma(X - \bar{X})^2}} = \sqrt{\frac{1.87}{1288.29}} = 0.038$$

  Remember, $s_{y.x}^2$ is estimated from the residual mean squares (error) term in the ANOVA.
  Therefore

$$D = b^2 - ts_b^2 = -0.64^2 - (2.09 \times 0.038^2) = 0.407$$

- *Calculation of K*

$$K = \frac{t}{D} \sqrt{s_{Y.X}^2 \left[D\left(1 + \frac{1}{N}\right) + \frac{(y - \bar{Y})^2}{\Sigma X^2} \right]}$$

  Inserting the relevant parameters into this equation,

$$K = \frac{2.09}{0.407} \sqrt{1.87\left[0.407\left(1 + \frac{1}{21}\right) + \frac{(90.00 - 94.73)^2}{3510.00}\right]} = 4.62$$

(iii) Calculation of the 95% confidence intervals

$$CI_{95\%} = \bar{X} + \frac{b(y - \bar{Y})}{D} \pm K = 10.29 + \frac{-064(90.00 - 94.73)}{0.407} \pm 4.62$$

$$= 17.73 \pm 4.62$$

Therefore the 95% confidence interval for the shelf-life of the pharmaceutical suspension is 13.11–22.35 months. Accordingly, there is a 95% chance that the true (population) shelf-life lies within this range.

12.1.7 Statistical comparisons of two slopes

In pharmaceutical experiments, an investigator may frequently wish to examine the similarity or differences between two slopes that have been obtained using linear regression analysis. For example, the comparative dose–response relationships of two therapeutic agents, or the comparative release rates of a named drug from two formulations, may be under investigation. In both of these experiments, it may be possible to mathematically describe the relationship between the independent variable (e.g. dose or time of release) and the dependent variable (pharmacological response or cumulative mass of drug released) using linear regression analysis. If this is the case it is logical to use the regression parameters as a means to compare the performance of the two treatments in the experimental design. Under these circumstances, the slopes of the lines of best fit associated with each treatment may be statistically compared by an independent-samples t test, using the generic formula for this type of analysis:

$$t = \frac{b_{\text{treatment 1}} - b_{\text{treatment 2}}}{s_{\text{treatment 1} - \text{treatment 2}}}$$

The standard error of the difference between slopes ($s_{\text{treatment 1} - \text{treatment 2}}$) must be independently calculated by firstly computing the pooled residual mean square ($s_{y.x}^2$) and then solving the following equation:

$$s_{\text{treatment 1} - \text{treatment 2}} = \sqrt{\frac{s_{Y.X}^2}{(\sum X_{\text{treatment 1}}^2)} + \frac{s_{Y.X}^2}{(\sum X_{\text{treatment 2}}^2)}}$$

where N is the number of pairs in each treatment group.

The mechanics of this analysis are further described in the following example.

EXAMPLE 12.12 *Two controlled-release formulations of an analgesic have been developed for the treatment of pain in patients with cancer. In a previous experiment, it was confirmed that the release of the analgesic from these systems was diffusion controlled, and the mass of drug release was a function of the square root of time. As a pharmaceutical scientist you have been asked to statistically examine the in vitro rates of release of the two formulations and comment on their similarities or differences. Therefore, the cumulative masses of therapeutic agent released as a function of time from the two formulations were examined at 37 °C using the USP dissolution test. The results are shown in Table 12.20. Are the rates of release of the analgesic (mg $h^{-0.5}$) from the two controlled-release formulations similar?*

The rate of release of therapeutic agent from the two formulations may be obtained by mathematical calculation of the slope of the relationship between the mass of drug released from the two formulations and the square root of time, using linear regression analysis. The outputs from

Table 12.20 Mass of an analgesic drug released from two controlled release formulations as a function of time

Time (h)	Cumulative mass of drug released from formulation 1 (mg $h^{-0.5}$)			Cumulative mass of drug released from formulation 2 (mg $h^{-0.5}$)		
	Sample 1	Sample 2	Sample 3	Sample 1	Sample 2	Sample 3
1	5.62	5.21	5.01	8.41	8.25	8.57
2	7.61	7.99	7.25	12.60	13.04	13.20
3	9.20	9.01	9.08	15.11	14.99	14.67
4	11.20	10.58	11.02	18.57	18.05	18.07
5	12.12	11.59	12.05	20.19	19.47	20.02
6	13.21	13.55	13.46	22.04	21.04	21.59

this are as follows:

Formulation 1:

- slope = 5.52 mg $h^{-0.5}$
- intercept = −0.26 mg
- line of best fit Y = 5.52X − 0.26

Formulation 2:

- slope = 9.02 mg $h^{-0.5}$
- intercept = −0.29 mg
- line of best fit Y = 9.02X − 0.29

The full calculation of these relationships has not been provided, but it may be useful for the reader to perform the regression calculations manually to gain further practice in this statistical technique.

The validity of the stated linear relationship may also be examined using an ANOVA, for which the experimental conditions are as follows.

(i) State the null hypothesis

The null hypothesis states that no linear relationship exists between the cumulative mass of drug released from either formulation 1 or formulation 2 and $t^{0.5}$:

$$H_0: \beta_{formulation\ 1} = 0$$
$$H_0: \beta_{formulation\ 2} = 0$$

(ii) State the alternative hypothesis

The alternative hypothesis states that the relationship between the cumulative mass of drug released from either formulation 1 or formulation 2 and $t^{0.5}$ is linear:

$$H_a: \beta_{\text{formulation 1}} \neq 0$$
$$H_a: \beta_{\text{formulation 2}} \neq 0$$

(iii) State the level of significance and the number of tails

In this example the level of significance will be accepted as 0.05 and, as there are two potential outcomes that will result in the null hypothesis being rejected, the experimental design is two-tailed.

(iv) Perform the statistical test

The reader will be aware from the previous sections in this chapter that the validity of the calculated line of best fit may be assessed using either an ANOVA or a two-samples t test. In this example, the latter test will be employed. The outputs of the two analyses of variance are shown in Tables 12.21 and 12.22. As before, the full details of the calculation have not been included, but the conscientious student may wish to perform the appropriate calculations in order to gain more experience of the mechanics of this analysis.

(v) Define the critical F statistic

The critical F statistic for each ANOVA is determined with reference to the critical values of the F distribution (Appendix 7) under the

Table 12.21 Summary of the output of the analysis of variance for the linear relationship between the cumulative mass of an analgesic drug released from a controlled release formulation (formulation 1) and $t^{0.5}$

Source	Sum of squares	df	Mean square	F statistic
Regression	132.92	1	132.92	1661.50
Residual	1.29	16	0.08	
Total	134.20	19		

Table 12.22 Summary of the output of the analysis of variance concerning the linear relationship between the cumulative mass of an analgesic drug released from a controlled release formulation (formulation 2) and $t^{0.5}$

Source	Sum of squares	df	Mean square	F statistic
Regression	354.84	1	354.84	1478.50
Residual	3.76	16	0.24	
Total	358.60	19		

conditions of the analysis. In this example, the conditions for each linear regression are identical and are as follows:

- $\alpha = 0.05$
- $df_{numerator}$ (regression sum of squares) = 1
- $df_{denominator}$ (residual sum of squares) = 16

The critical F statistic can therefore be identified as 4.49.

(vi) Interpret the outcome of the statistical analysis

As in other examples, the critical F statistic defines the regions of acceptance and rejection of the null hypothesis. Hence, the null hypothesis is accepted if the calculated F statistic is less than the critical F statistic, but rejected if the calculated F statistic is equal to or greater than the critical statistic. In this example, the two regressions will be considered independently.

- Formulation 1

$$F_{calculated} (1661.50) > F_{critical} (4.49)$$

  so the null hypothesis is rejected in favour of the alternative hypothesis.
- Formulation 2

$$F_{calculated} (1478.50) > F_{critical} (4.49)$$

  so the null hypothesis is rejected in favour of the alternative hypothesis

We may therefore conclude that a linear relationship exists between the cumulative mass of drug released from either formulation 1 or formulation 2 and $t^{0.5}$.

Having defined the nature of the relationship between the cumulative mass of drug released and $t^{0.5}$, the question of whether or not the release rates of drug from the two formulations are similar may be resolved using a two-samples t test. Once more, the conditions associated with the analytical procedure should be clarified.

(i) State the null hypothesis

The null hypothesis for this problem states that the release rates of the therapeutic agent from the two formulations, defined as the slopes of the linear relationship between the cumulative mass of therapeutic agent released from the two formulations and $t^{0.5}$ are similar:

$$H_0: \quad \beta_{formulation\ 1} = \beta_{formulation\ 2}$$

(ii) State the alternative hypothesis

The alternative hypothesis states that the release rates of the therapeutic agent from the two formulations are not identical:

$$H_a: \quad \beta_{\text{formulation 1}} \neq \beta_{\text{formulation 2}}$$

(iii) State the level of significance and the number of tails associated with the experimental design

In this example, the chosen level of significance (a) is 0.05 and there are two tails associated with the experimental design.

(iv) Perform the statistical test

In this example, a two-samples t test will be employed to compare the magnitudes of the two slopes. The use of the t test is valid as many of the assumptions of linear regression analysis (from which the regression parameters were derived) are similar to those imposed by the t test. The execution of the t test to resolve the current problem will be performed in a stepwise fashion.

Step 1   Calculate the pooled residual mean square
The pooled residual mean square $(s^2_{y.x})$ is estimated using the data derived from the two regression analyses:

$$(s^2_{Y.X})_p = \frac{(SS_{\text{residual/formulation 1}} + SS_{\text{residual/formulation 2}})}{(df_{\text{residual/formulation 1}} + df_{\text{residual/formulation 2}})}$$

The values of the above parameters are derived from the ANOVA table associated with each linear regression (Tables 12.20 and 12.21). Thus:

$$(s^2_{Y.X})_p = \frac{(SS_{\text{residual/formulation 1}} + SS_{\text{residual/formulation 2}})}{(df_{\text{residual/formulation 1}} + df_{\text{residual/formulation 2}})}$$

$$= \frac{(1.29 + 3.76)}{(16 + 16)} = 0.16$$

Step 2   Calculate the standard error of the difference between slopes
Previously it was shown that the standard error of the difference between slopes $(s_{\text{treatment 1 - treatment 2}})$ may be calculated using the following formula:

$$s_{\text{treatment 1-treatment 2}} = \sqrt{\frac{(s^2_{Y.X})_p}{(\Sigma X^2_{\text{treatment 1}})} + \frac{(s^2_{Y.X})_p}{(\Sigma X^2_{\text{treatment 2}})}}$$

Therefore, as $(s^2_{y.x})_p = 0.16$, $\Sigma X^2_{\text{treatment 1}} = 273.00$ and $\Sigma X^2_{\text{treatment 2}} = 273.00$, the standard error may be calculated:

$$s_{\text{treatment 1-treatment 2}} = \sqrt{\frac{0.16}{(273.00)} + \frac{0.16}{(273.00)}} = 0.03$$

Step 3   Calculate the t statistic

$$t = \frac{b_{\text{formulation 1}} - b_{\text{formulation 2}}}{s_{\text{treatment 1 - treatment 2}}} = \frac{(5.52 - 9.02)}{0.03} = -116.67$$

Step 4   Identify the critical t statistic
The critical t statistic is determined from the table of the distribution of the critical values of the t statistic (Appendix 2), on the basis of the following information:

- $\alpha = 0.05$
- two-tailed outcome
- 32 (i.e. 16 + 16) *df*

The critical t statistic is approximately ± 2.04.

Step 5   Interpret the outcome of the statistical analysis
The regions of acceptance and rejection of the null hypothesis may now be defined:

$$H_0: \quad -2.04 < t < +2.04$$
$$H_a: \quad t > +2.04 \text{ or } t < -2.04$$

Therefore, as the calculated t statistic (-116.67) is less than the critical t statistic (-2.04), the null hypothesis is rejected. Accordingly, we may conclude that there is a significant difference between the rates of release of the therapeutic agent from the two controlled-release formulations.

There are statistical tests, based on ANOVA, that may be used for the comparison of more than two slopes, but the theory and applications of these tests are outside the scope of this book.

12.2   Correlation analysis

In section 12.1, the term *correlation* was introduced as a method of characterising the relationship that exists between two variables. This chapter has already described a type of relationship, i.e. the linear relationship that may exist between an independent variable and a dependent variable. In defining this relationship it was stated that linear regression analysis is used to define the line of best fit between the two variables. If the line of best fit and the line defined by the experimental data are superimposable, then we may conclude that the regression equation is an exact representation of the relationship and accordingly, the variation in the measured y variable is exclusively dependent on the variation of the X variable. Unfortunately this ideal scenario is rarely observed in practice because other factors may contribute the measured value of the y variable. Therefore, when linear regression is performed on a set of data, the line of best fit has mathematically defined the mean relationship between the two variables. One problem associated with linear regression concerns the variability of data around the line of best fit. If the variation is low, then it is possible to accurately predict the value of one variable with knowledge of the other variable, but in situations in which the variability is marked, this process is not possible. Accordingly, although linear regression is a useful statistical technique by which the linear relationship between two sets of data may be defined, it does not provide any measurement of the reliability or strength of the relationship between the two variables. If the deviation of the data from the line of best fit is low, the relationship between the two variables may be considered to be reliable: the converse is true when the variation is high. Correlation analysis is therefore applied to determine the degree of association of two variables. There is a range of statistical tests that may be used to examine the correlation of two variables and, as with other statistical methods, these tests may be conveniently categorised into either parametric or non-parametric methods. The theory and applications of several of these tests will be described in the following sections, once more with the aid of pharmaceutical examples.

12.2.1 Parametric estimation of correlation: Pearson's product moment correlation and the coefficient of determination

The parametric measure of linear association (correlation) is referred to as Pearson's product moment correlation. The use of this test is restricted by many of the assumptions of parametric analyses that have been documented in previous chapters and, in particular, the requirement that the data must be measured on at least an interval scale. The correlation between two variables is expressed as a correlation coefficient (r) and this is calculated using the following equation:

$$r = \frac{(N \sum Xy) - (\sum X \sum y)}{\sqrt{[N \sum X^2 - (\sum X)^2][N \sum y^2 - (\sum y)^2]}}$$

As before, N is the number of pairs of data.

The magnitude of the correlation coefficient ranges from -1 through 0 to $+1$. As the value of the coefficient approaches ± 1 the strength of the relationship between the two variables is increasing, with values of either -1 or $+1$ indicating a perfect relationship. The reader may be slightly confused by the nature of the sign associated with the calculated coefficient. A correlation coefficient value of $+1$ indicates a *perfect directly proportional relationship* between the two variables, whereas a value of −1 is evidence of a *perfect inversely proportional relationship*.

Another method by which the strength of a (parametric) relationship may be expressed is the *coefficient of determination*, which is calculated as the square of the correlation coefficient. This is a statistic that is frequently employed to interpret the relevance of a calculated correlation coefficient. For example, in a clinical experiment, a research team have investigated the relationship between stress (X variable) and the incidence of migraine (y variable) and have calculated that the correlation coefficient is 0.85. Does a correlation coefficient of 0.85 represent a strong relationship? One method by which the significance of this value may be addressed is to examine the coefficient of determination, which, for the example concerning the incidence of migraine, may be calculated as $(0.85)^2$, i.e. 0.72. The coefficient of determination is an excellent estimate of the contribution of the variation associated with the y (dependent) variable that is mathematically explained by the line of best fit. If the variation of the X variable is explained perfectly by the line of best fit, the r^2 value is equal to 1 and the correlation coefficient is equal to either −1 or +1. Returning to the hypothetical example that described the relationship between migraine and stress, the calculated r^2 value (0.72) informs the analyst that the variation in stress accounts for 72% of the total variation in the incidence of migraine. Conversely, it may be estimated that 28% of the variation in the incidence in migraine is due to other extraneous factors, e.g. diet, consumption of alcohol, etc. When a linear relationship between two variables has been examined, it is therefore good statistical practice to provide details of either the correlation coefficient or the coefficient of determination.

As before, the mechanics and interpretation of the correlation coefficient will be explained with the aid of pharmaceutical examples.

EXAMPLE 12.13 *A clinician is interested in examining the relationship between the mechanical properties of a medical implant and the time of implantation in patients. This interest has arisen as a result of the reported in vivo failure of the medical implant. Therefore, in a clinical study, when the period of implantation was complete, the implant was removed and its mechanical properties were examined by tensile analysis. The results concerning the relationship between the percentage elongation at break and time of implantation of the implant are shown in Table 12.23. Using an appropriate statistical method, quantify the degree of association between the two variables.*

Table 12.23 Effect of time of implantation on the percentage elongation at break of a medical implant

Time of implantation (weeks)	% Elongation at break
0	90.1
0	92.1
0	85.9
1	85.9
1	96.7
1	100.2
3	79.5
6	95.8
6	78.5
6	75.4
12	68.5
12	70.8
12	78.9
12	86.9
16	84.1
16	80.7
20	95.6
20	90.4
20	80.5
24	84.9

The degree of association between two variables may be quantified with reference to the correlation coefficient and the coefficient of determination. The correlation coefficient is calculated, in a stepwise fashion, using the following formula:

$$r = \frac{(N \sum Xy) - (\sum X \sum y)}{\sqrt{[N \sum X^2 - (\sum X)^2][N \sum y^2 - (\sum y)^2]}}$$

Step 1   Calculate the relevant descriptive statistics (Table 12.24)

Step 2   Calculate the correlation coefficient
The correlation coefficient is calculated by inserting the appropriate descriptive statistics into the previous equation:

$$r = \frac{(20 \times 15\,685.1) - (188 \times 1701.4)}{\sqrt{[(20 \times 2984.0) - (188)^2][(20 \times 146\,161.1) - (1701.4)^2]}}$$

$$= \frac{-6161.2}{26\,317.4} = -0.23$$

Table 12.24 Effect of time of implantation on the percentage elongation at break of a medical implant, incorporating descriptive parameters that are employed in the calculation of the correlation coefficient

Time of implantation (weeks)	% Elongation at break	Product of X and y
0	90.1	0
0	92.1	0
0	85.9	0
1	85.9	85.9
1	96.7	96.7
1	100.2	100.2
3	79.5	238.5
6	95.8	574.8
6	78.5	471
6	75.4	452.4
12	68.5	822
12	70.8	849.6
12	78.9	946.8
12	86.9	1042.8
16	84.1	1345.6
16	80.7	1291.2
20	95.6	1912
20	90.4	1808
20	80.5	1610
24	84.9	2037.6
$\Sigma X = 188$	$\Sigma y = 1701.4$	$\Sigma Xy = 15\ 685.1$
$\Sigma X^2 = 2984$	$\Sigma y^2 = 146\ 161.1$	

Step 3   Calculate the coefficient of determination
The coefficient of determination is the square of the correlation coefficient, i.e. $(-0.23)^2$ or 0.05.

Step 4   Interpret the calculated coefficients
The correlation coefficient that describes the relationship between the time of implantation of a medical device and the resultant percentage elongation at break of the device has a negative sign, which may be attributed to the inverse nature of the relationship. Interestingly, the value of the correlation coefficient is low, indicating a poor relationship between the two variables. This may be further investigated by consideration of the coefficient of determination (0.05). The magnitude of this coefficient indicates that only 5% of the total variation associated with the measurement of the percentage elongation may be accredited to

variation in the time of implantation. Conversely, approximately 95% of the variation is due to other factors. Therefore, we may conclude that the degree of association (i.e. the strength of the relationship) between the time of implantation and percentage elongation of a medical implant is poor and is not clinically relevant.

Example 12.13 was designed to illustrate the calculation and application of the correlation coefficient in the characterisation of the relationship (or lack of it) between two variables. This is the primary application of the technique. However, one interesting use of the correlation coefficient is in the process of linear regression in which correlation analysis is employed in the selection of the line of best fit. As the reader is now aware, linear regression is a technique in which the line of best fit may be determined to mathematically define the (linear) relationship between two variables. Accordingly, the equation is selected to represent the linear characteristics of the relationship and linear regression analysis is used to provide details of the slope and intercept. However, in some cases, an improved linear relationship may be obtained by performing a mathematical transformation of the data. Therefore, as the relationship between two sets of data may be described by more than one linear equation, the statistical analyst requires a method by which the most appropriate linear relationship may be determined. This selection process may be facilitated by correlation analysis, as shown in Example 12.14.

EXAMPLE 12.14 *A medical device company has developed a novel technology for drug-impregnated medical implants and consequently wishes to define the mechanism of release of the therapeutic agent from this system. The release of the therapeutic agent from a candidate formulation has been examined using an* in vitro *method and the results are shown in Table 12.25. Using appropriate statistical methodology, determine whether the release of therapeutic agent from the medical implant is zero-order or diffusion controlled.*

Table 12.25 Cumulative mass of therapeutic agent (mg) released from a medical implant *in vitro* as a function of time

Time (months)	Sample 1	Sample 2	Sample 3
1	5.61	4.19	6.10
2	11.19	9.10	12.81
3	17.16	13.01	17.19
6	30.96	27.16	34.11
12	59.91	54.93	61.66

In this problem, the analyst has been asked to examine the mechanism of release to determine whether release is either zero-order or diffusion controlled. If the mechanism of release is zero-order, a plot of cumulative mass of therapeutic agent released against time will be linear. Conversely, if the release is diffusion controlled, a linear relationship exists between the cumulative mass of therapeutic agent released and $t^{0.5}$. Therefore, the first stage of the statistical analysis involves the application of linear regression to examine the validity of these two scenarios.

Relationship between the cumulative mass of therapeutic agent released and time

Computation of the slope and intercept

Step 1   Calculation of the descriptive statistics associated with the regression
The main parameters associated with the linear regression procedure are calculated (Table 12.26).

Step 2   Calculate the slope of the line of best fit
Using the equation that was defined previously, the slope of the

Table 12.26 Cumulative mass of therapeutic agent released from a medical implant *in vitro* as a function of time, incorporating important parameters that are employed in linear regression analysis

Time (months)	Cumulative mass of drug released (mg)	Product of X and y
1	5.61	5.61
1	4.19	4.19
1	6.10	6.10
2	11.19	22.38
2	9.10	18.20
2	12.81	25.62
3	17.16	51.48
3	13.01	39.03
3	17.19	51.57
6	30.96	185.76
6	27.16	162.96
6	34.11	204.66
12	59.91	718.92
12	54.93	659.16
12	61.66	739.92
$\Sigma X = 72.00, \bar{X} = 4.80$	$\Sigma y = 365.09, \bar{y} = 24.34$	$\Sigma Xy = 2895.56$
$\Sigma X^2 = 582.00$	$\Sigma y^2 = 14\ 485.73$	

regression may be calculated as:

$$b = \frac{N(\Sigma\,Xy) - (\Sigma\,X)(\Sigma\,y)}{N(\Sigma\,X^2) - (\Sigma\,X)^2}$$

$$= \frac{(15 \times 2895.56) - (72.00)(365.09)}{(15 \times 582.00) - (72.00)^2} = 4.84 \text{ mg/month}$$

Step 3   Calculate of the intercept
The intercept is calculated by rearranging the equation of a straight line:

$$a = \bar{y} - (b \times \bar{X})$$

$$= 24.34 - (4.84 \times 4.80)$$

$$= 1.11 \text{ mg}$$

Step 4   Summary
The slope (b) and intercept (a) of the line of best fit, as determined by linear regression of the relationship between the cumulative mass of therapeutic agent released and time, are 4.84 mg/month and 1.11 mg, respectively. This linear relationship is displayed in Figure 12.11.

Validity of linear relationship

(i) *State the null hypothesis*

The null hypothesis states that a linear relationship does not exist between the cumulative mass of therapeutic agent released and time:

$$H_0: \quad \beta = 0$$

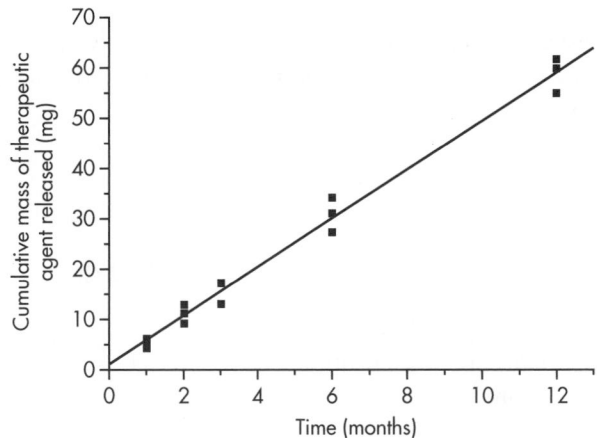

Figure 12.11 Cumulative mass of therapeutic agent released from a drug-impregnated medical implant as a function of time.

(ii) State the alternative hypothesis

The alternative hypothesis states that a linear relationship does exist between the cumulative mass of therapeutic agent released and time:

$$H_a: \quad \beta \neq 0$$

(iii) State the level of significance

In this example, it is assumed that the level of significance (α) is 0.05.

(iv) Perform the ANOVA

Step 1 Calculate the total sum of squares

$$SS_{total} = \Sigma\, y^2 - \frac{(\Sigma\, y)^2}{N} = 14\,485.73 - \frac{(365.09)^2}{15} = 5599.68$$

Step 2 Calculate the regression sum of squares

$$SS_{regression} = \frac{[(\Sigma\, Xy) - \Sigma\, X \, \Sigma\, y/n]^2}{\Sigma\, X^2 - (\Sigma\, X)^2/n}$$

$$= \frac{[(2895.56) - (72.00 \times 365.09)/15]^2}{582.00 - (72.00)^2/15} = 5527.67$$

Step 3 Calculate the residual sum of squares

$$SS_{residual} = SS_{total} - SS_{regression}$$
$$= 5599.68 - 5527.67$$
$$= 72.01$$

Step 4 Construct a summary table for the analysis of variance
The numbers of degrees of freedom associated with the regression parameters are:

- df_{total} = number of observations – 1 = 14
- $df_{regression}$ = 1
- $df_{residual}$ = 13

The summary table may now be created (Table 12.27).

Step 5 Define the critical F statistic
The critical F statistic is determined using Appendix 7 using the following information:

- level of significance (α) = 0.05
- $df_{regression}$ = 1
- $df_{residual}$ = 13

Table 12.27 Summary of the output of the analysis of variance concerning the linear regression of the cumulative mass of therapeutic agent released from a medical implant and time

Source	Sum of squares	df	Mean square	F statistic
Regression	5527.67	1	5527.67	997.77
Residual	72.01	13	5.54	
Total	5599.68	14		

Under these experimental conditions the critical value of the F statistic is 4.67.

Step 6 Interpret the outcome of the statistical analysis
In Example 12.14 $F_{calculated}$ (997.77) > $F_{critical}$(4.67) and, accordingly, the null hypothesis is rejected in favour of the alternative hypothesis. Therefore, it may be concluded that the linear relationship between the cumulative mass of therapeutic agent released and time, as defined by linear regression, is valid.

Correlation coefficient and coefficient of determination
The correlation coefficient and the coefficient of determination may be used to assess the strength of the relationship between the cumulative mass of drug released and time. The same mechanism is employed as in the previous example.

Step 1 Calculate the correlation coefficient
$$r = \frac{(15.00 \times 2895.56) - (72.00 \times 365.09)}{\sqrt{[(15 \times 582.00) - (72.00)^2][(15 \times 14\,485.73) - (365.09)^2]}}$$
$$= 0.994$$

Step 2 Calculate the coefficient of determination
The coefficient of determination is calculated as the square of the correlation coefficient, i.e. $(0.994)^2$ or 0.988.

Step 3 Interprete the calculated coefficients
The correlation coefficient is high, thereby implying that there is a strong association between the cumulative mass of therapeutic agent released and time. A further insight into this relationship may be obtained by reference to the coefficient of determination (0.988). This figure indicates that 98.8% of the total variation associated with the cumulative release of therapeutic agent may be accredited to variation in the time of release. This implies a strong relationship between the two variables.

Relationship between the cumulative mass of therapeutic agent released and $t^{0.5}$

Computation of the slope and intercept

Step 1   Calculate the descriptive statistics associated with the regression
Once more, the main parameters associated with the linear regression procedure are calculated and presented as a table (Table 12.28).

Step 2   Calculate the slope of the line of best fit

$$b = \frac{N(\Sigma Xy) - (\Sigma X)(\Sigma y)}{N(\Sigma X^2) - (\Sigma X)^2} = \frac{(15 \times 982.07) - (30.18)(365.09)}{(15 \times 72.00) - (30.18)^2}$$

$$= 21.95 \text{ mg/month}^{0.5}$$

Step 3   Calculate the intercept
The intercept is calculated by rearranging the equation of a straight line:

$$a = \bar{y} - (b \times \overline{X})$$
$$= 24.34 - (21.95 \times 2.01)$$
$$= -19.78 \text{ mg}$$

Table 12.28 Cumulative mass of therapeutic agent released from a medical implant in vitro as a function of $t^{0.5}$, incorporating important parameters that are employed in linear regression analysis

Time (months)	$t^{0.5}$	Cumulative mass of drug released (mg)	Product of X and y
1	1.00	5.61	5.61
1	1.00	4.19	4.19
1	1.00	6.10	6.10
2	1.41	11.19	15.83
2	1.41	9.10	12.87
2	1.41	12.81	18.12
3	1.73	17.16	29.72
3	1.73	13.01	22.53
3	1.73	17.19	29.77
6	2.45	30.96	75.84
6	2.45	27.16	66.53
6	2.45	34.11	83.55
12	3.46	59.91	207.53
12	3.46	54.93	190.28
12	3.46	61.66	213.60
	$\Sigma X = 30.18$, $\overline{X} = 2.01$ $\Sigma X^2 = 72.00$	$\Sigma y = 365.09$, $\bar{y} = 24.34$ $\Sigma y^2 = 14\,485.73$	$\Sigma Xy = 982.07$

Step 4 Summary

The parameters associated with the linear regression of the relationship between the cumulative mass of therapeutic agent released and $t^{0.5}$ are 21.95 mg/month$^{0.5}$ (slope) and −19.78 mg (intercept). This linear relationship is displayed in Figure 12.12.

Validity of the linear relationship

(i) State the null hypothesis

The null hypothesis states that a linear relationship does not exist between the cumulative mass of therapeutic agent released and $t^{0.5}$:

$$H_0: \quad \beta = 0$$

(ii) State the alternative hypothesis

The alternative hypothesis states that a linear relationship does exist between the cumulative mass of therapeutic agent released and $t^{0.5}$:

$$H_a: \quad \beta \neq 0$$

(iii) State the level of significance

In this example, it is assumed that the level of significance (α) is 0.05.

(iv) Perform the ANOVA

Step 1   Calculate the total sum of squares

$$SS_{total} = \Sigma y^2 - \frac{(\Sigma y)^2}{N} = 14\,485.73 - \frac{(365.09)^2}{15} = 5599.68$$

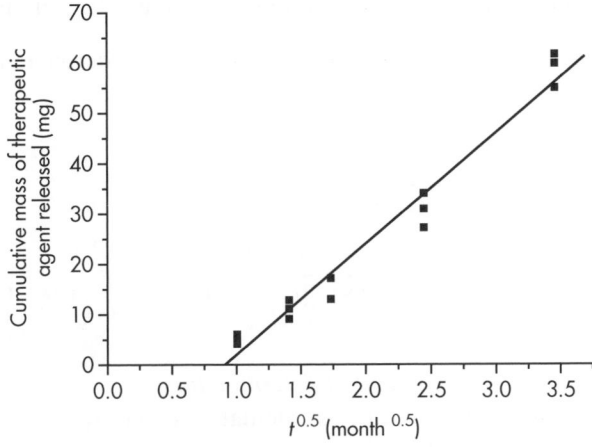

Figure 12.12   Cumulative mass of therapeutic agent released as a function of $t^{0.5}$.

Step 2   Calculate the regression sum of squares

$$SS_{\text{regression}} = \frac{[(\Sigma\, Xy) - \Sigma\, X \Sigma\, y/n]^2}{\Sigma\, X^2 - (\Sigma\, X)^2/n}$$

$$= \frac{[(982.07) - (30.18 \times 365.09)/15]^2}{72.00 - (30.18)^2/15} = 5431.95$$

Step 3   Calculate the residual sum of squares

$$SS_{\text{residual}} = SS_{\text{total}} - SS_{\text{regression}}$$

$$= 5599.68 - 5431.95$$

$$= 167.73$$

Step 4   Construct a summary table for the analysis of variance
The numbers of degrees of freedom associated with the regression parameters are:

- df_{total} = number of observations − 1 = 14
- $df_{\text{regression}}$ = 1
- df_{residual} = 13

The summary table may now be created (Table 12.29).

Step 5   Define the critical F statistic
The critical F statistic is identical to that defined for the previous part of this example, i.e. 4.67.

Step 6   Interpret the outcome of the statistical analysis
In Example 12.6 $F_{\text{calculated}}$ (421.08) > F_{critical} (4.67) and, accordingly, the null hypothesis is rejected in favour of the alternative hypothesis. Therefore, we may be conclude that there is a valid linear relationship between the cumulative mass of therapeutic agent released and $t^{0.5}$.

Calculate the correlation coefficient and coefficient of determination

Step 1   Calculate the correlation coefficient

$$r = \frac{(N\, \Sigma\, Xy) - (\Sigma\, X \Sigma\, y)}{\sqrt{[N\, \Sigma\, X^2 - (\Sigma\, X)^2][N\, \Sigma\, y^2 - (\Sigma\, y)^2]}}$$

$$= \frac{(15.00 \times 982.07) - (30.18 \times 365.09)}{\sqrt{[(15 \times 72.00) - (30.18)^2][(15 \times 14\,485.73) - (365.09)^2]}}$$

$$= 0.985$$

Step 2   Calculate the coefficient of determination
The coefficient of determination is calculated as the square of the correlation coefficient, i.e. $(0.985)^2$ or 0.970.

Table 12.29 Summary of the output of the analysis of variance for the linear regression of the cumulative mass of therapeutic agent released from a medical implant and $t^{0.5}$

Source	Sum of squares	df	Mean square	F statistic
Regression	5431.95	1	5431.95	421.08
Residual	167.73	13	12.90	
Total	5599.68	14		

Step 3 Interpret the calculated coefficients
Once more, the correlation coefficient is high, thereby implying a strong association between the cumulative mass of therapeutic agent released and $t^{0.5}$. Calculation of the coefficient of determination allows the sources of the variability to be assessed. Subsequently, it may be concluded that 97.0% of the total variation associated with the cumulative release of therapeutic agent may be accredited to variation in the square root of time of release.

Conclusions

In the above example linear regression analysis has been used to examine the relationships between the cumulative mass of therapeutic agent released and time (t), and also between the cumulative mass and $t^{0.5}$. In both scenarios, the lines of best fit were mathematically characterised in terms of the slope and intercept and the validity of the application of linear regression to the data sets was confirmed using ANOVA. However, if one follows this logic, then the conclusion to the analysis is that the mechanism of release of therapeutic agent from the medical device is both zero-order and diffusion controlled. Obviously this cannot be so, and the analyst must decide which linear regression is more appropriate by examination and comparison of the correlation coefficients of each relationship. As the correlation coefficient of the regression associated with the zero-order assumption is closer to unity than the correlation coefficient associated with the diffusion-controlled scenario, it is appropriate to conclude that the zero-order model is more appropriate than the diffusion-controlled model.

12.2.2 Statistical evaluation of zero correlation

As described in the previous section, the correlation coefficient (and the related coefficient of determination) is used to assess the strength of the relationship between two variables. Accordingly, as the correlation coefficient approaches ±1, or the coefficient of determination approaches

+1, it is assumed that the association between the two variables is progressively stronger. Conversely, a calculated correlation coefficient of zero represents no association. In many of the examples that have been described in this chapter, it was apparent that the calculated coefficient was sufficiently close to unity to represent a significant correlation. However, if the calculated value of r is not close to 1, the statistical analyst may wish to inquire whether the calculated correlation coefficient is evidence of association (albeit rather weak in nature) or whether the calculated value of the correlation coefficient does not represent association, i.e. it is not significantly different from zero. This question may be addressed using a t test with the general formula

$$t_{(a, N-2\ df, \text{two-tailed})} = \frac{(r\sqrt{N-2})}{\sqrt{1-r^2}}$$

where r is the experimentally calculated correlation coefficient and N is the number of pairs of data.

The use of this equation to examine the statistical relevance of the correlation coefficient is described in the following examples.

EXAMPLE 12.15 *In Example 12.13, the relationship between the time of implantation of a medical device* in vivo *and the resultant percentage elongation at break was examined. In particular, the association between these variables was characterised in terms of a correlation coefficient (−0.23). Using an appropriate statistical technique, examine whether this calculated coefficient is valid, or, alternatively, is due to random error.*

In correlation analysis, a valid relationship between two variables is represented by a correlation coefficient that is either greater than or less than zero. Conversely, a correlation coefficient of 0 is indicative of no correlation. Therefore, the null and alternative hypotheses of the t test are based on these concepts.

(i) State the null hypothesis

The null hypothesis of this example states that the population correlation coefficient, represented by the sample correlation coefficient, is equal to zero, indicating a lack of interaction between the time of implantation of a medical device *in vivo* and the resultant percentage elongation at break:

H_0: $r = 0$

(ii) State the alternative hypothesis

The alternative hypothesis states that the population correlation coefficient is not equal to zero, indicating a valid relationship between the time of implantation of a medical device *in vivo* and the resultant percentage elongation at break:

H_a: $r \neq 0$

(iii) State the level of significance and the number of tails associated with the experimental design

In this example it will be assumed that the level of significance (α) is 0.05. As there are two outcomes ($r > 0$ and $r < 0$) that will allow the null hypothesis to be rejected, the experimental design is two-tailed.

(iv) Perform the statistical test

Step 1   Calculate the t statistic

$$t = \frac{(r\sqrt{N-2})}{\sqrt{1-r^2}} = \frac{(-0.23\sqrt{20-2})}{\sqrt{1-(-0.23)^2}} = \frac{-0.976}{0.973} = 1.003$$

Step 2   Define the critical t statistic

The critical t statistic is determined from the table of critical values of the t distribution (Appendix 2) with knowledge of the following parameters:

- level of significance (α) = 0.05
- number of tails = 2
- df ($N_{total} - 2 = 20 - 2$) = 18

The critical t statistic is therefore 2.10.

Step 3   Interpret the outcome of the statistical analysis

The critical t statistic defines the regions of acceptance and rejection of the null hypothesis. In this example, the region of acceptance of the null hypothesis is defined as $-2.10 < t < +2.10$. Conversely, the regions of rejection of the null hypothesis in the two-tailed experimental design are $t < -2.10$ and $t > +2.10$. Therefore, as the calculated t statistic (1.003) lies within the region of acceptance of the null hypothesis, we may conclude that there is no relationship between the time of implantation of the medical implant *in vivo* and the resultant percentage elongation at break.

This example illustrates the need to examine the relevance of the calculated correlation coefficient using the t test, as this will confirm the absence or presence of a significant relationship between the two variables. The next example illustrates the application of the technique to examine the significance of a relationship that has been defined by a correlation coefficient close to unity.

EXAMPLE 12.16 *In Example 12.14 the relationship between the cumulative mass of release of a therapeutic agent from a medical implant and time was defined using correlation analysis (r = 0.994). Using an appropriate statistical technique, examine whether this calculated coefficient is valid, or, alternatively, is due to random error.*

The parameters relevant to the experimental design are defined as in the previous example.

(i) State the null hypothesis

The null hypothesis of this example states that the population correlation coefficient, represented by the sample correlation coefficient, is equal to zero. Therefore, there is no relationship between the cumulative mass of therapeutic agent released and time:

$$H_0: \quad r = 0$$

(ii) State the alternative hypothesis

The alternative hypothesis states that the population correlation coefficient is not equal to zero, indicating a valid relationship between the cumulative mass of therapeutic agent released and time:

$$H_a: \quad r \neq 0$$

(iii) State the level of significance and the number of tails associated with the experimental design

In this example it will be assumed that the level of significance (α) is 0.05 and the experimental design is two-tailed.

(iv) Perform the statistical test

Step 1   Calculate the t statistic

$$t = \frac{(r\sqrt{N-2})}{\sqrt{1-r^2}} = \frac{(0.994\sqrt{15-2})}{\sqrt{1-(0.994)^2}} = \frac{3.58}{0.11} = 32.55$$

Step 2   Define the critical t statistic
The critical t statistic is determined from the table of critical values of the t distribution with knowledge of the following parameters:

- level of significance (α) = 0.05
- number of tails = 2
- df ($N_{total} - 2 = 15 - 2$) = 13

The critical t statistic is therefore either <-2.16 or $+2.16$, i.e. ±2.16.

Step 3   Interpret the outcome of the statistical analysis
The regions of the t distribution relating to the null and alternative hypotheses are:

H_0: $-2.16 < t < +2.16$

H_a: $t < -2.16$ and $t > 2.16$

Therefore, as the calculated t statistic (32.55) lies within the region of rejection of the null hypothesis, we may conclude that there is a valid relationship between the cumulative mass of therapeutic agent released and time.

12.2.3   Correlation analysis using non-parametric methods

In the previous section the theory and applications of the Pearson product moment correlation coefficient to define the degrees of association of two variables were described. This method is parametric in origin and in particular, assumes that the data have been measured on at least an interval scale and have been sampled from a bivariate normal population. When these assumptions are invalid, alternative (non-parametric) methods must be used to examine the strength of the relationship between the variables. These tests may be applied to all data types (nominal, ordinal, interval and ratio) and do not require the population from which the samples have been derived to be normally distributed. In this section, the theory and applications of two non-parametric tests that may be used to determine the strength of a relationship between two variables, namely the *contingency coefficient* ϕ and the *Spearman rank correlation coefficient*, will be explained, once more with reference to pharmaceutical examples.

12.2.3.1   *Assessment of the degree of association between two variables using the contingency coefficient or the ϕ coefficient*

The contingency coefficient is commonly used to examine the degree of correlation or dependence between variables in the χ^2 analysis. In Chapter 8 it was stressed that the null hypothesis for a χ^2 analysis assumes that there is no correlation between the variables and conversely, the alternative hypothesis assumes that there is a correlation. Therefore, in situations where the null hypothesis has been rejected, it may be of interest to the analyst to obtain a measure of the correlation between the variables. There are two coefficients that are employed for this purpose, namely the ϕ coefficient and the contingency coefficient

(C). The ϕ coefficient is employed when the null hypothesis has been rejected in a 2×2 contingency experiment, whereas the contingency coefficient is used for higher experimental designs. Therefore, these methods are primarily employed to examine correlation between two variables in which the data have been measured on a nominal scale.

The ϕ coefficient and the contingency coefficient (C) are calculated using the following formulae:

$$\phi = \sqrt{\frac{\chi^2_{\text{calculated}}}{n}}$$

$$C = \sqrt{\frac{\chi^2_{\text{calculated}}}{\chi^2_{\text{calculated}} + n}}$$

where $\chi^2_{\text{calculated}}$ is the calculated χ^2 statistic and N is the total number of observations.

Both coefficients provide a measure of the correlation or dependence between the variables with an experimental design. The use of these coefficients is explained using the following examples.

EXAMPLE 12.17　*A clinical study has been designed to examine the comparative performances of two brands of steroid inhalers. Asthmatic volunteers were asked to use each inhaler as directed by the manufacturer and to record the number of asthma attacks suffered over a 6-month period. The results from the study are shown in Table 12.30. Using an appropriate statistical method, comment on the validity of the relationship between the type of inhaler and the incidence of asthma attacks.*

As before, it is important to established the criteria on which the statistical model will be formulated. This should be done before the collection of data.

Table 12.30 Observed incidences and severity of asthma attacks associated with two inhaled steroid formulations

Inhaler	Number of recorded observations (O_i)			
	No attacks	1–10 attacks	10–20 attacks	Total
Inhaler A	174	55	18	247
Inhaler B	65	121	70	256
Total	239	176	88	503

(i) State the null hypothesis

A suitable null hypothesis for this scenario is that there is no relationship between the type of inhaler and the incidence of asthma attacks.

(ii) State the alternative hypothesis

A suitable alternative hypothesis for the above example is that there is a relationship between the type of inhaler and the incidence of asthma attacks.

(iii) State the level of significance

In this example, it is assumed that the level of significance (α) is 0.05.

(iv) Select an appropriate statistical test

This is an example of a 2×3 experimental design in which the data have been recorded as frequencies (incidences). The data is therefore nominal in nature and, as a result, the examination of the independence or dependence of the two variables is most appropriately performed using a 2×3 χ^2 analysis.

(v) Compute the χ^2 statistic

The χ^2 statistic is calculated in a stepwise fashion, as follows.

Step 1   Calculate the expected frequencies associated with each cell
The expected frequencies associated with each cell are found by multiplying the row total associated with a cell by the column total associated with the cell and dividing by the total number of observations in the study. The expected frequencies for the four cells are calculated and expressed in tabular form (Table 12.31).

Step 2   Calculate the corrected χ^2 statistic
Calculating and adding the ratios of the squared differences between the observed and expected frequencies for each cell and the expected

Table 12.31   Expected incidences and severity of asthma attacks associated with two inhaled steroid formulations, as defined by the null hypothesis

Inhaler	Expected numbers of observations (E_f)			
	No attacks	1–10 attacks	10–20 attacks	Total
Inhaler A	117.36	86.43	43.21	247.00
Inhaler B	121.64	89.57	44.79	256.00
Total	239.00	176.00	88.00	503.00

frequencies, determine the χ^2 statistic:

$$\chi^2 = \left[\frac{[(174.00 - 117.36)]^2}{117.36} + \frac{[(65.00 - 121.64)]^2}{121.64} \right.$$

$$+ \frac{[(55.00 - 86.43)]^2}{86.43} + \frac{[(121.00 - 89.57)]^2}{89.57}$$

$$\left. + \frac{[(18.00 - 43.21)]^2}{43.21} + \frac{[(70.00 - 44.79)]^2}{44.79} \right]$$

$$= 105.07$$

Step 3 Define the critical χ^2 statistic
The critical χ^2 statistic is determined from the table in Appendix 3 with knowledge of the following information:

- $\alpha = 0.05$
- $df = (\text{rows} - 1)(\text{columns} - 1) = 1 \times 2 = 2$

Under these experimental conditions, the critical value of χ^2 is 5.99.

Step 4 Interpret the outcome of the statistical analysis
The region associated with acceptance of the null hypothesis is $\chi^2 < 5.99$. Conversely, the region associated with rejection of the null hypothesis is $\geqslant 5.99$. In this example the calculated χ^2 statistic (105.07) is greater than the critical χ^2 statistic (5.99) and, accordingly, the two variables are dependent. Therefore, it may be concluded that the incidence of asthma attacks is dependent on the type of inhaler used.

Step 5 Calculate the strength of the relationship
Having identified a relationship between the above variables, the statistical analyst should examine their degree of association (correlation). The choice of the most appropriate method of doing this is dependent on the nature of the data and the type of experimental design. In this example the data has been measured in a nominal scale and the experimental design is a 2×3 contingency table. The most appropriate method to examine the correlation between the two variables is therefore the contingency coefficient, which is calculated as follows:

$$C = \sqrt{\frac{\chi^2_{calculated}}{\chi^2_{calculated} + n}} = \sqrt{\frac{105.07}{105.07 + 503}} = 0.42$$

This value may seem to indicate that there is a moderate association between the two variables. However; this betrays one of the problems associated with the use of the contingency coefficient (and indeed the ϕ coefficient), i.e. a perfect correlation is not denoted by a coefficient value of unity. The value of perfect correlation is dependent on the experimental design, in particular the number of categories. In an experimental design composed of two categories, maximum correlation is reflected by a coefficient value of approximately 0.7, whereas for a design containing three categories this value increases to approximately 0.82. Therefore, in light of this, the calculated value of 0.42 represents a good correlation.

The square of the contingency coefficient may be used to examine the nature of the association. In this example C^2 is 0.18, which means that knowing the type of inhaler increases the accuracy of predicting the incidence of asthma attacks by 18%.

The next example describes the use of this technique to examine the relationship between two variables in which the experimental design is in the form of a 2×2 contingency table.

EXAMPLE 12.18 *It is accepted that the initial step in the process of infection is the adherence of microorganisms to the host epithelial cells. A microbiologist wishes to examine whether treatment of epithelial cells with a non-antibiotic antimicrobial agent (a normal component of mouthwash formulations) increases the number of cells that are devoid of pathogenic microorganisms. Therefore, in a laboratory experiment, epithelial cells were collected by scraping the buccal mucosa of several human volunteers, pooled and treated with either sterile water or a defined concentration of the non-antibiotic antimicrobial agent for 30 s. The epithelial cells were then exposed to a defined number of viable* Candida albicans *and the numbers of cells that either did or did not have attached microbial cells after a defined period were recorded using light microscopy. The results are shown in Table 12.32. Using appropriate statistical methods, examine whether there is a relationship between the type of treatment used and the subsequent nature of microbial attachment to epithelial cells.*

Table 12.32 Effects of treatment of epithelial cells with either sterile water or a non-antibiotic antimicrobial agent on the subsequent adherence of *Candida albicans*, expressed as the number of cells with and without attached yeast cells

Treatment	Categorisation of microbial adherence		Totals
	Cells without attached yeast cells	Cells with attached yeast cells	
Sterile water	26	178	204
Antimicrobial agent	121	45	166
Totals	147	223	370

As before, it is important to establish the criteria on which the statistical model will be formulated before collecting data.

(i) State the null hypothesis

A suitable null hypothesis for this scenario is that there is no relationship between the type of treatment used and the subsequent nature of microbial attachment to epithelial cells.

(ii) State the alternative hypothesis

A suitable alternative hypothesis for the above example is that there is a relationship between the type of treatment used and the subsequent nature of microbial attachment to epithelial cells.

(iii) State the level of significance

In this example, it is assumed that the level of significance (α) is 0.05.

(iv) State the number of tails associated with the experimental design

As there are two ways in which the null hypothesis may be rejected – the number of cells without attached microorganisms after treatment with the non-antibiotic antimicrobial agent may be greater or less than that after treatment with sterile water – the experimental design associated with this example is two-tailed.

(v) Select an appropriate statistical test

This is an example of a 2×2 experimental design in which the data have been recorded as frequencies (incidences). The data is therefore nominal in nature and, as a result, the examination of the independence or dependence of the two variables is most appropriately performed using a 2×2 χ^2 analysis.

(vi) Computation of the χ^2 statistic

The equation for the calculation of the χ^2 statistic for a 2×2 experimental design has been previously presented in Chapter 8 as

$$\chi^2 = \sum \frac{[(O_f - E_f) - 0.5]^2}{E_f}$$

The χ^2 statistic is calculated as follows.

Step 1   Calculate the expected frequencies associated with each cell
The expected frequency associated with each cell is performed by multiplying the row total associated with a cell by the column total associated

with the cell and dividing the product by the total number of observations in the study. The expected frequencies for the four cells are calculated and expressed in tabular form (Table 12.33).

Step 2   Calculate the corrected χ^2 statistic
The χ^2 statistic is determined by calculating and adding the ratios of the squared differences between the observed and expected frequencies for each cell (corrected for continuity) and the expected frequencies:

$$\chi^2 = \left[\frac{[(26.00 - 81.05) - 0.5]^2}{81.05} + \frac{[(121.00 - 65.95) - 0.5]^2}{65.95} \right.$$

$$\left. + \frac{[(178.00 - 122.95) - 0.5]^2}{122.95} + \frac{[(45.00 - 100.05) - 0.5]^2}{100.05} \right]$$

$$= 138.23$$

Step 3   Define the critical χ^2 statistic
The critical χ^2 statistic is determined from the table of the critical values of the χ^2 statistic with knowledge of the following information:

- $\alpha = 0.05$
- $df = (\text{rows} - 1)(\text{columns} - 1) = 1 \times 1 = 1$.

Under these experimental conditions, the critical value of χ^2 is 3.84 (from Appendix 3).

Step 4   Interpret the outcome of the statistical analysis
The region associated with acceptance of the null hypothesis is $\chi^2 < 3.84$, whereas the region associated with rejection of the null hypothesis is $\geqslant 3.84$. In Example 12.18 the calculated χ^2 statistic (138.23) is greater than the critical χ^2 statistic (3.84) and, accordingly, it may be concluded that the two variables are dependent. Therefore, the number of cells that have no attached *Candida albicans* is dependent on the nature of the pre-treatment, i.e. sterile water or the non-antibiotic antimicrobial agent.

Table 12.33 Expected incidences of the effects of treatment type on microbial adherence, as defined by the null hypothesis

Treatment	Categorisation of microbial adherence		Totals
	Cells without attached yeast cells	Cells with attached yeast cells	
Sterile water	81.05	122.95	204
Antimicrobial agent	65.95	100.05	166
Totals	147	223	370

Step 5   Calculate the strength of the relationship

Once a relationship is identified between the number of cells without attached microorganism and the nature of the pre-treatment, the next step involves the calculation of the degree of association (correlation) between these variables. The choice of the most appropriate method to perform this task is dependent on the nature of the data and the type of experimental design. In this example the data has been measured in a nominal scale and the experimental design is a 2×2 contingency table. Therefore, in this scenario, the most appropriate method to examine the correlation between the two variables is the ϕ coefficient, which is calculated as follows:

$$\phi = \sqrt{\frac{\chi^2_{\text{calculated}}}{n}} = \sqrt{\frac{138.23}{370}} = 0.61$$

As before, the ϕ coefficient associated with perfect correlation in this experimental design would be approximately 0.7 and therefore the calculated value of 0.61 indicates that there is good association between the two variables. In a similar fashion to the contingency coefficient, the square of the ϕ coefficient may be used to examine the nature of the association. In this example ϕ^2 is 0.37, so it may be estimated that the accuracy of estimating the number of epithelial cells with no attached microorganisms is improved by 37% if we know the nature of the pre-treatment of the epithelial cells.

12.2.3.2 Assessment of the degree of association between two variables using the Spearman rank correlation coefficient

The Spearman rank correlation coefficient (r_S) is statistical measure of association between two variables that have been measured on an ordinal (ranking) scale, or in situations in which one variable has been measured on an ordinal scale and the second variable in an interval or ratio scale. As with the correlation coefficient (but not the contingency coefficient), perfect correlation between two variables is denoted by a value of +1 or −1, dependent on the nature of the association (i.e. direct or inverse). In this statistical method, the difference between the ranks of each pair of data (d) is calculated, squared and summed. Subsequently, the Spearman rank correlation coefficient is calculated using the following formula:

$$r_S = 1 - \left(\frac{6 \sum d^2}{n(n^2 - 1)} \right)$$

As before, n refers to the number of pairs of data.

The mechanics of this statistical method are illustrated in the following examples.

EXAMPLE 12.19 *A laboratory that specialises in skin irritancy studies has been asked to perform a clinical study to determine the skin irritancy of a pharmaceutical ingredient. A clinical study has therefore been defined in which the pharmaceutical ingredient is applied to the forearm of volunteers and the degree of irritancy is measured using two analytical methods. The first method involves a visual analogue scale in which the degree of irritation is assigned a rank (0–10) commensurate with the redness at the site of application. A value of 0 indicates no irritancy whereas a value of 10 is indicative of extreme irritancy, values in between these limits showing increasing levels of redness. The second method involves the measurement of the degree of redness at the site of application using an instrumental probe (laser Doppler velocimetry). The results from the clinical study are shown in Table 12.34. Using an appropriate analytical technique, examine whether there is a good correlation between the two methods for the quantification of irritancy.*

To examine the correlation between these two variables, one must initially select the most appropriate method, considering the nature of the data associated with the variables. The data associated with the visual scale is ordinal in nature, whereas the instrumental method has employed a ratio scale of measurement. It is therefore appropriate to use Spearman's rank correlation coefficient to examine the relationship between the variables, but the ratio data must first be converted into ordinal data. This is performed by assigning the smallest value a rank score of one, subsequent scores being assigned larger ranks in increasing order of magnitude (Table 12.35).

Spearman's rank correlation coefficient is then calculated in a stepwise fashion.

Table 12.34 Assessment of the skin irritancy of a pharmaceutical ingredient using a visual method and an instrumental method

Patient ID number	Visual method	Instrumental method (arbitrary units)
1	1	0.15
2	4	0.61
3	5	0.66
4	3	0.59
5	8	0.71
6	7	0.69
7	9	0.70

Table 12.35 Assessment of the skin irritancy of a pharmaceutical ingredient using a visual method and an instrumental method (expressed as a rank score)

Patient ID number	Visual method	Instrumental method (arbitrary units)
1	1	1
4	3	2
2	4	3
3	5	4
6	7	5
7	9	6
5	8	7

Step 1   Calculate the difference between the ranks and the square of the difference between the ranks

The differences between the ranks of each pair of data are calculated, squared and presented in tabular form (Table 12.36). In this example, the rank score of the instrumental method is subtracted from the rank score of the visual method.

Step 2   Calculate the Spearman rank correlation coefficient

$$r_S = 1 - \left(\frac{6 \sum d^2}{n(n^2 - 1)} \right) = 1 - \left(\frac{6 \times 17}{7(7^2 - 1)} \right) = 1 - \frac{102}{336} = 0.70$$

Perfect correlation is defined by a Spearman rank correlation coefficient of unity, and consequently, the calculated value of 0.7 is indicative of a correlation between the two methods for the evaluation of skin irritancy.

Table 12.36 Assessment of the skin irritancy of a pharmaceutical ingredient using a visual method and an instrumental method (expressed as a rank score), incorporating parameters that will be employed in the calculation of the Spearman's rank correlation coefficient

Patient ID number	Visual method	Instrumental method (arbitrary units)	Difference in ranks (d)	d²
1	1	1	0	0
4	3	2	+1	1
2	4	3	+1	1
3	5	4	+1	1
6	7	5	+2	4
7	9	6	+3	9
5	8	7	+1	1
				$\sum d^2 = 17$

Step 3 Determination of the significance of the calculated Spearman rank correlation coefficient

There are two methods by which the significance of the calculated Spearman coefficient may be calculated, the choice being dependent on sample size. As in other statistical methods, the conditions of the experimental design should be clarified.

(i) State the null hypothesis

The null hypothesis states that there is no relation between the two methods for the evaluation of skin irritancy.

(ii) State the alternative hypothesis

The alternative hypothesis states that there is a relation between the two methods for the evaluation of skin irritancy.

(iii) State the level of significance

In this example, it is assumed that the level of significance (α) is 0.05.

(iv) State the number of tails associated with the experimental design

In this analysis the number of tails relates to the nature of the correlation as defined by the alternative hypothesis. If there are two possible reasons for the null hypothesis to be rejected, namely a negative correlation and a positive correlation, the outcome is two-tailed. However, in this analysis it is assumed that if a correlation exists it will be positive and therefore, as only one outcome is specified, the design is one-tailed.

(v) Perform the statistical analysis

There are two possible methods by which the significance of the calculated Spearman rank correlation coefficient may be examined, the choice being dependent on the size of the sample. As the sample size is small in this example (i.e. <30), the significance of the calculated r_S value may be directly ascertained with reference to the table of critical values of the Spearman rank correlation coefficient (Appendix 18). As before, this table defines the critical r_S statistic associated with a defined level of significance ($\alpha = 0.05$), one-tailed experimental design and the number of pairs of observations in the analysis. In this example the critical r_S statistic ($N = 7$, one-tailed outcome, $\alpha = 0.05$) is 0.71. If the calculated value of r_S is either greater than or equal to this critical value, the null hypothesis is rejected in favour of the alternative hypothesis. As $r_{S\,\text{calculated}}$ (0.70) $< r_{S\,\text{critical}}$, the null hypothesis is accepted and it may be concluded that there is no correlation between the methods for the evaluation of skin irritancy.

Before leaving this example, it is important to highlight a couple of points concerning this outcome.

- The null hypothesis has been accepted of the basis of a selected significance level of 0.05. The calculated r_S value corresponds to a probability value that is greater than 0.05 but less than 0.1. The null hypothesis should therefore be accepted only with extreme caution, in light of the marginal nature of the outcome.
- The sample size in this study was small, so it would be appropriate (cost permitting) to repeat the clinical study with a greater number of volunteers. This would clarify the statistical outcome.

The final example to be considered in this section addresses an additional concept that must be understood concerning the use of Spearman's rank correlation coefficient for the examination of the relationship between two variables, namely the presence of tied values. In the calculation of the Spearman rank correlation coefficient, tied values are defined as values possessing the same rank order within the same variable. As in previous non-parametric tests, tied ranks must share the same rank score and therefore the average rank for each tied score is allocated. If the presence of tied values is overlooked, the calculated r_S is incorrect and therefore mathematical corrections must be performed to overcome this problem. In these circumstances, the Spearman rank correlation coefficient is calculated using the following formula:

$$r_S = \frac{\Sigma x^2 + \Sigma y^2 - \Sigma d^2}{2\sqrt{\Sigma x^2 \times \Sigma y^2}}$$

where d^2 is the square of the difference of the rank scores of paired values,

$$\Sigma x^2 = \left(\frac{N^3 - N_x}{12}\right) - \Sigma\left(\frac{t_x^3 - t_x}{12}\right)$$

$$\Sigma y^2 = \left(\frac{N^3 - N_y}{12}\right) - \Sigma\left(\frac{t_y^3 - t_y}{12}\right)$$

where N is the number of paired observations and t is the number of ties in any rank score in either the x or y variable.

The use and interpretation of this calculation are described in Example 12.20.

EXAMPLE 12.20 *A physiology department has developed a novel means of evoking pain using ultrasound, which is more rapid and more* *economical than the current method used to examine pain. The researchers wish to examine whether there is a correlation between the two methods. Therefore, in a clinical study, 15 volunteers were recruited and exposed to each method of evoking pain. The degrees of pain associated with each model were then recorded using a visual analogue scale in which 1 represented no pain and 10 represented extreme pain. Rank scores between 1 and 10 represented increasing pain. The results from the study are shown in Table 12.37. Using an appropriate statistical method, examine whether there is a correlation between the two methods.*

The evaluation of the relationship between these two variables requires an initial examination of the most appropriate statistical method for this purpose. The data has been measured on an ordinal ranking scale in which pain has been assigned a numerical rank commensurate with severity, so the most appropriate coefficient to examine the relationship between these two variables is Spearman's rank correlation coefficient. The calculation of this coefficient is illustrated in a stepwise fashion.

Step 1   Correct the rank scores for tied values
The rank scores associated with the x and y variables are corrected for the presence of tied values and retabulated (Table 12.38).

Table 12.37 Clinical comparison of evoked pain using two models

Patient ID number	New (ultrasound) model	Current model
1	1	2
2	2	1
3	2	6
4	3	5
5	3	5
6	4	5
7	4	5
8	5	4
9	5	8
10	6	5
11	6	4
12	8	6
13	8	7
14	9	7
15	10	8

Table 12.38 Clinical comparison of evoked pain using two models, showing rank scores that have been corrected for the presence of tied ranks

Patient ID number	New (ultrasound) model		Current model	
	Rank scores	Rank scores corrected for ties	Rank scores	Rank scores corrected for ties
1	1	1	2	2
2	2	2.5	1	1
3	2	2.5	6	10.5
4	3	4.5	5	7
5	3	4.5	5	7
6	4	6.5	5	7
7	4	6.5	5	7
8	5	8.5	4	3.5
9	5	8.5	8	14.5
10	6	10.5	5	7
11	6	10.5	4	3.5
12	8	12.5	6	10.5
13	8	12.5	7	12.5
14	9	14	7	12.5
15	10	15	8	14.5

Table 12.39 Clinical comparison of evoked pain using two models, incorporating parameters that will be employed in the calculation of the Spearman's rank correlation coefficient

Patient ID number	New (ultrasound) model	Current model	Difference in ranks (d)	d^2
1	1	2	−1.0	1.00
2	2.5	1	1.5	2.25
3	2.5	10.5	−8.0	64.00
4	4.5	7	−2.5	6.25
5	4.5	7	−2.5	6.25
6	6.5	7	−0.5	0.25
7	6.5	7	−0.5	0.25
8	8.5	3.5	5.0	25.00
9	8.5	14.5	−6.0	36.00
10	10.5	7	3.5	12.25
11	10.5	3.5	7.0	49.00
12	12.5	10.5	2.0	4.00
13	12.5	12.5	0.0	0.00
14	14	12.5	1.5	2.25
15	15	14.5	0.5	0.25
				$\Sigma\, d^2 = 209.00$

Step 2   Calculate the difference between the corrected ranks and the square of the difference between the ranks (see Table 12.39)

Step 3   Calculate Σx^2 (New ultrasound model)
The term Σx^2 is calculated using the following equation, remembering that N the number of pairs of observations is 15 and, furthermore, there are six sets of tied observations, each composed of two cases. Therefore:

$$\Sigma x^2 = \left(\frac{N^3 - N_x}{12}\right) - \Sigma\left(\frac{t_x^3 - t_x}{12}\right)$$

$$= \left(\frac{15^3 - 15}{12}\right) - \left[\left(\frac{2^3 - 2}{12}\right) + \left(\frac{2^3 - 2}{12}\right) + \left(\frac{2^3 - 2}{12}\right) + \left(\frac{2^3 - 2}{12}\right)\right.$$

$$\left. + \left(\frac{2^3 - 2}{12}\right) + \left(\frac{2^3 - 2}{12}\right)\right]$$

$$= 280 - 3 = 277$$

Step 4   Calculate Σy^2 (Current model)
The term Σy^2 is calculated in an analogous fashion to Σx^2. In this calculation $N = 15$ and there are five sets of tied rank scores, four of which are composed of two ranks and the other is composed of five ranks.

$$\Sigma y^2 = \left(\frac{N^3 - N_y}{12}\right) - \Sigma\left(\frac{t_y^3 - t_y}{12}\right)$$

$$= \left(\frac{15^3 - 15}{12}\right) - \left[\left(\frac{2^3 - 2}{12}\right) + \left(\frac{2^3 - 2}{12}\right) + \left(\frac{2^3 - 2}{12}\right) + \left(\frac{2^3 - 2}{12}\right)\right.$$

$$\left. + \left(\frac{5^3 - 5}{12}\right)\right] = 280 - 12 = 268$$

Step 5   Calculate Spearman's rank correlation coefficient (r_S)

$$r_S = \frac{\Sigma x^2 + \Sigma y^2 - \Sigma d^2}{2\sqrt{\Sigma x^2 \times \Sigma y^2}} = \frac{(277 + 268) - 209}{2\sqrt{(277 \times 268)}} = 0.62$$

A rank correlation coefficient of 0.62 indicates correlation between the two pain models.

Step 6   Determine the significance of the calculated Spearman rank correlation coefficient
As in other statistical methods, the conditions of the experimental design should be clarified:

- *State the null hypothesis.* The null hypothesis states that there is no relationship between the two pain models.

- *State the alternative hypothesis.* The alternative hypothesis states that there is a relationship between the two pain models.
- *State the level of significance.* In this example, it is assumed that the level of significance (α) is 0.05.
- *State the number of tails associated with the experimental design.* In this analysis it is assumed that if a correlation exists it will be positive, so, as only one outcome is specified, it is assumed that this analysis is one-tailed.
- *Perform the statistical analysis.* In this example, there are two possible methods by which the significance of the calculated Spearman rank correlation coefficient may be examined. These are addressed individually.

Small sample size

As the sample size is small (<30), the table of critical values of the Spearman rank correlation coefficient may be used to determine the significance of the calculated r_S value (Appendix 18). The critical r_S statistic associated with this experimental design is determined from this table with knowledge of the following parameters:

- $\alpha = 0.05$
- one-tailed design
- $N = 15$

In this example the critical r_S statistic ($N = 15$, one-tailed outcome, $\alpha = 0.05$) is approximately 0.44. If the calculated value of r_S is either greater than, or equal to this critical value, the null hypothesis is rejected in favour of the alternative hypothesis. As $r_{S \text{ calculated}}$ $(0.62) > r_{S \text{ critical}}$, the null hypothesis is rejected and it may be concluded that there is a significant association between the two pain models.

Large sample size

When the sample size is large (> 10 pairs of observations), the t distribution may be employed to statistically evaluate the significance of the calculated Spearman rank correlation coefficient. The t statistic is calculated using the following equation:

$$t = r_S \sqrt{\frac{(N-2)}{(1 - r_S^2)}}$$

where r_S is the calculated Spearman rank correlation coefficient and n is the number of pairs of data. The t statistic associated with this example is therefore:

$$t = r_S \sqrt{\frac{(N-2)}{1 - r_S^2}} = 0.61 \sqrt{\frac{(15-2)}{(1 - 0.61^2)}} = 2.78$$

To interpret the significance of this calculated t statistic, one must first identify the critical t statistic that relates to the experimental design from the critical values of the t distribution (Appendix 2). From this table the critical t statistic for a one-tailed outcome at a defined level of significance (0.05) and a defined number of degrees of freedom ($15 - 2 = 13$) is 1.77. The regions of acceptance and rejection of the null hypothesis may be defined with respect to this critical t statistic as $H_0 < 1.771$ and $H_a > 1.77$. Therefore, as the calculated t statistic (2.78) is greater than the critical t statistic (1.77), the null hypothesis is rejected in favour of the alternative hypothesis. It can be concluded that there is a strong relationship between the two pain models.

12.3 Conclusions

This chapter has concentrated on statistical methods that may be employed to examine and quantify the relationship between two variables, namely linear regression analysis and correlation analysis. The former is a statistical technique that is used to characterise the relationship between an independent variable and a dependent variable in terms of a straight line, termed the line of best fit. This mathematical relationship may then be used to predict the response of the dependent variable with knowledge of the magnitude of the independent variable. Inverse prediction and methods by which confidence intervals may be applied to linear regression have also been described.

In addition, this chapter described methods by which the strength of the relationship, i.e. the degree of association between two variables may be examined (correlation analysis). For this purpose, the theory and application of four methods were described, namely Pearson's product moment correlation coefficient, the contingency coefficient, the ϕ coefficient and Spearman's rank correlation coefficient. Pearson's product moment correlation coefficient is used to examine the correlation between two variables if the data are measured on an interval or ratio scale and derived from a bivariate normal population. The other statistical methods are used when the assumption of the normal distribution is invalid, and the choice of each individual test is largely dependent on the nature of the data associated with the variables. The contingency coefficient and the ϕ coefficient are employed to examine the correlation between variables that have been measured in a nominal scale within a contingency-table experimental design. These coefficients are calculated after the identification of dependence between the two variables by χ^2 analysis, i.e. after rejection of the null hypothesis. The ϕ coefficient is employed to determine the significance of the dependence between the two variables in a 2×2 design, whereas the contingency coefficient is used when the experimental design is more complex, e.g. 2×3, 3×3, etc.

Finally, the use of Spearman's rank correlation coefficient was described to examine the nature of the relationship between two variables in which the data have been measured on an ordinal (ranking) scale, or when one variable has been measured on an ordinal scale and the other on an interval or ratio scale. In all cases, statistical methods were described to quantify the relevance of the calculated correlation coefficients.

References

Draper N R, Smith H (1981). *Applied Regression Analysis*, 2nd edition. New York: Wiley.

Peppas N A (1985) Analysis of Fickian and non-Fickian drug release from polymers. *Acta Pharm Helv* 60(4): 110–11.

Appendix 1

Standardised normal distribution

z	$\phi(x)$	z	$\phi(x)$	z	$\phi(x)$	z	$\phi(x)$	z	$\phi(x)$	z	$\phi(x)$
0.00	0.5000	0.40	0.6554	0.80	0.7881	1.20	0.8849	1.60	0.9452	2.00	0.97725
0.01	0.5040	0.41	0.6591	0.81	0.7910	1.21	0.8869	1.61	0.9463	2.01	0.97778
0.02	0.5080	0.42	0.6628	0.82	0.7939	1.22	0.8888	1.62	0.9474	2.02	0.97831
0.03	0.5120	0.43	0.6664	0.83	0.7967	1.23	0.8907	1.63	0.9484	2.03	0.97882
0.04	0.5160	0.44	0.6700	0.84	0.7995	1.24	0.8925	1.64	0.9495	2.04	0.97932
0.05	0.5199	0.45	0.6736	0.85	0.8023	1.25	0.8944	1.65	0.9505	2.05	0.97982
0.06	0.5239	0.46	0.6772	0.86	0.8051	1.26	0.8962	1.66	0.9515	2.06	0.98030
0.07	0.5279	0.47	0.6808	0.87	0.8078	1.27	0.8980	1.67	0.9525	2.07	0.98077
0.08	0.5319	0.48	0.6844	0.88	0.8106	1.28	0.8997	1.68	0.9535	2.08	0.98124
0.09	0.5359	0.49	0.6879	0.89	0.8133	1.29	0.9015	1.69	0.9545	2.09	0.98169
0.10	0.5398	0.50	0.6915	0.90	0.8159	1.30	0.9032	1.70	0.9554	2.10	0.98214
0.11	0.5438	0.51	0.6950	0.91	0.8186	1.31	0.9049	1.71	0.9564	2.11	0.98257
0.12	0.5478	0.52	0.6985	0.92	0.8212	1.32	0.9066	1.72	0.9573	2.12	0.98300
0.13	0.5517	0.53	0.7019	0.93	0.8238	1.33	0.9082	1.73	0.9582	2.13	0.98341
0.14	0.5557	0.54	0.7054	0.94	0.8264	1.34	0.9099	1.74	0.9591	2.14	0.98382
0.15	0.5596	0.55	0.7088	0.95	0.8289	1.35	0.9115	1.75	0.9599	2.15	0.98422
0.16	0.5636	0.56	0.7123	0.96	0.8315	1.36	0.9131	1.76	0.9608	2.16	0.98461
0.17	0.5675	0.57	0.7157	0.97	0.8340	1.37	0.9147	1.77	0.9616	2.17	0.98500
0.18	0.5714	0.58	0.7190	0.98	0.8365	1.38	0.9162	1.78	0.9625	2.18	0.98537
0.19	0.5733	0.59	0.7224	0.99	0.8389	1.39	0.9177	1.79	0.9633	2.19	0.98574
0.20	0.5793	0.60	0.7257	1.00	0.8413	1.40	0.9192	1.80	0.9641	2.20	0.98610
0.21	0.5832	0.61	0.7291	1.01	0.8438	1.41	0.9207	1.81	0.9649	2.21	0.98645
0.22	0.5871	0.62	0.7234	1.02	0.8461	1.42	0.9222	1.82	0.9656	2.22	0.98679
0.23	0.5910	0.63	0.7357	1.03	0.8485	1.43	0.9236	1.83	0.9664	2.23	0.98713
0.24	0.5948	0.64	0.7389	1.04	0.8508	1.44	0.9251	1.84	0.9671	2.24	0.98745
0.25	0.5987	0.65	0.7422	1.05	0.8531	1.45	0.9265	1.85	0.9678	2.25	0.98778
0.26	0.6026	0.66	0.7454	1.06	0.8554	1.46	0.9279	1.86	0.9686	2.26	0.98809
0.27	0.6064	0.67	0.7486	1.07	0.8577	1.47	0.9292	1.87	0.9693	2.27	0.98840
0.28	0.6103	0.68	0.7517	1.08	0.8599	1.48	0.9306	1.88	0.9699	2.28	0.98870
0.29	0.6141	0.69	0.7549	1.09	0.8621	1.49	0.9319	1.89	0.9706	2.29	0.98899
0.30	0.6179	0.70	0.7580	1.10	0.8643	1.50	0.9332	1.90	0.9713	2.30	0.98928
0.31	0.6217	0.71	0.7611	1.11	0.8665	1.51	0.9345	1.91	0.9719	2.31	0.98956
0.32	0.6255	0.72	0.7642	1.12	0.8686	1.52	0.9357	1.92	0.9726	2.32	0.98983
0.33	0.6293	0.73	0.7673	1.13	0.8708	1.53	0.9370	1.93	0.9732	2.33	0.99010
0.34	0.6331	0.74	0.7704	1.14	0.8729	1.54	0.9382	1.94	0.9738	2.34	0.99036
0.35	0.6368	0.75	0.7734	1.15	0.8749	1.55	0.9394	1.95	0.9744	2.35	0.99061

z	$\phi(x)$	z	$\phi(x)$	z	$\phi(x)$	z	$\phi(x)$	z	$\phi(x)$	z	$\phi(x)$
0.36	0.6406	0.76	0.7764	1.16	0.8770	1.56	0.9406	1.96	0.9750	2.36	0.99086
0.37	0.6443	0.77	0.7794	1.17	0.8790	1.57	0.9418	1.97	0.9756	2.37	0.99111
0.38	0.6480	0.78	0.7823	1.18	0.8810	1.58	0.9429	1.98	0.9761	2.38	0.99134
0.39	0.6517	0.79	0.7852	1.19	0.8830	1.59	0.9441	1.99	0.9767	2.39	0.99158
0.40	0.6554	0.80	0.7881	1.20	0.8849	1.60	0.9452	2.00	0.9772	2.40	0.99180
2.40	0.99180	2.55	0.99461	2.70	0.99653	2.85	0.99781	3.00	0.99865	3.15	0.99918
2.41	0.99202	2.56	0.99477	2.71	0.99664	2.86	0.99788	3.01	0.99869	3.16	0.99921
2.42	0.99224	2.57	0.99492	2.72	0.99674	2.87	0.99795	3.02	0.99874	3.17	0.99924
2.43	0.99245	2.58	0.99506	2.73	0.99683	2.88	0.99801	3.03	0.99878	3.18	0.99926
2.44	0.99266	2.59	0.99520	2.74	0.99693	2.89	0.99807	3.04	0.99882	3.19	0.99929
2.45	0.99286	2.60	0.99534	2.75	0.99702	2.90	0.99813	3.05	0.99886	3.20	0.99931
2.46	0.99305	2.61	0.99547	2.76	0.99711	2.91	0.99819	3.06	0.99889	3.21	0.99934
2.47	0.99324	2.62	0.99560	2.77	0.99720	2.92	0.99825	3.07	0.99893	3.22	0.99936
2.48	0.99343	2.63	0.99573	2.78	0.99728	2.93	0.99831	3.08	0.99896	3.23	0.99938
2.49	0.99361	2.64	0.99585	2.79	0.99736	2.94	0.99836	3.09	0.99900	3.24	0.99940
2.50	0.99379	2.65	0.99598	2.80	0.99744	2.95	0.99841	3.10	0.99903	3.25	0.99942
2.51	0.99396	2.66	0.99609	2.81	0.99752	2.96	0.99846	3.11	0.99906	3.26	0.99944
2.52	0.99413	2.67	0.99621	2.82	0.99760	2.97	0.99851	3.12	0.99910	3.27	0.99946
2.53	0.99430	2.68	0.99632	2.83	0.99767	2.98	0.99856	3.13	0.99913	3.28	0.99948
2.54	0.99446	2.69	0.99643	2.84	0.99774	2.99	0.99861	3.14	0.99916	3.29	0.99950
2.55	0.99461	2.70	0.99653	2.85	0.99781	3.00	0.99865	3.15	0.99918	3.30	0.99952

The term $\phi(x)$ denotes the area under the standardised normal distribution from $-\infty$ to a particular z value (x axis).

Reproduced from Lindley D V, Scott W F, *New Cambridge Elementary Statistical Tables*, Cambridge: Cambridge University Press, 1984.

Appendix 2

Critical values of the *t* distribution

df	Two-tailed test			One-tailed test		
	α = 0.10	α = 0.05	α = 0.01	α = 0.10	α = 0.05	α = 0.01
1	6.314	12.706	63.657	3.078	6.314	31.821
2	2.920	4.303	9.925	1.886	2.920	6.965
3	2.353	3.182	5.841	1.638	2.353	4.541
4	2.132	2.776	4.604	1.533	2.132	3.747
5	2.015	2.571	4.032	1.476	2.015	3.365
6	1.943	2.447	3.707	1.440	1.943	3.143
7	1.895	2.365	3.499	1.415	1.895	2.998
8	1.860	2.306	3.355	1.397	1.860	2.896
9	1.833	2.262	3.250	1.383	1.833	2.821
10	1.812	2.228	3.169	1.372	1.812	2.764
11	1.796	2.201	3.106	1.363	1.796	2.718
12	1.782	2.179	3.055	1.356	1.782	2.681
13	1.771	2.160	3.012	1.350	1.771	2.650
14	1.761	2.145	2.977	1.345	1.761	2.624
15	1.753	2.131	2.947	1.341	1.753	2.602
16	1.746	2.120	2.921	1.337	1.746	2.583
17	1.740	2.110	2.898	1.333	1.740	2.567
18	1.734	2.101	2.878	1.330	1.734	2.552
19	1.729	2.093	2.861	1.328	1.729	2.539
20	1.725	2.086	2.845	1.325	1.725	2.528
21	1.721	2.080	2.831	1.323	1.721	2.518
22	1.717	2.074	2.819	1.321	1.717	2.508
23	1.714	2.069	2.807	1.319	1.714	2.500
24	1.711	2.064	2.797	1.318	1.711	2.492
25	1.708	2.060	2.787	1.316	1.708	2.485
26	1.706	2.056	2.779	1.315	1.706	2.479
27	1.703	2.052	2.771	1.314	1.703	2.473
28	1.701	2.048	2.763	1.313	1.701	2.467
29	1.699	2.045	2.756	1.311	1.699	2.462
30	1.697	2.042	2.750	1.310	1.697	2.457
40	1.684	2.021	2.704	1.303	1.684	2.423
60	1.671	2.000	2.660	1.296	1.671	2.390
120	1.658	1.980	2.617	1.289	1.658	2.358
∞	1.645	1.960	2.576	1.282	1.645	2.326

α denotes the level of significance and df the number of degrees of freedom.
Adapted from Murdoch J, Barnes J A, *Statistical Tables for Students of Science, Engineering, Psychology, Business, Management and Finance*, 4th edition, Basingstoke: Macmillan, 1998.

Appendix 3

Critical values of the χ^2 distribution

df	$\alpha = 0.10$	$\alpha = 0.05$	$\alpha = 0.01$
1	2.706	3.841	6.635
2	4.605	5.991	9.210
3	6.251	7.815	11.345
4	7.779	9.488	13.277
5	9.236	11.070	15.086
6	10.645	12.592	16.812
7	12.017	14.067	18.475
8	13.362	15.507	20.090
9	14.684	16.919	21.666
10	15.987	18.307	23.209
11	17.275	19.675	24.725
12	18.549	21.026	26.217
13	19.812	22.362	27.688
14	21.064	23.685	29.141
15	22.307	24.996	30.578
16	23.542	26.296	32.000
17	24.769	27.587	33.409
18	25.989	28.869	34.805
19	27.204	30.144	36.191
20	28.412	31.410	37.566
21	29.615	32.671	38.932
22	30.813	33.924	40.289
23	32.007	35.172	41.638
24	33.196	36.415	42.980
25	34.382	37.652	44.314
26	35.563	38.885	45.642
27	36.741	40.113	46.963
28	37.916	41.337	48.278
29	39.087	42.557	49.588
30	40.256	43.773	50.892
40	51.805	55.759	63.691
50	63.167	67.505	76.154
60	74.397	79.082	88.379
70	85.527	90.531	100.425
80	96.578	101.880	112.329
90	107.565	113.145	124.116
100	118.498	124.342	135.807

α denotes the level of significance and df the number of degrees of freedom.

Modified from Murdoch J, Barnes J A, *Statistical Tables for Students of Science, Engineering, Psychology, Business, Management and Finance*, 4th edition, Basingstoke: Macmillan Press, 1998.

Appendix 4

Probabilities associated with the binomial distribution

N	X = 0	1	2	3	4	5	6	7	8	9	10	11	12	13
2	0.250	0.750	–	–	–	–	–	–	–	–	–	–	–	–
3	0.125	0.500	0.875	–	–	–	–	–	–	–	–	–	–	–
4	0.0625	0.3125	0.6875	0.9375	–	–	–	–	–	–	–	–	–	–
5	0.0313	0.1875	0.5000	0.8125	0.9688	–	–	–	–	–	–	–	–	–
6	0.0156	0.1094	0.3438	0.6562	0.8906	0.9844	–	–	–	–	–	–	–	–
7	0.0078	0.0625	0.2266	0.5000	0.7734	0.9375	0.9922	–	–	–	–	–	–	–
8	0.0039	0.0352	0.1445	0.3633	0.6367	0.8555	0.9648	0.9961	–	–	–	–	–	–
9	0.0020	0.0195	0.0898	0.2539	0.5000	0.7461	0.9102	0.9805	0.9980	–	–	–	–	–
10	0.001	0.0107	0.0547	0.1719	0.3770	0.6230	0.8281	0.9453	0.9893	0.9990	–	–	–	–
11	0.0005	0.0059	0.0327	0.1133	0.2744	0.5000	0.7256	0.8867	0.9673	0.9941	0.9995	–	–	–
12	0.0002	0.0032	0.0193	0.0730	0.1938	0.3872	0.6128	0.8062	0.9270	0.9807	0.9968	0.9998	–	–
13	0.0001	0.0017	0.0112	0.0461	0.1334	0.2905	0.5000	0.7095	0.8666	0.9539	0.9888	0.9983	0.999	–
14	0.0001	0.0009	0.0065	0.0287	0.0898	0.2120	0.3953	0.6047	0.7880	0.9102	0.9713	0.9935	0.9991	0.9999
15	–	0.0005	0.0037	0.0176	0.0592	0.1509	0.3036	0.5000	0.6964	0.8491	0.9408	0.9824	0.9963	0.9995

N denotes the total number of independent observations and X the number of successes.

Modified from Lindley D V, Scott W F, *New Cambridge Elementary Statistical Tables*, 2nd edn. Cambridge: Cambridge University Press, 1995.

Appendix 5

Critical values in the Kolmogorov–Smirnov one-sample test

$\alpha = 0.05$

k	N	D_{crit}	k	N	D_{crit}
3	3	3	4	44	8
3	6	3	4	48	8
3	9	4	4	52	9
3	12	4	4	56	9
3	15	5	4	60	9
3	18	5	4	64	9
3	21	6	4	68	10
3	24	6	4	72	10
3	27	6	4	76	10
3	30	7	4	80	10
3	33	7	4	84	10
3	35	7	4	88	10
3	39	7	4	92	10
3	42	8	4	96	10
3	45	8	4	100	11
3	48	8	5	5	3
3	51	8	5	10	4
3	54	9	5	15	5
3	57	9	5	20	6
3	60	9	5	25	6
3	63	9	5	30	7
3	66	9	5	35	7
3	69	9	5	40	8
3	72	9	5	45	8
3	75	10	5	50	9
3	78	10	5	55	9
3	81	10	5	60	9
3	84	10	5	65	10
3	87	10	5	70	10
3	90	10	5	75	10
3	93	10	5	80	11
3	95	10	5	85	11

k	N	D_{crit}	k	N	D_{crit}
3	99	10	5	90	11
4	4	3	5	95	11
4	8	4	5	100	11
4	12	5	6	6	4
4	15	5	6	12	5
4	20	6	6	18	6
4	24	6	6	24	6
4	28	7	6	30	7
4	32	7	6	36	8
4	36	7	6	42	8
4	40	8	6	48	9

α denotes the level of significance, D_{crit} the critical value of the Kolmogorov–Smirnov statistic, k the number of categories and N the number of samples.
Adapted from Zar J H, *Biostatistical Analysis*, 3rd edition, Englewood Cliffs, NJ: Prentice-Hall International, 1984.

Appendix 6

Critical difference in the fractional observed and fractional expected frequencies in the Kolmogorov–Smirnov one-sample test

	α	
N	0.05	0.01
1	0.975	0.995
2	0.842	0.929
3	0.708	0.828
4	0.624	0.733
5	0.565	0.669
6	0.521	0.618
7	0.486	0.577
8	0.457	0.543
9	0.432	0.514
10	0.410	0.490
11	0.391	0.468
12	0.375	0.450
13	0.361	0.433
14	0.349	0.418
15	0.338	0.404
16	0.328	0.392
17	0.318	0.381
18	0.309	0.371
19	0.301	0.363
20	0.294	0.356
25	0.270	0.320
30	0.240	0.290
35	0.230	0.270

α denotes the level of significance associated with the difference between the fractional observed and fractional expected frequencies, and N denotes the sample size.
Modified from Massey F J, The Kolmogorov–Smirnov test for goodness of fit, *J Amer Statist Assoc*, 1951; 46: 68–78.

Appendix 7

Critical values of the F distribution

$\alpha = 0.05$

df_2	df_1 1	2	3	4	5	6	7	8	10	12	24	∞
1	161.4	199.5	215.7	224.6	230.2	234.0	236.8	238.9	241.9	243.9	249.0	254.3
2	18.5	19.0	19.2	19.2	19.3	19.3	19.4	19.4	19.4	19.4	19.5	19.5
3	10.13	9.55	9.28	9.12	9.01	8.94	8.89	8.85	8.79	8.74	8.64	8.53
4	7.71	6.94	6.59	6.39	6.26	6.16	6.09	6.04	5.96	5.91	5.77	5.63
5	6.61	5.79	5.41	5.19	5.05	4.95	4.88	4.82	4.74	4.68	4.53	4.36
6	5.99	5.14	4.76	4.53	4.39	4.28	4.21	4.15	4.06	4.00	3.84	3.67
7	5.59	4.74	4.35	4.12	3.97	3.87	3.79	3.73	3.64	3.57	3.41	3.23
8	5.32	4.46	4.07	3.84	3.69	3.58	3.50	3.44	3.35	3.28	3.12	2.93
9	5.12	4.26	3.86	3.63	3.48	3.37	3.29	3.23	3.14	3.07	2.90	2.71
10	4.96	4.10	3.71	3.48	3.33	3.22	3.14	3.07	2.98	2.91	2.74	2.54
11	4.84	3.98	3.59	3.36	3.20	3.09	3.01	2.95	2.85	2.79	2.61	2.40
12	4.75	3.89	3.49	3.26	3.11	3.00	2.91	2.85	2.75	2.69	2.51	2.30
13	4.67	3.81	3.41	3.18	3.03	2.92	2.83	2.77	2.67	2.60	2.42	2.21
14	4.60	3.74	3.34	3.11	2.96	2.85	2.76	2.70	2.60	2.53	2.35	2.13
16	4.49	3.63	3.24	3.01	2.85	2.74	2.66	2.59	2.49	2.42	2.24	2.01
18	4.41	3.55	3.16	2.93	2.77	2.66	2.58	2.51	2.41	2.34	2.15	1.92
20	4.35	3.49	3.10	2.87	2.71	2.60	2.51	2.45	2.35	2.28	2.08	1.84
22	4.30	3.44	3.05	2.82	2.66	2.55	2.46	2.40	2.30	2.23	2.03	1.78
24	4.26	3.40	3.01	2.78	2.62	2.51	2.42	2.36	2.25	2.18	1.98	1.73
26	4.23	3.37	2.98	2.74	2.59	2.47	2.39	2.32	2.22	2.15	1.95	1.69
28	4.20	3.34	2.95	2.71	2.56	2.45	2.36	2.29	2.19	2.12	1.91	1.65
30	4.17	3.32	2.92	2.69	2.53	2.42	2.33	2.27	2.16	2.09	1.89	1.62
40	4.08	3.23	2.84	2.61	2.45	2.34	2.25	2.18	2.08	2.00	1.79	1.51
60	4.00	3.15	2.76	2.53	2.37	2.25	2.17	2.10	1.99	1.92	1.70	1.39
120	3.92	3.07	2.68	2.45	2.29	2.18	2.09	2.02	1.91	1.83	1.61	1.25
∞	3.84	3.00	2.60	2.37	2.21	2.10	2.01	1.94	1.83	1.75	1.52	1.00

α denotes the level of significance, df_1 the degrees of freedom in the numerator and df_2 the degrees of freedom in the denominator.

Modified from Murdoch J, Barnes J A, *Statistical Tables for Students of Science, Engineering, Psychology, Business, Management and Finance*, 4th edition, Basingstoke: Macmillan, 1998.

Appendix 8

Critical values of the Mann–Whitney U statistic

$\alpha = 0.05$ for a two-tailed test or 0.10 for a one-tailed test

N_1 \ N_2	1	2	3	4	5	6	7	8	9	10	11	12	13	14	15	16	17	18	19	20
1	—	—	—	—	—	—	—	—	—	—	—	—	—	—	—	—	—	—	—	—
2	—	—	—	—	—	—	—	0	0	0	0	1	1	1	1	1	2	2	2	2
3	—	—	—	—	0	1	1	2	2	3	3	4	4	5	5	6	6	7	7	8
4	—	—	—	0	1	2	3	4	4	5	6	7	8	9	10	11	11	12	13	13
5	—	—	0	1	2	3	5	6	7	8	9	11	12	13	14	15	17	18	19	20
6	—	—	1	2	3	5	6	8	10	11	13	14	16	17	19	21	22	24	25	27
7	—	—	1	3	5	6	8	10	12	14	16	18	20	22	24	26	28	30	32	34
8	—	0	2	4	6	8	10	13	15	17	19	22	24	26	29	31	34	36	38	41
9	—	0	2	4	7	10	12	15	17	20	23	26	28	31	34	37	39	42	45	48
10	—	0	3	5	8	11	14	17	20	23	26	29	33	36	39	42	45	48	52	55
11	—	0	3	6	9	13	16	19	23	26	30	33	37	40	44	47	51	55	58	62
12	—	1	4	7	11	14	18	22	26	29	33	37	41	45	49	53	57	61	65	69
13	—	1	4	8	12	16	20	24	28	33	37	41	45	50	54	59	63	67	72	76
14	—	1	5	9	13	17	22	26	31	36	40	45	50	55	59	64	67	74	78	83
15	—	1	5	10	14	19	24	29	34	39	44	49	54	59	64	70	75	80	85	90
16	—	1	6	11	15	21	26	31	37	42	47	53	59	64	70	75	81	86	92	98
17	—	2	6	11	17	22	28	34	39	45	51	57	63	67	75	81	87	93	99	105
18	—	2	7	12	18	24	30	36	42	48	55	61	67	74	80	86	93	99	106	112
19	—	2	7	13	19	25	32	38	45	52	58	65	72	78	85	92	99	106	113	119
20	—	2	8	13	20	27	34	41	48	55	62	69	76	83	90	98	105	112	119	127

α denotes the level of significance, N_1 the number of observations in group 1 and N_2 the number of observations in group 2. Modified from the Bulletin of the Institute of Educational Research at Indiana University 1, No. 2.

Appendix 9

Probabilities associated with values as small as observed values of U in the Mann–Whitney test

$N_2 = 3$

U	N_1		
	1	2	3
0	0.250	0.100	0.050
1	0.500	0.200	0.100
2	0.750	0.400	0.200
3	–	0.600	0.350
4	–	–	0.500
5	–	–	0.650

$N_2 = 4$

U	N_1			
	1	2	3	4
0	0.200	0.067	0.028	0.014
1	0.400	0.133	0.057	0.029
2	0.600	0.267	0.114	0.057
3	–	0.400	0.200	0.100
4	–	0.600	0.314	0.171
5	–	–	0.429	0.243
6	–	–	0.571	0.343
7	–	–	–	0.443
8	–	–	–	0.557

$N_2 = 5$

U	N_1				
	1	2	3	4	5
0	0.167	0.047	0.018	0.008	0.004
1	0.333	0.095	0.036	0.016	0.008
2	0.500	0.190	0.071	0.032	0.016
3	0.667	0.286	0.125	0.056	0.028
4	–	0.429	0.196	0.095	0.048
5	–	0.571	0.286	0.143	0.075
6	–	–	0.393	0.206	0.111
7	–	–	0.500	0.278	0.155
8	–	–	0.607	0.365	0.210
9	–	–	–	0.452	0.274
10	–	–	–	0.548	0.345
11	–	–	–	–	0.421
12	–	–	–	–	0.500
13	–	–	–	–	0.579

$N_2 = 6$

U	N_1					
	1	2	3	4	5	6
0	0.143	0.036	0.012	0.005	0.002	0.001
1	0.286	0.071	0.024	0.010	0.004	0.002
2	0.428	0.143	0.048	0.019	0.009	0.004
3	0.571	0.214	0.083	0.033	0.015	0.008
4	–	0.321	0.131	0.057	0.026	0.013
5	–	0.429	0.190	0.086	0.041	0.021
6	–	0.571	0.274	0.129	0.063	0.032
7	–	–	0.357	0.176	0.089	0.047
8	–	–	0.452	0.238	0.123	0.066
9	–	–	0.548	0.305	0.165	0.090
10	–	–	–	0.381	0.214	0.120
11	–	–	–	0.457	0.268	0.155
12	–	–	–	0.545	0.331	0.197
13	–	–	–	–	0.396	0.242
14	–	–	–	–	0.465	0.294
15	–	–	–	–	0.535	0.350
16	–	–	–	–	–	0.409
17	–	–	–	–	–	0.469
18	–	–	–	–	–	0.531

N_1 and N_2 denote the sample sizes.
Reproduced from Siegel S, *Non-Parametric Statistics for the Behavioral Sciences*, New York: McGraw-Hill, 1956.

Appendix 10

Critical values of the Wilcoxon
signed-rank statistic (T)

One-tailed test

N	$\alpha = 0.05$	$\alpha = 0.01$	N	$\alpha = 0.05$	$\alpha = 0.01$
5	0	–	28	130	101
6	2	–	29	140	110
7	3	0	30	151	120
8	5	1	31	163	130
9	8	3	32	175	140
10	10	5	33	187	151
11	13	7	34	200	162
12	17	9	35	213	173
13	21	12	36	227	185
14	25	15	37	241	198
15	30	19	38	256	211
16	35	23	39	271	224
17	41	27	40	286	238
18	47	32	41	302	252
19	53	37	42	319	266
20	60	43	43	336	281
21	67	49	44	353	296
22	75	55	45	371	312
23	83	62	46	389	328
24	91	69	47	407	345
25	100	76	48	426	362
26	110	84	49	446	379
27	119	92	50	466	397

Two-tailed test

N	$\alpha = 0.05$	$\alpha = 0.01$	N	$\alpha = 0.05$	$\alpha = 0.01$
5	–	–	28	116	91
6	0	–	29	126	100
7	2	–	30	137	109
8	3	0	31	147	118
9	5	1	32	159	128
10	8	3	33	170	138
11	10	5	34	182	148
12	13	7	35	195	159
13	17	9	36	208	171
14	21	12	37	221	182
15	25	15	38	235	194
16	29	19	39	249	207
17	34	23	40	264	220
18	40	27	41	279	233
19	46	32	42	294	247
20	52	37	43	310	261
21	58	42	44	327	276
22	65	48	45	343	291
23	73	54	46	361	307
24	81	61	47	378	322
25	89	68	48	396	339
26	98	75	49	415	355
27	107	83	50	434	373

α denotes the level of significance and N the sample size.
Modified from Lindley D V, Scott W F, *New Cambridge Elementary Statistical Tables*, 2nd edn. Cambridge: Cambridge University Press, 1995.

Appendix 11

Critical values of the F_{max} test

$\alpha = 0.05$

$N-1$	k										
	2	3	4	5	6	7	8	9	10	11	12
4	9.60	15.50	20.60	25.20	29.50	33.60	37.50	41.40	44.60	48.00	51.40
5	7.15	10.80	13.70	16.30	18.70	20.80	22.90	24.70	26.50	28.20	29.90
6	5.82	8.38	10.40	12.10	13.70	15.00	16.30	17.50	18.60	19.70	20.70
7	4.99	6.94	8.44	9.70	10.80	11.80	12.70	13.50	14.30	15.10	15.80
8	4.43	6.00	7.18	8.12	9.03	9.78	10.50	11.10	11.70	12.20	12.70
9	4.03	5.34	6.31	7.11	7.80	8.41	8.95	9.45	9.91	10.30	10.70
10	3.72	4.85	5.67	6.34	6.92	7.42	7.87	8.28	8.66	9.01	9.34
12	3.28	4.16	4.79	5.30	5.72	6.09	6.42	6.72	7.00	7.25	7.48
15	2.86	3.54	4.01	4.37	4.68	4.95	5.19	5.40	5.59	5.77	5.93
20	2.46	2.95	3.29	3.54	3.76	3.94	4.10	4.24	4.37	4.49	4.59
30	2.07	2.40	2.61	2.78	2.91	3.02	3.12	3.21	3.29	3.36	3.39
60	1.67	1.85	1.96	2.04	2.11	2.17	2.22	2.26	2.30	2.33	2.36

α denotes the level of significance, k the number of samples in the study and N the number of observations in each column or treatment.

Adapted from Pearson E, Hartley H, *Biometrika Tables for Statisticians*, Volume 1, 3rd edition, Cambridge: Cambridge University Press, 1966.

Appendix 12

Critical values of the studentised range statistic (q)

$\alpha = 0.05$

df	k										
	2	3	4	5	6	7	8	9	10	11	12
1	18.00	27.00	32.80	37.10	40.40	43.10	45.40	47.40	49.10	50.60	52.00
2	6.09	8.30	9.80	10.90	11.70	12.40	13.00	13.50	14.00	14.40	14.70
3	4.50	5.91	6.82	7.50	8.04	8.48	8.85	9.18	9.46	9.72	9.95
4	3.93	5.04	5.76	6.29	6.71	7.05	7.35	7.60	7.83	8.03	8.21
5	3.64	4.60	5.22	5.67	6.03	6.33	6.58	6.80	6.99	7.17	7.32
6	3.46	4.34	4.90	5.31	5.63	5.89	6.12	6.32	6.49	6.65	6.79
7	3.34	4.16	4.69	5.06	5.36	5.61	5.82	6.00	6.16	6.30	6.43
8	3.26	4.04	4.53	4.89	5.17	5.40	5.60	5.77	5.92	6.05	6.18
9	3.20	3.95	4.42	4.76	5.02	5.24	5.43	5.60	5.74	5.87	5.98
10	3.15	3.88	4.33	4.65	4.91	5.12	5.30	5.46	5.60	5.72	5.83
11	3.11	3.82	4.26	4.57	4.82	5.03	5.20	5.35	5.49	5.61	5.71
12	3.08	3.77	4.20	4.51	4.75	4.95	5.12	5.27	5.40	5.51	5.62
13	3.06	3.73	4.15	4.45	4.69	4.88	5.05	5.19	5.32	5.43	5.53
14	3.03	3.70	4.11	4.41	4.64	4.83	4.99	5.13	5.25	5.36	5.46
16	3.00	3.65	4.05	4.33	4.56	4.74	4.90	5.03	5.15	5.26	5.35
18	2.97	3.61	4.00	4.28	4.49	4.67	4.82	4.96	5.07	5.17	5.27
20	2.95	3.58	3.96	4.23	4.45	4.62	4.77	4.90	5.01	5.11	5.20
24	2.92	3.53	3.90	4.17	4.37	4.54	4.68	4.81	4.92	5.01	5.10
30	2.89	3.49	3.84	4.10	4.30	4.46	4.60	4.72	4.83	4.92	5.00
40	2.86	3.44	3.79	4.04	4.23	4.39	4.52	6.43	4.74	4.82	4.91
60	2.83	3.40	3.74	3.98	4.16	4.31	4.44	4.55	4.65	4.73	4.81
120	2.80	3.36	3.69	3.92	4.10	4.24	4.36	4.48	4.56	4.64	4.72
∞	2.77	3.31	3.63	3.86	4.03	4.17	4.29	4.39	4.47	4.55	4.62

α denotes the level of significance, df the degrees of freedom within groups (degrees of freedom in denominator of F ratio) and k the number of means being compared.
Modified from Winer W J, *Statistical Principles in Experimental Design*, New York: McGraw-Hill, 1962.

Appendix 13

Critical values of Dunnett's statistic (t_d)

$\alpha = 0.05$

df_e	k								
	2	3	4	5	6	7	8	9	10
5	2.57	3.03	3.29	3.48	3.62	3.73	3.82	3.90	3.97
6	2.45	2.86	3.10	3.26	3.39	3.49	3.57	3.64	3.71
7	2.36	2.75	2.97	3.12	3.24	3.33	3.41	3.47	3.53
8	2.31	2.67	2.88	3.02	3.13	3.22	3.29	3.35	3.41
9	2.26	2.61	2.81	2.95	3.05	3.14	3.20	3.26	3.32
10	2.23	2.57	2.76	2.89	2.99	3.07	3.14	3.19	3.24
11	2.20	2.53	2.72	2.84	2.94	3.02	3.08	3.14	3.19
12	2.18	2.50	2.68	2.81	2.90	2.98	3.04	3.09	3.14
13	2.16	2.48	2.65	2.78	2.87	2.94	3.00	3.06	3.10
14	2.14	2.46	2.63	2.75	2.84	2.91	2.97	3.02	3.07
15	2.13	2.44	2.61	2.73	2.82	2.89	2.95	3.00	3.04
16	2.12	2.42	2.59	2.71	2.80	2.87	2.92	2.97	3.02
17	2.11	2.41	2.58	2.69	2.78	2.85	2.90	2.95	3.00
18	2.10	2.40	2.56	2.68	2.76	2.83	2.89	2.94	2.98
19	2.09	2.39	2.55	2.66	2.75	2.81	2.87	2.92	2.96
20	2.09	2.38	2.54	2.65	2.73	2.80	2.86	2.90	2.95
24	2.06	2.35	2.51	2.61	2.70	2.76	2.81	2.86	2.90
30	2.04	2.32	2.47	2.58	2.66	2.72	2.77	2.82	2.86
40	2.02	2.29	2.44	2.54	2.62	2.68	2.73	2.77	2.81
60	2.00	2.27	2.41	2.51	2.58	2.64	2.69	2.73	2.77
120	1.98	2.24	2.28	2.47	2.55	2.60	2.65	2.69	2.73
∞	1.96	2.21	2.35	2.44	2.51	2.57	2.61	2.65	2.69

df_e denotes the error degrees of freedom and k denotes the number of treatments.
Modified from Dunnett C W, New tables for multiple comparisons with a control, *Biometrics*, 1964; 20: 482–91

Appendix 14

Critical values of the non-central F distribution

$\alpha = 0.05$, $df_1 = 1$

df_e	φ									
	0.50	1.0	1.2	1.4	1.6	1.8	2.0	2.2	2.6	3.0
2	0.93	0.86	0.83	0.78	0.74	0.69	0.64	0.59	0.49	0.40
4	0.91	0.80	0.74	0.67	0.59	0.51	0.43	0.35	0.22	0.12
6	0.91	0.78	0.70	0.62	0.52	0.43	0.34	0.26	0.14	0.06
8	0.90	0.76	0.68	0.59	0.49	0.39	0.30	0.22	0.11	0.04
10	0.90	0.75	0.66	0.57	0.47	0.37	0.28	0.20	0.09	0.03
12	0.90	0.74	0.65	0.56	0.45	0.35	0.26	0.19	0.08	0.03
16	0.90	0.74	0.64	0.54	0.43	0.33	0.24	0.17	0.07	0.02
20	0.90	0.73	0.63	0.53	0.42	0.32	0.23	0.16	0.06	0.02
30	0.89	0.72	0.62	0.52	0.40	0.31	0.22	0.15	0.06	0.02
∞	0.89	0.71	0.60	0.49	0.38	0.28	0.19	0.12	0.04	0.01

$\alpha = 0.05$, $df_1 = 2$

df_e	φ									
	0.50	1.0	1.2	1.4	1.6	1.8	2.0	2.2	2.6	3.0
2	0.93	0.88	0.85	0.82	0.78	0.75	0.70	0.66	0.56	0.48
4	0.92	0.82	0.77	0.70	0.62	0.54	0.46	0.38	0.24	0.14
6	0.91	0.79	0.71	0.63	0.53	0.43	0.34	0.26	0.13	0.05
8	0.91	0.77	0.68	0.58	0.48	0.37	0.28	0.20	0.08	0.03
10	0.91	0.75	0.66	0.55	0.44	0.34	0.24	0.16	0.06	0.02
12	0.90	0.74	0.64	0.53	0.42	0.31	0.22	0.14	0.05	0.01
16	0.90	0.73	0.62	0.51	0.39	0.28	0.19	0.12	0.04	0.01
20	0.90	0.72	0.61	0.49	0.36	0.26	0.17	0.11	0.03	0.01
30	0.90	0.71	0.59	0.47	0.35	0.24	0.15	0.09	0.02	0.00
∞	0.89	0.68	0.56	0.43	0.30	0.20	0.12	0.06	0.01	0.00

$a = 0.05, df_1 = 3$

df_e	φ									
	0.50	1.0	1.2	1.4	1.6	1.8	2.0	2.2	2.6	3.0
2	0.93	0.89	0.86	0.83	0.80	0.76	0.73	0.69	0.60	0.52
4	0.92	0.83	0.77	0.71	0.63	0.55	0.47	0.39	0.25	0.14
6	0.91	0.79	0.71	0.62	0.52	0.42	0.33	0.24	0.11	0.04
8	0.91	0.76	0.67	0.57	0.46	0.35	0.25	0.17	0.06	0.02
10	0.91	0.75	0.65	0.53	0.41	0.30	0.21	0.13	0.04	0.01
12	0.90	0.73	0.62	0.50	0.38	0.27	0.18	0.11	0.03	0.01
16	0.90	0.71	0.60	0.47	0.34	0.23	0.14	0.08	0.02	0.00
20	0.90	0.70	0.58	0.45	0.32	0.21	0.13	0.07	0.01	0.00
30	0.89	0.68	0.55	0.42	0.29	0.18	0.10	0.05	0.01	0.00
∞	0.88	0.64	0.50	0.36	0.23	0.13	0.07	0.03	0.00	0.00

$a = 0.05, df_1 = 4$

df_e	φ									
	0.50	1.0	1.2	1.4	1.6	1.8	2.0	2.2	2.6	3.0
2	0.94	0.89	0.87	0.84	0.81	0.77	0.74	0.70	0.62	0.54
4	0.92	0.83	0.78	0.71	0.64	0.55	0.47	0.39	0.25	0.14
6	0.92	0.79	0.71	0.62	0.52	0.41	0.31	0.23	0.10	0.04
8	0.91	0.76	0.66	0.55	0.44	0.33	0.23	0.15	0.05	0.01
10	0.91	0.74	0.63	0.51	0.39	0.27	0.18	0.11	0.03	0.01
12	0.90	0.72	0.61	0.48	0.35	0.24	0.15	0.08	0.02	0.00
16	0.90	0.70	0.57	0.44	0.31	0.19	0.11	0.06	0.01	0.00
20	0.89	0.68	0.55	0.41	0.28	0.17	0.09	0.04	0.01	0.00
30	0.89	0.66	0.52	0.37	0.24	0.14	0.07	0.03	0.00	0.00
∞	0.88	0.60	0.45	0.29	0.17	0.08	0.04	0.01	0.00	0.00

Power = 1 − (table entry).
a denotes the level of signficance and df_e the error degrees of freedom.
Modified from Tiku M L, Tables of the power of the F test, J Amer Statist Assoc, 1967; 62: 525–39.

Appendix 15

Critical values of the Kruskal–Wallis statistic (H)

Three treatment groups; $\alpha = 0.05$

Number of observations in each group			
N_1	N_2	N_3	H_{crit}
2	2	2	–
3	2	1	–
3	2	2	4.714
3	3	1	5.143
3	3	2	5.361
3	3	3	5.600
4	2	1	–
4	2	2	5.333
4	3	1	5.208
4	3	2	5.444
4	3	3	5.791
4	4	1	4.967
4	4	2	5.455
4	4	3	5.598
4	4	4	5.692
5	2	1	5.000
5	2	2	5.160
5	3	1	4.960
5	3	2	5.251
5	3	3	5.648
5	4	1	4.985
5	4	2	5.273
5	4	3	5.656
5	4	4	5.657
5	5	1	5.127
5	5	2	5.338
5	5	3	5.705
5	5	4	5.666
5	5	5	5.780
6	2	1	4.822
6	2	2	5.345

N_1	N_2	N_3	H_{crit}
6	3	1	4.855
6	3	2	5.348
6	3	3	5.615
6	4	1	4.947
6	4	2	5.340
6	4	3	5.610
6	4	4	5.681
6	5	1	4.990
6	5	2	5.338
6	5	3	5.602
6	5	4	5.661
6	5	5	5.729
6	6	1	4.945
6	6	2	5.410
6	6	3	5.625
6	6	4	5.724
6	6	5	5.765
6	6	6	5.801
7	1	1	–
7	2	1	4.706
7	2	2	5.143
7	3	1	4.952
7	3	2	5.357
7	3	3	5.620
7	4	1	4.986
7	4	2	5.376
7	4	3	5.623
7	4	4	5.650
7	5	1	5.064
7	5	2	5.393
7	5	3	5.607
7	5	4	5.733
7	5	5	5.708
7	6	1	5.067
7	6	2	5.357
7	6	3	5.689
7	6	4	5.706
7	6	5	5.770
7	6	6	5.730
7	7	1	4.986
7	7	2	5.398
7	7	3	5.688
7	7	4	5.766
7	7	5	5.746

N_1	N_2	N_3	H_{crit}
7	7	6	5.793
7	7	7	5.818
8	1	1	–
8	2	1	4.909
8	2	2	5.356
8	3	1	4.881
8	3	2	5.316
8	3	3	5.617
8	4	1	5.044
8	4	2	5.393
8	4	3	5.623
8	4	4	5.779
8	5	1	4.869
8	5	2	5.415
8	5	3	5.614
8	5	4	5.718
8	5	5	5.769
8	6	1	5.015
8	6	2	5.404
8	6	3	5.678
8	6	4	5.743
8	6	5	5.750
8	6	6	5.770
8	7	1	5.041
8	7	2	5.403
8	7	3	5.698
8	7	4	5.759
8	7	5	5.782
8	7	6	5.781
8	7	7	5.802
8	8	1	5.039
8	8	2	5.408
8	8	3	5.734
8	8	4	5.743
8	8	5	5.761
8	8	6	5.779
8	8	7	5.791
8	8	8	5.805
9	9	9	5.845
∞	∞	∞	5.991

Four treatment groups; $\alpha = 0.05$

Number of observations in each group

N_1	N_2	N_3	N_4	H_{crit}
2	2	2	1	5.679
2	2	2	2	6.167
3	2	1	1	–
3	2	2	1	5.833
3	2	2	2	6.333
3	3	1	1	6.333
3	3	2	1	6.244
3	3	2	2	6.527
3	3	3	1	6.600
3	3	3	2	6.727
3	3	3	3	7.000
4	2	1	1	5.833
4	2	2	1	6.133
4	2	2	2	6.545
4	3	1	1	6.178
4	3	2	1	6.309
4	3	2	2	6.621
4	3	3	1	6.545
4	3	3	2	6.795
4	3	3	3	6.984
4	4	1	1	5.945
4	4	2	1	6.386
4	4	2	2	6.731
4	4	3	1	6.635
4	4	3	2	6.874
4	4	3	3	7.038
4	4	4	1	6.725
4	4	4	2	6.957
4	4	4	3	7.142
4	4	4	4	7.235
∞	∞	∞	∞	7.815

Five treatment groups; $\alpha = 0.05$

Number of observations in each group

N_1	N_2	N_3	N_4	N_5	H_{crit}
2	2	1	1	1	–
2	2	2	1	1	6.750
2	2	2	2	1	7.133
2	2	2	2	2	7.418
3	2	1	1	1	6.583
3	2	2	1	1	6.800
3	2	2	2	1	7.309
3	2	2	2	2	7.682
3	3	1	1	1	7.111
3	3	2	1	1	7.200
3	3	2	2	1	7.591
3	3	2	2	2	7.910
3	3	3	1	1	7.576
3	3	3	2	1	7.769
3	3	3	2	2	8.044
3	3	3	3	1	8.000
3	3	3	3	2	8.200
3	3	3	3	3	8.333
∞	∞	∞	∞	∞	9.488

Six treatment groups; $\alpha = 0.05$

Number of observations in each group

N_1	N_2	N_3	N_4	N_5	N_6	H_{crit}
2	2	1	1	1	1	–
2	2	2	1	1	1	7.600
2	2	2	2	1	1	8.018
2	2	2	2	2	1	8.455
2	2	2	2	2	2	8.846
3	2	1	1	1	1	7.467
3	2	2	1	1	1	7.945
3	2	2	2	1	1	8.348
3	2	2	2	2	1	8.731
3	2	2	2	2	2	9.033
3	3	1	1	1	1	7.909
3	3	2	1	1	1	8.303
3	3	2	2	1	1	8.615
3	3	2	2	2	1	8.923
3	3	2	2	2	2	9.190
∞	∞	∞	∞	∞	∞	11.07

α denotes the level of significance and H_{crit} the critical value of the Kruskal–Wallis statistic.
Modified from Lindley D V, Scott W F, New Cambridge Elementary Statistical Tables, 2nd edn.
Cambridge: Cambridge University Press, 1995.

Appendix 16

Critical values of Friedman's statistic (χ_r^2)

$\alpha = 0.05$

$N_{columns} = 3$		$N_{columns} = 4$		$N_{columns} = 5$		$N_{columns} = 6$	
N_{rows}	χ_r^2	N_{rows}	χ_r^2	N_{rows}	χ_r^2	N_{rows}	χ_r^2
3	6.000	3	7.400	3	8.533	3	9.857
4	6.500	4	7.800	4	8.800	4	10.290
5	6.400	5	7.800	5	8.960	5	10.490
6	7.000	6	7.600	6	9.067	6	10.570
7	7.143	7	7.800	7	9.143	∞	11.070
8	6.250	8	7.650	8	9.200		
9	6.222	9	7.667	9	9.244		
10	6.200	10	7.680	∞	9.488		
11	6.545	11	7.691				
12	6.500	12	7.700				
13	6.615	13	7.800				
14	6.143	14	7.714				
15	6.400	15	7.720				
16	6.500	16	7.800				
17	6.118	17	7.800				
18	6.333	18	7.733				
19	6.421	19	7.863				
20	6.300	20	7.800				
21	6.095	∞	7.815				
22	6.091						
23	6.348						
24	6.250						
25	6.080						
26	6.077						
27	6.000						
28	6.500						
29	6.276						
30	6.200						
31	6.000						
32	6.063						
33	6.061						
34	6.059						
∞	5.991						

α denotes the level of significance, $N_{columns}$ the number of columns and N_{rows} the number of rows.
Modified from Lindley D V, Scott W F, *New Cambridge Elementary Statistical Tables*, 2nd edn.
Cambridge: Cambridge University Press, 1995.

Appendix 17

Critical values of the Q statistic for non-parametric multiple comparison testing

	α	
k	0.05	0.01
2	1.960	2.576
3	2.394	2.936
4	2.639	3.144
5	2.807	3.291
6	2.936	3.403
7	3.038	3.494
8	3.124	3.570
9	3.197	3.635
10	3.261	3.692
11	3.317	3.743
12	3.368	3.789
13	3.414	3.830
14	3.456	3.868
15	3.494	3.902
16	3.529	3.935
17	3.562	3.965
18	3.593	3.993
19	3.622	4.019
20	3.649	4.044
21	3.675	4.067
22	3.699	4.089
23	3.722	4.110
24	3.744	4.130
25	3.765	4.149

α denotes the level of significance and k the number of treatments.
Adapted from Zar J H, *Biostatistical Analysis*, 3rd edition, Englewood Cliffs, NJ: Prentice-Hall International, 1984.

Appendix 18

Critical values of the Spearman rank correlation coefficient (r_S) for a one-tailed test

k	α	
	0.05	0.01
4	1.000	
5	0.900	1.000
6	0.829	0.943
7	0.714	0.893
8	0.643	0.833
9	0.600	0.783
10	0.564	0.746
12	0.506	0.712
14	0.456	0.645
16	0.425	0.601
18	0.399	0.564
20	0.377	0.534
22	0.359	0.508
24	0.343	0.485
26	0.329	0.465
28	0.317	0.448
30	0.306	0.432

α denotes the level of significance and k the number of pairs of observations.
Modified from Olds E G, Distributions of sums of squares of rank differences for small numbers of individuals, *Ann Math Statist*, 1938; 20: 117–18.

Index